BROCK'S

INJURIES OF THE BRAIN
AND SPINAL CORD

CONTRIBUTORS: CHARLES ABLER

BERNARD J. ALPERS

EMANUEL APPELBAUM

STANLEY M. ARONSON

RICHARD G. BERRY

ABRAM BLAU

KARL M. BOWMAN

MICHAEL J. BRESNAN

SAMUEL BROCK

JEFFERSON BROWDER

RANDOLPH BYERS

NIALL CARTLIDGE

LEO M. DAVIDOFF

ALFRED EBEL

FRANCIS A. ECHLIN

MILTON ELKIN

BERNARD EPSTEIN

EMANUEL H. FEIRING

E. S. GURDJIAN

PAUL F. A. HOEFER

J. TREVOR HUGHES

W. BRYAN JENNETT

HARRY KAPLAN

LIONEL R. KING

LOUIS LINN

ROBERT L. McLAURIN

HENRY MILLER

PABLO A. MORALES

JOE PENNYBACKER

THEODORE RASMUSSEN

ROBERT REICH

MANNIE M. SCHECHTER

KENNETH SHULMAN

J. L. SILVERSIDES

JOHN D. SPILLANE

SIR CHARLES SYMONDS

L. MURRAY THOMAS

EDMOND UHRY, JR.

ROBERT J. WHITE

DAVID YASHON

BROCK'S
INJURIES OF THE BRAIN AND SPINAL CORD
AND THEIR COVERINGS

Fifth Edition

Edited by

EMANUEL H. FEIRING
Albert Einstein College of Medicine, New York

SPRINGER SCIENCE+BUSINESS MEDIA, LLC

The brain is full of all sorts of little doors and chambers. Sometimes a knock on the head upsets the whole business. Still, all of it has to do with the soul. Without the soul, the head would be no wiser than the foot.

I. B. Singer

"The Chimney Sweep," in *A Friend of Kafka and Other Stories.* Farrar, Straus & Giroux, Inc., New York, 1970.

First Edition, 1940
Second Edition, 1943
Third Edition, 1949
Fourth Edition, 1960
Fifth Edition, 1974

ISBN 978-3-662-38997-3   ISBN 978-3-662-39966-8 (eBook)
DOI 10.1007/978-3-662-39966-8

Library of Congress Catalog Card Number 72-81247

PREFACE TO FIFTH EDITION

Trauma in general and injuries of the brain and spinal cord in particular continue to burden society to an inordinate degree. This is evident from statistical data accumulated since the fourth edition of this book was published over a decade ago, and from the extensive literature on the subject that has appeared since then. In most countries throughout the world trauma is one of the principal causes of death at all ages and the leading cause in young people. Traffic accidents continue to increase in number and account for a high proportion of serious injuries. The head is frequently involved in automobile accidents, and craniocerebral injury is the decisive factor in well over half of the fatal cases. Unfortunately the full potential of preventive measures in automotive design is yet to be realized.

Many of the problems pertaining to injuries of the brain and spinal cord remain unresolved; there have been no recent major innovations relative to treatment in either area. The outlook following serious spinal cord trauma remains as dismal as ever. In view of the incidence and gravity of craniovertebral trauma and the limitations of current therapeutic methods, an intensified program of accident prevention is urgently required if this major health problem is to be brought under control.

While the basic format of earlier editions has been retained, the subject matter has been substantially revised and, in many instances, new contributors have provided a fresh viewpoint. The material on head trauma has been expanded to include sections on metabolic alterations and injuries during infancy and childhood. Two other subjects, the diagnosis and treatment of uncomplicated head trauma and brain injuries in boxers, are considered in separate, additional chapters. Contributions on orthopedic management, radiology, and rehabilitation have been added to broaden the perspective relative to spinal cord trauma. It seemed insufficiently rewarding to recapitulate at length the largely speculative discussions of the relationship of brain and spinal cord injury to other diseases of the nervous system and accordingly these chapters have been deleted.

It is a pleasure to acknowledge the help of Mrs. Hilda Feiring in the preparation of this book.

E. H. F.

LIST OF CONTRIBUTORS

ABLER, CHARLES, M.D.
Associate Clinical Professor of Pediatrics, Albert Einstein College of Medicine, Bronx, N. Y.; Attending Pediatrician, Bronx-Lebanon Hospital Center, Bronx, N. Y.

ALPERS, BERNARD J., M.D.
Emeritus Professor of Neurology, Jefferson Medical College, Thomas Jefferson University, Philadelphia, Pa.

APPELBAUM, EMANUEL, M.D.
Professor of Clinical Medicine, New York University School of Medicine, New York, N. Y.; Visiting Physician, Bellevue Hospital, New York, N. Y.

ARONSON, STANLEY M., M.D.
Professor of Medical Science and Chief, Section of Pathology, Brown University; Pathologist-in-Chief, the Miriam Hospital, Providence, R. I.

BERRY, RICHARD G., M.D.
Professor of Neurology (Neuropathology) and Professor of Pathology (Neuropathology), Jefferson Medical College, Thomas Jefferson University, Philadelphia, Pa.

BLAU, ABRAM, M.D.
Clinical Professor of Psychiatry, The Mount Sinai School of Medicine of the University of the City of New York; Attending Psychiatrist-in-Charge, the Child Psychiatry Division, Department of Psychiatry, The Mount Sinai Medical Center; New York, N. Y.

BOWMAN, KARL M., M.D.
Formerly Professor of Psychiatry, University of California Medical School; Formerly Medical Superintendent, The Langley Porter Clinic, San Francisco, Cal.

BRESNAN, MICHAEL J., M.D.
Assistant in Neurology, Children's Medical Center, Boston, Mass.

BROCK, SAMUEL, M.D.
Formerly Professor of Neurology, New York University School of Medicine, New York, N. Y.

vii

BROWDER, JEFFERSON, M.D.
Professor Emeritus of Neurosurgery, State University of New York, Downstate Medical Center; Professor of Neurosurgery, College of Medicine and Dentistry of New Jersey at Newark; Staff Surgeon, Veterans Administration Hospital, East Orange, N. J.

BYERS, RANDOLPH K., M.D.
Consultant Neurologist, Children's Medical Center, Boston, Mass.

CARTLIDGE, NIALL, M.B., M.R.C.P.
Research Associate in Neurology, The Royal Victoria Infirmary, Newcastle upon Tyne, England.

DAVIDOFF, LEO M., M.D.
Emeritus Professor of Neurosurgery, Albert Einstein College of Medicine, Bronx, N. Y.

EBEL, ALFRED, M.D., F.A.C.P.
Professor of Rehabilitation Medicine, Albert Einstein College of Medicine, Bronx, N. Y.; Chief, Clinical Services, Department of Rehabilitation Medicine, Montefiore Hospital Medical Center, Bronx, N. Y.

ECHLIN, FRANCIS A., M.D., Med. Sc.D., F.A.C.S
Consulting Neurosurgeon, Lenox Hill and Bellevue Hospitals, New York, N. Y.; Research Fellow in Neurosurgery, New York University Medical Center, New York, N. Y.

ELKIN, MILTON, M.D., F.A.C.R.
Professor and Chairman, Department of Radiology, Albert Einstein College of Medicine, Bronx, N. Y.; Director of Radiology, Bronx Municipal Hospital Center, Bronx, N. Y.

EPSTEIN, BERNARD, M.D.
Clinical Professor of Radiology, Albert Einstein College of Medicine, Bronx, N. Y.; Director, Department of Radiology, Long Island Jewish Hospital, New Hyde Park, N. Y.; Radiologist-in-Chief, Long Island Jewish Hospital, Queens Hospital Center affiliation.

FEIRING, EMANUEL H., M.D.
Clinical Professor of Neurosurgery, Albert Einstein College of Medicine, Bronx, N. Y.; Attending Neurosurgeon, Montefiore Hospital and Medical Center, Bronx, N. Y.

GURDJIAN, E. S., M.D., Ph.D.
Professor Emeritus, Department of Neurosurgery, Wayne State University School of Medicine, Detroit, Mich.

HOEFER, PAUL F. A., M.D.
Professor Emeritus of Neurology, College of Physicians and Surgeons, Columbia University, New York, N. Y.; Consultant in Neurology, Presbyterian Hospital, New York, N. Y.

HUGHES, J. TREVOR, M.D., D. Path. (Eng.)
Consultant Neuropathologist, United Oxford Hospitals, Oxford, England.

JENNETT, W. BRYAN, M.D., F.R.C.S.
Professor of Neurosurgery, Institute of Neurological Sciences and the University of Glasgow, Glasgow, Scotland.

KAPLAN, HARRY, M.D.
Professor of Surgery and Director of Division of Neurosurgery, College of Medicine and Dentistry of New Jersey at Newark, Newark, N. J.

KING, LIONEL R., M.D.
Assistant Clinical Professor of Medicine, University of Cincinnati College of Medicine, Cincinnati, Ohio.

LINN, LOUIS, M.D.
Clinical Professor of Psychiatry, The Mount Sinai School of Medicine of the University of the City of New York; Attending Psychiatrist, The Mount Sinai Hospital and Medical Center, New York, N. Y.

McLAURIN, ROBERT L., M.D.
Professor of Surgery, Director of Division of Neurosurgery, University of Cincinnati College of Medicine, Cincinnati, Ohio.

MILLER, HENRY, M.D., F.R.C.P., D.P.M.
Vice-Chancellor, University of Newcastle upon Tyne, England; Honorary Consulting Neurologist, The Royal Victoria Infirmary, Newcastle upon Tyne, England.

MORALES, PABLO A., M.D.
Professor of Urology, New York University School of Medicine, New York, N. Y.

PENNYBACKER, JOE, M.D., F.R.C.S.
Neurological Surgeon, Radcliffe Infirmary, Oxford, England.

RASMUSSEN, THEODORE, M.D.
Professor of Neurology and Neurosurgery, Montreal Neurological Institute, McGill University, Montreal, Canada.

REICH, ROBERT, M.D.
Instructor in Psychiatry, The Mount Sinai School of Medicine of the University of the City of New York; Chief Psychiatrist, Department of Social Services of the City of New York.

SCHECHTER, MANNIE M., M.D.
Professor of Radiology, Albert Einstein College of Medicine, Bronx, N. Y.

SHULMAN, KENNETH, M.D.
Professor and Chairman, Department of Neurosurgery, Albert Einstein College of Medicine, Bronx, N. Y.; Attending Neurosurgeon, Montefiore Hospital and Medical Center, Bronx, N. Y.

SILVERSIDES, J. L., B.Sc., M.D., F.R.C.P. (C.)
Professor of Medicine, University of Toronto, Toronto Western Hospital, Toronto, Canada.

SPILLANE, JOHN D., M.D., F.R.C.P.
Consultant Neurologist, The United Cardiff Hospitals and the Welsh Hospital Board; Lecturer in Neurology in the Welsh National School of Medicine.

SYMONDS, CHARLES, K.B.E., D.M., F.R.C.P.
Consultant Emeritus for Nervous Diseases, Guy's Hospital; Honorary Consulting Physician, National Hospital for Nervous Diseases, Queen Square, London, England.

THOMAS, L. MURRAY, M.D.
Professor and Chairman, Department of Neurosurgery, Wayne State University School of Medicine, Detroit, Mich.

UHRY, EDMOND, JR., M.D.
Attending Orthopedic Surgeon, Montefiore Hospital and Medical Center, Bronx, N. Y.

WHITE, ROBERT J., Ph.D., M.D., F.A.C.S.
Professor of Neurosurgery, School of Medicine, Case Western Reserve University, Cleveland, Ohio.

YASHON, DAVID, M.D., F.A.C.S., F.R.C.S. (C.)
Associate Professor of Neurosurgery, College of Medicine, Ohio State University Hospitals, Columbus, Ohio.

CONTENTS

GENERAL CONSIDERATIONS IN INJURIES OF THE BRAIN AND SPINAL CORD AND THEIR COVERINGS

EMANUEL H. FEIRING, M. D.
AND
SAMUEL BROCK, M. D.

The appalling number of accidents in modern life makes the subject of injury as important as that of any pandemic scourge. Data for the three-year period between 1966 and 1968 show that an estimated 114,000 accidental deaths occur each year in the United States (U. S. Dept. of Health, Education and Welfare, 1970). According to the National Safety Council (1970) disabling injuries in 1969 totalled almost 11 million, of which 115,000 were fatal; motor vehicle accidents accounted for 2 million injuries of which 56,400 were fatal; over 2 million people sustained injuries at work and, of these, 14,200 died. Accidents in 1969 cost the nation 25 billion dollars.

Each year 50 million are injured – approximately one person in four of the total U.S. population. About 44 million of the injured receive medical care; 11 million are so disabled that they are confined to bed, and 2 million are hospitalized. Annual losses resulting from these injuries include about 550 million days of restricted activity, 141 million days of disability in bed, and 97 million days lost from work.

Over 22 million people are injured in and about their homes each year, and these account for about one-quarter of all accidental deaths. About 21 million children (under 17 years of age) are injured each year, over half at home. Accidents are the leading cause of death between the ages of one and 37 years.

Since 1958 the number of accidents has risen 11 percent; automobile accidents have increased 28 percent in the same period of time. About 4 million people two-thirds of whom are between the ages of 17 and 44 years, are injured annually in moving motor vehicle accidents. In 1969 motor vehicles were responsible for 49 percent of all accidental deaths. The incidence of deaths caused by motor vehicle accidents is distinctly higher in males. Thirty percent of all motor vehicle deaths occur among males between the ages of 15 and 24. About 9300 pedestrians are killed annually by motor vehicles.

Of the 50 million accidental injuries incurred each year, about 3 million involve the head, and of these over half a million are caused by motor vehicles (U. S. Dept. of Health, Education and Welfare, 1969). Head trauma occurs in about 70 percent of the injured occupants involved in automobile accidents (Kihlberg, 1966); usually multiple injuries are incurred (Kihlberg, 1970). Most commonly impact is made with the windshield. Ejection substantially increases the frequency and severity of the head injury.

Automobile accidents being so numerous and devastating in their consequences, there has been much speculation concerning the factors related to the high incidence of such mishaps. To what extent is driver carelessness a factor and, if it is a factor, what is the basis of this carelessness? Are some individuals more "accident prone" because of their personality quirks? There is ample reason to believe that, in the hands of some, the automobile may serve as an outlet for feelings of revolt, hostility, and aggression (Mark and Ervin, 1970). Those inclined to flaunt authority might be expected to violate traffic laws. Undoubtedly, the automobile provides some with a sense of power and status, otherwise lacking. Suicidal intent may underlie some vehicular accidents (Hamburger, 1969). An excellent example is afforded by the career of T. E. Lawrence (Lawrence of Arabia) who was killed while driving a motorcycle at 80 miles an hour. Those acquainted with his life will readily perceive that a masked suicidal drive was responsible for such careless driving. Physical defects caused by disease play a relatively minor role in comparison with psychologic factors.

A determined effort must be made to conquer the aggressive qualities of the ego which underlie the desire to "get ahead of the other fellow" or to "burn up the road" in order to conquer time and space. One-third of the fatal accidents in 1969 involved vehicles driven too fast. Excessive use of alcohol also contributes to automobile accidents by impairing judgment and ability to drive well and by permitting freer play of aggresive and suicidal drives. Equally important is its dulling effect on those quick, automatic acts that are so vital in dealing with traffic problems that may suddenly arise on the road. Alcohol is a factor in at least half of the fatal motor accidents (National Safety Council, 1970). Various "stimulating" drugs in common use today constitute another hazard to those under their influence while operating a vehicle (Waller, 1971). Unfortunately, in recent years, the number of defective cars has risen appreciably, thereby compounding the problems created by human shortcomings. The causes of carelessness among pedestrians are probably similar to those among drivers.

Modifications in the design of automobiles, including the use of headrests, laminated windshields, padded instrument panels, seat belts, energy-absorbing bumpers and rear-end body structures, restraint systems, and changes in the steering assembly — such as the collapsible column, for example — have been suggested or introduced as means of reducing the incidence and severity of injuries resulting from accidents (Lange and Van Kirk, 1970; Snyder, 1970; States et al, 1970). Expansion of the biomechanics research program is essential in this era of high-speed transportation. The crash helmet has already proved its usefulness to motorcyclists. It has been estimated that if safety belts were used at all times, eight to ten thousand lives might be saved annually, since it is believed that there were about 3000 fewer fatalities in 1969 as a result of their use.

HISTORY AND RECORD OF ACCIDENT

In most accident cases, the history that is elicited by the physician is much too casual and too often inadequate; the same may be said of the records kept by physicians. It must be realized that the history and record, including progress notes, laboratory data, and operative findings in cases of accident, are always likely to become part of legal evidence and, for this reason, have great importance. When more than one history has been elicited the essential details should not be at variance. If there are discrepancies, these should be noted. Some uncertainties in the history may be due to faulty memory; on the other hand, a very smooth narration may be the result of "coaching."

In the case of a fall, the distance involved should be determined, as well as what part of the body received the impact, and the nature of the surface on which the patient landed. If the patient was struck by a falling object, how far did it fall, and what was its shape, consistency, and weight? Was the patient's head moving or stationary? Contrecoup injuries are more apt to occur when the head is in motion at the time of impact. Whether the patient lost consciousness is of considerable importance. Did he remain standing or did he fall to the floor? An attempt should be made to determine the duration of the period of amnesia. Was the patient merely dazed and able to proceed home or to a doctor's office, or was assistance required? How did he react upon arriving home or at a hospital? Did he vomit? Did the vomitus contain blood and, if so, had it been swallowed or was it evidence of visceral injury? Was there bleeding from any of the cranial orifices? Did blood in the mouth stem from local cuts or abrasions? Were injuries of the

3

auricle or external canal, or a ruptured eardrum responsible for the appearance of blood within the ear? If there was bleeding from the nose, was it caused by local trauma? Answers to all of these questions must be taken into consideration before concluding that bleeding from these orifices is indicative of skull fracture. Did clear fluid (cerebrospinal) escape from the nose or ears? Did a "black eye" appear soon after injury or did it come on hours later, suggesting a fracture of the anterior fossa? The time of appearance of other ecchymoses, such as those overlying the mastoid (Battle sign) should be noted.

Scalp Lacerations. The location, depth, extent, and state of contamination of the wound must be noted; also, how soon after injury surgical treatment was administered, whether antibiotics were prescribed, and the specific prophylactic measures taken against tetanus.

Skull Fracture. While the presence of a fracture may be suspected on clinical grounds, the diagnosis is usually established or confirmed on the basis of the x-ray findings. Coexisting fractures of the facial bones and of the vertebral column, especially of the cervical region, must not be overlooked. Radiologic examination may be deferred unless one is dealing with a compound fracture or penetrating wound, or is concerned over the possibility of an extradural hemorrhage. In the event the fracture involves a sinus, the patient should be questioned with regard to previous attacks of sinusitis. Should the fracture extend into the mastoid region, the possibility of past middle-ear disease should be explored.

As complete a neurologic examination as is feasible should be performed at the earliest possible time after injury. Especially to be noted are the patient's state of consciousness, the size and reaction of the pupils, focal deficits, pathologic reflexes, and the presence of nuchal rigidity which is indicative of blood in the cerebrospinal fluid.

The long bones, spine, chest, and abdomen must be examined for coexisting injuries.

The blood pressure, pulse, respiratory rate, and temperature should be recorded at frequent intervals for at least 48 hours. Motor function should be tested frequently and the eyes examined for pupillary changes. The physician must be constantly alert to the possibility of intracranial bleeding.

PHYSICAL FACTORS IN HEAD INJURY

The skull, the meninges and their partitions, the subarachnoid layer of cerebrospinal fluid, and the highly organized brain with its unique

4

vascular supply and ventricular system form a structure of unusual complexity. Injuries affecting this structure involve a number of physical factors which require special consideration. This aspect of head trauma has been studied in recent years by a number of investigators, including Denny-Brown and Russell, Gurdjian and his co-workers, Holbourn, Ommaya, Lindenberg, and Unterharnscheidt and Sellier.

Head injuries are most commonly caused by blows, objects dropped from a height, falls, and moving vehicles; those caused by penetrating (gunshot) wounds occur less often. The offending agent may be a blunt or sharp object or a compressing force. Blunt injuries result in acceleration or deceleration of the head, depending on whether a moving object strikes a relatively immobile head, thereby causing it to be set in motion (acceleration), or whether it is a head in motion that comes in contact with a stationary, unyielding object that brings it to an abrupt stop (deceleration). In either case the skull may be momentarily deformed (compressed) and, if sufficient force has been applied, fractured. The importance of acceleration and deceleration in the pathogenesis of concussion was first revealed by the studies of Denny-Brown and Russell (1941). Concussion was produced in the monkey and cat when the head was struck by a heavy mass with a velocity of approximately 28 feet per second. Experiments in monkeys led Ommaya (1966) to conclude that the production of concussion can be correlated with only two parameters, impulse of the impact and linear acceleration of the head; the best index of the concussive effect of a blow is the impulse; the force of the blow, the tangential velocity of the head, and the levels of intracranial pressure change are not significantly related to the occurrence of concussion.

Compression injuries of the head occur infrequently. Considerable damage may be inflicted by such injuries, even without loss of consciousness (Russell and Schiller, 1949). In drawing a distinction between acceleration concussion and compression concussion, Denny-Brown and Russell emphasized the difficulty in producing concussion of the fixed head without fracturing the skull. Head trauma may also occur as a consequence of force applied to another part of the body, as in the case of a fall on the buttocks, the stress being transmitted along the vertebral column to the base of the skull. Indirect stress resulting from stretching movements of the neck produced by hyperflexion or hyperextension at the craniospinal junction (so-called "whiplash" injury) is still another cause of head injury. Experimental whiplash injury in the monkey induced by rotational displacement of the head on the neck without significant direct head impact, has caused cerebral concussion, together with hemorrhages and contusions over the surface of the brain and upper cervical cord and breakdown of the blood-brain barrier to Evans blue (Ommaya et al, 1968).

The surface area involved as a result of a sharp injury is relatively small, and the effect of such trauma localized, depending on the nature of the mechanical agent and its velocity.

It has been demonstrated that blunt trauma causes an indentation (inward bending) at the site of impact and the very opposite effect (outward bending) in the surrounding bone (Gurdjian et al, 1950; Gurdjian and Webster, 1958.) The fractures induced by the stress resulting from such distortion arise in the bone adjacent to the site of impact (area bent outward) and radiate both towards and away from it. The pattern of the fracture depends on the area of the skull struck and the strain resulting therefrom. In general, fracture lines tend to circumvent bony buttresses unless their direction is perpendicular to the latter. Both tables of the skull are most commonly affected, the inner frequently to a greater degree. Trauma to the midfrontal region results in fractures affecting the frontal sinus, cribriform plate, and orbital roofs; the fracture line may extend into the temporal regions following blows higher in the frontal region. Lateral frontal injuries tend to produce fractures directed towards the frontotemporal region and base of the skull. Fractures resulting from parietal blows radiate inferiorly towards the middle fossa implicating the temporal region. The dehiscences produced by posterolateral trauma tend to involve the temporal region or to radiate towards the base behind the petrous bone. Occipital injuries cause fractures directed towards the foramen magnum or jugular foramen, and may even extend across the petrous bone into the middle fossa. Midline blows at the vertex produce linear fractures extending towards the base and crossing the middle fossa in the direction of the sella turcica and optic foramen.

Involvement of the base of the skull usually, though not invariably, is an accompaniment of fractures of the vault. Basilar skull fractures may occur independently as the result of a force applied directly or indirectly. In the anterior fossa, the central region is mainly affected; fractures may also radiate obliquely across the orbital roof towards the optic foramen. In the middle fossa, the fracture lines run along the anterior border of the petrous bone towards the foramen lacerum to the opposite side. Posterior basilar fractures tend to gravitate towards the large foramina; they may also extend through the petrous

6

bone into the middle fossa and occasionally may be present about the foramen magnum.

Compression fractures induced by force applied in an anteroposterior direction affect the frontal sinuses, cribriform plate, ethmoid sinuses and, rarely, extend around the clivus to the foramen magnum. Lateral compression results in fractures of the middle fossa extending around the sella turcica to the opposite side (Hooper, 1969).

The type and extent of the fracture varies with the age of the patient, the nature of the offending agent, and the amount of force applied. Thus fractures may be linear, comminuted, depressed or compound. In newborn infants the skull may be indented without disrupting the continuity of the bone, and in young children trauma may cause a separation of sutures. Owing to the absence of buttresses and to immaturity of the skull, fractures in infants do not conform to any pattern.

The extent of injury inflicted by a penetrating missile is dependent on its velocity. In addition to the trauma caused by penetration, a missile that strikes the head imparts energy in a direction radial to its trajectory (Butler et al, 1945). The bone may be shattered by the resultant explosive force and, depending on the mass and velocity of the missile, extensive "bursting" fractures may be produced.

Brain. As a consequence of trauma, various factors are brought into play which may affect the intracranial contents. At the moment of impact a temporary deformation of the skull occurs, associated with a sharp, transient rise of intracranial pressure (Scott, 1940; Walker et al, 1944; Gurdjian and Lissner, 1944; Gurdjian et al, 1966). Gurdjian and Lissner observed an increase in intracranial pressure on the side of the impact and a decreased pressure on the opposite side. According to Gurdjian, Webster, and Lissner (1955), the increase in pressure may reach 750 to 5,000 mm of mercury. The elevation of cerebrospinal fluid pressure inmediately following experimental concussion in the monkey was attributed by Grubb et al (1970) almost entirely to engorgement of intracranial vessels, the degree of pressure elevation corresponding to the duration of the postconcussive apnea.

The deformation of the skull produces a flattening of the brain at the site of trauma and a shortening of its axis in the line of direction of the applied force. Simultaneously, a corresponding elongation and stretching of the brain occurs in a plane at right angles to the line of force. The effects of such physical force may be seen, for example, following trauma to the vertex, in which case contusion of the corpus

7

callosum may occur as a consequence of stretching and downward displacement (Lindenberg et al, 1955).

Both compression and acceleration affect the intracranial pressure at the moment of impact. The factor of acceleration is responsible for a pressure gradient, highest at the site of impact and lowest directly opposite it (Thomas et al, 1967; Thomas, 1970). It has been suggested that, in the event the negative pressure becomes sufficiently pronounced, cavitation of nervous tissue may occur in the affected area and that this is the mechanism whereby cortical contusions are produced (Gross, 1958; Unterharnscheidt and Sellier, 1966). The concept of a "central cavitation effect" has also been proposed by Unterharnscheidt and Sellier to explain the central hemorrhages in the subependyma of the ventricles and the adjacent parts of the corpus callosum. Deformation of the skull resulting from a blow to the vertex suddenly increases its bitemporal diameter, causing a negative pressure and cavitation effect in the ventricular system and structures in the immediate proximity (see also Unterharnscheidt, 1970).

As a consequence of the pressure wave caused by acceleration of the head, the brain is subject to compression and shear stresses. According to Gurdjian et al (1955, 1966, 1968), maximum shear strains occur in the region of the brain stem and craniospinal junction, and provide the physical basis for concussion (see also Thomas, 1970 and Hodgson, 1970).

Whenever the head is struck, the brain is set into motion. This was well demonstrated experimentally in monkeys with lucite calvaria by Pudenz and Shelden (1946). Employing high-speed cinematography, rotatory movements of the brain within the cranial cavity were observed following trauma. Brain displacement (and skull deformation) has also been revealed by a flash x-ray technique (Hodgson et al, 1966). When the frontal or occipital regions are the site of impact, the brain tends to rotate about a coronal axis. The tips of the frontal and temporal lobes may be contused and cortical veins in the parasagittal region torn with resultant subdural bleeding. Lateral blows tend to cause rotation about the sagittal plane. The brain stem and the medial aspect of the hemisphere may be injured, the former as it strikes the free edge of the tentorium, the latter as it makes contact with the inferior margin of the falx. Holbourn (1943) in particular has emphasized rotation as the causative factor in the production of shear strains leading to brain damage. The widespread degenerative changes in the white matter of the cerebrum and brain stem following head trauma, described by Strich (1961), were attributed to the

8

stresses resulting from rotational acceleration of the head at the time of the accident.

The various mechanical explanations that have been suggested as the modus operandi in head trauma have been critically analyzed (Ommaya, 1970; Ommaya et al, 1971). He questioned the significance of the evidence in support of the concept of intracranial pressure gradients and resultant shear stresses in the brain stem, purported to be responsible for concussion, and of "cavitation" as a cause of hemorrhage and other brain lesions. His own experimental observations in monkeys support Holbourn's theory that brain concussion is related to the shearing strains developed by severe rotational motions of the brain. His data further indicate that local skull deformation is a significant contributing factor. He and his co-workers conclude that "when the freely movable head is subject to an impact, there are two injurious mechanisms immediately responding: rotation of the head and deformation of the skull, each contributing about equal amounts to the injury potential of the blow. When the head is suddenly accelerated indirectly as in a 'whiplash', skull deformation effects may probably be neglected and rotational effects become highly significant. When the relatively immobile head is subjected to impact, skull deformation effects predominate, and head rotation becomes the minor factor" (Hirsch et al, 1970). These conclusions were criticized by Gurdjian (1970), who believes that rotational and linear acceleration occur in most impact injuries, together with deformation of the skull. He further pointed out that as a rule whiplash injuries in humans do not result in concussion.

Contrecoup lesions, i.e., contusions and lacerations sustained by parts of the brain remote from the point of impact but in line with its force, occur most commonly when the moving head is suddenly decelerated. The advancing surfaces of the brain corresponding to the direction of motion imparted to it impinge on bone or dural septa as the movement of the brain is arrested. Various parts of the brain, both supratentorial and infratentorial in location, may suffer injury, depending on the forcefulness of the impact. Most commonly, contrecoup lesions involve the poles of the frontal and temporal lobes, owing to the structural characteristics of the adjacent bone. The analysis of the mechanism of cerebral contusions, both coup and contrecoup, by Lindenberg and Freytag (1960) is noteworthy. They observed that the occurrence and location of such contusions is dependent not only upon the magnitude and direction of the impact and the physical characteristics of the region of the skull affected, but also upon

9

certain other factors — whether the head is movable or in motion at the time of injury, or whether it is fixed in position. Local lesions at the site of trauma in cases in which the head is free to move are believed to be caused by the combined action of the positive acceleration pressure and the positive pressure due to depression of the skull. Contrecoup lesions in such cases are usually less prominent than the contusions suffered on the side of the blow, and, when present, indicate that severe depression of the skull occurred, causing a positive shifting pressure of sufficient intensity to traumatize the opposite side of the brain. Lesions at the site of trauma in cases in which the head is in motion at the moment of impact (e.g., falls on the head) are attributed to circumscribed skull indentations producing local pressure in excess of the negative acceleration pressure. To explain the contralateral lesions that are more conspicuous in such cases, it is assumed that a larger area of skull is flattened at the time of injury; this exerts pressure on the brain and shifts it towards the opposite side; and, since a positive acceleration pressure already exists on the opposite side, the combined pressure effects are thought to account for the contrecoup lesion. Unless considerable force is applied, coup and contrecoup lesions are uncommon following trauma when the head is rigidly fixed in position and not subject to acceleration. (See also Lindenberg, 1971.)

According to Lindenberg (1966), the tentorium and its opening are a determining factor in the distribution of contusions affecting the deeper structures of the brain provided the force of the trauma is of sufficient magnitude to deform the skull and that it is directed towards the tentorium. Anatomic factors limit the displacement of the intracranial contents in the direction of the tentorial opening to the central parts of the brain. The effect of such deformation and downward displacement on the corpus callosum has already been indicated. The location of the hippocampal gyri relative to the tentorial edge makes them especially vulnerable to herniation and contusion. Hemorrhagic lesions may also appear near the mammillary bodies, in the corpus callosum, thalamus, floor of the third ventricle, upper midbrain, pontine tegmentum, and brachium conjunctivum. Displacement of the brain stem in an upward direction may occur following the application of force at the base of the skull, with resultant contusion of the upper pons, midbrain, and thalamus.

The tentorium is also significant in the development of secondary lesions that result from supratentorial pressure and transtentorial herniation. The idea of a tentorial pressure cone was introduced by

10

Meyer (1920) and subsequently elaborated upon by others. Cerebral edema or intracranial hemorrhage causes a protrusion of the hippocampal gyrus on one or both sides through the tentorial opening compressing and displacing the midbrain and the blood vessels and nerves in proximity to it and blocking the circulation of cerebrospinal fluid. The cerebral peduncle on the side opposite a unilateral uncal herniation becomes indented by the free edge of the tentorium (Kernohan's notch). As a result of tentorial herniation, lesions are produced in the midbrain and pons and in the areas supplied by blood vessels that have suffered compression (e.g., calcarine infarction caused by compression of the posterior cerebral artery or its branches). Ammon's horn, the pallidum, thalamus and rostral cerebellum may also be the site of lesions (Lindenberg, 1966, 1971). Veins as well as arteries are compressed and hemorrhages within the brain stem often occur as a consequence of tentorial herniation.

The more important factor in the production of such lesions, according to Scheinker (1945), is frank herniation of the rostral brain stem through the tentorial opening. Howell (1959), who reviewed the findings in a series of 150 cases of upper brain-stem compression secondary to intracranial space-occupying lesions and brain swelling, found that in almost half of the cases, there was no significant herniation of the temporal lobe. He too concluded that downward movement of the midbrain alone adequately explained the clinical manifestations referable to the upper brain stem, and viewed temporal lobe herniation as an additional cause of compression and distortion of the midbrain. Transtentorial herniation accounts for the phenomenon of the fixed dilated pupil (oculomotor paralysis) resulting from ipsilateral cerebral compression.

Pontine and medullary hemorrhages have been produced experimentally in the dog by mechanical compression of the cerebral cortex (Dill and Isenhour, 1939). Vertical compression of the brain tending to cause herniation of the pons and medulla towards the foramen magnum has been invoked as the responsible mechanism.

Compression of the lower brain stem as a result of displacement of the cerebellar tonsils through the foramen magnum ("pressure cone" or foraminal impaction) is a well-known complication of expanding intracranial lesions. Herniation of the cingulate gyrus beneath the free edge of the falx may also occur as a consequence of unilateral cerebral swelling or intracranial hemorrhage. Additional effects include displacement of the frontal lobes into the middle cranial fossae and of the gyri recti of the orbital lobes toward the optic chiasm and sella turcica.

Abrupt movement of the head relative to the cervical spine is an invariable accompaniment of cranial trauma and may be a factor in determining the occurrence of concussion. Thus, Ommaya et al (1964) found that immobilization of the neck by means of a collar was an effective means of preventing concussion in the monkey. Further evidence was provided by Hollister et al (1958) and by Friede (1961) who produced concussion in cats by stretching the cervical cord at the craniovertebral junction. Friede observed cellular changes in the brain stem which were thought to result from damage to nerve fibers in the ventral spinal cord at the odontoid level. These lesions were similar to those he observed following trauma to the head. He suggested that the upper cervical cord lesions were primarily responsible for concussion, a view not generally accepted (Denny-Brown, 1961). It would appear more likely, as indicated by Ommaya (1966), that rotational acceleration of the brain and stretching forces acting primarily on the brain stem rather than distortion at the craniospinal level are responsible for the occurrence of concussion. The protective effect of immobilization of the neck of the experimental animal on consciousness is attributed by Ommaya (1964, 1970) to a reduction of the rotational or angular acceleration imparted to the head and a diminished shear strain acting on the brain stem.

PATHOLOGY

Primary Effects. When the head is struck, the forces that act upon the brain subject it to varying degrees of compression, expansion, acceleration, deceleration, and rotation. Diffuse or local effects or both, including contusion, laceration, disseminated neuronal injury, and hemorrhage — both parenchymal and subarachnoid — may result from blunt trauma. Ischemic changes and areas of infarction are not uncommon.

Injuries to the front of the head most often produce coup lesions alone. The incidence of contrecoup contusions is highest following blows to the back of the head. Lateral impacts produce either coup or contrecoup lesions. The frontotemporal basal and lateral temporal areas are involved most frequently regardless of the site of trauma.

The wounds caused by missiles are of varying complexity, depending on the shape, mass and velocity of the offending agent (radial effects), its site of entrance (and exit, if perforating), its course within the brain, and its depth of penetration. Contrecoup lesions are almost non-existent in missile wounds (Russell, 1968).

The most common forms of head trauma are those in which the scalp alone is injured and consciousness is retained and those in which consciousness is briefly lost but there is no other evidence of cerebral dysfunction (concussion). As is indicated elsewhere in this volume (Chapter 4), it should not be assumed that concussion, defined as a transient state of unconsciousness following trauma seemingly with full recovery, is not associated with some degree of neuronal damage.

It has been observed that when the head of an experimental animal is struck, changes occur in the smaller blood vessels (Walker, 1970). Following a mild blow, the pial circulation of the cat increases. Within 2 minutes of a mild impact, and within 5 minutes of a moderately severe one, the flow returns to the pre-traumatic level. Following a severe blow, disturbances of blood flow persist for 10 to 15 minutes, during which time arteriolar constriction and dilatation may develop, often with sludging of blood and reversal of flow.

The occurrence of intracranial spasm in association with craniocerebral trauma has been reported by a number of observers (Wilkins and Odom, 1970).

Secondary Effects. In addition to its immediate effects, head trauma may induce a number of other pathologic processes that become manifest after some delay. These include intracranial hemorrhage, edema, sepsis and, at a still later stage, arteriovenous fistula and both obstructive and normal pressure hydrocephalus. Thrombosis of dural venous sinuses producing intracranial hypertension may also occur following blunt trauma (Martin, 1955; Kinal, 1967). Intracranial hemorrhage — whether epidural, subdural, or intracerebral — raises the intracranial pressure and, by its compressing and displacing effects, can irreversibly damage the brain stem. Similar untoward effects may be caused by cerebral edema. Swelling of the brain (cerebral edema) has been studied intensively in recent years and merits further consideration.

Cerebral edema implies an increase in the volume of brain tissue as a result of excessive accumulation of fluid. The pathogenesis of this condition is not fully understood. Klatzo (1967) has suggested that there are two types of edema, vasogenic and cytotoxic. It is postulated that in the vasogenic variety, injury to blood vessels causes an escape of plasma into the extracellullar spaces; the edema involves predominantly the white matter. Brain tissue parenchyma is believed to be primarily affected in the cytotoxic variety; intracellular swelling occurs, vascular permeability remaining relatively unaffected; gray or

13

white matter may be involved depending on the cytotoxic agent.

Cerebral edema has been produced experimentally by various means, including cortical freezing and compression. In traumatic experimental edema it is the white matter that is mainly affected, presumably as a result of increased permeability of the blood-brain barrier. The edema induced by a combination of hypoxia and hypercapnea results from cellular damage which interferes with normal ionic homeostasis and from injury to blood vessels that permits plasma to escape into the tissues.

Brain swelling is not uncommon after head trauma. While its frequency and clinical significance have been disputed, its occurrence in both localized and generalized forms is well recognized. Vasomotor paralysis has been suggested as the important etiologic factor (Evans and Scheinker, 1945), and evidence in support of this hypothesis has been presented by Langfitt and his collaborators (1966, 1966) and by Ishii and his co-workers (1966, 1967). Vasomotor atony leads to an increase in the volume of the cerebrovascular bed, and the resultant congestion causes edema and a rise in intracranial pressure. Possibly, as suggested by Ishii, injury to the hypothalamus is responsible for the loss of vasomotor tone. The elevation of intracranial pressure may activate the medullary vasopressor mechanism, thus producing a rise in systemic blood pressure and augmenting intracranial blood flow. Intracranial pressure is further increased and a vicious cycle ensues. In the event respiratory function is inadequate, carbon dioxide retention and hypoxia cause further vascular dilatation. According to Tomlinson (1964), in the absence of hemorrhage or widespread contusion, anoxia is the most likely cause of generalized cerebral edema. While there is no pathologic evidence that generalized edema follows uncomplicated trauma in adults, it does occasionally occur in children (Strich, 1969). No significant degree of brain swelling was reported by Fass and Ommaya (1968) following experimental concussion in the monkey. For a comprehensive account of current knowledge concerning cerebral edema, the reader is referred to the monograph by Bakay and Lee (1965) and the publication edited by Klatzo and Seitelberger (1967).

Head injuries, usually of a severe nature and often occurring in association with fractures of the temporal or occipital bone, may cause considerable contusion of the temporal lobe (McLaurin and Helmcr, 1965; Lewin, 1968). The resultant hemorrhage, infarction, necrosis, and reactionary edema combine to act as an expanding lesion which is clinically manifested by increasing lethargy and con-

14

tralateral hemiparesis. Neurologic deterioration is most pronounced about 72 hours after injury. Anterior temporal lobectomy for the purpose of removing the pulped, necrotic brain has been recommended.

Hydrocephalus following head trauma may be an ex vacuo phenomenon resulting from loss of cerebral substance, or it may develop as a consequence of interference with the circulation of cerebrospinal fluid. Obstruction to the outflow of cerebrospinal fluid from the ventricular system causes high pressure hydrocephalus, whereas interference with the absorptive mechanism is responsible for so-called occult or normal pressure hydrocephalus.

Associated Lesions. Occasionally, the pituitary gland is injured when a basal fracture occurs. Hemorrhage into the posterior lobe or damage to the pituitary stalk may give rise to diabetes insipidus. Massive ischemic necrosis of the anterior lobe may also occur following trauma. Lesions of the pituitary gland are often present in fatal cases. In a study of 100 such cases, one or more lesions, including capsular hemorrhage, hypophyseal stalk hemorrhage or laceration, posterior lobe involvement, and ischemic necrosis of the anterior lobe were found in 62 (Kornblum and Fisher, 1969). According to Lewin (1966), the signs that suggest pituitary or hypothalamic injury include hypothermia, bradycardia, hypotension, and flaccidity of the limbs. Coma may result from pituitary failure.

Thrombosis of the intracranial or cervical internal carotid artery is an uncommon complication of head and neck trauma (Lewin, 1968; Trevor Hughes and Brownell, 1968; Mastaglia et al, 1969; Zilkha, 1970; Olafson and Christoferson, 1970). Intracranial occlusion has been reported in association with fractures of the middle fossa as well as after relatively minor head injuries. Thrombosis of the cervical segment has occurred following blunt trauma and after penetrating wounds. Recognition of this condition is important since clinically it may be confused with an epidural hematoma. The main branches of the carotid artery may also thrombose after injury. Rarely, a traumatic aneurysm may occur.

Petechial hemorrhages in the upper segments of the cervical cord may occur as a consequence of cerebral trauma (Schneider at al, 1970). Such lesions have also been observed following experimental head injury (Denny-Brown and Russell, 1941; Gosch et al, 1970).

Erosions of the gastrointestinal tract are known to occur in association with intracranial lesions and may develop following cerebral trauma. Eleven such cases were observed by Heiskanen and Törmä (1968) in a series of 960 severe head injuries. In eight of the 11 cases symptoms appeared within two weeks following trauma. No particular area of the brain could be implicated in the production of the gastrointestinal lesion.

INJURY OF THE BRAIN STEM

The effects of head injury on the brain stem are of great importance. This is evident from clinical and pathologic observation (Freytag, 1963) and from the experimental work of Denny-Brown and Russell (1941), Gurdjian and Webster (1945), and Ommaya (1966).

In their study of experimental concussion, Denny-Brown and Russell observed "transient reflex paralysis of the respiratory and vasomotor mechanism, corneal and pinna reflexes, reflex deglutition, and of the reflex motor mechanisms of the pons and medulla." Blood pressure rose sharply following concussion. Subconcussive blows often stimulated the vagoglossopharyngeal system, causing temporary depression of cardiac, vasomotor, and respiratory function; it was suggested that these effects might account for the "knockout" blow in boxing. Experimental concussion in the decerebrate preparation produced effects similar to those observed in the intact animal, indicating that the reaction of the brain stem was not dependent on influences originating in higher centers. Gurdjian and Webster found that moderate and severe head injuries in dogs usually resulted in a sudden rise in blood pressure, respiratory paralysis, coma, loss of palpebral and corneal reflexes, and often rigidity followed by loss of muscle tone. The changes in blood pressure, respiration, and reflexes were attributed to stimulation or paralysis of medullary centers. Ommaya observed that in monkeys a concussive blow induced transient apnea, areflexia, bradycardia, and a fall in blood pressure. Bilateral vagotomy minimized the hypotensive effect, which was followed by a rapid elevation of blood pressure. The cardiopulmonary effects following uncomplicated experimental concussion in the monkey were found to be wholly reversible (Grubb et al, 1970).

Clinically, loss of consciousness represents the most common effect of trauma on the brain stem, being related in all probability to a disturbance of function of the reticular activating system. This concept is discussed further in Chapter 4, where reference is also made to the cytologic changes observed in the brain stem following experimental concussion.

The brain stem may be injured immediately upon impact or in the aftermath of transtentorial herniation. Lesions may be caused by

16

shearing forces that result from acceleration and deformation of the skull (Gurdjian and Lissner, 1961; Gurdjian et al, 1966), or as a consequence of sudden physical changes that involve the cervico-medullary junction. Contusion of the brain stem may follow a sudden thrust against the clivus or the edge of the tentorium. Interference with its blood supply as a result of stretching and avulsion of penetrating arteries produces ischemic changes.

According to Crompton (1971) most primary brain-stem lesions that occur in closed head injuries are caused by occipital impacts. Unilateral tegmental infarcts and hemorrhages together with lesions involving the vestibular nuclei and inferior olive in an undistorted brain stem are the characteristic findings at necropsy. On the other hand, the secondary lesions that result from shift and distortion of the brain stem are paramedian hemorrhages and necrosis that affect the midbrain and pons.

Tears and hemorrhages in the pyramids at the junction of the medulla and pons following traumatic hyperextension of the head have been described by Lindenberg and Freytag (1970). Such lesions of the rostral pyramids might be expected to produce tetraplegia without loss of consciousness or sensory deficit.

The ischemic and hemorrhagic lesions of the brain stem that occur fellowing transtentorial herniation are believed to be due to stretching and compression of blood vessels. Both veins and arteries have been implicated as the source of the hemorrhage (Moore and Stern, 1938; Scheinker, 1945; Lindenberg, 1955, and Johnson and Yates, 1956). The peduncle on the side opposite the hippocampal herniation may suffer compression against the rigid edge of the tentorium. This accounts for the occurrence of ipsilateral hemiplegia, a "false localizing" sign.

The clinical manifestations of brain stem injury comprise alterations of consciousness, changes in muscle tone and posture, disturbances of vital functions including temperature and respiration, cranial nerve palsies, and evidence of involvement of pyramidal and cerebellar pathways. Flaccidity, corresponding physiologically to a transection just below the vestibular nucleus, is a transient phenomenon that accompanies concussion, though it may reappear at a terminal stage. Decerebrate rigidity characterized by retraction of the head, opisthotonos, extension of the limbs, and pronation of the hands is an ominous sign. Experimentally it is observed when the brain stem is transected at the intercollicular level. Decorticate rigidity, manifested by extension of the lower limbs and flexion of the arms, implies a lesion above the midbrain interrupting the influence of the cerebral cortex. Hyper-

17

thermia combined with a rapid pulse and respiratory rate usually presages a fatal outcome. Oculomotor paralysis, manifested by pupillary dilatation and varying degrees of external ophthalmoplegia, is characteristic of upper brain-stem injury. A midbrain syndrome following head injury was described by Kremer, Russell, and Smyth (1947). The outstanding features were ataxia of the limbs and dysarthria. In addition, there was often a parkinsonian-like tremor, pupillary and oculomotor disorders, loss of balance, and pyramidal tract signs.

Two clinical patterns of brain-stem dysfunction secondary to tentorial herniation — a central and an uncal syndrome — have emerged from the study of McNealy and Plum (1962). Patients who exhibited the central syndrome were often found at necropsy to have no significant uncal herniation. This syndrome occurs more commonly and results from progressive impairment of diencephalic function. In the early (diencephalic) stage, consciousness becomes increasingly depressed, respiration at first normal may develop a Cheyne-Stokes pattern, the pupils are miotic, caloric stimulation evokes tonic deviation of the eyes, vertical gaze is defective, a generalized motor hypertonus (paratonia) appears, both plantar responses are commonly extensor, and decerebrate or decorticate postural effects may be elicited. At this stage, recovery is still possible provided appropriate therapy is promptly instituted. Otherwise further deterioration inevitably occurs with the development of signs indicative of progressive rostral-caudal brain stem failure (midbrain and pontine stages). Hyperthermia may give way to hypothermia, the pupils dilate and fail to react, hyperventilation develops, caloric stimulation elicits a tonic deviation only of the homolateral eye, the tendon reflexes are suppressed, and decerebrate phenomena appear in response to painful stimuli. Eventually, in the terminal medullary phase, flaccidity supervenes, hyperpnea may alternate with periods of apnea, the pupils dilate widely, the pulse rate varies, blood pressure falls, vestibular stimulation fails to evoke any ocular response and, finally, respiration ceases.

The syndrome of uncal herniation and lateral brain-stem compression is initiated by ipsilateral pupillary dilatation. Consciousness is not consistently impaired at the outset. As additional signs appear, the patient's condition may deteriorate rapidly. External ophthalmoplegia and stupor followed by coma ensue. Bilateral motor signs and decerebrate phenomena become demonstrable. Treatment at this stage is imperative if a fatal issue is to be avoided. As decompensation continues, eupnea changes to neurogenic hyperventilation, both pupils dilate and fail to react to light, and vestibular stimulation elicits either a monocular

18

tonic deviation or no response. The pupils may eventually fix in mid-position. In the final stage, the manifestations of the uncal syndrome are indistinguishable from those of the central syndrome. A more detailed account of the sequence of events that occur in the course of progressive brain-stem deterioration may be found in the article by McNealy and Plum (1962) and in the monograph by Plum and Posner (1966).

RESPIRATION AND OXYGEN SUPPLY TO THE BRAIN

The necessity for providing the brain with an adequate and unobstructed supply of oxygen is clearly indicated in the following comments by Peet :

"Intracranial pressure is greatly increased by any obstructions to respiration. This is due to the back pressure through the jugular veins and dural sinuses to the cortical and deeper veins of the brain. Such increased pressure may develop very rapidly, in fact almost instantaneously, with respiratory obstruction. It may, if the skull and dura are open as in an extensive compound skull fracture, or during an intracranial operation, cause such a rapid and marked herniation of the brain with rupture of the cortex and tearing of veins that death quickly ensues. Even if the skull is intact, the increased pressure in the dural sinuses resulting from respiratory obstruction may cause death from cortical and sub-cortical venous hemorrhages. The results of respiratory obstruction are also evident in the milder cases of head trauma, the increased intracranial pressure causing an elevation of blood pressure, sufficient in some cases to start arterial bleeding from vessels which had been temporarily thrombosed. There is probably increasing brain edema and certainly the oxygen supply to the brain is diminished. This latter is a vital factor which has not received the attention it deserves. The coma, which may be causing deep concern, may be due solely to brain anoxia, the result of respiratory obstruction. Clearing the pharynx and trachea often results in immediate improvement of the patient's general condition, with a return to semi- or full consciousness, a lowering of the blood pressure, and a change from stertorous to normal respirations. Muscular twitchings, even convulsions, may cease after correcting respiratory obstruction.

"It is therefore evident that special and continued attention to

19

the airways must be given in all cases of head trauma. In comatose patients lying upon their backs it is exceedingly common for the tongue to drop back, obstructing the posterior pharynx and seriously interfering with respiration. It scarcely seems necessary to call attention to this and the simple expedient of pulling the angle of the lower jaw forward to relieve the obstruction, but the author has time and again had to demonstrate this manoeuvre to residents and nurses. Turning the body slightly so the head will naturally lie on the side helps greatly in preventing the tongue from falling back.

"Alcoholic patients are particularly prone to vomit and have particles of food obstruct the pharynx and often the larynx. At the first sign of vomiting immediate steps must be taken to prevent any of the vomitus being aspirated into the larynx and trachea. The head should be forcibly turned to the side and if vomiting is profuse or there is evidence that some material has been aspirated the general rule to keep the head elevated in all cases of cerebral trauma is reversed and the head quickly lowered below the level of the abdomen. At times sudden, drastic action is necessary to prevent actual or impending suffocation from aspiration of vomitus. It is necessary to pull the patient half out of bed and hold the thorax and head in an almost vertical head-down position. Suction of the posterior pharynx is of great help in clearing the air passage. The horizontal position is restored as soon as the crisis has passed. It is remarkable how quickly a deeply cyanosed patient may have normal color restored, and respirations and pulse greatly improved by such apparently simple, but immediately necessary manoeuvres."

Respiratory insufficiency, whatever the cause, leads to hypoxia and hypercapnea which, in turn, induce cerebral vasodilatation and increased intracranial pressure. Cerebral edema is aggravated and the likelihood of hemorrhage increased; neurologic deficits may be accentuated and consciousness depressed further.

Respiratory depression may be caused by lesions that involve the brain stem. Aside from the respiratory hazards indicated by Peet, ventilation may be inadequate as a result of associated injuries of the chest and cervical cord, or as a consequence of tracheal obstruction brought about by trauma to the head and neck. Shock, occurring in patients with multiple injuries, increases cerebral ischemia by virtue of its hypotensive and hypoxic effects.

To combat respiratory insufficiency, a mechanical respirator and/or tracheotomy (or endotracheal intubation) may be required. The respirator will assure adequate ventilation, the tracheotomy a patent airway. An endotracheal tube may be safely left in place for 48 hours. Suction must be performed as often as necessary to clear the nasopharynx or trachea, employing a sterile technique to avoid infection. Supplementary administration of oxygen may be indicated in the face of anoxia.

CHEMICAL CHANGES

Little information is available concerning the chemical changes in the nervous system resulting from trauma. Significant elevation of brain and cerebrospinal fluid serotonin following experimental trauma has been demonstrated by Osterholm et al (1969, 1971). It was postulated that serotonin in the free state produces serious neurologic deficits. In cats the intracerebral injection of serotonin caused severe edema.

Excessive accumulation of acetylcholine in the cerebrospinal fluid and in traumatized brain tissue has been reported following experimental injury (Bornstein 1946; Metz, 1971). Tower and McEachern (1948) found a high concentration of acetylcholine and a low cholinesterase level in the cerebrospinal fluid of humans who had sustained cerebral trauma. The significance of the high concentration of acetylcholine lies in the fact that it can block synaptic transmission.

An increase in the acidity of the cerebrospinal fluid and elevation of its lactate content following trauma have also been reported (Fisher, 1966; Kurze et al, 1966). Changes in the phospholipids and glycolipids, including a reduction in lecithin and gangliosides, were found by Ishii (1966) following experimental compression in the cat. Fass and Ommaya (1968) reported no significant alterations in the sodium, potassium, and water content of the frontal and parietal gray and white matter of the monkey after experimental concussion; the chloride content of the white matter was decreased.

By measuring the major components of the energy reserve, ATP (adenosine triphosphate), P-creatine, glucose, and glycogen, Nelson et al (1966) found a 50 percent increase in metabolic rate following a lethal blow to the decapitated mouse head. The extra energy expenditure was derived mainly from ATP and P-creatine.

Walker's summary of the chemical alterations occurring in the brain tissue of animals following severe head trauma (1970) listed a decrease in oxygen, ATP and P-creatine; an increase in lactate and carbon dioxide; and a lowered pH. Similar changes with regard to oxygen, carbon dioxide, lactate, and pH occurred in the cerebrospinal fluid; in

21

addition, potassium and acetylcholine were increased.

Metabolic studies by Zupping (1970) in 45 cases of severe head trauma within the first 12 days after injury revealed a considerable decrease of CSF bicarbonate, Pco_2 and pH, and an increase of CSF lactate and pyruvate concentrations. Most commonly, the cerebral venous Pco_2 and Po_2 were appreciably diminished. Arterial blood studies disclosed a respiratory alkalosis with hypocapnia, hypoxemia, and elevated pH. A close correlation was noted between the severity of the brain injury and the degree of CSF metabolic acidosis and arterial and venous hypocapnia.

CAUSES OF DEATH IN HEAD INJURY

Lewin (1966) divided the causes of death resulting from head injury into six categories:

1. Severe brain injury with damage to vital areas (posterior hypothalamus, midbrain, and medulla) as a result of concussion, contusion, or secondary effects (Freytag, 1963).
2. Cerebral compression, including epidural and subdural hemorrhage, edema, and infection.
3. Chest complications which, aside from the primary and secondary effects of head trauma, pose the most serious threat to the patient. Aspiration is most commonly responsible for pulmonary complications, including bronchopneumonia and lung abscess. Complications may also occur as a result of chest trauma incurred at the time of injury, and fat emboli that arise in a fracture of a long bone. Pulmonary edema of cerebral origin may be an additional factor (Ducker, 1968; Ducker and Simmons, 1968). It is well to keep in mind the fact that, in addition to causing pulmonary manifestations, fat embolism may be responsible for a deterioration of consciousness.
4. Metabolic disturbances, including such disorders of water and electrolyte balance as cerebral salt retention which is attributed to dehydration, and cerebral salt wasting which is believed to be due to an inappropriate secretion of antidiuretic hormone causing water retention (Matthews, 1965; McLaurin, 1966). Diabetes insipidus may develop and, when overlooked in an unconscious patient, may result in severe water depletion and hypernatremia. In addition, various disorders of acid-base balance, of renal function, and of carbohydrate metabolism may appear. Such metabo-

22

lic disturbances may have considerable bearing on the ultimate outcome. This subject is considered at length in Chapter 6.

5. Multiple injuries involving other parts of the body, which in the comatose patient may be hard to recognize. Early diagnosis of such concomitant injuries, particularly those of the chest, abdomen, and spine, may be of critical importance. In this connection it should be borne in mind that shock caused by head trauma is most unusual. As a rule, the explanation for its occurrence will be found in injuries affecting other parts of the body.

6. Coincidental vascular lesions affecting the coronary and cerebral blood vessels, hypertension, and congestive heart failure may play an important role in the eventual outcome, especially in older individuals.

CRANIOCEREBRAL INJURIES IN EARLY LIFE

Head injuries in the newborn and during infancy and childhood are discussed at length in Chapters 14 and 15. Only certain highlights will be considered at this point.

During birth the fetal head is subjected to considerable stress and undergoes changes in shape as it descends through the maternal pelvis. Excessive trauma to the head may occur as a result of cephalopelvic disproportion, precipitous delivery, prolonged labor, or injudicious obstetric management. Prematurity increases the susceptibility of the infant to birth injury. The alterations in shape of the head, termed "molding," stretch the dural septa to a degree sufficient at times to tear the tentorium and, less often, the falx. Veins leading into dural sinuses may also be stretched and torn, with resultant intracranial hemorrhage. Among the vessels which may be injured are the cortical veins leading into the superior sagittal sinus, small tentorial vessels, the internal cerebral veins, the vein of Galen, and the superior longitudinal, transverse, and straight sinuses. While there is considerable overlap, the hemorrhages have been classified by Dekaban (1970) as subdural, intracerebral, subarachnoid, predominantly intraventricular or subependymal, and multiple small lesions. Compression of the intracranial contents as a result of molding may affect the brain stem, particularly the respiratory center, through the intermediary of a pressure cone at the foramen magnum. Venous compression caused by a rise in intracranial pressure may lead to hemorrhagic extravasation.

According to Towbin (1970) four basic types of head injury involve the nervous system in the fetus and newborn: 1) Subdural hematoma due to dural venous laceration that is caused by excessive cranial molding. 2) Spinal cord and brain-stem injury, mechanically induced. 3) Periventricular cerebral (venous) infarction with intraventricular hemorrhage, occurring especially in prematures. 4) Cortical cerebral infarction, found mainly in term infants.

Fractures of the cranium are rare in the neonate, the most common variety being an indentation ("Ping-Pong fracture") that results from the application of obstetrical forceps.

Although it is well known that anoxia may cause severe damage to the brain, the importance of asphyxia neonatorum (or apnea neonatorum, i.e., apnea at birth) in this respect is still unsettled (Ford, 1966). With regard to its etiology, various factors have been implicated, including maternal disorders (e.g. anemia, toxemia), placental defects, depression of the respiratory center as a result of intracranial pathology or the administration of a pharmacologic agent, prematurity, and pulmonary disease (e.g., hyaline membrane disease). According to Walsh and Lindenberg (1961), in most cases asphyxia neonatorum does not cause ill effects, though at times it may damage the brain stem and basal ganglia. They suggest that "since hypoxia is a normal state during the birth process, an immediate subsequent period of anoxia such as occurs in asphyxia neonatorum is infinitely less dangerous than a brief period of oxygen lack after adequate respiration has been established." Davison and Snaith (1964) believe that "anoxia as a major factor in the production of cerebral damage is probably usually initiated before the actual onset of labor, the result of relative insufficiency of the placenta." This degree of anoxia in itself is insufficient to be injurious but it renders the fetus more susceptible to other factors, such as uterine contractions that interrupt the placental circulation, produce further anoxia and, eventually, brain damage.

In experiments with newborn monkeys, Windle (1968) has shown that asphyxiation of the fetus for more than seven minutes invariably caused permanent brain damage. Most vulnerable were the nerve cells of the inferior colliculus and ventrolateral thalamic nuclei. More extensive lesions followed more prolonged asphyxiation. The neurologic deficits were of varied severity and duration. The experimental data led Windle to conclude that birth asphyxia lasting long enough to make resuscitation necessary always damages the brain and that the incidence of minimal brain damage in humans due to asphyxia is greater than commonly believed.

Towbin (1969, 1971) also emphasizes the vulnerability of the central nervous system of the fetus and newborn to the effects of hypoxia.

The resulting damage may be extensive and manifested by major neurologic disability, or, more often, limited and related to the subsequent development of the syndrome of minimal brain dysfunction. According to Towbin, most hypoxic cerebral lesions are of venous infarctional origin. The periventricular subependymal matrix is most frequently damaged in the fetus and premature newborn; intraventricular hemorrhage may occur as a consequence. In the term fetus and newborn, it is mainly the cerebral cortex that is affected by hypoxia.

Of the three major possible causes of brain damage at birth — trauma, anoxia, and disturbances of circulation — Courville (1971) considered paranatal anoxia to be by far the most important factor. This thesis is developed at length in his monograph, *Birth and Brain Damage*.

Asphyxia may occur before labor (due to maternal or obstetrical abnormalities), during delivery (obstetrical causes), or after birth. Whatever the mechanism of its production, the ultimate ill effect of cerebral anoxia is neuronal injury. As a result of damage to the respiratory center, breathing is affected and anoxia made worse. Anoxia leads to venous congestion which in turn may cause bleeding.

With regard to the clinical manifestations of birth injury, so-called "asphyxia pallida," which occurs in the immediate postpartum period, is characterized by profound stupor, pallor, flaccidity, a weak cry, feeble pulse, subnormal temperature, soft fontanels, and a markedly abnormal respiratory rhythm. The outcome is invariably fatal. Less seriously injured infants are apathetic and exhibit varying degrees of cyanosis and irregularity of respiration, hypertonicity, a shrill weak cry, inability to nurse, twitchings, convulsions, and fullness of the fontanels. Less severe degrees of asphyxia are referred to as "asphyxia livida." Massive intracranial hemorrhage usually results in death at birth or during the early neonatal period.

The management of cerebral birth trauma is largely supportive and involves the initiation and maintenance of respiration utilizing a respirator if necessary, establishment of a clear airway and administration of oxygen, and the use of an incubator. Parenteral vitamin K may be advisable and anticonvulsant medication may be necessary. Lumbar puncture is of doubtful therapeutic value. In the presence of a bulging fontanel, subdural puncture is indicated in search of a hematoma. Operation should be performed in the event subdural puncture alone is unsuccessful in the treatment of subdural hematoma (Hooper, 1969).

Infants who survive cerebral birth trauma seemingly recover fully in most instances. Permanent sequelae are deemed more likely to result from cerebral anoxia.

25

A subdural hematoma that may manifest itself clinically after some weeks or months of life may have had its inception at birth. The following comments by Matson (1954) are significant in this regard: "Extensive bilateral subdural bleeding dating from birth may be compatible with life and with normal development if it is recognized early enough and properly treated. This, however, is not an acute, but a subacute or chronic lesion. Subdural bleeding severe enough to cause increased intracranial pressure and serious symptomatology immediately after delivery is apt to be promptly fatal. In chronic subdural hematoma dating from birth, the findings may be quite obscure — nothing more than failure to eat well and gain, together with slight head enlargement, irritability, and perhaps a single convulsion. Localizing signs are not common and diagnosis can be made only by puncture of the subdural space through the coronal suture."

Of common occurrence in the newborn is cephalhematoma, an accumulation of blood beneath the pericranium, usually in the parietal region on one side and bounded by suture lines. No treatment is necessary in most cases.

Postnatal craniocerebral trauma requires little in the way of special comment here. In children the skull may undergo appreciable molding without sustaining a fracture. Epidural hemorrhage is relatively uncommon during infancy but may occur in the absence of a demonstrable skull fracture or in association with diastasis of a suture. The clinical presentation in infants may be considerably modified as a result of the rapid diminution of blood volume caused by the relatively large amount of bleeding into the epidural space. Severe anemia and signs of profound shock may be the outstanding features.

Courville (1965) found that the incidence of contrecoup lesions is very low in children under the age of three years and that it increases rapidly thereafter. During early life (six weeks to five years) contrecoup injuries occurred most often following lateral or multiple impacts of the moving skull. No ipsilateral coup lesions were observed in this group of cases, presumably owing to the shallow convolutional markings on the inner surface of the temporal region of the skull.

Leptomeningeal cysts (growing skull fractures) are infrequent complications of skull fractures incurred during infancy and early childhood. Rupture of the dura and herniation of the arachnoid into the fracture occur at the time of injury. Cerebrospinal fluid continues to accumulate within the arachnoid herniation, the dural defect enlarges, and the margins of the fracture are increasingly expanded. Fits, a progressive neurologic deficit, and an enlarging lump at the site of trauma are the usual manifestations. The radiologic findings are diagnostic. Treatment is surgical, consisting of excision of the leptomeningeal cyst and repair of the dural defect followed by cranioplasty.

THE AFTERMATH OF HEAD AND BRAIN INJURY.
ORGANIC VERSUS NEUROTIC DISEASE

Headache, dizziness, undue fatigability, inability to concentrate, irritability, and insomnia are common complaints following head injury and constitute the basic elements of the posttraumatic (post-concussion) syndrome. Its manifestations are essentially or exclusively subjective, abnormal neurologic signs as a rule not being evident. The preceding head injury need not necessarily have been associated with loss of consciousness. Headache, the most frequent symptom, is of variable intensity, location, character, and duration. Dizziness, another common complaint, is not usually a truly vertiginous sensation, but rather a feeling of unsteadiness or faintness.

The nature of this condition has been the subject of much controversy. The problem of evaluation of the respective parts played by organic brain disease, compensation, and neurotic illness has never been fully resolved, so that, viewed both from a medical and legal standpoint, the posttraumatic syndrome remains in large measure a dilemma. Questions of compensation and neurotic invalidism almost invariably arise and are the cause of much medicolegal friction. If the patient's posttraumatic symptoms are to be evaluated in their proper perspective, it is obviously important to elicit a detailed account of his physical condition and behavioral pattern prior to injury, and of his socioeconomic background. After analyzing 1,925 cases of head injury, Muller (1969) concluded: "The psychological, social, and economic setting seems far more important than the initial gravity of the head trauma in determining permanent disability. The incidence of permanent disability is remarkably high in slight head trauma and remarkably low in severe head injuries." According to Miller (1966), "The post-concussional syndrome of headache, postural dizziness, irritability and failure of concentration is sanctified by tradition, graven on the heart of every claimant for compensation, and attributed by some whose authority cannot be doubted to molecular neuronal damage. A moment's consideration of the epidemiology and natural history of the condition is enough to indicate that such damage, if it exists at all, must be of the most remarkable kind." Elsewhere, Miller (1969) states: "It (i.e., the post-concussional syndrome) is hardly ever seen

27

after injuries sustained in sports such as football or steeplechasing, or even in the home, but is conspicuous amongst cases where compensation is concerned. More significantly still, it is very much commoner after trivial injury without skull fracture or prolonged unconsciousness than in severe cases." (See also Cook, 1969). Hooper (1969) too subscribes to the idea that the post-concussion syndrome is largely neurotic in origin. This problem is considered further in Chapter 19.

The question of causal relationship may arise in connection with the diagnosis of posttraumatic epilepsy. Answers to the following queries should help resolve this problem (Walker, 1969):

Did the alleged accident actually cause brain damage?

Did the patient have any predisposing disease — cerebral or systemic — which may have given rise to the alleged posttraumatic condition?

Did the patient have any evidence of the alleged posttraumatic condition before the accident?

Has the alleged posttraumatic condition been verified?

Was the time interval between injury and the onset of symptoms appropiate?

Is the alleged posttraumatic condition compatible with the available data, including the site of injury and the clinical and laboratory (EEG) evidence?

THE PROVOCATION OR AGGRAVATION OF ORGANIC NON-TRAUMATIC DISEASES OF THE NERVOUS SYSTEM BY INJURY OF THE BRAIN AND SPINAL CORD

Whether trauma bears any relation to other diseases of the nervous system is a moot question. Much has been written on the subject but, in most instances, what has been adduced as proof of causal relationship represents no more than speculation based on a temporal sequence of events. Often the etiology of the condition under consideration is unknown so that only inferences of a conjectural nature can be drawn. Even in cases in which the cause of the diseases is known, its relation to trauma is often no less obscure. The insistence on positive opinions which the facts may not warrant and the conflicting testimony of medical experts in the course of litigation cloud the issues still further.

The question whether head trauma can cause a brain tumor cannot be categorically denied or affirmed. Considering the frequency of occurrence of head injuries and the infrequency with which tumors develop thereafter, a causal relationship appears highly unlikely. Among the many soldiers who have sustained cerebral injuries in combat, the incidence of brain tumor has been no greater than that of the population at large. Admittedly, there is some evidence that occasionally meningiomas have developed at the site of previous trauma. Similar claims with regard to the gliomas have met with greater skepticism. Probably the effect of trauma in most such cases has been to unmask a tumor already existent.

Trauma has also been implicated as a causative agent in multiple sclerosis, another disease of unknown etiology. The evidence cited, however, is inadequate to justify such claims. On the contrary, in our present state of knowledge, it appears highly probable that trauma is not related to multiple sclerosis.

The cerebral blood vessels may be affected by trauma and, while cerebral arteriosclerosis as such is of non-traumatic origin, a severe blow to the head may, in all likelihood, further damage a vessel already diseased. The possibility of an inverse relationship must not be overlooked — that is, the initial event may have been a cerebral vascular accident and the injury was sustained as a result of a fall caused by the underlying disease.

With regard to paralysis agitans, trauma bears no relationship to the idiopathic or postencephalitic forms of the disease. Symptomatic parkinsonism may, however, appear as a consequence of damage to the midbrain or after repeated head injuries, such as occur in prize fighters.

There is no unequivocal evidence linking trauma to other diseases of the spinal cord.

CONCUSSION

In accordance with Trotter's definition (1924), the term concussion is generally employed to denote "an essentially transient state due to head injury which is of instantaneous onset, manifests widespread symptoms of purely paralytic kind, does not as such comprise any evidence of structural cerebral injury, and is always followed by amnesia for the actual moment of the accident." It is a transitory and reversible phenomenon (Denny-Brown, 1945), loss of consciousness of brief duration being its most conspicuous feature.

A more elaborate concept of concussion is advocated by Symonds based on the belief that neuronal injury is an accompaniment of all grades of trauma. Transient loss of consciousness without clinical residua is regarded as indicative of the mildest degree of concussion. In the more severe degrees of concussion, coma is of longer duration and neuronal damage proportionately greater. In such cases recovery may be incomplete (see Chapter 4). The concept that the severity of neuronal damage in head injury may be expressed in terms of varying grades of concussion, as measured by the degree and duration of impaired consciousness, is an important one. The degree of disturbed consciousness varies from mild drowsiness to deep stupor; its duration refers to the length of time during which "current events have not been stored," and is synonymous with the period of posttraumatic amnesia (Russell, 1932; Symonds, 1937; Russell and Smith, 1961).

The period of posttraumatic amnesia (P.T.A.) may then be taken as a yardstick of the severity of head trauma. By itself it is not a perfect measuring device since it is indicative only of the degree of diffuse cerebral dysfunction and takes no account of the focal or diffuse effects resulting from injuries which do not cause "acceleration concussion." Thus, amnesia is often absent in penetrating and crushing injuries (Russell, 1951; Russell and Schiller, 1949). Allowance must also be made for the factor of age which tends to lengthen the duration of the P.T.A. (Russell and Smith, 1961). Notwithstanding these limitations, the duration of the P.T.A. remains the best criterion of prognosis currently available (Russell, 1971).

With regard to the mechanism of concussion, Russell (1932) has offered the following comment: "My conception of the mechanism of concussion is that at the moment of injury the whole of the brain tissue undergoes mechanical agitation. This causes molecular disturbance within the nerve elements (probably in the myelin sheaths) which brings about an interruption in the conducting functions of the nerve-cell processes, and leads to the instantaneous loss of consciousness." Various other causes, such as cerebral anemia (Trotter), have been suggested but there is little evidence in their support and it appears more likely that commotion of nerve elements is responsible for the abrupt loss of consciousness.

INJURIES OF THE VERTEBRAL COLUMN AND SPINAL CORD

Spinal cord injuries usually occur in association with traumatic lesions of the vertebral column. The injury may be caused by a penetrating or stab wound or, more commonly, as a result of indirect trauma producing a spinal fracture or dislocation. Compression fractures most often involve the thoracolumbar junction; dislocations are most frequent

30

in the cervical region. Most fractures and fracture dislocations of the spine are the result of flexion-rotation forces. Extension injuries are not uncommon in the cervical region and may traumatize the cord without producing any demonstrable skeletal lesion. A dislocation of transient duration is thought to be the responsible mechanism in such cases (Taylor and Blackwood, 1948). Inward bulging of the ligamentum flavum impinging on the cord has also been suggested as the causative factor (Taylor, 1951). The disc and anterior longitudinal ligament may rupture in such cases but the posterior ligaments are unaffected; as a rule, the resultant dislocation reduces spontaneously. A similar clinical picture may result from a flexion injury causing acute retropulsion of an intervertebral disc. Cervical cord trauma produced by hyperextension occurs frequently in older people with spondylosis.

The usual mechanism of vertebral injury involves a flexion-rotation force, rotation being the more important factor responsible for displacement (Roaf, 1960; Holdsworth, 1963). A pure flexion force will produce a compression fracture before rupturing the spinal ligaments, the latter being extremely resistant to simple flexion. This is the mechanism of production of the common anterior wedge fracture in the thoraco-lumbar region. The addition of a rotatory element to the flexion force results in a rupture of spinal ligaments and this leaves the spine vulnerable to dislocation since its stability is then wholly dependent on the articular facets. Whether the spinal ligaments maintain their integrity or not is a most important consideration and is the basis of the concept of stable and unstable fractures (Nicoll, 1949). In consequence of flexion-rotation injury in the cervical region with rupture of the posterior ligament complex, the articular facets slide off one another, the disc ruptures, and a pure dislocation results; in the thoracolumbar region this type of injury more often produces a fracture of one or both articular facets with a dislocation in flexion and rotation, and a slice fracture of the vertebral body. Forcible extension combined with compression or compression and rotation in the cervical region may result in a hyperextension or rotary hyperextension fracture dislocation. Landing on the feet after a fall from a height may be the cause of a vertical compression fracture. Fractures of the ring of the atlas occur in this manner. Some injuries of the cervical spine and cord are caused mainly by lateral flexion (Roaf, 1963). The application of a powerful force directly to the back, especially in the thoracic region, may cause a shearing fracture with disruption of articular processes and ligaments and displacement of one vertebra on the other. Shear fractures invariably are associated with paraplegia. The subject of vertebral fractures and dislocations is

31

very well reviewed in a recent article by Holdsworth (1970).

Neonatal injuries of the spinal cord involve most commonly the cervical and upper thoracic region, and are mainly caused by excessive longitudinal traction, combined with flexion, hyperextension, or torsion of the spinal axis during delivery (Towbin, 1970). Contributing factors are precipitous delivery, prematurity, primiparity, and intrauterine fetal malposition (cervical hyperextension). In the course of a breech delivery, or following forceps traction in a cephalic delivery, spinal nerve roots may be avulsed and injuries may also be sustained by the vertebral column, brain stem and, at times, even the vertebral arteries. According to Towbin the commonest form of spinal injury in the newborn is epidural hemorrhage.

The pathologic changes following trauma range from mild contusion to complete transection. Petechial hemorrhages and, less often, massive bleeding involving several segments of the cord (hematomyelia) may be observed. Edema is a frequent occurrence. Cavitation and secondary degeneration of fibers within the white matter take place at a later date. The anatomic basis of spinal concussion, a condition characterized clinically by a rapid recovery of function, is not known.

The neurologic manifestations depend on the location and severity of the lesion. A partial lesion of the spinal cord results in a variable degree of weakness and sensory loss of those parts of the body innervated by cord segments situated below the level of injury. Hemisection of the spinal cord leads to a Brown-Séquard syndrome which is characterized by an upper motor neuron paralysis and loss of position and vibratory sense on the same side, and an inability to appreciate pain and temperature changes on the opposite side, below the level of the lesion; involvement of the anterior horn cells of the spinal cord at the site of injury produces an ipsilateral segmental lower motor neuron lesion. Usually, variants of this syndrome are encountered. Injuries of the cauda equina are manifested by flaccid paralysis and sensory loss affecting the lower extremities, inability to control the bladder and rectum, and impotence.

Compression or destruction of the anterior spinal cord results in a syndrome characterized by an immediate complete paralysis with hypalgesia below the level of the lesion, touch and position sense being spared (syndrome of acute anterior spinal cord injury; Schneider, 1955). Hyperextension injuries of the cervical region with compression of the spinal cord both anteriorly and posteriorly may result in a clinical picture consisting of disproportionately greater weakness of the upper than the lower limbs, bladder dysfunction, and varying degrees of sen-

32

sory impairment (syndrome of acute central cervical spinal cord injury; Schneider et al, 1954).

Transection of the cord is immediately followed by a state of "spinal shock." Power and sensation are lost below the level of the lesion and the bladder and rectum are paralyzed; the muscles are flaccid and the superficial and deep reflexes abolished. Blood pressure falls temporarily because of the interruption of flow of vasomotor impulses to the thoracolumbar level of the cord. This condition persists for a period of several days to six or eight weeks. Infection and toxic states tend to retard the recovery of reflex function. The stage of spinal shock is followed by a period of minimal reflex activity. Thereafter, tone increases, flexor spasms develop, and the Babinski toe reflex becomes demonstrable. Eventually, extensor activity appears and constitutes the dominant reflex pattern in most instances (Kuhn, 1950). The view that paraplegia in flexion is pathognomonic of complete transection of the cord, while paraplegia in extension indicates an incomplete lesion has been shown to be erroneous. Spinal shock may occur in association with partial lesions of the cord, in which case some degree of improvement is evident within a matter of hours or days. For a detailed account of the symptomatology of spinal cord lesions, the article by Guttmann in the Handbook of Clinical Neurology (1969) is highly recommended.

In general, the prognosis in cases of severe injury of the spinal cord is serious. Injuries involving the upper cervical region are often immediately fatal due to respiratory paralysis. When the clinical picture is one of an incomplete lesion, considerable return of function may be anticipated. Much less favorable is the prognosis in patients with evidence of a complete transverse lesion who fail to exhibit some improvement within 24 hours. It is improbable that any degree of recovery will ensue in such cases (Kahn, 1959; Holdsworth, 1965).

A spinal fracture should be suspected whenever an individual who has been injured complains of pain in the back. Unless the condition is recognized at the scene of the accident and appropriate precautions observed, the spinal cord may be inadvertently damaged, or additional injury inflicted as a result of ill-advised first aid measures. After the the patient has been examined in detail and the extent of neurologic involvement ascertained, the exact nature of the vertebral lesion is determined by roentgenographic studies. Normal alignment of the spine should be restored as soon as possible. Stable wedge fractures require no special treatment. Unstable fractures and fracture dislocations must be reduced and either immobilized or fused. Treatment must often be modified in cases in which the cord has been injured. For example, the

33

use of plaster is contraindicated because of the hazard of pressure sores, and operative treatment is inadvisable in the event paraplegia is complete and there is no likelihood of recovery. A vexing problem arises in connection with the role of laminectomy in the treatment of closed spinal-cord injuries. Undoubtedly, operation is indicated when there is evidence that a bony fragment or extruded disc is exerting pressure on the cord and in the very rare case in which the neurologic deficit progresses. More controversial is the issue of laminectomy in cases of cord trauma in which vertebral malalignment has been corrected, a neurologic deficit persists, and the Queckenstedt test reveals a block of the subarachnoid space. While opinions differ, it is generally believed that operation in such cases is not likely to prove beneficial.

Rehabilitation of the paraplegic patient entails an intensive program of physiotherapy, including measures to achieve bowel and bladder control. This subject is considered in detail in Chapter 26.

BIBLIOGRAPHY

Bakay, L. and Lee, J. C. *Cerebral Edema,* Springfield, Ill.: Charles C Thomas, 1965.

Bornstein, M. B. Presence and Action of Acetylcholine in Experimental Brain Trauma. *J. Neurophysiol., 9,* 349, 1946.

Butler, E. G., Puckett, W. O., Harvey, E. N., and McMillen, J. H. Experiments in Head Wounding by High Velocity Missiles. *J. Neurosurg., 2,* 358, 1945.

Cook, J. B. The Effects of Minor Head Injuries Sustained in Sport and the Post-concussional Syndrome. In A. E. Walker, W. F. Cavaness, and M. Critchley (Eds.), *The Late Effects of Head Injury.* Springfield, Ill.: Charles C Thomas, 1969. Pp. 408-413.

Courville, C. B. Contrecoup Injuries of the Brain in Infancy. *Arch. Surg. 90,* 157, 1965.

Courville, C. B. Birth and Brain Damage. Privately published by M. F. Courville, Pasadena, Calif., 1971.

Crompton, M. R. Brainstem Lesions Due to Closed Head Injury. *Lancet, 1,* 669, 1971.

Davison, G. and Snaith, L. Cerebral Birth Injuries. In G. F. Rowbotham, *Acute Injuries of the Head.* 4th ed. Baltimore: Williams and Wilkins, 1964. Pp. 510-526.

Dekaban, A. *Neurology of Early Childhood.* Baltimore: Williams and Wilkins, 1970.

Denny-Brown, D. Cerebral Concussion. *Physiol. Rev., 25,* 296, 1945.

Denny-Brown, D. Brain Trauma and Concussion (Editorial). *Arch. Neurol., 5,* 1, 1961.

Denny-Brown, D. and Russell, W. R. Experimental Cerebral Concussion. *Brain, 64,* 93, 1941.

Dill, L. V. and Isenhour, C. E. Etiological Factors in Experimentally Produced

Pontile Hemorrhages. *Arch. Neurol.* & *Psych.*, *41*, 1146, 1939.

Ducker, T. B. Increased Intracranial Pressure and Pulmonary Edema. Part 1: Clinical Study of 11 Patients. *J. Neurosurg.*, *28*, 112, 1968.

Ducker, T. B. and Simmons, R. L. Increased Intracranial Pressure and Pulmonary Edema. Part 2: The Hemodynamic Response of Dogs and Monkeys to Increased Intracranial Pressure. *J. Neurosurg.*, *28*, 118, 1968.

Evans, J. P. and Scheinker, I. M. Histologic Studies of the Brain Following Head Trauma. I. Posttraumatic Cerebral Swelling and Edema. *J. Neurosurg.*, *2*, 306, 1945.

Fass, F. H. and Ommaya, A. K. Brain Tissue Electrolytes and Water Content in Experimental Concussion in the Monkey. *J. Neurosurg.*, *28*, 137, 1968.

Fisher, R. H. The Acid-Base Balance of the Cerebrospinal Fluid in the Head Injured Patient. In W. F. Caveness and A. E. Walker (Eds.), *Head Injury.* Conference Proceedings. Philadelphia: J. B. Lippincott Co., 1966. Pp. 249-253.

Ford, F. R. *Diseases of the Nervous System in Infancy, Childhood and Adolscence.* 5th ed. Springfield. Ill.: Charles C Thomas, 1966.

Freytag, E. Autopsy Findings in Head Injuries From Blunt Forces. *Arch. Pathol.*, *75*, 402, 1963.

Friede, R. L. Experimental Acceleration Concussion. *Arch. Neurol.*, *4*, 150, 1961.

Gosch, H. H., Gooding, E., and Schneider, R. C. Cervical Spinal Cord Hemorrhages in Experimental Head Injuries. *J. Neurosurg.*, *33*, 640, 1970.

Gross, A. G. A New Theory on the Dynamics of Brain Concussion and Brain Injury. *J. Neurosurg.*, *15*, 548, 1958.

Grubb, R. L., Jr., Naumann, R. A., and Ommaya, A. K. Respiration and the Cerebrospinal Fluid in Experimental Cerebral Concussion. *J. Neurosurg.*, *32*, 320, 1970.

Gurdjian, E. S. Discussion, Tolerance of Subhuman Primate Brain to Cerebral Concussion. In E. S. Gurdjian, W. A. Lange, L. M. Patrick, and L. M. Thomas (Eds.), *Impact Injury and Crash Protection.* Springfield, Ill.: Charles C Thomas, 1970. Pp. 370-371.

Gurdjian, E. S., Hodgson, V. R., Thomas, L. M., and Patrick, L. M. Significance of Relative Movements of Scalp, Skull and Intracranial Contents During Impact Injury of the Head. *J. Neurosurg.*, *29*, 70, 1968.

Gurdjian, E. S. and Lissner, H. R. Mechanism of Head Injury as Studied by the Cathode Ray Oscilloscope. Preliminary Report. *J. Neurosurg.*, *1*, 393, 1944.

Gurdjian, E. S. and Lissner, H. R. Deformation of the Skull in Head Injury. *Surg. Gyn. Obstet.*, *81*, 679, 1945.

Gurdjian, E. S. and Lissner, H. R. Photoelastic Confirmation of the Presence of Shear Strains at the Craniospinal Junction in Closed Head Injury. *J. Neurosurg.*, *18*, 58, 1961.

Gurdjian, E. S., Lissner, H. R., Hodgson, V. R., and Patrick, L. M. Mechanism of Head Injury. *Clinical Neurosurgery, 12*, 112-128. Baltimore: Williams and Wilkins, 1966.

Gurdjian, E. S. and Webster, J. E. Experimental and Clinical Studies on the Mechanism of Head Injury, In *Trauma of the Central Nervous System.* A.R.N.M.D., *24*, 48-97. Baltimore: Williams and Wilkins, 1945.

Gurdjian, E. S. and Webster, J. E. Head Injuries. *Mechanisms, Diagnosis and Management. Boston*: Little Brown & Co., 1958.

Gurdjian, E. S., Webster, J. E., and Lissner, H. R. The Mechanism of Skull Fracture. *J. Neurosurg.*, 7, 106, 1950.

Gurdjian, E. S., Webster, J. E., and Lissner, H. R. Observations on the Mechanism of Brain Concussion, Contusion and Laceration. *Surg. Gyn. Obstet.*, 101, 680, 1955.

Guttman, Sir L. Clinical Symptomatology of Spinal Cord Lesions. In A. Biemond (Ed.), Localization in Clinical Neurology in *Handbook of Clinical Neurology*, Vol. 2, pp. 178-216. New York: Amer. Elsevier, 1969.

Hamburger, E. Vehicular Suicidal Ideation. *Milit. Med.*, 134, 441, 1969.

Heiskanen, O. and Törmä, T. Gastrointestinal Ulceration and Hemorrhage Associated with Severe Brain Injury. *Acta Chir. Scand.*, 134, 562, 1968.

Hirsch, A. E., Ommaya, A. K., and Mahone, R. H. Tolerance of Subhuman Primate Brain to Cerebral Concussion. In E. S. Gurdjian, W. A. Lange, L. M. Patrick, and L. M. Thomas (Eds.), *Impact Injury and Crash Protection*. Springfield, Ill.: Charles C Thomas), 1970. Pp. 352-369.

Hodgson, V. R. Physical Factors Related to Experimental Concussion. In E. S. Gurdjian, W. A. Lange, L. M. Patrick, and L. M. Thomas (Eds.), *Impact Injury and Crash Protection*. Springfield, Ill.: Charles C Thomas, 1970. Pp. 275-302.

Hodgson, V. R., Gurdjian, E. S., and Thomas, L. M. Experimental Skull Deformation and Brain Displacement Demonstrated by Flash X-ray Technique. *J. Neurosurg.*, 25, 549, 1966.

Holbourn, A. H. S. Mechanics of Head Injuries. *Lancet*, 2, 438, 1943.

Holdsworth, F. W. Fractures, Dislocations and Fracture-Dislocations of the Spine. *J. Bone Joint Surg.*, 45 B, 6, 1963.

Holdsworth, F. W. Acute Injuries of the Cervical Spine with Cord Damage. *Excerpta Medica International Congress Series* No. 93, 85. Amsterdam, Third International Congress of Neurological Surgery Excerpta Medical Foundation, 1965.

Holdsworth, F. W. Fractures, Dislocations, and Fracture-Dislocations of the Spine. *J. Bone Joint Surg.*, 52 A, 1534, 1970.

Hollister, N. R., Jolley, W. P., and Horne, R. G. Biophysics of Concussion. *Wright Air Development Center Technical Report*, 1958. Pp. 58-193.

Hooper, R. Patterns of Acute Head Injury. Baltimore: Williams and Wilkins, 1969.

Howell, D. A. Upper Brain-stem Compression and Foraminal Impaction with Intracranial Space-occupying Lesions and Brain Swelling. *Brain*, 82, 525, 1959.

Ishii, S. Brain Swelling. Studies of Structural Physiologic and Biochemical Alterations. In W. F. Caveness and A. E. Walker (Eds.), *Head Injury*. Conference Proceedings. Philadelphia: J. B. Lippincott Co., 1966. Pp. 276-299.

Ishii, S., Tsuji, H., Ozawa, K., Kundo, Y. and Evans, J. P. Brain Edema. Some Clinical and Experimental Correlations. In I. Klatzo and F. Seitelberger, *Brain Edema*. New York: Springer-Verlag, 1967. Pp. 32-66.

Johnson, R. T. and Yates, P. O. Brain Stem Hemmorrhages in Expanding Supratentorial Conditions. *Acta Radiol.*, 46, 250, 1956.

Kahn, E. A. Editorial on Spinal Cord Injuries. *J. Bone Joint Surg.*, 41 A, 6, 1959.

Kihlberg, J. K. Head Injury in Automobile Accidents. In W. F. Caveness and A. E. Walker (Eds.), *Head Injury*. Conference Proceedings. Philadelphia: J. B. Lippincott Co., 1966. Pp. 27-36.

Kihlberg, J. K. Multiplicity of Injury in Automobile Accidents. In E. S. Gurdjian, W. A. Lange, L. M. Patrick, and L. M. Thomas (Eds.), *Impact Injury and Crash Protection*. Springfield, Ill.: Charles C Thomas, 1970. Pp. 5-24.

Kinal, M. E. Traumatic Thrombosis of Dural Venous Sinuses in Closed Head Injuries. *J. Neurosurg.*, 27, 142, 1967.

Klatzo, I. Neuropathological Aspects of Brain Edema. J. *Neuropath. Exp. Neurol.*, 26, 1, 1967.

Klatzo, I. and Seitelberger, F. (Eds.), *Brain Edema*. New York: Springer-Verlag, 1967.

Kornblum, R. N. and Fisher, R. S. Pituitary Lesions in Craniocerebral Injuries. *Arch. Pathol.*, 88, 242, 1969.

Kremer, M., Russell, W. R., and Smith, G. E. A Mid-brain Syndrome Following Head Injury. *J. Neurol. Neurosurg. Psychiatry*, 10, 49, 1947.

Kuhn, R. A. Functional Capacity of the Isolated Human Spinal Cord. *Brain*, 73, 1, 1950.

Kurze, T., Tranquada, R. E., and Benedict, K. Spinal Fluid Lactic Acid Levels in Acute Cerebral Injury. In W. F. Caveness and A. E. Walker (Eds.), *Head Injury*. Conference Proceedings. Philadelphia: J. B. Lippincott Co., 1966. Pp. 254-259.

Lange, W. A. and Van Kirk, D. J. The Effectiveness of Current Methods and Systems Used to Reduce Injury. In E. S. Gurdjian, W. A. Lange, L. M. Patrick, and L. M. Thomas (Eds.), *Impact Injury and Crash Protection*. Springfield, Ill.: Charles C Thomas, 1970. Pp. 475-493.

Langfitt, T. W., Tannanbaum, H. M., and Kassell, N. F. The Etiology of Acute Brain Swelling Following Experimental Head Injury. *J. Neurosurg.*, 24, 47, 1966.

Langfitt, T. W., Weinstein, Y. D., and Kassell, N. F. Vascular Factors in Head Injury. Contribution to Brain-Swelling and Intracranial Hypertension. In W. F. Caveness and A. E. Walker, (Eds.), *Head Injury*. Conference Proceedings. Philadelphia: J. B. Lippincott Co., 1966. Pp. 172-194.

Lewin, W. *The Management of Head Injuries*. London: Baillière, Tindall & Cassell, 1966.

Lewin, W. Vascular Lesions in Head Injuries. *Brit. J. Surg.*, 55, 321, 1968.

Lindenberg, R. Compression of Brain Arteries as Pathogenetic Factor for Tissue Necroses and Their Areas of Predilection. *J. Neuropath. Exp. Neurol.*, 14, 223, 1955.

Lindenberg, R. Significance of the Tentorium in Head Injuries from Blunt Forces. *Clinical Neurosurgery*, 12, 129-142. Baltimore: Williams and Wilkins, 1966.

Lindenberg, R. Trauma of Meninges and Brain. In J. Minckler (Ed.), *Pathology of the Nervous System*. Vol. 2, New York: McGraw Hill Book Co., 1971. Pp. 1705-1765.

Lindenberg, R., Fisher, R. S., Durlacher, S. H., Lovitt, W. V., Jr., and Freytag, E. Lesions of the Corpus Callosum Following Blunt Mechanical Trauma to the Head. *Amer. J. Pathol.*, 31, 297, 1955.

Lindenberg, R. and Freytag, E. The Mechanism of Cerebral Contusions. A Pathologic-Anatomic Study. *Arch. Pathol.*, 69, 440, 1960.

Lindenberg, R. and Freytag, E. Brain Stem Lesions Characteristic of Traumatic Hyperextension of the Head. *Arch. Pathol.*, 90, 509, 1970.

37

Mark, V. H. and Ervin, F.R. *Violence and the Brain*. New York: Harper & Row, 1970.

Martin, J. P. Signs of Obstruction of the Superior Longitudinal Sinus Following Closed Head Injuries (Traumatic Hydrocephalus). *Br. Med, J.*, 2, 467, 1955.

Mastaglia, F. L., Savas, S., and Kakulas, B. A. Intracranial Thrombosis of the Internal Carotid Artery After Closed Head Injury. *J. Neurol. Neurosurg. Psychiatry*, 32, 383, 1969.

Matson, D. D. Intracranial Hemorrhage in Infancy and Childhood. *Neurology and Psychiatry in Childhood*. A.R.N.M.D. 34, 59-67. Baltimore: Williams and Wilkins, 1954.

Matthews, D. M. Biochemical Aspects of Head Injury. In J. N. Cumings and M. Kramer (Eds.), *Biochemical Aspects of Neurological Disorders*, 2nd series. Oxford: Blackwell Scientific Publications, 1965. Pp. 199-213.

McLaurin, R. L. Metabolic Changes Accompanying Head Injury. *Clinic.:l Neurosurgery*, 12, 143-160. Baltimore: Williams and Wilkins, 1966.

McLaurin, R. L. and Helmer, F. The Syndrome of Temporal-Lobe Contusion. *J. Neurosurg.*, 23, 296, 1965.

McNealy, D. E. and Plum, F. Brain Stem Dysfunction with Supratentorial Mass Lesions. *Arch. Neurol.*, 7, 10, 1962.

Metz, B. Acetylcholine and Experimental Brain Injury. *J. Neurosurg.*, 35, 523, 1971.

Meyer, A. Herniation of the Brain. *Arch. Neurol. & Psychiat.*, 4, 387, 1920.

Miller, H. Mental After-effects of Head Injury. *Proc. R. Soc. Med.*, 59, 257, 1966.

Miller, H. Problems of Medicolegal Practice. In A. E. Walker, W. F. Caveness, and M. Critchley (Eds.), *The Late Effects of Head Injury*. Springfield, Ill.: Charles C Thomas, 1969. Pp. 429-430.

Moore, M. T. and Stern K. Vascular Lesions of the Brain Stem and Occipital Lobe Occurring in Association with Brain Tumours. *Brain*, 61, 70, 1938.

Muller, G. E. Early Clinical History, EEG Controls and Social Outcome in 1925 Head Injury Patients. In A. E. Walker, W. F. Caveness, and M. Critchley, (Eds.) *The Late Effects of Head Injury*. Springfield, Ill.: Charles C Thomas, 1969. Pp. 414-422.

National Safety Council. *Accident Facts*. Chicago: National Safety Council, 1970.

Nelson, S. R., Lowry, O. H., and Passonneau, J. V. Changes in Energy Reserves in Mouse Brain Associated with Compressive Head Injury. In W. F. Caveness and A.E. Walker (Eds.), *Head Injury*. Conference Proceedings. Philadelphia: J. B. Lippincott Co., 1966. Pp. 444-447.

Nicoll, E A. Fractures of the Dorso-Lumbar Spine. *J. Bone Joint Surg.*, 31 B, 376, 1949.

Olafson, R. A. and Christoferson, L. A. The Syndrome of Carotid Occlusion Following Minor Craniocerebral Trauma. *J. Neurosurg.*, 33, 636, 1970.

Ommaya, A. K. Discussion, Injury Mechanisms. In W. F. Caveness and A. E. Walker (Eds.), *Head Injury*. Conference Proceedings. Philadelphia: J. B. Lippincott Co., 1966. P. 505.

Ommaya, A. K. Discussion, Physical Factors Related to Experimental Concussion. In E. S. Gurdjian, W. A. Lange, L. M. Patrick, and L. M. Thomas (Eds.), *Impact Injury and Crash Protection*. Springfield, Ill.: Charles C Thomas, 1970. Pp. 303-307.

Ommaya, A. K., Faas, F., and Yarnell, P. Whiplash Injury and Brain Damage. An Experimental Study. *J.A.M.A.*, *204*, 285, 1968.

Ommaya, A. K., Grubb, R. J., Jr., and Naumann, R. A. Coup and Contre-coup Injury: Observations on the Mechanics of Visible Brain Injuries in the Rhesus Monkey. *J. Neurosurg.*, *35*, 503, 1971.

Ommaya, A. K., Rockoff, S. D., and Baldwin, M. Experimenal Concussion. *J. Neurosurg.*, *21*, 249, 1964.

Osterholm, J. L., Bell, J., Meyer, R., and Pyenson, J. Experimental Effects of Free Serotonin on the Brain and Its Relation to Brain Injury. *J. Neurosurg.*, *31*, 408, 1969.

Osterholm, J. L., Black, W. A., Jr., Bonner, R. A., and Angelakos, E. T. Cerebral Serotonin Metabolism Following Severe Cerebral Trauma. In D. B. Skinner and P. A. Ebert (Eds.), *Current Topics in Surgical Research*, Vol. 3, New York: Academic Press, 1971. Pp. 147-156.

Peet, M. M. Personal Communication, 1948.

Plum, F. and Posner, J. B. *Diagnosis of Stupor and Coma*. Philadelphia: F. A. Davis Co., 1966.

Pudenz, R. H., and Shelden, C. H. The Lucite Calvarium — A Method for Direct Observation of the Brain. II. Cranial Trauma and Brain Movement. *J. Neurosurg.*, *3*, 487, 1946.

Roaf, R. A Study of the Mechanics of Spinal Injuries. *J. Bone Joint Surg.*, *42 B*, 810, 1960.

Roaf, R. Lateral Flexion Injuries of the Cervical Spine. *J. Bone Joint Surg.*, *45 B*. 36, 1963.

Russell, W. R. Cerebral Inolvement in Head Injury. *Brain*, *55*, 549, 1932.

Russell, W. R. The Development of Grand Mal after Missile Wounds of the Brain. *J. Hopkins Med. J.*, *122*, 250, 1968.

Russell, W. R. *The Traumatic Amnesias*. London: Oxford, 1971.

Russell W. R. and Schiller, F. Crushing Injuries to the Skull: Clinical and Experimental Observations. *J. Neurol. Neurosurg. Psychiatry*, *12*, 52, 1949.

Russell, W. R. and Smith, A. Post-traumatic Amnesia in Closed Head Injury. *Arch. Neurol.*, *5*, 4, 1961.

Scheinker, I. M. Transtentorial Herniation of the Brain Stem. A Characteristic Clinicopathologic Syndrome; Pathogenesis of Hemorrhages in the Brain Stem. *Arch. Neurol. & Psychiat.* *53*, 289, 1945.

Schneider, R. C. The Syndrome of Acute Anterior Spinal Cord Injury. *J. Neurosurg.*, *12*, 95, 1955.

Schneider, R. C., Cherry, G., and Pantek, H. The Syndrome of Acute Central Cervical Spinal Cord Injury. *J. Neurosurg.*, *11*, 546, 1954.

Schneider, R. C., Gosch, H. H., Norrell, H., Jerva, M., Combs, L. W., and Smith, R. A. Vascular Insufficiency and Differential Distortion of Brain and Cord Caused by Cervicomedullary Football Injuries. *J. Neurosurg.*, *33*, 363, 1970.

Scott, W. W. Physiology of Concussion. *Arch. Neurol. & Psychiat.* *43*, 270, 1940.

Snyder, R. G. Occupant Restraint Systems of Automotive Aircraft and Manned Space Vehicles. In E. S. Gurdjian, W. A. Lange, L. M. Patrick, and L. M. Thomas (Eds.), *Impact Injury and Crash Protection*. Springfield, Ill.: Charles C Thomas, 1970. Pp. 496-561.

States, J. D., Korn, M. W., and Masengill, J. B. The Enigma of Whiplash Injury. *New York State J. Med.*, *70*, 2971, 1970.

Strich, S. J. Shearing of Nerve Fibers as a Cause of Brain Damage Due to Head Injury. *Lancet, 2,* 443, 1961.

Strich, S. J. The Pathology of Brain Damage Due to Blunt Head Injuries. In A. E. Walker, W. F. Caveness, and M. Critchley (Eds.), *The Late Effects of Head Injury.* Springfield, Ill.: Charles C Thomas, 1969. Pp. 501-524.

Symonds, C. P. The Assessment of Symptoms Following Head Injury. *Guy's Hosp. Gaz., 51,* 461, 1937.

Taylor, A. R. The Mechanism of Injury to the Spinal Cord in the Neck Without Damage to the Vertebral Column. *J. Bone Joint Surg., 33 B,* 543, 1951.

Taylor, A. R., and Blackwood, W. Paraplegia in Hyperextension Cervical Injuries with Normal Radiographic Appearances. *J. Bone Joint Surg., 30 B,* 245, 1948.

Thomas, L. M. Mechanisms of Head Injury. In E. S. Gurdjian, W. A. Lange, L. M. Patrick, and L. M. Thomas (Eds.), *Impact Injury and Crash Protection.* Springfield, Ill.: Charles C Thomas, 1970. Pp. 27-42.

Thomas, L. M., Roberts, V. L., and Gurdjian, E. S. Impact-Induced Pressure Gradients Along Three Orthogonal Axes in the Human Skull. *J. Neurosurg., 26,* 316, 1967.

Tomlinson, B. E. Pathology. In G. F. Rowbotham, *Acute Injuries of the Head.* 4th ed. Baltimore: Williams and Wilkins, 1964. Pp. 93-158.

Towbin, A. Mental Retardation Due to Germinal Matrix Infarction. *Science, 164,* 156, 1969.

Towbin, A. Central Nervous System Damage in the Human Fetus and Newborn Infant. *Amer. Jour. Dis. Child., 119,* 529, 1970.

Towbin, A. Neonatal Damage of the Central Nervous System. In C. G. Tedeschi (Ed.), *Neuropathology Methods and Diagnosis.* Boston: Little Brown & Co., 1970. Pp. 609-653.

Towbin, A. Organic Causes of Minimal Brain Dysfunction. *J.A.M.A., 217,* 1207, 1971.

Tower, D. B. and McEachern, D. Acetylcholine and Neuronal Activity in Craniocerebral Trauma. *J. Clin. Invest., 27,* 558, 1948.

Trevor Hughes, J. and Brownell B. Traumatic Thrombosis of the Internal Carotid Artery in the Neck. *J. Neurol. Neurosurg. Psychiatry, 31,* 307, 1968.

Trotter, W. Certain Minor Injuries of the Brain. *Lancet, 206* (1), 935, 1924.

U. S. Department of Health, Education, and Welfare. *Types of Injuries. Incidence and Associated Disability. U. S. July 1965 - June, 1967.* Public Health Service Publication No. 1000 — Series 10 — No. 57. October, 1969.

U. S. Department of Health, Education, and Welfare. *Reports on Epidemiology and Surveillance of Injuries.* (No. FY 70 - R4.) *How Accidents Affect the Nation's Health.* Cincinnati: Environmental Epidemiology Branch, U. S. Department of Health, Education and Welfare, June 1970.

Unterharnscheidt, F. J. Discussion, Mechanisms of Head Injury. In E. S. Gurdjian, W. A. Lange, L. M. Patrick, and L. M. Thomas (Eds.), *Impact Injury and Crash Protection.* Springfield, Ill.: Charles C Thomas, 1970. Pp. 43-62.

Unterharnscheidt, F. and Sellier, K. Mechanics and Pathomorphology of Closed Brain Injuries. In W. F. Caveness and A. E. Walker (Eds.), *Head Injury.* Conference Proceedings. Philadelphia: J. B. Lippincott Co., 1966. Pp. 321-341.

Walker, A. E. Medicolegal Problems of the Head Injured: Critique. In A. E. Walker, W. F. Caveness, and M. Critchley (Eds.), *Late Effects of Head Injury,* Springfield, Ill.: Charles C Thomas, 1969. Pp. 494-497.

Walker, A. E. The Pathogenesis and Pathology of Head Injuries. In *Proceedings VI International Congress of Neuropathology*. Paris: Masson et Cie, 1970. Pp. 155-175.

Walker, A. E., Kollros, J. J., and Case, T. J. The Physiological Basis of Concussion. *J. Neurosurg., 1*, 103, 1944.

Waller, J. A. Drugs and Highway Crashes. *J. A. M. A., 215*, 1477, 1971.

Walsh, F. B. and Lindenberg, R. Hypoxia in Infants and Children: A Clinical-Pathological Study Concerning the Primary Visual Pathways. *Bull. J. Hopkins Hosp., 108*, 100, 1961.

Wilkins, R. H. and Odom, G. L. Intracranial Arterial Spasm Associated wtih Craniocerebral Trauma. *J. Neurosurg., 32*, 626, 1970.

Windle, W. F. Brain Damage at Birth. *J. A. M. A., 206*, 1967, 1968.

Windle, W. F. Brain Damage by Asphyxia at Birth. *Sci. Am., 221*, 76, 1969.

Zilkha, A. Traumatic Occlusion of the Internal Carotid Artery. *Radiology, 97*, 543, 1970.

Zupping, R. Cerebral Acid-Base and Gas Metabolism in Brain Injury. *J. Neurosurg., 33*, 498, 1970.

CHAPTER 2

PATHOLOGIC CONSIDERATIONS IN HEAD INJURY

STANLEY M. ARONSON, M. D.

The pathology of head injury does not lend itself to analysis on the basis of obvious cause and effect. In many instances the resulting intracranial lesion seems inappropriate to the trauma that initiated it. Both subjectively and objectively, the reconstruction of a valid sequence of events is difficult. Subjectively, the patient is only dimly aware of the true angle of contact or the physical magnitude of the injuring force. When there has been a symptom-free interval of several hours or days between the injury and the appearance of symptoms, accurate recall is even more unreliable. Objectively, there are striking differences in the clinical and pathological responses of the child, the young adult, and the senior adult exposed to the same mode of injury. These factors combine to create an aura of unpredictability both in prognosis and in the development of firm concepts of pathogenesis regarding head injury.

While acknowledging that the outcome of head trauma is frequently unpredictable, there are, nevertheless, certain parameters which have a modest degree of correlation with underlying pathologic lesions. The nature and severity of the head injury can be related to several factors, including the force and direction of the blow, the attitude and movement of the head at the moment of impact, the surface contour of the traumatizing instrument, the area of the cranium struck and, ultimately, the vector of forces within the cranial cavity. Generally speaking, a blow with a sharp instrument results in focal cranial perforation, setting up a severe but localized cerebral maceration, and carrying with it the critical danger of secondary infection through communication with the contaminated exterior. Trauma caused by a bluntly surfaced force usually produces a more diffuse form of craniocerebral injury and is, not infrequently, of more serious import. When the clinical counterpart of blunt craniocerebral injury is more intense and diffuse than the local hemorrhage or laceration appears to warrant, it may be the damaging effects of the transmitted impulse through the brain that are responsible.

Many of the delayed effects of craniocerebral injury may be ascribed to the combined effects of progressive intracranial bleeding, cellular reaction, and the accumulation of edema fluid within a space of unyielding capacity. The intracranial hypertension so generated may, by compressing critical intracranial veins and arteries, ultimately produce lesions which at autopsy are histologically indistinguishable from ischemic or occlusive vascular disease of non-traumatic origin.

CONCUSSION

Concussion is the most common form of definable head injury and, by definition, is associated with the least degree of gross structural change. The difficulties in assessing concussive alterations, particularly in the human brain, are virtually insurmountable since these lesions of themselves are seldom fatal, and only rarely are they subjected to pathologic scrutiny. The term "concussion" is often somewhat loosely based upon the presumption of absent gross structural change. Windle and his associates (1944) have suggested that concussion is a "transient state which sets in immediately upon application of an adequate force to the brain." They suggested further that the histopathologic counterpart of this transitory state is a subtle disorganization of the neuronal cytoplasm, without any gross pathologic change.

Careful experimental studies of concussive injury have been designed not only to obviate the problems of capricious fixation, perfusion, and staining, but also to maintain control circumstances and to eliminate, where possible, those cytologic changes of an artefactual nature (Windle et al, 1944; Chason et al, 1958, 1966; Friede, 1961; Hamberger and Rinder, 1966).

It has been convincingly demonstrated that a succession of histopathologic changes occur within the brain as early as 12 to 15 hours after a controlled blow to the head has been sustained. These changes consist of a chromatolysis of infratentorial neurons which is frequently progressive, and which sometimes culminates in complete neuronal destruction. It has been felt that the chromatolytic change of head injury could be distinguished from the chromatolysis of axonal section. Posttraumatic specimens have a more rapid onset, featuring a more homogenous alteration of the chromatin material. In contrast, the lesions which follow axonal section show a tendency toward selective chromatolysis in a perinuclear location. Nuclear eccentricity, frequently observed after damage, is rarely encountered in the posttraumatic ganglion cells.

The neurons most likely to display chromatolytic alteration are the larger ganglion cells of the reticular substance of the brain stem, par-

43

ticularly the retro-olivary cells of the medulla, the neurons of the lateral vestibular nuclei, and scattered ganglion cells of the midbrain and pontine tegmentum. Of considerable importance is the lack of any consistent hemorrhage, local edema, inflammation, or glial reaction in association with these early neuronal changes, and the fact that neurons of the cerebral and cerebellar cortex do not participate in this early process.

Histochemical studies have shown that even minimal cerebral trauma is capable of inducing significant metabolic change in cellular elements proximal to the injury (Robinson, 1969). The metabolic activity of oxidative enzymes within ganglion cell mitochondria is substantially elevated within 24 hours of damage to neighboring tissue. The elevated dehydrogenase reactions are presently used as indicators of increased oxidative metabolism of the altered tissue. Acetylcholinesterase and monamine oxidase have not been shown to exhibit any significantly altered response to local injury. Increases in acid phosphatase of lysosomal origin are coincident with glial cell reaction to the altered environment. Nerve cells isolated from the lateral vestibular nucleus in experimentally concussed animals have demonstrated a markedly elevated in vitro respiratory activity (Hamberger and Rinder, 1966).

Experimentalists have correlated the effect of acute pressure pulses to the brain with alterations in intracellular enzyme activity. Analysis of neurons and glial cells, isolated ten minutes after a series of short pressure pulses, showed a striking increase in succinoxidase activity. The degree of augmented activity is proportionate, within a certain range, to the force of the provoking mechanical pulse. Currently it is believed that mechanical pressure, exerted upon the entire nervous system, is responsible for the disruption of intraneuronal organelles such as the cytoplasmic chromatin bodies. Chason and his colleagues (1966) go even farther and suggest that physical trauma to the cell may indeed alter the cytoplasmic microsomes bearing nucleotidase. By causing an enzymatic inactivation of mitochondrial diphosphopyridine and triphosphopyridine nucleotides (coenzymes vital to the utilization of neuronal carbohydrates), extensive cytoplasmic damage ensues, particularly within the ribosomal clusters of the Nissl bodies.

Rinder and Olsson (1968) have studied the effects of transitory concussion upon intracranial vasculature permeability. They have noted that brief pressure pulses exerted against the lateral cranium were followed by distinctly increased vascular permeability (as exemplified by extravasation of circulating fluorescent indicators). The augmented permeability was particularly evident below the tentorium in the alt-

44

eral part of the brain stem and upper cervical spinal cord segments. One concept, as yet unverified, is that caudally directed nerve root traction, provoked by the concussive wave, may determine the selective localization of both vascular permeability and chromatolytic changes. Indeed, Friede (1961) has ascribed the acute chromatolytic changes in reticular substance neurons of experimentally traumatized animals to primary radicular axonal damage within the upper cervical cord.

CONTUSION

The adult brain is confined to a rigid, non-spherical chamber with numerous ventrolateral buttresses and intervening cul-de-sacs. The cranial interior is further divided by relatively inflexible dural septa which serve to increase the depth of each fossa. Ventrally, the housed brain is selectively tethered to the bony walls by means of arteries, veins, and cranial nerves, and mid-dorsally by veins. In addition to the possibility of causing local fracture, the absorption and transfer of mechanical energy which is exerted against one portion of the calvarium initiates radiating vectors of pressure through the softer cerebral tissues. As a result of the peculiar limitations of tissue mobility caused by the non-spherical and septate character of the cranial cavity and the non-random distribution of rigid vascular and cranial nerve attachments, the mechanical stresses occurring at the moment of physical impact are selectively channeled through only certain cerebral tissues. The combined acceleration-deceleration creates shearing forces that are responsible for surface bruises which are referred to as contusions. These lesions must be distinguished pathogenetically from local cerebral lacerations that are caused by the direct movement of foreign fragments or spicules of bone driven into the soft cerebral parenchyma (Lindenberg and Freytag, 1960).

Typically, contusions are superficial lesions involving the cerebral cortex. They are usually less than 3 centimeters in surface diameter and are confined to one or two neighboring gyri. Location at the crest of the involved cerebral gyrus is characteristic. Contusions show a predilection for the ventral aspects of the frontal lobes, particularly the mesial orbital gyri and the gyrus rectus. In this location it is common to find the olfactory bulb and tract lacerated or even destroyed (Fig. 1). An orbital contusion is sometimes, but not necessarily, accompanied by linear fracture of the underlying cribriform plate of the anterior

45

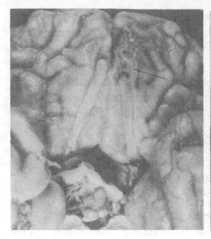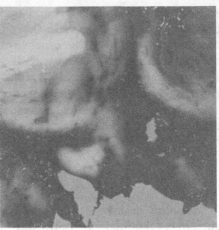

Fig. 1. Ventral surface of frontal lobe showing old contusion of both gyri recti, with destruction of left olfactory bulb (arrow).

Fig. 2. Cross section of cerebrum at chiasmatic level. There are multiple contusions involving the temporal lobe and optic chiasm, accompanied by diffuse subarachnoid hemorrage.

fossa. Still another common site for traumatic contusions is the rostro-lateral aspects of the temporal poles.

Contusions are frequently bilateral and may occasionally be associated with similar but smaller lesions at the diagonal extremity of the cerebrum (contrecoup lesions).

When viewed in cross section, the contusion is hemorrhagic, and tends to be triangular in shape with the apex extending to, or through, the superficial gyral white matter. The pial membrane is not preserved and there is, therefore, a continuity between the hemorrhagic laceration of the cortical tissues and the overlying leptomeningeal space, with variable amounts of subarachnoid blood accumulated in the vicinity of the tissue bruise.

The older contusion presents as a well-circumscribed, usually shallow, excavation of the ventrally located cortical tissues. The walls are often bright orange-brown in color, the result of residual hemosiderin pigment. Myelin preparations disclose an ill-defined zone of partial demyelination extending into the deep white matter, typically with severence of the arcuate fiber system. A glial zone of appropriate

46

astrocytosis creates a poorly defined limit to the lesion. Occasionally, the glial reaction intermixes to a very limited degree with some perivascular fibrosis at the pial margin of the lesion. The preserved neurons at the edges of the necrotic zone show varying degrees of cell sclerosis, agglutination of Nissl substance, and cell membrane ferrugination. Not until months after the traumatic episode can these latter neurocellular changes be found. Introduction of dura mater into the contused tissues is more typical of cerebral lacerations caused by depressed skull fracture. In such instances, the interdigitation of astrocytic and fibroblastic reaction is often very striking.

The first and second cranial nerves are occasionally incorporated into areas of basilar contusion (Fig. 2). Tissue disruption, presumably caused by the stress of a shearing force or basilar fracture, may traverse the olfactory tract and optic chiasm, inexorably extending dorsally, and ultimately breaking through the inferior margin of the lateral ventricle. Lacerations that create abnormal communication between subarachnoid and ventricular space invariably lead to hemorrhage into the ventricle. Such injuries are frequently found to be associated with linear or comminuted fractures of the orbital plate of the anterior fossa and the lesser wing of the sphenoid, extending caudally toward the tuberculum sellae, and traversing one or more of the cranial nerve foramens. In large series of head injuries associated with skull fracture, about 15 percent were extensively comminuted with depressed fragments and about 85 percent were simple linear fractures (LeCount and Apfelbach, 1920). Comminution is more typical of anterior fossa fractures than it is of posterior or middle fossa fractures. In addition, anterior fossa fractures often enter the nasal or frontal sinuses. This fact explains the increased risk of posttraumatic leptomeningitis in cases with anterior fossa fracture (21.3 percent) as opposed to cases with middle fossa (4.2 percent) or posterior fossa (8.4 percent) fracture.

Contusion-lacerations of Infancy

Certain notable features distinguish cerebral contusions in infancy from those sustained in adulthood. The careful studies of Lindenberg and Freytag (1969) have shown that the characteristic lesion of infancy consists of orbital and temporal cleft-like tissue tears without extensive hemorrhage. Those of the temporal lobes frequently begin opposite to the tentorial margins. The orbital tears dissect dorsally, circumventing the corpus striatum to enter the lateral ventricle. The laceration is associated with little necrosis and appears to incite only slight phagocytic and glial reaction. No capillary proliferation or perivascular reticulin production is seen in neighboring tissues.

Freytag (1963) noted another age-related distinction in that the volume of subarachnoid bleeding issuing from cortical contusions is notably greater in patients over 30 years of age.

Hypophyseal and Pituitary Laceration

Systematic studies have shown that traumatically induced lesions of the pituitary gland are common despite the paucity of clinical evidence of posttraumatic pituitary insufficiency (Ceballos, 1966). Hypophyseal stalk laceration has been shown to be a fairly common event following severe head injury, frequently causing amputation of the axonal system as well as the pituitary portal venous plexus. The most commonly encountered lesion of the pituitary gland consists of zones of coagulative infarction of the anterior lobe, occasionally resulting in a massive coalescing necrosis. In patients who survive for more than ten days after head injury, considerable reactive inflammatory cell infiltration, phagocytosis, and marginal fibroblastic proliferation are noted. Most observers agree that hypophyseal transection is rarely seen in the absence of basal skull fracture of the middle fossa. Statistical analyses also indicate that pituitary necrosis is more prone to ensue in head injury among persons in younger age groups.

Cerebral Contusion and Posttraumatic Epilepsy

The relationship between the location of the cerebral contusion and the frequency of subsequent seizures in retrospective collections of head injury data make certain predictions possible. Group statistics show an impressive concordance between the risk of future fits and the proximity of the lesion to the precentral gyrus. There are, however, enough individual exceptions to make us look elsewhere for other factors in the ultimate determination of seizure-risk. Most of the compiled data derive from follow-up studies upon living, war-injured populations and some inaccuracy in pinpointing the precise location of the contusion-laceration is, therefore, inevitable. Undoubtedly, numerous biophysical, and perhaps genetic, factors determine the ultimate likelihood of posttraumatic epilepsy.

Some generalizations, however, are permissible: Contusions associated with penetrating wounds of the dura, for example, have a higher frequency of posttraumatic epilepsy than similarly located contusions with intact neighboring dural membranes. The site of injury is also a major determining factor (Russell, 1951; Walker, 1962; Caveness, 1963). Contusions in the parietal and posterior frontal areas are associated with a higher frequency of posttraumatic seizures than those incurred in a prefrontal, occipital, or basilar location. Caveness (1963) demonstrated that about 72 percent of patients who survived parietal lobe wounds associated with penetration of dura mater, eventually developed fits. Other local factors that influence the likelihood of posttraumatic seizures include the depth of wound penetration, the volume of cortical tissue destruction, and the presence of bone fragments or foreign bodies within the cerebral parenchyma, as well as the introduction of viable dura into deep cerebral tissue. This deeply imbedded dura promotes the development of extensive fibroglial scars leading to sequestered collections of marginally viable neurons. The typical lesion consists of a variably broad zone of old, ischemic necrosis surrounded by margins of partially atrophic and ischemic gray matter which contains numbers of altered, shrunken, distorted, and presumably epileptogenic neurons. Both collagen fibers (derived from invaginated dura) and astrocytic glial fibers abound in conjunction with capillary proliferation; there is extensive ferric salt deposition over the perikaryons and proximal axons of scattered, subviable, or dead neurons.

PARENCHYMAL HEMATOMA

Some head injuries, usually those involving frontal or occipital areas, may result in a cerebral shearing lesion which extends beyond the cortical gray mantle. These injuries are typically associated with extensive occipital or frontal fracture. The softer cranial tissues may be the site of disrupted pia, broad zones of confluent cortical maceration, perivascular hemorrhages in the depths of the subjacent white matter, and a plane of tissue separation which may extend up to 5 centimeters in depth. Blood commonly pools within the disrupted tissues sometimes culminating in a large hematoma, in excess of 50 ml, within the white matter. Deep hematomata of this kind are most commonly found in the ventral frontal white matter or in the temporal white matter (rostral to the temporal horn of the lateral ventricle) and may not only dissect into the ventricular cavity, but may also extend laterally along the subcortical arcuate fibers of the neighboring, intact, cerebral cortex.

When the patient dies within 24 hours of head injury, the white

49

matter adjacent to the hematoma shows little gross change. As the posttraumatic interval lengthens, an obvious demyelination and tissue swelling supervenes, sometimes spreading into the neighboring ipsilateral lobe. This reactive edema may cause secondary brain-stem hemorrhages (see below) or, in rare instances, sufficient intracranial pressure to collapse the middle cerebral artery within the S·lvian fissure causing encephalomalacia in the area of distribution of this vessel. In theory, the ambient pressure required to collapse a vessel would be a function both of the lumenal pressure to be overcome and the physical properties of the vascular wall (Shapiro et al, 1966). However, in their study of the relationships between experimental intracranial hypertension and cerebral vessel compression, Shapiro and his colleagues observed that certain cerebral arteries (as well as veins) may be collapsed in the face of augmented intracranial pressures that are lower than diastolic arterial levels.

The chronologic sequence of events leading to the escape of fluid into interstitial tissues following local brain injury has been carefully documented by Klatzo and co-workers (1958). They have shown that edema commences as early as six hours after experimental injury, coincident with altered vascular permeability.

EPIDURAL HEMORRHAGE

In the majority of instances, the accumulation of enough extradural blood to produce clinical symptoms occurs as a sequel to traumatic laceration of one or more branches of the middle meningeal artery in its temporal course (Fig. 3). The artery, typically accompanied by two parallel veins, flows in a series of canyon-like channels between the inner calvarial periosteum and the underlying bone. The fixation of the artery between the rigid bone and the dura makes a shearing laceration of the artery a common sequel to temporal bone fracture.

Middle Meningeal Artery

The external carotid artery divides terminally into two branches, the larger one being the internal maxillary artery. This vessel passes between the mandible and the neighboring sphenomandibular ligament and divides into numerous branches. Proximally, its largest component is the middle meningeal artery. This vessel commences at the level of the mandibular ramus and passes superiorly through the foramen

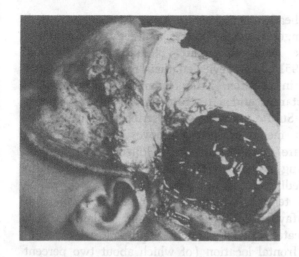

FIG. 3. Epidural hemorrhage in the left temporal region in a child who died shortly after an automobile accident. Note the sharply delimited margins of the extradural clot.

spinosum to enter the cranial cavity. Within the cranial chamber, it ascends between the inner calvarial table and the lateral dura mater. Its anterior branch travels over the greater sphenoid wing and eventually arborizes over the parietal bone. The osseous groove that harbors the anterior branch is more prominent than that of the posterior branch and deepens in its course – at times, enough to permit the walls to converge into a bony septum. Terminally, the anterior branch ramifies into a number of orbital branches at the level of the superior orbital fissure.

The posterior branch of the middle meningeal artery travels a more caudad course, extending over the inner surface of the squamous portion of the temporal bone. This vessel is characterized by relatively few branches until it reaches the posterior portion of the parietal bone when it subdivides and sends branches as far dorsally as the superior longitudinal sinus.

Relation to Skull Fracture and Age of Patient

In the absence of any demonstrable fracture, the occurrence of extradural bleeding is regarded as unusual. Mealey (1960) gathered published reports of 21 cases of extradural hematoma without skull fracture, seven of which involved patients ten years of age or younger, indicating that epidural hematoma without preceding fracture occurs more frequently in children than in adults. This may be the result of the greater resilience of children's skulls. Freytag's (1963) review of 1,367

51

autopsied cases of fatal head injury shows a lower frequency of skull fracture in patients younger than ten years, indirectly corroborating the suggestion that the skull has greater pliability in childhood. Campbell and Cohen (1951) have reviewed their records of 20 cases of epidural hemorrhage in children. X-ray examination of the skull was performed in 17 instances and a fracture (nearly always linear) was noted in 11 patients. Suture diastasis was described in ten patients. The fact that the middle meningeal artery grooves within the inner table of the calvarium are more shallow in childhood must also be regarded as a contributing factor affecting the relationship between fracture and epidural bleeding in this age group.

Extradural hematomas tend to be unilateral in about 96 percent of cases (Maurer and Mayfield, 1965; Jamieson and Yelland, 1968). About 70 percent are located upon the lateral supratentorial calvarial surface, 11 percent in a frontal location (of which about two percent are situated over the vertex), six percent are basilar, seven percent occipital and the remaining approximately seven percent situated in the posterior fossa (Kosary et al, 1966). Posterior fossa epidural hemorrhages generally pursue a less acute course and may not become clinically overt until days after the provoking injury. This difference in clinical evolution has been attributed to the fact that the bleeding arises from a venous rather than arterial source. An occipital fracture, typically intersecting the transverse sinus or torcular Herophili is demonstrated in over 90 percent of cases of infratentorial epidural hemorrhage (Kosary et al, 1966).

In an extensive, retrospective study of skull fractures, Vance (1927) showed that about 24 percent (56 of 233) of lateral skull fractures culminate in demonstrable epidural hematoma, a figure remarkably similar to Freytag's (1963) data which showed that epidural bleeding occurred in 22 percent of her cases with skull fracture. The posterior branch of the middle meningeal artery was implicated as the source of the bleeding twice as often as the anterior branch of this vessel. In fact, bleeding from the rostral branches of the anterior branch of the middle meningeal artery is quite rare. Whittaker (1960) has found less than a score of cases of anterior fossa extradural clot. It must be noted that these figures also reflect the fact that middle fossa skull fractures constitute 32.9 percent of all skull fractures, while but 12.1 percent are found in the anterior fossa (LeCount and Apfelbach, 1920).

Another uncommon locus of extradural hemorrhage is the calvarial vertex. Hematomas in this area are commonly associated with a simple, linear fracture intersecting the sagittal suture (Columella et al, 1968). The superior longitudinal sinus is stripped from the inner table of the skull and depressed. The expanding collection of blood typically dissects the periosteum from its calvarial attachment, creating a disc-shaped hematoma with a sharp rim. The margin of the hematoma rarely reaches the anterior or posterior suture lines which commonly act as deterrents to further spread of the hemorrhage.

The average weight of the epidural hematoma is about 110 grams (Vance's 1927 data indicate a mean weight of 122 grams, or an average volume of 115 ml.). In the extensive series of LeCount and Apfelbach (1920), containing data on 504 cases of fatal skull fracture, 199 showed some autopsy evidence of extradural bleeding. In 95 cases, the volume was negligible. In the remaining 104 cases, from 20 to 246 gm of blood were encountered.

Dissection of the cerebral hemispheres frequently discloses a shift of the structures to the contralateral side, which has been caused by the cumulative effects of the epidural hemorrhage as well as by selective cerebral swelling of the ipsilateral hemisphere (Fig. 4). The ipsilateral ventricle is commonly found to be compressed and partially rotated. Hippocampal herniation around the tentorial margin is frequently encountered, and may sometimes create the conditions responsible for hippocampal incarceration and hemorrhagic necrosis of both hippocampal and mesencephalic tissues. Distortion and caudal displace-

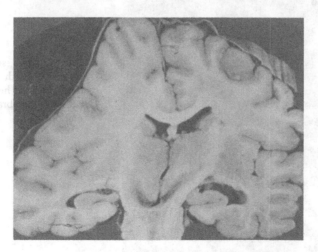

Fig. 4. Epidural hemorrhage, in cross section. Note the displacement of midline structures to the contralateral side, but no hippocampal herniation.

ment of the midbrain together with secondary brain-stem hemorrhages, are also commonly present.

SUBDURAL HEMATOMA

Subdural accumulation of blood is a commonly observed phenomenon, whether it is the clinically innocent dural staining seen at autopsy in patients without any record of head injury; or the laminated *pachymeningitis hemorrhagica interna* (probably the residue of repeated, small, traumatically induced subdural bleedings); or the posttraumatic hematoma of volume sufficient to initiate neurological changes.

In large series of trauma cases such as those recorded by Vance (1927), subdural hemorrhage was the commonest hemorrhagic manifestation of serious head injury. Gurdjian and colleagues (1968) studied the data from 900 consecutive cases of impact head injury and uncovered 83 instances of subdural hematoma (of which 14 were also associated with multiple epidural and intracerebral clots). In a 24-year review of 41,549 Kings County Hospital patients who had sustained craniocerebral injury, Aronson and Kaplan (1957) gathered

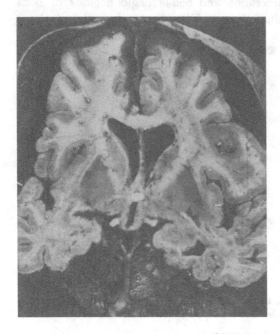

FIG. 5. Cross section of cerebrum with a bilateral subdural hematoma, without membrane formation.

data on 822 (frequency, 5.1 percent) verified instances of subdural hematoma.

The typical acute, subdural hematoma is unilateral (less than 8 percent are bilateral) and supratentorial in location (Fig. 5). The most extensive clots are usually formed over the lateral posterior frontal and anterior parietal lobes. The blood is typically of venous origin, derived from the traumatically opened veins bridging the superior longitudinal sinus and the dorsal parasagittal leptomeninges, or from the lacerated veins which drain the anterior component of the Sylvian fissure and bridge the subdural space to enter the sphenoparietal venous sinus.

Prior to encapsulation, the subdural collection of blood tends to diffuse over the entire dorsolateral hemispheric surface, its spread being limited only in the midline by the falx. The range of volume is considerable, although records indicate that the hemorrhagic mass rarely exceeds 200 ml (Laudig et al, 1941; Aronson and Okazaki, 1963). It is difficult to determine the volumetric threshold beyond which neurologic abnormalities may be confidently anticipated, because the majority of subdural hematomas are accompanied by multiple contusions and lacerations of the hemispheric cortical surfaces, and there is no clear assignment of responsibility for the abnormal clinical state to any one of the intracranial lesions. In the review of their experience with acute subdural hematomas, McLaurin and Tutor (1961) stated that the size of the hematoma is not prognostically significant and that the presence or absence of associated intracranial traumatic lesions (e.g., parenchymal clots, cerebral contusions, epidural hematomas) is more pertinent in predicting mortality rates.

In *uncomplicated* subacute subdural hemorrhage, some estimates that relate hematoma volume to clinical outcome may be made. The autopsy evaluation of cases without other intracranial injuries makes it possible to correlate the volume of subdural bleeding with the frequency of neurologic signs. Thus, very few patients with subdural bleeding of less than 25 ml showed any clinical signs which might have been attributed to the hematoma (Laudig et al, 1941; Aronson and Okazaki, 1963). Of the patients whose hematomas measured between 26 and 50 ml, about half showed signs which, in retrospect, were caused by the hematoma. When the hematoma exceeded 50 ml, neurologic symptoms had been evident in the overwhelming majority of appropriately examined patients. When the volume of subdural blood was larger than 150 ml (and in the absence of preexistent cerebral atrophy), most patients have died.

There is some data to indicate that the volume threshold necessary to induce neurologic signs is not constant, but may indeed vary with the age of the patient (Aronson and Okazaki, 1963). A number of factors contribute to this variance, preeminent among which is the existing ratio between the volume of central nervous system tissue and total intracranial volume. Intracranial volume is essentially unchanged beyond the second decade of life; nervous system tissue volume, however, diminishes with advancing age. There is, for example, an average 5.5 percent brain weight loss in males and 4.2 percent loss in females between the ages of 55 and 75 years, which results in an increase in the free intracranial space of about 65 ml. Thus it is apparent that the inevitable atrophy which accompanies increasing age permits the cranium to contain progressively larger subdural hemorrhages before the underlying hemisphere will be subjected to critical compressive forces.

Reactive Membrane Formation

The normal cerebral dura is composed of two fused layers, an outer component (the internal calvarial periosteum) and an inner membrane (the true cerebral dura). Under normal circumstances, the dural blood vessels are confined largely to the outer lamina. The vessels are, for the

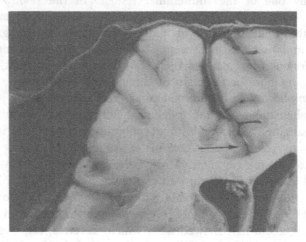

Fig. 6. Cross section of cerebrum showing the site of a a left subdural hematoma. The hematoma was evacuated at the time of autopsy to demonstrate the inner and outer reactive membranes. The mesial angle typically begins about two centimeters from the sagittal plane. Note the herniation of the cingulate gyrus (arrow) to the contralateral side.

56

most part, made up of arterial branches of the external carotid circulation and companion veins but with virtually no capillary bed. The inner dura is almost completely avascular. After subdural bleeding there is a rapid proliferation of capillaries through the previously avascular inner dura, accompanied by perithelial fibroblastic activity. A granulation tissue layer is thus established at the interface between the dura and hematoma. Somewhat belatedly, another membrane is formed over the ventral (arachnoid) surface of the hematoma, thinner and less vascularized than the dorsal membrane (Fig. 6). The origin of the cells which give rise to this membrane facing the arachnoid surface is in dispute. It is most unlikely that they are derived from the layer of granulation tissue at the dural surface of the clot, since a definable margin of reactive tissue is not observed advancing over the inferior surface of the hematoma. It is possible that the membrane between the hematoma and the arachnoid surface is formed by mesothelial cells which have been mobilized from multipotential cells within the clot.

Chronic, encapsulated subdural hematomas may, in time, be obliterated by reactive fibrous tissue. Secondary calcification, and even ossification with hematopoietic foci, have been noted in long-standing subdural hematomas.

The course of patients with clinically evident subdural hematomas makes it obvious that the effects of the hematoma are not constant. In some patients, there is total regression of signs and a return to a neurologically normal state. Others appear to undergo progressive clinical deterioration. Serial angiographic and pneumoencephalographic studies that clearly demonstrate a continuing shift of midline structures to the contralateral side, signify either continuing expansion of the hematoma or an enlargement of the subjacent hemisphere.

The earlier speculation that enlargement of subdural hematomas occurred as a result of the osmotic absorption of fluids through the membrane that encapsulates the hemorrhage was not an adequate explanation, particularly of those cases in which no membrane could be demonstrated at autopsy (Laudig et al, 1941; Goodell and Mealey, 1963). Subsequent, careful scrutiny of autopsy-derived specimens has provided a more rational basis for the appearance of progressive neurologic symptoms. There is no significant difference in hemispheric volume among patients who have died with acute, uncomplicated, subdural hematomas. However, as survival time is prolonged, differences do emerge. Typically, the white matter of the cerebral hemisphere on the side of the subdural hematoma becomes visibly swollen and its volume greater than that of the contralateral hemisphere. The involved white matter is softened, pallid, and frequently discolored, suggesting early demyelination. Histologic examination shows that the vessels of the deep transcerebral venous system (a network of collateral veins within hemispheric white matter that form an extensive intercommunicating system between the cortical and deep internal cerebral veins) (Kaplan, 1959) are variably dilated and their walls focally necrotic and typically infiltrated with inflammatory cells. When post-trauma survival is prolonged beyond a few days, the white matter in the immediate vicinity of these venous channels shows interstitial fluid accumulation, breakdown of myelin sheaths, some inflammatory response, and frequently an intense macrophagocytic reaction (Aronson and Kaplan, 1957). The reactive expansion of the compressed hemisphere appears to reach a peak between seven and ten days following the apparent onset of subdural bleeding. At this stage, specimens show compression of the ipsilateral ventricle, contralateral deviation of the third ventricle and midsagittal plane, and a clockwise rotation of the corpus callosum. The contralateral ventricle tends to be dilated. The hemispheric expansion is accompanied by herniation of the cingulate gyrus beneath the falx and a temporal lobe uncinate herniation over the free, mesial edge of the tentorial membrane.

In most uncomplicated subdural hematomas that develop during presenile adulthood, there is a striking correlation between the posttraumatic interval and the extent of regional brain swelling. In cases in which death has occurred soon after the injury, no significant subcortical swelling has been recorded. As the interval between trauma and death increases, however, the hemisphere subjacent to the hematoma increases in weight and volume, with the surface convolutions becoming progressively more flattened and the intervening sulci more narrowed. In addition to the diffuse perivenous demyelinating pattern and the transudative edema of the centrum semiovale, the ipsilateral corpus callosum becomes asymmetrically wider than its contralateral ramus. Frequently, there is a dramatic enlargement of the anterior limb of the ipsilateral internal capsule, a swelling which at times extends inferiorly through the cerebral peduncle of the midbrain. This cerebral swelling may assume an independent existence of its own, since surgical evacuation of the hematoma may not necessarily reverse the prevailing depression of consciousness or other symptoms referable to hemispheric disease.

It has been argued that the cerebral swelling coincident with subdural hemorrhage is the result of the inciting head injury rather than the compressive effects of the hematoma. Langfitt and colleagues (1966) have suggested that the pathophysiologic mechanism of brain swelling after head injury is generated through a direct concussive effect upon the internal cerebral vasculature, producing vasodilatation and secondarily increased intracranial pressure (which by diminishing effective arterial pressures results in a decreased cerebral blood flow), and culminating in irreversible cerebral vascular dilatation and cerebral edema. Ishii and colleagues (1959), employing an experimentally implanted extradural sac capable of controlled distension, demonstrated unequivocally that increased pressure upon the hemisphere without the accompanying shock of acute injury is sufficient to provoke a reactive swelling of the compressed hemisphere. This unilaterally augmented volume has been demonstrated by both planimetric and volumetric methods. Histologic preparations in these experimental animals have shown perivenous changes remarkably similar to those noted in human patients dying of subdural hematoma (Aronson and Kaplan, 1957). Using radioactive diiodofluorescein, these observers also demonstrated a selective uptake of radioactive isotopes by the affected hemispheric white matter, thus substantiating the histologic observation of a striking disturbance in permeability of the traversing blood vessels within the compressed white matter (Ishii et al, 1959).

Unusual Locations of Subdural Hematomas

The overwhelming majority of subdural hemorrhages accumulate over the lateral frontoparietal surfaces. Those over the posterior fossa are most rare, constituting only about 0.6 percent of all the subdural hematomas recorded in large, retrospective series (Fisher et al, 1958; McKissock et al, 1960; Ciembroniewicz, 1965). Most of the posterior fossa hematomas are found to be associated with direct occipital injury, and occipital fracture has been observed in about 30 percent of reported cases (Ciembroniewicz, 1965). Hemorrhage in this location is relatively more common in childhood (about 35 percent of cases have been in patients under 10 years of age). The source of bleeding may be from bridging veins which enter the neighboring dural sinuses, or from lacerated cerebellar cortical veins. Ciembroniewicz (1965) states that the subdural blood may extend below the foramen magnum and compress the spinal cord. Obstructive internal hydrocephalus, presumably caused by compression of the foramina of Lushka and Magendie, has also been noted.

Interhemispheric subdural hematomas have been described as infrequent complications of head injury. The inadequate number of cases which have been documented does not warrant any generalizations about the pathogenetic forces by which bleeding confined to this location is produced (Wollschlaeger and Wollschlaeger, 1964; Clein and Bolton, 1969). Data on the pneumoencephalographic (Clein and Bolton, 1969) and angiographic (Wollschlaeger and Wollschlaeger, 1964) features of this unique lesion have been published.

A major prognostic determinant in a patient with a subdural hematoma is the degree to which the white matter of the ipsilateral hemisphere becomes enlarged through the process of reactive cerebral edema. When this process has increased the volume of the hemisphere by an estimated 75 to 100 ml, a number of secondary changes supervene.

Calcarine Cortex Encephalomalacia

The basilar artery bifurcates into the two posterior cerebral arteries which curve around the cerebral peduncles and proceed caudally, crossing the edge of the tentorium, to enter the middle fossa. Proximal branches supply the posterior choroidal tissues, and perforating branches irrigate the medial portion of the optic thalamus. The main stream of the artery continues posteriorly, progressively ramifying to supply most of the ventromedial temporal lobe and the entire ventromedial occipital lobe.

The posterior cerebral artery is uniquely vulnerable to increases in pressure within the cranium as it traverses the space between the tentorium and the lateral margin of the cerebral peduncle. In instances of transtentorial herniation, this vessel may be compressed resulting in secondary infarction within its terminal zone of distribution. At times, the entire occipital and posterior temporal lobes may be converted into a zone of infarction. More commonly, however, the area of encephalomalacia is confined to the calcarine portion (visual cortex) of the occipital lobe (Fig. 7). This secondary lesion is encountered in approximately 28 percent of autopsied patients whose subdural hematomas were larger than 25 ml in volume (Aronson and Okazaki, 1963).

Secondary Brain-Stem Hemorrhage

A deteriorating state of consciousness, accompanied by the clinical attitudes of decerebration and a depression of the vital signs are the clinical representations of significant caudad displacement of the upper brain stem and transtentorial herniation. The outstanding effects of this

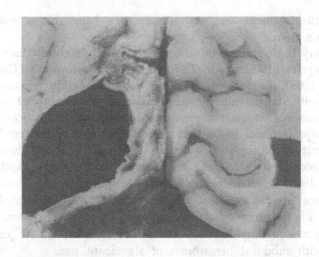

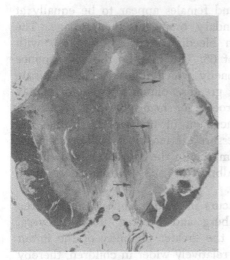

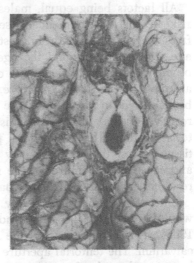

FIG. 7. Occipital lobes, in cross section, from a patient with a large left subdural hematoma. Transtentorial herniation of the temporal lobe, with compression of the left posterior cerebral artery, causing calcarine cortex encephalomalacia.

FIG. 8. Photomicrograph of midbrain showing an area of encephalomalacia and demyelination (arrows) caused by transtentorial herniation and lateral compression of midbrain (Weil myelin stain).

FIG. 9. Cross section of upper brain stem, at tentorial level, showing secondary brain-stem hemorrhage encroaching upon the aqueduct. Note also tentorial groove and hippocampal herniation. Patient had a 150 gram subdural hematoma.

61

physical displacement and compression are hemorrhages within the upper brain stem.

Secondary brain-stem hemorrhages are found in about three percent of all autopsies (199 cases in 7,110 consecutive autopsies) (Cohen and Aronson, 1968). In general, they are most frequently encountered in patients with large, rapidly accumulating, supratentorial space-occupying masses. Non-traumatic cerebral hemorrhage is the most common primary supratentorial lesion that causes secondary brain-stem bleeding (57 percent of patients with lethal, apoplectic cerebral hemorrhage showed secondary brain-stem hemorrhage at autopsy) (Cohen and Aronson, 1968). Secondary brain-stem hemorrhage also occurs as a consequence of the cerebral edema which has inevitably followed occlusion of the internal carotid artery (15 percent of such cases showing the secondary lesion); and it occurs in about 20 percent of patients with subdural hematomas of significant size.

All factors being equal, males and females appear to be equally at risk in the development of secondary brain-stem hemorrhage. The frequency of secondary brain-stem bleeding seems to diminish with age, particularly beyond the age of 65. This may be the consequence of an increase in pericerebral capacity which follows cerebral tissue atrophy. In the aged, therefore, a greater volume of hematoma may be required to inaugurate the process of hemispheric compression, reactive edema, and caudal displacement of tissue through the tentorial opening. However, lateral pressure exerted by herniated temporal tissue against the midbrain may compromise the regional blood supply and cause a local infarct of the midbrain (Fig. 8), without necessarily resulting in brain-stem hemorrhage.

Brain-stem hemorrhage rarely occurs in infants and young children who die of head injury (Lindenberg and Freytag, 1969; Freytag, 1963). This may be partly due to the greater pliability of the infant calvarium. The tentorial aperture is relatively wider in children, thereby lessening the risk of incarcerating a transtentorial herniation (a prominent factor in the production of secondary midbrain and pontine bleeding).

The lesion consists of multiple hemorrhages of variable volume, which infiltrate the tissues of the midbrain and pons. Within the midbrain, the hemorrhage is typically linear, extending from the inferior periaqueductal margin to the dorsal extremity of the interpeduncular fossa, and rarely exceeds 3 mm in width (Fig. 9). Posteriorly, within the pons, hemorrhages are more commonly confined to the tegmentum and are both multiple and bilateral. They are circular

62

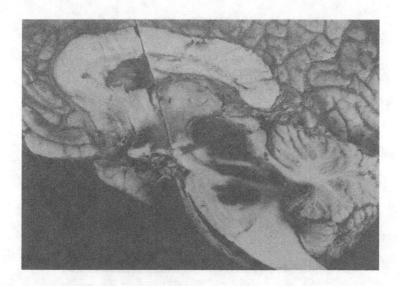

Fig. 10. Secondary brain-stem hemorrhage as viewed in midsaggital plane. Note the angulation of blood in a dorsocaudal direction. Compare with midsagittal angiogram in Figure 12.

when viewed in cross section but, when serially studied or viewed sagittally, they tend to be fusiform (Fig. 10). At times, the extravasation of blood is considerable, and results in a rupture into the aqueduct of Sylvius or the rostral fourth ventricle.

Most observers agree that sudden caudal displacement of the brain stem is the initiating force in secondary brain-stem bleeding. Occasionally, the lateral compression generated by the transtentorial prolapse of temporal lobe tissue appears to contribute to the bleeding tendency within the upper brain stem, although Klintworth's (1968) postmortem observations signify that there is no linear correlation between the degree of paratentorial grooving and the frequency of secondary brain-stem hemorrhage. His data are more consistent with downward brain-stem displacement as the effective variable.

Despite earlier conjectures, most current studies seem to indicate that brain-stem bleeding is of arterial origin and that its distribution coincides with the ramifications of the mesencephalic perforating arteries

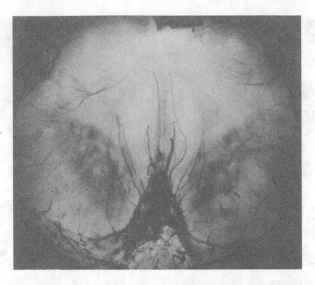

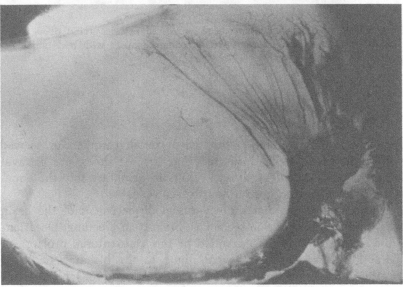

Fig. 11. Cross section of normal midbrain demonstrating, by postmortem angiographic injection technics, the distribution of the mesencephalic perforating arteries, the vessels held to be the source of secondary brain-stem bleeding.

Fig. 12. Midsagittal section of midbrain (right) and pons (left) following injection of an opaque solution into the basilar artery. The mesencephalic perforating arteries proceed dorsocaudally from the interpeduncular fossa.

(parasagittal branches of the terminal basilar artery) which enter the midbrain via the interpeduncular fossa and curve posteriorly to supply the pontine tegmentum (Figs. 11, 12).

NECK INJURY AND VASCULAR OCCLUSION

The four major arteries upon which the brain is dependent for sustenance are vulnerable to various forms of neck and head injury. The vertebral arteries pass through a series of lateral vertebral foramens and, by virtue of their partial fixation, become susceptible to transient closure and possible intimal damage after lateral-hyperextension movements of the neck or fracture of the cervical vertebrae. The carotid arteries, while not similarly tethered, may nevertheless be injured by various forms of penetrating and non-penetrating cervical trauma.

Vertebral Artery

Numerous studies on the biophysical status of the vertebral artery have demonstrated that the lumen of this vessel can be transiently obliterated by sudden and forced lateral rotation of the head. Instances of basilar-vertebral artery insufficiency have been noted in association with chiropractic manipulation, tong traction blunt, injury to the lateral neck, and vertebral fracture (Simeone and Goldberg, 1968; Green and Joynt, 1959; Carpenter, 1961; Husni et al, 1966). Because vital tissues are supplied by these vessels, a high mortality rate has resulted from such traumatic occlusions.

Postmortem examinations in many of these patients have shown the existence of dissecting hematomas of the vertebral artery media which are believed to have arisen from an intimal laceration secondary to the stretching of the artery over the bony foramen transversarium of the sixth cervical vertebra (Simeone and Goldberg, 1968). In other patients, the intimal and subintimal injury provokes secondary thrombus formation and arterial occlusion. A flap of exfoliated intima is sometimes found in the core of the thrombus.

Carpenter (1961) has stated that the primary site of posttraumatic vertebral artery thrombosis is the plane of the atlas and the atlanto-occipital membrane.

Typically, blood dissects through the intimal rent and burrows within the subintimal tissues both rostral and caudal to the area of initial endothelial damage. The site of endothelial laceration does not appear to be influenced by the existence of preceding atheromatous changes.

However, the extent of cervical vertebral osteoarthritis (with possible osteophyte compression of vertebral arteries) may be a factor contributing to the risk of vertebral artery thrombosis following neck injury.

It is likely that the actual number of cases of vertebral artery thrombosis resulting from hyperextension injury to the neck far exceeds the number of clinical examples that are acknowledged. When the contralateral vertebral artery is adequate to perfuse the basilar artery, unilateral vertebral artery closure may go unnoticed (Husni et al, 1966).

Posttraumatic thrombi in the vertebral arteries tend to propagate distally and may cause occlusion of the posterior inferior cerebellar artery or even the basilar artery (Simeone and Goldberg, 1968; Carpenter, 1961).

Yates (1959) has performed anatomic studies upon the vertebral arteries of infants who died shortly after birth and has found a very high frequency of adventitial hemorrhage which he felt could be ascribed to birth trauma.

Basilar Artery

In contrast to the relative vulnerability of the vertebral artery, the basilar artery is in a relatively protected site. Nevertheless, rare instances of direct trauma to the basilar artery have been reported. One such case resulted from a fracture of the clivus (an industrial accident in a 59-year-old man) (Loop et al, 1964). The fracture had caught the proximal two-thirds of the basilar artery, and the hemostatic action of the fracture occluded the artery. Blood clots were found in the subjacent sphenoid sinuses, and the mid-sagittal section of the pons disclosed a large area of very recent encephalomalacia.

Innominate Artery

The rare instances of innominate artery injury which have been reported are typically associated with superior mediastinal injury (Heggtveit et al, 1964). Some penetrating wounds of the innominate artery produce arteriovenous fistulas. In other cases blood dissects through the wall of the injured vessel into the adventitia, forming a false circumferential aneurysmal mass; if the patient survives, the hematoma is subjected to fibroblastic organization and collagenization.

Internal Carotid Artery

The craniocervical artery most susceptible to traumatically-induced injury is the internal carotid artery (Trevor Hughes and Brownell, 1968; Hockaday, 1959; Goldring, 1968; Gurdjian et al, 1963). In both world wars, military surgeons were familiar with the hazards of carotid artery thrombosis following penetrating neck wounds. It was a common experience to find that a missile fragment that had penetrated the neck, but had not actually perforated the internal carotid artery, was able nevertheless to induce some form of intimal damage which predisposed toward local thrombus formation. Indeed, it was suggested that it was the sudden neck movement associated with the penetrating injury, along with the secondary soft tissue laceration, hemorrhage, and swelling of the neighboring voluntary musculature, that was responsible for the carotid thrombosis. The fact that there were numerous cases, both in military and civilian circumstances, in which thrombosis of the internal carotid artery had followed non-penetrating cervical injury, lent strength to this supposition. It is the opinion of some observers that specific modes of injury selectively increase the risk of carotid thrombosis. They suggest that when the vector of forces is directed to the angle of the jaw and also associated with sternal injury, a stretching damage to the carotid intima might ensue. Indeed, Trevor Hughes and Brownell have shown that the stretching effect upon the carotid arteries which occurs with forcible backward head movement, is augmented by the presence of a sternal fracture, because the fracture serves to immobilize the innominate artery (1968).

The commonest site of intimal and medial damage to the internal carotid artery is the segment about two to three centimeters above the bifurcation of the common carotid. In many instances there is a dissecting extravasation of the blood within the carotid sheath, forming a fusiform, false aneurysm.

Carotid occlusion at a somewhat higher level is more frequently associated with fracture of the cranial base which extends through both petrous ridges and traverses the carotid foramens. Careful studies have sometimes demonstrated the impingement of bony spicules upon the interosseous segment of the internal carotid artery. Some of these cases have shown bilateral internal carotid artery occlusion Yashon et al, 1964). Basilar skull fracture may result in mural damage to the intracranial extradural segment of the internal carotid artery with the formation, within a few months, of a traumatic aneurysm. Clinically, such

67

a lesion is manifested by cranial bruit, blindness and delayed, massive epistaxis (Araki et al, 1965).

Thrombosis of the internal carotid artery has also been found in association with soft palate injuries, and with penetrating or blunt damage to the paratonsillar region (typically following a forward fall and the forceful upward thrust of a foreign object carried in the mouth). This type of injury occurs mainly during childhood (Pitner, 1966; Martin and Warren, 1969).

Trauma to the carotid artery, penetrating or otherwise, may result in a pseudoaneurysm consisting of laminated fibrous connective tissue which encapsulates the adventitial clot. There may, therefore, be an aneurysmal reservoir with a pulsating, progressively expansile mass in the neck. The occurrence of delayed occlusive thrombosis in such vessels has been described.

Severe head injury without apparent trauma to the neck may also precipitate thrombosis of intracranial arteries. Bots and Kramer (1964) have recorded four cases of severe head injury which showed thrombosis of both carotids and the basilar artery at autopsy. They conjectured that the initial injury caused some intimal damage, and that the hypotension, respiratory arrest, and impaired circulation promoted thrombus deposition upon the previously damaged vascular intima.

Middle Cerebral Artery

This artery is very rarely the site of direct traumatic injury. DeVeer and Browder (1942) have described possibly the first instance of a posttraumatic middle cerebral artery thrombosis superimposed upon a focal intimal disruption. They felt that the 12 hours of relative lucidity before the emergence of neurologic impairment was analogous to the phenomenon of *Spätapoplexie*. Further examples of posttraumatic middle cerebral artery obstruction have been recorded (Duman and Stephens, 1963). Where careful pathologic studies have been carried out, intimal breaks that formed the mural hiatus for subintimal dissection have been identified. The low incidence of post-injury dissecting aneurysm of the middle cerebral artery suggests that a preexisting mural anomaly or an arteritis is required to permit a concussive force to traumatize this artery effectively.

Traumatic Aneurysms of Cerebral Arteries

Injury to intracranial arteries (the result of closed cranial trauma or direct manipulation) may cause blood to dissect through the intimal and medial laminae, and to pool in the perivascular space. The clot may become organized by connective tissue hyperplasia and ultimately form an aneurysmal reservoir that communicates with the parent vessel (Raimondi et al, 1968). These traumatic aneurysms have been noted in the middle meningeal artery, the internal carotid artery, and peripheral branches of the anterior and middle cerebral arteries (Raimondi et al, 1968; Smith and Bardenheier, 1968; Eichler et al, 1969). The angiographic appearances of these aneurysms may be indistinguishable from those of a congenital nature. Occlusive thrombosis, possibly hastened by the perivascular tamponade, is a common sequel to traumatic aneurysm.

REFERENCES

Araki, C., Handa, H., Handa, J., and Yoshida, K. Traumatic Aneurysm of the Intracranial Extradural Portion of the Internal Carotid Artery. *J. Neurosurg.*, 23, 64-67, 1965.

Aronson, S. M., and Kaplan, H. A. Pathogenesis of Cerebral Lesions Resulting from Contact Trauma to the Head. *Bull. N. Y. Acad. Med.*, 33, 450-454, 1957.

Aronson, S. M., and Okazaki, H. A Study of Some Factors Modifying Response of Cerebral Tissue to Subdural Hematomata. *J. Neurosurg.*, 20, 89-93, 1963.

Bots, G. and Kramer, W. Traumatic Thrombosis of Intracranial Arteries and Extensive Necrosis of the Brain Developed During Reanimation. *Acta Neuropathol.*, 3, 416-427, 1964.

Campbell, J. B., and Cohen, J. Epidural Hemorrhage and the Skull of Children. *Surg. Gynec. Obstet.*, 92, 257-280, 1951.

Carpenter, S. Injury of Neck as Cause of Vertebral Artery Thrombosis. *J. Neurosurg.*, 18, 849-853, 1961.

Caveness, W. F. Onset and Cessation of Fits Following Craniocerebral Trauma. *J. Neurosurg.*, 20, 570-583, 1963.

Ceballos, R. Pituitary Changes in Head Trauma. *Ala. J. Med. Sc.*, 3, 185-198, 1966.

Chason, J. L., Fernando, O., Hodgson, V., Thomas, L., and Gurdjian, E. Experimental Brain Concussion: Morphologic Findings and a New Cytologic Hypothesis. *J. Trauma*, 6, 767-779, 1966.

Chason, J. L., Hardy, W., Webster, J., and Gurdjian, E. S. Alterations in Cell Structure of the Brain Associated with Experimental Concussion. *J. Neurosurg.*, 15, 135-139, 1958.

Ciembroniewicz, J. E. Subdural Hematoma of the Posterior Fossa. *J. Neurosurg.*, 22, 465-473, 1965.

Clein, L. J., and Bolton, C. F. Interhemispheric Subdural Hematoma: A Case Report. *J. Neurol. Neurosurg. Psychiatry*, *32*, 389-392, 1969.

Cohen, S., and Aronson, S. M. Secondary Brain-Stem Hemorrhages. Predisposing and Modifying Factors. *Arch. Neurol.*, *19*, 257-263, 1968.

Columella, F., Gaist, G., Piazzo, G., and Caraffa, T. Extradural Hematoma at the Vertex. *J. Neurol. Neurosurg. Psychiatry*, *31*, 315-320, 1968.

DeVeer, J. A., and Browder, J. Post-traumatic Cerebral Thrombosis and Infarction. *J. Neuropathol. Exper. Neurol.*, *1*, 24-31, 1942.

Duman, S., and Stephens, J. W. Post-traumatic Middle Cerebral Artery Occlusion. *Neurology*, *13*, 613-616, 1963.

Eichler, A., Story, J. L., Bennett, D. E., and Galo, M. V. Traumatic Aneurysm of a Cerebral Artery. *J. Neurosurg.*, *31*, 72-76, 1969.

Fisher, R. G., Kim, J. K., and Sachs, E., Jr. Complications in Posterior Fossa Due to Occipital Trauma — Their Operability. *J. A. M. A.*, *167*, 176-182, 1958.

Freytag, E. Autopsy Findings in Head Injuries from Blunt Forces. *Arch. Pathol.*, *75*, 402-413, 1963.

Friede, R. L. Experimental Concussion Acceleration. *Arch. Neurol.*, *4*, 449-462, 1961.

Goldring, S. Traumatic Occlusion of the Carotid Artery. *J. Neurosurg.*, *28*, 78-80, 1968.

Goodell, C. L., and Mealey, J., Jr. Pathogenesis of Chronic Subdural Hematoma. *Arch. Neurol.*, *8*, 429-437, 1963.

Green, D., and Joynt, R. J. Vascular Accidents to the Brain Stem Associated with Neck Manipulation. *J. A. M. A.*, *170*, 522-524, 1959.

Gurdjian, E. S., Hardy, W. G., Lindner, D. W., and Thomas, L. M. Closed Cervical Cranial Trauma Associated with Involvement of Carotid and Vertebral Arteries. *J. Neurosurg.*, *20*, 418-427, 1963.

Gurdjian, E. S., Thomas, L. M., Hodgson, V. R., and Patrick, L. M. Impact Head Injury. *GP*, *37*, 78-87, 1968.

Hamberger, A., and Rinder, L. Experimental Brain Concussion. *J. Neuropath. Exp. Neurol.*, *25*, 68-75, 1966.

Heggtveit, H. A., Campbell, J. S., and Hooper, G. D. Innominate Arterial Aneurysms Occurring After Blunt Trauma. *Am. J. Clin. Path.*, *42*, 69-74, 1964.

Hockaday, T. Traumatic Thrombosis of the Internal Carotid Artery. *J. Neurol. Neurosurg. Psychiatry*, *22*, 229-231, 1959.

Husni, E. A., Bell, H. S., and Storer, J. Mechanical Occlusion of the Vertebral Artery. *J. A. M. A.*, *196*, 475-478, 1966.

Ishii, S., Hayner, R., Kelly, W., and Evans, J. P. Studies of Cerebral Swelling. II. Experimental Cerebral Swelling Produced by Supratentorial Extradural Compression. *J. Neurosurg.*, *26*, 152-166, 1959.

Jamieson, K. G., and Yelland, J. D. Extradural Hematoma. Report of 167 Cases. *J. Neurosurg.*, *29*, 13-23, 1968.

Kaplan, H. A. The Transcerebral Venous System. *Arch. Neurol.*, *1*, 148-152, 1959.

Klatzo, I., Piraux, A., and Laskowski, E. J. The Relationship Between Edema, Blood-Brain Barrier and Tissue Elements in a Local Brain Injury. *J. Neuropath. Exp. Neurol.*, *17*, 548-564, 1958.

Klintworth, G. K. Paratentorial Grooving of Human Brains with Particular Reference to Transtentorial Herniation and the Pathogenesis of Secondary Brainstem Hemorrhages. *Am. J. Pathol.*, *53*, 391-408, 1968.

Kosary, I. Z., Goldhammer, Y., and Lerner, M. A. Acute Extradural Hematoma of the Posterior Fossa. *J. Neurosurg.*, *24*, 1007-1012, 1966.

Langfitt, T. W., Tannanbaum, H. M., and Kassell, N. F. The Etiology of Acute Brain Swelling Following Experimental Head Injury. *J. Neurosurg.*, *24*, 47-56, 1966.

Laudig, G., Browder, E. J., and Watson, R. A. Subdural Hematoma. *Ann. Surg.*, *113*, 170-188, 1941.

LeCount, E. R., and Apfelbach, C. W. Pathologic Anatomy of Traumatic Fractures of Cranial Bones. *J. A. M. A.*, *74*, 501-511, 1920.

Lindenberg, R., and Freytag, E. The Mechanism of Cerebral Contusions. *Arch. Pathol.*, *69*, 440-469, 1960.

Lindenberg, R., and Freytag, E. Morphology of Brain Lesions from Blunt Trauma in Early Infancy. *Arch. Pathol.*, *87*, 298-305, 1969.

Loop, J. W., White, L. E., Jr., and Shaw, C. M. Traumatic Occlusion of the Basilar Artery Within a Clivus Fracture. *Radiology*, *83*, 36-40, 1964.

Martin, N., and Warren, G. Thrombosis of the Internal Carotid Artery Due to Intra-oral Trauma. *South. Med. J.*, *62*, 103-107, 1969.

Maurer, J. J., and Mayfield, F. H. Acute Bilateral Extradural Hematomas. *J. Neurosurg.*, *23*, 63, 1965.

McKissock, W., Richardson, A., and Bloom, W. Subdural Hematoma. A Review of 389 Cases. *Lancet*, *1*, 1365-1369, 1960.

McLaurin, R. L., and Tutor, F. T. Acute Subdural Hematoma. *J. Neurosurg.*, *18*, 61-67, 1961.

Mealey, J. Acute Extradural Hematomas Without Demonstrable Skull Fractures. *J. Neurosurg.*, *17*, 27-34, 1960.

Pitner, S. Carotid Thrombosis Due to Intraoral Trauma. *New Engl. J. Med.*, *274*, 764-767, 1966.

Raimondi, A. J., Yashon, D., Reyes, C., and Yarzagaray, L. Intracranial False Aneurysms. *Neurochirurg.*, *11*, 219-233, 1968.

Rinder, L. and Olsson, Y. Studies on Vascular Permeability Changes in Experimental Brain Concussion. I. Distribution of Circulating Flourescent Indicators in Brain and Cervical Cord After Sudden Mechanical Loading of the Brain. *Acta Neuropathol.*, *11*, 183-200, 1968.

Robinson, N. Histochemical Changes in Neocortex and Corpus Callosum After Intracranial Injection. *J. Neurol., Neurosurg. Psychiatry*, *32*, 317-323, 1969.

Russell, W. R. Disability Caused by Brain Wounds. A Review of 1,166 Cases. *J. Neurol., Neurosurg.. Psychiatry*, *14*, 35-39, 1951.

Shapiro, H. M., Langfitt, T. W., and Weinstein, J. D. Compression of Cerebral Vessels by Intracranial Hypertension. II. Morphological Evidence for Collapse of Vessels. *Acta Neurochir.*, *15*, 223-233, 1966.

Simeone, F. and Goldberg, H. Thrombosis of the Vertebral Artery from Hyperextension Injury to the Neck. *J. Neurosurg*, *29*, 540-544, 1968.

Smith, K. R., Jr. and Bardenheier, J. A. Aneurysm of the Pericallosal Artery Caused by Closed Cranial Trauma. *J. Neurosurg.*, *29*, 551-554, 1968.

Trevor Hughes, J. and Brownell, B. Traumatic Thrombosis of the Internal Carotid Artery in the Neck. *J. Neurol. Neurosurg. Psychiatry*, *31*, 307-314, 1968.

71

Vance, B. M. Fractures of the Skull. *Arch. Surg.*, *14*, 1023-1092, 1927.

Walker, A. E. Post-traumatic Epilepsy. *World Neurol.*, *3*, 185-194, 1962.

Whittaker, K. Extradural Hematoma of the Anterior Fossa. *J. Neurosurg.*, *17*, 1089-1092, 1960.

Windle, W. F., Groat, R. A., and Fox, C. A. Experimental Structural Alterations in the Brain During and After Concussion. *Surg. Gynec. Obstet.*, *79*, 561-572, 1944.

Wollschlaeger, P. B. and Wollschlaeger, G. The Interhemispheric Subdural or Falx Hematoma. *Amer. J. Roentgenol. Rad. Ther. Nucl. Med.* *42*, 1252-1254, 1964.

Yashon, D., Johnson, H. B., and Jane, J. A. Bilateral Internal Carotid Artery Occlusion Secondary to Closed Head Injuries. *J. Neurol. Neurosurg. Psychiatry*, *27*, 547-552, 1964.

Yates, P. O. Birth Trauma to the Vertebral Arteries. *Arch Dis. Child.* *34*, 436-441, 1959.

CHAPTER 3

FRACTURE OF THE SKULL

JEFFERSON BROWDER, M.D.

In patients with craniocerebral injuries the attention of the surgeon is directed for the most part toward the effects of the trauma on the structures within the cranial cavity. For this reason, little consideration is now given to a fracture of the skull except in instances in which the injury has opened the cranial cavity to potential infection, has altered the intracranial capacity by a depression of the cranial bones, has compressed a cranial nerve at its foramen of exit from the skull, or has lacerated a dural vessel with resultant epidural hemorrhage. In many instances this lesion is accompanied by clinical findings indicative of alteration in brain function, consequently the term "fracture of the skull" has been frequently, but incorrectly, used synonymously with craniocerebral injuries. While the brain is the most important structure in the head that may be altered anatomically and physiologically by a traumatic insult, the significance of the bony injury should not be underestimated. The principal function of the skull is to protect the brain. The cranial bones are denser and thicker over exposed parts and thinner in most cases where they are covered by muscle, as in the temporal and inferior occipital areas. The rounded shape of the vault, the resiliency of the bones, and the formation of the secondary arches make the skull moderately resistant to external trauma. The buttresses at the base (petrous part of the temporal bone and the sphenoidal ridge in particular), situated as they are between thin bone perforated with foramina, frequently cause convergence of fracture lines toward the region of the sella turcica.

The anatomical interruption of any part of the bony cranium by violence may be considered a "fracture of the skull." The fracture may be described according to the mechanism of its production, the region involved, or the character of the bony interruption. As estimated by the external evidence of violence, the parietal bosses are the most common sites struck, the frontal aspect of the head next in order of frequency, and the posterior area least often. The fracture may extend across one or more of the several bony foramina in the base of the skull, damaging cranial nerves at this level. Observations at autopsy do not support the oft-heard clinical differentiation between fractures of the

73

vault and those of the base of the skull. Infrequently are there fractures limited in their extent to one or the other of these locations; most so-called fractures of the vault extend into the base and the majority of those in the base may be traced into a part of the vault. The age of the patient, contour of the skull, thickness of the cranial bones, resiliency of the cranium, site of the trauma, shape of the traumatizing object, estimated amount of force employed in the production of the injury, whether struck by a moving object or whether the head has forcefully come in contact with a stationary structure — all are factors to be considered when evaluating a fracture of the skull.

The present discussion is limited to the various traumatic lesions of the skull; the damage to the intracranial contents receives brief consideration only when the two connot be dissociated. The following classification will be used as a basis for description and discussion.

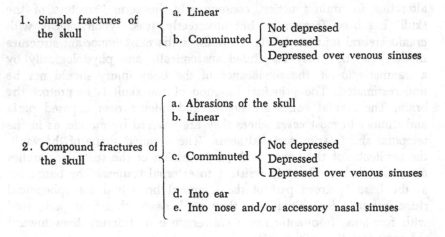

SIMPLE LINEAR FRACTURES

A simple linear fracture is by far the most common type of fracture of the skull. The line or lines of fracture may vary from a mere fissure in the orbital plate, scarcely demonstrable at autopsy, to a fracture extending from the vault across the base to the opposite side of the cranium. No part of the skull is exempt, although most frequently implicated are the bones of the middle fossae. Fractures of this variety are usually produced when the head comes violently in contact with

74

a broad, flat surface of an object, the head and/or the object or both being in motion. The clinical findings (excluding the abnormal physical signs that indicate an injury of the brain) that lend support to the diagnosis of linear fracture of the skull generally receive scant attention, owing to the facility of examination by roentgen ray. The *late* appearance of ecchymosis directly behind the external ear or in an upper eyelid following a blow to the head is presumptive evidence that a fracture is present through or adjacent to the petrous part of the temporal bone in the former instance or in the roof of the orbit in the latter. An elongated finger-like zone of scalp edema likewise is suggestive of an underlying fracture especially when it extends from a circular or oval swelling of the scalp surmounted by an abrasion. The presence of free blood in the middle ear, as disclosed by a bluish-black tympanic membrane, is sometimes associated with a fracture through or adjacent to the petrous part of the temporal bone. On the other hand, any or all of these abnormal physical findings may be present without a fracture being demonstrable even at autopsy. Although the presumptive evidence may be strong that a simple linear fracture is present, a properly conducted roentgen-ray examination is the most reliable means of disclosing this lesion. However, the results of this method of examination are not necessarily conclusive, since fractures limited in their extent to the floor of the anterior and middle cranial fossae are difficult to demonstrate. Unless there are reasons, other than the mere detection of a fracture, the roentgen-ray examination should be deferred until the manipulation of the patient incident to such an examination will not unfavorably alter the clinical course. If, however, there is clinical evidence of brain dysfunction indicative of a possible epidural hemorrhage, then the position of the fracture in relation to the course of the meningeal arteries should be determined without delay.

There is no treatment for simple linear fracture of the skull as such. The fracture only indicates that an injury has been sustained. All therapeutic efforts should be directed toward the brain injury, if present. In children, linear fractures demonstrable by roentgen-ray examination usually heal within a period of four to five months, whereas in adults healing of the fracture is commonly completed within one year after the accident. A linear fracture of the skull in some instances, especially in elderly people, may be demonstrable by roentgen-ray examination for many years after the injury, indicating fibrous (non-bony) healing of the lesion.

Simple comminuted fractures, unless depressed, present practically the same physical findings as simple linear fractures. Associated large hematomas situated between the scalp and the skull are commonly observed but these subside spontaneously except in rare cases in which it may become necessary to evacuate a liquefied blood clot by aspiration or incision. Multiplicity of fracture lines and the possibility that an edge of the comminuted bone may have been slightly depressed at the time of injury increase the likelihood of the subsequent formation of an epidural hemorrhage. The comminution may produce several small to large islands of bone and these fragments may become separated one from the other, giving a mosaic appearance. The margins may be separated fully 5 mm and one can readily understand that these seldom unite by bony bridging except in young individuals. As in simple linear fractures, no therapy directed at the fracture itself is indicated.

SIMPLE COMMINUTED DEPRESSED FRACTURES

The simple comminuted depressed fractures of clinical significance are encountered in the vault of the skull and are more frequently observed in the frontal half. The trauma is often produced by a blow with a rounded blunt object (as the face of a hammer) or less commonly by the cranial vault striking a small convex surface. The overlying scalp may be macerated. The area of skull implicated is frequently circular in outline and sharply depressed, but the bony deformity may be obscured by an overlying extravasation of blood. The force of the blow is often dissipated at the site of the impact without production of evident brain injury. Another type of this fracture results from a blow by a large flat-surfaced object, which usually produces a bashed-in area composed of several fair-sized fragments of bone. In such instances suture lines are not uncommonly opened, especially the sagittal suture, which may participate in the comminution. Other types of comminuted fractures with bizarre configurations are encountered less frequently but in general these present much the same clinical features. In most instances, a depressed fracture of the skull is suggested from the evidence derived from physical examination. Examination by roentgen-ray is necessary to disclose the extent of the injury and the position of the bone fragments. Palpation of the soft center of an extracranial blood clot with its firm margins may be mistaken for a depressed fracture by the inexperienced. These hemorrhagic extravasations of the scalp are aptly termed "doughnut hematomas." Firm pressure in the center of such a hematoma in the absence of a depressed fracture will disclose the normal contour of the underlying skull. Here again roentgen-ray examination may be necessary to establish the diagnosis. In fact all patients with evidence of a depressed fracture of the skull should have stereoscopic roentgen-ray films taken in both the anteroposterior and lateral positions before the surgeon embarks upon operative interference.

The treatment of a simple comminuted depressed fracture consists in elevation of the involved bone and restoration of the normal contour of the skull. The instances in which the extent of the depression of the inner table is estimated to be only a few millimeters require only conservative measures unless there is clinical evidence of an intracranial complication. In children, much larger areas of bony depression may be unassociated with evidence of brain dysfunction, and these cases should likewise be treated in a conservative manner unless restoration of the contour of the skull is indicated for cosmetic effect. Sharply defined areas of depression of the skull are more frequently associated with a circumscribed intracranial hemorrhage than are the larger and more diffuse types of depression. In the frontal region all comminuted depressed fractures should be elevated if for no other reason than to obtain a good cosmetic result. The operative procedure to be followed in the treatment is not difficult, if certain fundamental principles are adhered to. The area of depressed bone should be widely exposed by outlining a scalp flap which extends at least 2 cm beyond the margin of depression. For fractures in the region of the forehead, a transverse, curvilinear incision just within the hairline extending from one anterotemporal area to a corresponding site on the opposite side gives a good cosmetic result. After reflecting the scalp from the depressed bone, a flap of periosteum should be outlined and dissected from the fragments. A small burr opening is made just beyond the margin of depression and the fragments elevated piecemeal and removed. If the dura is bluish in color, it should be opened and underlying clots or pulpified brain tissue removed. After closing the dura and effecting complete hemostasis, the bone fragments are replaced in such a manner that the entire cranial defect including the burr hole is filled. Careful resuturing of the periosteal flap insures the maintenance of the bone fragments in the position in which they were placed. If the pericranium is badly lacerated, the aponeurosis may be utilized to maintain the position of the fragments. Drains should never be used. Bony union between the fragments rarely occurs, except in very young individuals; however, the interposition of fibrous tissue between the bone chips makes for a solid structure.

The observation that in some instances the replaced bone fragments become completely decalcified has led to a modification of the operation for comminuted depressed fracture in selected cases. Whenever the depressed area of bone is sharply defined and there are no radiating fracture lines, a bone flap is cut with the area of depression in its center. After reflecting the flap, the depressed fragments are manually pressed into position thereby producing minimal disturbance of the periosteal attachment of the fragments.

The treatment for simple comminuted depressed fractures as above outlined should not be followed if this type of fracture overlies the sagittal or transverse venous sinuses. Under these conditions a conservative regimen should be followed. If the peripheral border of a large zone of depressed skull lies over a venous sinus, the bone may be elevated with the exception of that part immediately over the sinus. There are two major reasons for a conservative attitude in the treatment of comminuted depressed fractures in these particular situations: firstly, if the wall of the venous sinus has been lacerated by a sharp-edged fragment of bone at the time of the accident or if the sinus is inadvertently opened during the process of elevating a bone fragment, air may be sucked into the venous circulation and result in sudden death. Once observed, such a dramatic calamity is not easily forgotten. Secondly, if the area of depressed bone should be situated over the posterior half of the sagittal sinus, and upon elevating the depression there is no ingress of air, the control of hemorrhage by reflecting a portion of the dura and suturing it over the venous sinus may be followed by a thrombotic occlusion. Likewise thrombosis may ensue if a laceration of a venous sinus is occluded at operation by a piece of transplanted muscle or Gelfoam. In any event occlusion of the sagittal snus in its posterior half is attended with cerebral venous stasis and in certain instances the resultant thrombosis of cerebral veins may produce extensive paralysis of the extremities.

COMPOUND FRACTURES OF THE SKULL

The term *compound fracture of the skull* is applied to a fracture of the bony cranium that communicates with the exterior by virtue of a break in the continuity of the cutaneous and other tissue coverings of the vault ot the skull, a rent in the mucous membrane of the nasopharynx or a rupture of the lining of the middle ear. Except for compound frac-

78

tures of the skull that communicate with the nasal accessory sinuses or the upper nasal cavity and those that open into the middle ear, the recognition of this lesion is seldom difficult. A break in the continuity of the scalp should be considered a compound fracture of the skull until proved otherwise by careful physical and roentgen-ray examination, particularly if the laceration of the scalp has been produced by other than an incisional type of injury. Fractures involving the base of the skull are not uncommonly associated with a rent in the adjacent dura, since this structure is firmly attached to bone, especially in the mesial part of the anterior cranial fossa and over the petrous part of the temporal bone. Compound fractures of the vault of the skull are frequently depressed. The extent of the involvement of the intracranial structures depends to a certain degree on the type of fracture. All patients with clinical evidence suggesting that a compound fracture has been sustained should receive antimicrobial therapy (antibiotics or chemotherapy) for a minimum of ten days. This treatment should be instituted without delay.

ABRASIONS OF THE SKULL

This type of injury is most often sustained in an automobile accident in which the individual is thrown or dragged along the surface of the street. The scalp is torn and dirt and sometimes gravel are ground into the outer table of the skull. The implicated bone has a blanched appearance with interspersed blackened pinpoint areas representing dirt-filled foramina. This lesion may be followed by osteomyelitis which in some instances remains localized to the involved area although the infection may become widespread in the skull. The scalp wound should be cleansed by excising all devitalized tissue and the involved bone surface scrubbed with a stiff bristle brush. If the foreign material cannot be dislodged from the small bony foramina then the surface of the external table of the skull should be chiseled away until bleeding bone is encountered. The traumatized area may be drained and if infection supervenes the wound should be opened widely and allowed to heal by granulation. A more radical surgical approach in the instances in which osteomyelitis ensues is reopening of the wound and complete excision of the infected bone. It has been my experience that this is not necessary. Adequate antibiotic therapy should be instituted in all patients with contaminated wounds.

79

Many unrecognized compound linear fractures of the vault of the skull would be visualized if all lacerations of the scalp were carefully inspected. The majority of these fractures heal without suppuration following proper treatment of the scalp wound. There are instances in which the healed wound of the scalp subsequently presents signs of infection, spontaneously opens and discharges a small piece of some foreign material. The wound again heals after the extrusion of the foreign body but if additional foreign material is retained, may reopen repeatedly. Exacerbations of the infection with eventual discharge of a bony sequestrum may occur, making it appear that a radical removal of all potentially diseased bone is indicated, yet even this form of therapy does not always result in a cure. A conservative therapeutic regimen is more effective and will be less frequently associated with intracranial complications than the attempted radical removal of all the infected bone. Osteomyelitis of the skull is largely preventable if all scalp wounds in the fresh state are carefully inspected and correctly treated. When it appears that foreign material has been driven into the fracture line, the margins of the scalp should be sharply excised, the wound enlarged, a small burr opening made in the middle of the exposed fracture, and a groove 3 to 4 mm in width cut along the fracture line. The dura is rarely opened by such an accident and should not be opened at the time of operation. After the wound is thoroughly cleansed, the scalp is closed without drainage and antibiotic therapy instituted. This method of treatment should be reserved for those cases in which foreign material is present within the fracture line, or the scalp is grossly contaminated. It may also be indicated in cases in which there is a suspicion of an underlying dural laceration. If the scalp overlying the area of bone excision is macerated or has been torn away completely, a flap of scalp should be cut with a broad pedicle, rotated, and sutured over the defect.

COMPOUND COMMINUTED FRACTURES

Lesions of this type without depression of the fragments are infrequently encountered. When observed the lines of fracture radiate in an irregular manner from a point where a relatively small scalp wound has been sustained. Some of the lines of fracture may join a few centimeters distant from their common point of origin, thereby creating one or more islands of bone which may retain their pericranial attachment and therefore some blood supply. The dura mater may or may not be lacerated. The treatment for this type of compound fracture is essentially the same as that suggested for the compound linear fractures. The likelihood of hemorrhage occurring in the epidural space at the site of a comminuted fracture must also be entertained.

Compound comminuted depressed fractures of the skull are of three well-defined types. The first type is a rounded or oval sharply defined depression markedly comminuted and usually produced by the impact of a relatively small blunt object. The force of the blow causing this fracture is often dissipated at the site of impact, the scalp generally presenting a small macerated area and the bone being sharply depressed. The dura may or may not be torn and frequently the cerebral surface directly beneath the depression is contused or lacerated. The clinical evidence that indicates serious general brain insult is absent in most cases. The second type consists of a large area of depressed bone made up of fair-sized fragments with a more or less extensive laceration of the overlying scalp. Often the edge of one or more fragments is displaced inward, lacerating the dura, brain and cortical vessels. Blood admixed with macerated brain and cerebrospinal fluid may be draining from the wound in considerable quantities if the normal capacity of the intracranial cavity has been greatly encroached upon or if the intracranial contents are increased in volume by hemorrhage and edema. The third type of compound fracture of the vault of the skull is produced by a penetrating missile. This will be discussed as a separate entity in another section. The diagnosis of compound depressed fracture of the vault of the skull is seldom difficult if the scalp wound is carefully investigated. The full extent of the injury cannot be determined prior to exposure at operation. The dura may be lacerated or intact, the brain badly macerated or merely contused. An unrecognized hemorrhage, situated in an epidural, subdural, or intracerebral location or various combinations of these lesions, may cause a fatal outcome. A state of "traumatic shock" characterized by a fast pulse, low systolic blood pressure, pallor and sweating is seldom observed unless a considerable quantity of blood has been lost or injury of other organs sustained. The alterations in vital signs that may be produced by intracranial lesions are discussed elsewhere. Unless exigency demands immediate treatment, operation may be deferred until four to eight hours have elapsed from time of injury. The scalp should be shaved by the surgeon and each stroke of the razor performed in such a manner that surface dirt and hair are carried away from the open wound. Gross foreign material not attached to the bone fragments is removed. The cutaneous surfaces are cleansed with antiseptic solution, care being taken not to allow the entrance of any of the solution into the wound. The lacerated scalp edges are sharply excised and all devitalized portions removed. The scalp wound should be increased in extent if necessary in order to visualize the entire area of bony depression, and the incisions made in a manner to facilitate complete closure. The depressed bone fragments may be "locked" and if so a burr opening is made in the intact skull just beyond the border of the depression. Through this opening the separate fragments are dislodged and laid aside. If there is gross contamination of the margins of the intact bone, this is cut away. The dura is inspected and if a laceration is found it should be sutured. In instances of compound depressed fractures in which a subdural hemorrhage is demonstrable beneath an intact dura, the dura should be incised, the blood clot evacuated and the dura closed. When the dura has been badly lacerated, the edges are cut away and the cerebral cortex carefully inspected. All macerated brain tissue and foreign material is removed. It is preferable, if possible, not to excise or damage the soft meninges, for by preserving these structures, the cerebral circulation is not compromised by the operative procedure. The dura is closed whenever possible. In the event a laceration of the dura cannot be made watertight, consideration should be given to the use of a transplant of fascia lata, pericranium, or freeze-dried dura to close the defect so as to seal off the intracranial contents and prevent cerebrospinal fluid from escaping. Depending on the estimated contamination of the wound, provided the dural rent has been repaired, the bone fragments may be replaced and secured with sutures if necessary, to preserve the contour of the skull. At other times it may be more judicious to discard all loose fragments and plan to repair the cranial defect at some future date. The galea aponeurotica is approximated with fine interrupted silk sutures closely set to insure against leaking of cerebrospinal fluid. If for any reason it seems advisable to drain the area for 24 hours, a small scalp opening is made a short distance away from the traumatized area and the drain placed in a tunnel (made between the galea and the pericranium) extending from the cranial defect through the opening in the scalp. The surgical principles that should be followed in the treatment of a compound fracture of the vault of the skull are the same as those applicable to any fresh wound caused by accidental trauma. All devitalized tissue must be sharply excised, foreign material removed, complete hemostasis secured, and antibiotic therapy judiciously employed. There is one factor that must be dealt with in wounds of the skull that is not encountered elsewhere in the body, namely, the cerebrospinal fluid. To avoid a leak of cerebrospinal fluid, the wound must be closed meticulously in layers. The prognosis following proper surgical treatment of a compound fracture of the vault of the skull should be excellent.

A compound depressed fracture over either the posterior half of the sagittal or one of the transverse venous sinuses presents a difficult therapeutic problem. When the involved area is grossly contaminated with debris, generous washing with saline solution and removal of the foreign material with a small curette, leaving the depressed bone in place over the venous sinus, may be preferable to removal of the fragments. If it is possible to determine that the underlying venous sinus has not been lacerated, there should be no hesitancy in elevating the depressed bone. When the outer margin of a zone of depressed bone is over a venous sinus, the involved bone, with the exception of that over the sinus, may be rongeured away. As stated in the discussion of the treatment of simple depressed fractures, the surgical manipulation of depressed bone over one of the large cranial venous sinuses may be followed by an ingress of air through a rent in the sinus wall. If such a depression of the skull is to be elevated, the patient should be placed on the operating table with the head lower than the heart in order to maintain a slightly positive pressure in the sinus and therefore prevent the entrance of air sufficient to cause sudden death. With the patient in the head-down position, profuse hemorrhage may occur following the elevation of the depressed fragments of bone; however, this can be brought under control by applying a muscle graft or by reflecting and suturing over the rent in the sinus a flap of dura cut so that its attached base parallels the border of the sinus. The technical difficulties encountered following the elevation of the bone fragments under these conditions make the procedure a questionable one and indicate that better results would be obtained by leaving the depressed bone in the position produced by the accident.

The principles underlying the surgical treatment of compound comminuted depressed fractures of the vault of the skull have been set forth on the basis that adequate antimicrobial (antibiotic) therapy has been instituted and that the operation is to be performed not later than 24 hours after the accident. If the wound has been neglected or the scalp has been sutured over an unrecognized area of depressed bone, there may be evidence at some later date of local infection with or without systemic reaction. Under these conditions the area of the skull that is involved is widely exposed and all bone fragments removed. If the dura and brain have been lacerated, the dura is opened over the full extent of the laceration and the traumatized, infected brain removed by suction. Following complete hemostasis, the contaminated area may be treated by King's method for brain abscess. It should be clearly understood that this form of treatment is to be considered only in cases of old untreated wounds with frank cerebritis. There will be copious drainage of blood-stained cerebrospinal fluid and rarely a generalized invasion of the subarachnoid space with bacteria will ensue. Whenever meningitis does not ensue, the subarachnoid space about the wound becomes occluded in three or four days and the zone of exposed brain, dura, bone, and lacerated scalp is slowly covered with a layer of granulation tissue. Usually the involved area bulges; the degree of herniation will depend upon the increased intracranial pressure resulting from both the trauma and the superimposed encephalitis. Excessive herniation of the brain may be kept under control by repeated withdrawal of cerebrospinal fluid by lumbar puncture. Slowly the protrusion of the damaged surface of the brain will recede to the level of the skull and when the wound surface is covered with granulations, grafting of skin should be carried out. After the area has been epithelialized for several weeks and all possible infection has been eliminated, the zone of grafted skin may be excised, the dura closed with a graft of fascia lata or freeze-dried dura, the cranial defect filled with a bone graft or other type of prosthesis, and the scalp securely closed by cutting appropiate flaps that can be sutured into position with their circulation intact. While this surgical approach may be regarded by some as a long-term, inappropriate procedure that is associated with excessive morbidity, more patients will be saved by it than by primary closure of the wound.*

COMPOUND FRACTURES INTO THE MIDDLE EAR

The linear fractures that traverse the posterior aspect of the middle fossa frequently cross the petrous part of the temporal bone. The dura overlying this part of the temporal bone is thin and firmly attached by numerous trabeculae. Linear fractures that implicate the temporal bone at the level of the middle ear not infrequently establish a communication between this cavity and the cerebral subarachnoid space. The force that produces the fracture may lacerate the tympanic membrane. In this manner, a pathway is established from the subarachnoid space to the external auditory canal through which cerebrospinal fluid may escape. Trauma of a similar nature may cause hemorrhage within the cavity of

*For additional comments on the treatment of old and infected wounds, see Chapter 9.

84

the middle ear without the tympanic membrane being lacerated, or the membrane may be ruptured without there having been an adjacent fracture of the skull. In other words, *a bloody discharge from the external auditory canal may result from a traumatic laceration of this canal, a rupture of the tympanic membrane alone, or a compound fracture of the skull into the middle ear with rupture of the tympanic membrane.* Therefore, "bleeding from the ear" is suggestive but not conclusive evidence that a fracture of the skull has been sustained. A comparison of the red cell count of the blood-stained discharge from the aural canal with that of the peripheral blood will establish the presence or absence of cerebrospinal fluid in the discharge from the ear. If a compound fracture of the skull into the middle ear has been sustained, the watery discharge from the involved ear when observed soon after the accident is usually contaminated with blood, but if the discharge continues for several hours the draining fluid tends to become clear. While the average aural cerebrospinal fluid "leak" ceases in 36 to 48 hours following the accident, there are instances in which large quantities of fluid continue to drain for many days without evidence of infection. This long continued discharge of cerebrospinal fluid may cause a whitish membrane to form over the part of the external ear that is being constantly bathed by the discharge. Cultures taken from this membrane have shown both staphylococci and streptococci. The critical situation produced by a compound fracture into the middle ear is not dependent upon the fracture as such nor the presence of a discharge of cerebrospinal fluid but on the complications that arise in an open wound that cannot be surgically closed. Attempts have been made to close the laceration of the dura usually found over the anterior surface of the petrous part of the temporal bone but uniform success has not been attained. Irrigating the external auditory canal with antiseptic solutions is a questionable procedure; in fact, the results indicate that infection may be introduced into the middle ear by this method. It seems best to follow a conservative course. Antimicrobial therapy is instituted and the patient maintained in a position that permits free drainage, preferably with the affected ear dependent so that "pooling" of the fluid in the external auditory canal is prevented. Repeated daily observations of the character of the fluid will give valuable information regarding the occurrence of infection since the aural discharge sometimes becomes turbid. If meningitis becomes established, the cerebrospinal fluid leak from the ear may abruptly cease. Blood may be present in the mastoid air cells and subsequent infection may extend into these cells or along the fracture line of the vault of the skull. Rarely, signs of an epidural abscess, a subdural abscess, or thrombophlebitis of the adjacent sinus appear.

The facial muscles supplied by the seventh cranial nerve on the affected side may become paretic or paralyzed as a result of a fracture through the petrous part of the temporal bone. Facial paralysis may be observed immediately after the injury, probably produced by a displacement of the bone fragments at the time of trauma. The appearance of the paralysis three or four days after the injury suggests that edema secondary to hemorrhage about the nerve is the causative factor. When the paralysis of the face appears eight or ten days after the injury, there is frequently an associated thin purulent discharge from the external auditory canal. This suggests that edema secondary to infection may be the etiological factor producing physiological interruption of nerve function. Except in rare instances in which facial paralysis results from direct trauma to the facial nerve, surgical intervention is contraindicated. Satisfactory recovery may be expected to follow physiotherapy of the affected part.

Many types of dysfunction of both the auditory and vestibular apparatus of the inner ear may result from a compound fracture of the skull into the middle ear. The one encountered most frequently is deafness due to faulty conduction of sound via middle ear structures because of the presence of hemorrhage alone or hemorrhage with superimposed infection. An infection established in this manner may extend into the inner ear and cause irreparable damage of either the cochlea or the vestibular apparatus or both. Such an extension of an infection may lead to meningitis. The entire auditory nerve may be damaged, with complete loss of hearing, or there may be partial loss of hearing associated with "noises" in the ear. Variable physiological alterations of the vestibular apparatus have been observed; usually functional adjustment follows. Singly or in combination, the fracture line itself, associated hemorrhage or subsequent infection may produce a variety of lesions of the structures within the petrous part of the temporal bone.

A compound depressed fracture of the squamous part of the temporal bone with a line of fracture extending into the cavity of the middle ear and perforation of the tympanic membrane may be encountered. The depressed area should be treated in the same manner as advocated for the care of other types of compound fractures of the vault of the skull, that part implicating the ear being treated conservatively.

Fractures of the skull that involve the accessory air sinuses, especially the ethmoid, sphenoid, and frontal air cells and those that are compounded into the nasopharynx, may be the result of direct injury over the frontal region or of a blow over the lateral or posterior aspect of the head causing a basilar fracture. The fracture may be linear in type or there may be an obvious depression of the frontal bone implicating the frontal and ethmoidal air cells. Occasionally subcutaneous crepitations are demonstrable over the forehead or the upper eyelids. In the few instances in which this has been observed, the air rapidly disappeared and suppuration did not follow. While a depressed fracture of the frontal region of the skull is easily recognized, great difficulty is at times encountered in determining whether a linear fracture has disrupted the mucous membrane at some site within the nose or its communicating sinuses. Bleeding from the nose or mouth immediately after a blow on any part of the head suggests the possibility of a compound fracture of the skull into the nasal cavity. A scanty discharge of bright red blood from the nose continuing for several hours following an accident lends support to this impression. A positive diagnosis of fracture from the character of the discharge alone can be made only when the *rhinorrhea* is copious clear fluid. The admixture of nasal secretion with blood must not be confused with a true leak of cerebrospinal fluid. Evidence of hemorrhage into the soft tissue of the upper eyelid appearing several hours after an injury to the head and unassociated with indications of trauma about the face is highly suggestive of a fracture through the roof of the orbit on the side of the hemorrhage. Examination by roentgen ray is not altogether satisfactory for the demonstration of fractures limited in their extent to the base of the anterior cranial fossa. This area can be visualized by an examination of stereoscopic roentgen-ray films of the head but a fracture line may be easily overlooked.

Roentgen-ray examination of the skull following trauma occasionally shows a collection of air within either the subdural or subarachnoid space while more rarely the ventricles of the brain are outlined. The presence of air within the intracranial cavity immediately after a head injury indicates that a compound fracture is present, the injury having produced at least a temporary communication between the nose or the nasal accessory sinuses and the intracranial cavity. Many patients with this roentgen-ray finding who present no evidence of cerebrospinal fluid leak from the nose recover without complications. Occasionally a patient who seems well along the road to recovery after a compound fracture through the floor of the anterior cranial fossa will complain of severe headache and vomit immediately after sneezing violently or forcefully blowing the nose. Focal signs, such as one-sided paresis or paralysis, convulsive seizures, and aphasia, may appear. At times advancing stupor is evident. Examination of the head by roentgen ray often discloses a large collection of air within a frontal lobe of the brain. Repeated examination may show a progressive increase in the size of the air pocket and the clinical course indicates that surgical intervention is necessary. Repair of the dural defect should be carried out and the air-containing cavity within the brain exposed and its contents evacuated.

In some instances, clinical evidence denoting meningitis is the first indication of a compound linear fracture involving the anterior fossa of the skull. Theoretically a traumatic opening in the dura that accompanies a compound linear fracture through the base of the anterior cranial fossa should be closed by operation. However, the fact that less than 1 percent of the patients with this lesion succumbed to meningitis limits the usefulness of this surgical procedure. Furthermore, when the fracture line traverses the cribriform plate of the ethmoid bone and the rent in the dura is in this region, both olfactory bulbs must be sacrificed if the dural opening is to be securely closed. A profuse flow of cerebrospinal fluid from the nose that continues for more than ten days after an injury or frequent recurrences of such episodes are both indications for surgical closure of the dural opening. The surgical procedure consists of exposure of the rent in the dura, which is usually found adjacent to an olfactory bulb on one or both sides. The crista galli is rongeured flush with the base of the skull and the implicated olfactory bulbs removed. Flaps of dura are cut with their bases short of the traumatic opening. The dural flaps are sutured over the traumatic opening. The bone flap is wired and the wound closed in layers with silk.*

Compound depressed fractures of the skull that implicate the nose and the air sinuses may be associated with various degrees of laceration of the skin over the forehead. Whether or not the cutaneous surface is lacerated, the surgical problem is essentially the same and demands immediate attention. There may be an associated local and/or general brain injury which is of primary importance and must be appropriately

---

*See section on CSF rhinorrhea and spontaneous pneumocephalus, Chapter 9.

treated. The operative procedure directed at the compound fracture itself should not be delayed. In contrast to compound fractures of the vault of the skull in which closure of the dura is of less importance, in all instances of compound depressed fractures over the frontal region of the head that communicate with the nose or the accessory sinuses, the lacerated dura must be closed primarily or repaired with a patch of fascia lata or other graft. First, the depressed area of bone is exposed either by an incision enlarging the original opening produced by the traumatic laceration or by appropiate skin flaps with the incision made high on the forehead within the hairline. Loose fragments are removed and depressed areas of bone are elevated. The extent of the fracture lines should be determined especially with regard to possible implication of the air sinuses. The dura should be inspected for lacerations and if such be present the frontal lobes of the brain should be carefully examined. All devitalized tissues are removed (scalp, bone, dura, brain). The dura must be securely closed or if this is technically impossible, the opening must be repaired with a graft. The involved accessory sinuses may be drained externally and the remainder of the wound closed without direct drainage. In some patients with grossly contaminated wounds, it may be advisable to sacrifice a large area of bone, the resultant cranial defect being corrected with a prosthesis at a later operation.

REPAIR OF CRANIAL DEFECTS DUE TO FRACTURES OF THE SKULL

Compound fractures of the skull must be converted into simple fractures by proper surgical treatment, the cosmetic results for the most part being of secondary importance. The use of modern antibiotic drugs has limited the sacrifice of portions of the cranial vault in the immediate treatment of certain fractures. In any event the patient may be left with a cranial defect which requires repair either because of its location or size. In order to obviate infection, several months should be permitted to elapse after the wound has completely healed before introducing foreign material to repair the cranial defect.

Small cranial defects with the underlying dura intact may be satisfactorily closed by "chipping" an adjacent area of the outer table of the skull, leaving each fragment of bone attached to the pericranium and shifting this sheet of bone fragments to fill the cranial defect. Stainless steel wire mesh molded to conform to the contour of the skull and sutured to pericranium is an eminently satisfactory subtitute.

For large openings free bone grafts may be utilized. Various alloplastic materials have proved valuable for use in cranioplasty. Tantalum, stainless steel, and the acrylic resins are currently preferred. The overlying scalp must be in healthy condition and the suturing of the galea aponeurotica should be meticulously performed. It may be necessary to excise scars of the scalp; however, if this is carried out, a flap of scalp is outlined and shifted into place in order to cover the area of graft with a full thickness of scalp. The operative area should never be drained. Rigid asepsis is essential if success is to be expected. This subject has also been referred to in Chapter 9.

BIBLIOGRAPHY

Browder, J. Craniocerebral Wounds — Exteriorization Method of Treatment. *Amer. J. Surg.*, *62*, 3, 1943.

Coleman, C. C. Fractures of the Skull Involving the Paranasal Sinus and Mastoids. *J.A.M.A.*, *109*, 1613, 1937.

Dandy, W. E. Pneumocephalus (Intracranial Pneumatocele or Aerocele). *Arch. Surg.*, *12*, 949, 1926.

Gurdjian, E. S. and Webster, J. E. *Head Injuries. Mechanisms, Diagnosis and Management*. Boston: Little Brown and Co., 1958. P. 482.

Hough, J. V. D., Ward, P. H., Barber, H. O., Schuknecht, H. F., Wright, J. W., Jr., Taylor, C. E., Bizal, J. A., and Fox, M. C.: Symposium on Auditory and Vestibular Disorders in Head Trauma. *Ann. Otol. Rhinol. Laryngol.*, *78*, 210-284, 1969.

Kriss, J. F., Taren, J. A., and Kahn, E. A. Primary Repair of Compound Skull Fractures by Replacement of Bone Fragments, *J. Neurosurg.*, *30*, 698, 1969.

Lewin, W. *The Management of Head Injuries*. London: Balliere, Tindall & Cassell, 1966. P. 318. (Chapter 9. Fractures of the Skull and Their Complications; Otorrhoea and Rhinorrhea.)

Lewin, W. Cerebrospinal Fluid Rhinorrhea in Nonmissile Head Injuries. In *Clinical Neurosurgery, Vol. 12*. Baltimore: Williams and Wilkins, 1966. P. 237.

Meirowsky, A. M. Compound Fractures of Convexity of the Skull. In A. M. Meirowsky (Ed.), *Neurological Surgery of Trauma*. Washington, D. C.: Office of Surgeon General, Dep't. of the Army, 1965. P. 604.

Miller, J. D. and Jennett, W. B. Complications of Depressed Skull Fracture. *Lancet*, *2*, 991, 1968.

Reeves, D. L. Repair of Cranial Defects. In A. M. Meirowsky (Ed.), *Neurological Surgery of Trauma*. Pp. 233-256. Washington, D. C. Office of Surgeon General, Dep't. of the Army, 1965. P. 604.

Rowbotham, G. F. *Acute Injuries of the Head*. 4th ed. Baltimore: Williams and Wilkins, 1964. P. 584. (Chapter 8. Fractures of the Skull, by Ramamurthel; Chapter 9. Open or Compound Wounds of the Head, by K. Kristiansen).

Scheibert, C. D. Cerebrospinal Fluid Fistula. In A. M. Meirowsky (Ed.). *Neuro-*

logical Surgery of Trauma. Pp. 213-219. Washington, D. C. Office of Surgeon General, Dep't. of the Army, 1965. P. 604.

Stöwsand, D., and Geile, G. Zur Frage der operativen Behandlung von Impressionsfrakturen. Acta Neurochirur. 13, 237, 1965.

Vance, B. M. Fracture of the Skull. Arch. Surg., 14, 1023, 1927.

OSTEOMYELITIS OF THE SKULL

The pyogenic infections of the skull that follow trauma may be divided into two groups, namely, osteomyelitis manifesting itself at the site of injury without a preceding open scalp wound (Pott's puffy tumor) and osteomyelitis due to direct implantation of bacteria through an open wound. The second group embraces a variety of pathological conditions from which several clinical syndromes may be delineated. As has been previously stated, the judicious use of antibiotic agents has greatly reduced the frequency of infections following craniocerebral injuries. As yet the employment of these agents has not entirely eliminated such complications; however, it may be fairly stated that seldom does one encounter, except in neglected instances, a rapid advance of the inflammatory process within the skull as formerly observed. Briefly stated, the same entities are still observed but in a less virulent form. Once established, however, a virulent organism may advance rapidly along the large and communicating venous channels of the diploë. One rarely encounters osteomyelitis following trauma, comparable in extent to the widespread involvement of the skull observed either as a direct extension of a frontal or ethmoidal sinusitis or as a complication of bacteremia.

The *diagnosis* of traumatic osteomyelitis of the skull can be made when an *open* skull fracture has become infected, as evidenced by long-continued drainage associated with signs of chronic cellulitis of the adjacent scalp. Bone destruction is seen in the x-ray, and sequestration occurs. If the skull fracture involves an infected sinus, then retrograde thrombophlebitis may infect the diploë, with further spread to other parts of the skull.

For convenience of presentation the following classification, arrived at on the basis of therapeutic considerations, will be employed: (1) osteomyelitis arising at the site of cranial trauma with the overlying scalp intact (Pott's puffy tumor); (2) osteomyelitis secondary to direct implantation of bacteria through an open wound; (a) exfoliative or desquamative; (b) circumscribed; (c) spreading; (d) associated with

91

compound fractures into the middle ear; (e) associated with compound fractures into the nose and/or accessory nasal sinuses.

POTT'S PUFFY TUMOR

This type of osteomyelitis of the skull was first described in detail by Sir Percival Pott in his book entitled "Observations on the Nature and Consequence of Wounds and Contusions of the Head, Fractures of the Skull, Concussion of the Brain," etc., published by C. Hitch and L. Haws in London in 1760. Reports by subsequent authors have added little to his excellent observations. The lesion is rare as shown by the fact that it has been observed by me only four times in a series of 46,574 craniocerebral injuries. It is encountered in patients who have sustained a localized trauma of the head without laceration of the scalp and with or without evidence of damage to the intracranial structures. On roentgen-ray examination the skull may or may not be fractured. At the site of the blow the scalp is swollen, owing to a hemorrhagic extravasation which rapidly resolves, although in some instances the swelling may persist unduly long. Two to three weeks after the accident and in some cases later, the traumatized area rather insidiously becomes more tender and painful. Untreated, the scalp may swell to large proportions and become widely edematous. The dome of the elevated area may present a bluish, mottled appearance. If the infection has existed for several weeks, roentgen-ray examination may show evidence of an underlying area of irregular bone destruction. In other cases the infected skull overlies a collection of pus in the epidural space. Signs of meningitis or brain abscess may appear before the patient seeks medical aid. Either or both of these conditions may occur after the infected bone has been surgically removed. Because of the rarity of the lesion it is seldom entertained in differential diagnosis. Once the diagnosis has been established, antimicrobial therapy followed by wide exposure and excision of all involved bone is indicated. A newly formed layer of granulation and connective tissue will be commonly found covering the dura that has been stripped from the involved bone. This newly formed connective tissue should be carefully preserved since it serves as a barrier against intradural invasion. Intracranial complications are treated according to indication.

The scalp over a large area of the skull may be destroyed by burns or torn away by violence leaving an exposed outer table of bone deprived of its periosteum. Not infrequently the denuded area is so large that it cannot be covered by surgically cut flaps of scalp or by other methods of skin grafting. Thus deprived of its external blood supply, the bone at first presents a pinkish hue, but gradually the color becomes livid and eventually the bone assumes a desiccated grayish-yellow appearance. If left undisturbed, a part or all of the exposed outer table will become detached, leaving a surface of granulation tissue. This surface may then be covered with pinch grafts of skin. The process of bony desquamation here described is a slow one. In an attempt to save the outer table of the skull, it has become common practice to make small, closely set perforations in this table through which new connective tissue will grow. Slowly granulation tissue arising from the multiple openings will coalesce, thereby covering the entire area of exposed bone. Small sequestra are frequently discharged during the healing process. When the area has been covered completely by the new tissue, epithelialization may be hastened by grafts of skin. The method is a safe one provided the perforations made in the outer table do not damage the inner table of the skull. A perforation made too deeply may be followed by an intracranial infection. In one such instance the operation was performed in another hospital and a chronological account of the clinical course could not be accurately ascertained. Postmortem examination disclosed an area in which both the inner and outer tables of the skull had been perforated and beneath the cranial opening a small zone of epidural granulation was present. Two large intracerebral abscesses were found, contiguous to the zone of dura covered with granulation tissue.

Burns, especially those produced by high voltage electric current, may produce death of the entire thickness of the skull over an area of considerable size. In such cases conservative treatment usually results in a slow demarcation of the dead from the living bone and the sequestrated part is spontaneously cast off. Necrosis of the underlying dura has never been observed under these circumstances. When the sequestrum has separated, a surface layer of granulation tissue forms. Grafts of skin will hasten epithelialization. Whenever feasible, destructive lesions of the scalp and skull produced by burns should be excised and flaps of scalp reflected over the implicated zone.

CIRCUMSCRIBED OSTEOMYELITIS

A localized area of infection of the skull may follow a laceration of the scalp with contusion of the adjacent bone or compound linear fracture of the skull.

Organisms transplanted directly into the skull through an open wound seldom cause a widespread suppurative process. Commonly, the infection becomes a smouldering one and the limited reactive process within the bone about it is characterized by excessive calcium deposition, demonstrable by roentgen-ray examination. Following antibiotic therapy such a circumscribed area of bone infection may undergo spontaneous resolution without producing gross structural changes in the skull, but often it is followed by the extrusion of small sequestra. Recurrent episodes of this nature, irregularly spaced, may eventually result in spontaneous cure. Rarely does a chronic osteomyelitis of this type break the surrounding cellular barrier and become widespread. If surgical intervention is to be undertaken, great care must be exercised to prevent damage of the dura mater.

SPREADING OSTEOMYELITIS

Theoretically the wide intercommunicating venous channels of the diplöe offer an ideal situation for the advance of infection when once implanted. The clinical evidence indicates that this is not the case except in rare instances in which contaminated material has been forced through the small foramina of the outer table of the skull. Rather extensive bone necrosis has been observed to follow this mode of inoculation. The appearance of a small tender swelling of the scalp some distance from the point of contamination of the bone, together with signs of systemic reaction, should arouse suspicion of a spreading infection. Under these circumstances the structural changes in the skull due to the infection cannot be demonstrated by roentgen-ray examination until loss of bone calcium has occurred, nor can one determine the extent of the pathological process even with the skull exposed at operation. It therefore becomes almost impossible to eradicate the process by attempting to cut away all infected bone. For several years I have maintained that the removal of large areas of the skull, presumably for cure of osteomyelitis, was unsound. Regardless of previous opinions expressed by me and others, it would seem that the excellent results now obtained by the use of present-day antibiotic agents and ultra-conservative surgical procedures should deter the advocates of radical removal of bone. The skull grossly implicated may be removed in order to permit adequate drainage of the epidural space, but the removal of large areas of normal bone about a zone of osteomyelitis is to be condemned. Cranial defects resulting from osteomyelitis may be repaired, if necessary, no sooner than 12 months after all evidence of infection has disappeared.

OSTEOMYELITIS ASSOCIATED WITH COMPOUND FRACTURE INTO THE
MIDDLE EAR

This is by far the commonest type of cranial bone infection following trauma of the head, although during recent years it has been largely eradicated by antibiotic therapy. The clinical picture of this complication is so constant that once observed it is not readily mistaken. A typical example of this syndrome is as follows: a patient who has sustained a compound fracture of the skull that implicates the middle ear, with attending perforation of the tympanic membrane and bloody or cerebrospinal fluid discharge from the affected ear, is making satisfactory improvement when, rather insidiously, slight mental confusion occurs, the temperature rises a few degrees and the scanty clear yellowish aural discharge becomes turbid and of foul odor. At this time examination usually discloses a mild to moderate amount of edema over the mastoid region of the affected side and, in some instances, a fingerlike prolongation of the edema over the course of an underlying fracture of the vault. The neck may be moderately rigid and Kernig's sign may also be present. Spinal puncture commonly discloses an increase in the cell content of the cerebrospinal fluid and in some instances of rapidly advancing infection, microorganisms are demostrated by culture of the fluid. If untreated there is extension of the inflammatory process, which ultimately invades the intracranial cavity, and one or more of the following conditions may ensue: epidural abscess, subdural abscess, meningitis, lateral sinus thrombophlebitis, and brain abscess. Not infrequently during the course of the infection, paralysis of all the facial muscles on the involved side appears. Early recognition of this lesion, institution of antibiotic treatment and immediate operation will be followed by recovery in the majority of cases. The mastoid cells should be exenterated, the cavity of the middle ear widely opened, the bony roof of the middle ear removed if the fracture line traverses this area, and any fissure fracture of the vault leading away from the mastoid region widened to 5 or 6 mm. The dura mater, even though lacerated, should not be disturbed. Many modifications of this operative

95

procedure will of necessity be required in order to deal with the variable pathological processes encountered. The principle to be followed is adequate drainage of all involved epidural structures. Far too often operation is deferred and in such instances intracranial complications may occur. These are discussed in another chapter.

OSTEOMYELITIS OF THE SKULL ASSOCIATED WITH COMPOUND FRACTURE INTO THE NOSE AND/OR THE ACCESSORY NASAL SINUSES

Many anatomical structures may be involved in a compound fracture of the skull that extends across the floor of the anterior cranial fossa or in one that is limited to the more external frontal region of the head. Furthermore, the frontal, ethmoidal, and sphenoidal air cells have such small ostia for drainage that once a fracture in this region is invaded by bacteria, infection may ensue in spite of adequate antibiotic therapy. When established in this location, infection resists treatment with surprising obstinacy. Osteomyelitis of the cranial bones adjacent to the upper nasal cavity and the accessory sinuses seldom follows a properly treated compound fracture of the skull produced by a blow to the frontal region of the head. If infection has supervened, the inflammatory process usually remains localized to a small area and sequestration of the destroyed bone should be awaited unless evidence of intracranial extension develops. Any operative procedure should be limited in scope and should be designed to drain the infected zone.

POSTTRAUMATIC EPIDURAL AND SUBDURAL ABSCESS

Any variety of compound fracture of the skull may result in an intracranial extension of an inflammatory process even though adequate antibiotic therapy has been carried out. In some instances, however, bacteria have entered the epidural, subdural, or subarachnoid spaces, or the intracerebral tissues without obvious implication of the bone itself. Epidural abscesses have been observed more commonly in the vicinity of the middle ear and about the region of the frontal air sinuses but they may be a sequel to either an unrecognized or an imperfectly treated compound fracture of any part of the cranial vault. A suppurative process in this epidural position unassociated with osteomyelitis of the skull or evidence of extension into the intradural structures is frequently difficult to diagnose with certainty. The occurrence of low grade fever, increasing drowsiness, headache, localized edema of the scalp, stiffness

96

of the neck and increased cellular content and protein of the cerebrospinal fluid without demonstrable microorganisms in a patient who
previously seemed to be recovering from the immediate effects of a head
injury should arouse strong suspicion that an epidural abscess is present. The electroencephalogram may point to a focus. There may be
focal signs including focal convulsive seizures. Generalized seizures
may occur. These findings and the demonstration by roentgen ray of
a fracture of the skull that has implicated either the middle ear or the
frontal air cells are sufficient evidence to warrant surgical intervention.

The presence of a subdural abscess is suggested by a sudden onset
of severe headache, increasing drowsiness progressing to stupor, and
such signs as rigidity of the neck and hemiparesis, focal or generalized
convulsive seizures, and evidences of increased pressure, including
papilledema. Meningitis is apt to occur. Arteriography and radioactive
scanning may provide confirmatory evidence. The only example of
this lesion subsequent to trauma that I have ever observed occurred
following a compound fracture of the skull into the middle ear. In
spite of what was considered proper antibiotic therapy instituted shortly
after the accident, symptoms and signs developed that were interpreted
as representing a subdural hematoma. At operation a large subdural
collection of pus was evacuated. The area was unroofed and the patient recovered. More detailed accounts of subdural abscess may be
found in the references listed in the bibliography. Meningitis and brain
abscess are discussed in Chapters 12 and 13.

SEPTIC THROMBOPHLEBITIS OF THE DURAL VENOUS SINUSES

The cavernous, longitudinal, or lateral dural venous sinuses may be
invaded by microorganisms that have gained entrance by way of a suppurative process previously established within or adjacent to a compound fracture of the skull. Staphylococcus aureus is the organism
most frequently recovered. In cavernous sinus thrombophlebitis, the
portal of entry for the offending organism is, as would be expected, a
compound fracture in a part of the anterior cranial fossa involving the
nasopharynx and/or the accessory nasal air cells. In some instances
proptosis of one eye, indicating a thrombophlebitis and periphlebitis of
the ophthalmic veins, appears several days after the original trauma
and precedes the actual invasion of the cavernous sinus. Eye manifestations appear bilaterally in other cases, suggesting retrograde involvement of the orbital structures from a septic thrombophlebitis of the
cavernous sinus. The portal of entry in the former case is more ante-

97

rior, while in the latter the bacteria have usually gained entrance through a fracture in the vicinity of the sphenoidal air cells.

In full-blown cavernous sinus thrombophlebitis, one finds swelling of the eyelids and adjacent tissues, congestion of the orbital and periorbital veins, cyanosis of the orbital tissues, and proptosis of the affected eye, together with swelling and thrombosis of the retinal veins. Involvement of the oculomotor nerves (third, fourth and sixth) may cause ophthalmoplegia — internal (i.e., pupillary) as well as external. Involvement of the ophthalmic division of the trigeminal nerve accounts for the loss of the corneal reflex and pains in the affected orbit and supraorbital regions. The above signs may be more or less confined to one side, or there may be bilateral involvement. Fever and other signs of infection are evident.

Surgical intervention was previously advocated for the prevention of cavernous sinus thrombophlebitis that frequently followed bacterial implication of the ophthalmic veins. The results obtained by the use of antibiotics have been so superior that operative procedures for these lesions have been abandoned.

Thrombophlebitis of the superior sagittal sinus may follow an infected compound fracture of the vault of the skull if this lesion directly overlies the sinus. This complication is rare if appropriate antibiotic therapy is employed. Thrombophlebitis of the superior sagittal sinus presents the usual general signs of infection, together with headache and vomiting. One is likely to detect congestion of adjacent frontotemporal scalp veins, associated with edema and some localizing signs as paraplegic weakness and cortical sensory defects, and bladder disturbance may develop. Papilledema is not infrequent. Jacksonian seizures, involving the foot, or beginning in the foot, may direct attention to the parasagittal region. Generalized convulsions have been described and a variety of other cortical disturbances. Some degree of subarachnoid bleeding may occur, with resultant xanthochromia and increased protein content of the spinal fluid. Fortunately, the advent of antibiotic therapy has made a full-blown septic superior sagittal sinus syndrome a rare occurrence.

Thrombophlebitis of the lateral sinus occurs in association with an inflammatory process that has followed a compound fracture of the skull into the middle ear. Such a lesion may establish itself even though the tympanic membrane of the affected ear had not been ruptured by the original trauma. Thrombophlebitis of the lateral sinus may cause edema of the scalp overlying the mastoid area, accompanied by venous congestion. Internal jugular vein tenderness, with swelling and pain in the neck, point to spread into that venous channel. Vomiting, headache, a spiking temperature with the usual accompaniments of severe infection (chills, sweats, etc.) were frequent in the pre-antibiotic days, as was the occurrence of positive blood cultures. Since the availability of antibiotic therapy this complication has been practically eliminated.

BIBLIOGRAPHY

Adelstein, L. J. and Courville, C. B. Traumatic Osteomyelitis of Cranial Vault with Particular Reference to Pathogenesis and Treatment. *Arch. Surg., 26*, 539, 1933.

French, L. A. and Chou, S. N. Osteomyelitis of the Skull and Epidural Abscess. In E. S. Gurdjian (Ed.), *Cranial and Intracranial Suppuration*. Springfield, Ill.: Charles C Thomas, 1969. P. 59.

Gurdjian, E. S. and Thomas, L. M. Surgical Treatment of Cranial and Intracranial Suppuration. In E. S. Gurdjian (Ed.), *Cranial and Intracranial Suppuration*. Springfield, Ill.: Charles C Thomas, 1969. P. 3.

Harsh, G. R., III. Infection Complicating Penetrating Craniocerebral Trauma. In A. M. Meirowsky (Ed.), *Neurological Surgery of Trauma*. Washington, D. C.: Office of the Surgeon General, Dept. of the Army, 1965. P. 135.

Hitchcock, E. and Andreadis, A. Subdural Empyema: A Review of 29 Cases. *J. Neurol. Neurosurg. Psychiatry, 27*, 422, 1964.

Keith, W. S. Subdural Empyema. *J. Neurosurg., 6*, 127, 1949.

King, J. E. J. Treatment of Osteomyelitis of the Cranial Vault. *Surgery, 1*, 401, 1937.

Kubik, C. S. and Adams, R. D. Subdural Empyema. *Brain, 66*, 18, 1943.

List, C. F. Interhemispheral Subdural Suppuration. *J. Neurosurg., 7*, 313, 1950.

McLaurin, R. L. Subdural Infection. In E. S. Gurdjian (Ed.), *Cranial and Intracranial Suppuration*. Springfield, Ill.: Charles C Thomas, 1969. P. 73.

Peyser, E. Subdural Empyemas. *Ann. Surg., 146*, 215, 1957.

Rowbotham, G. F. *Acute Injuries of the Head*. Baltimore: Williams and Wilkins Co., 1964. P. 584. (Chapter 10. Traumatic Osteomyelitis.)

Schiller, F., Cairns, H., and Russell, D. S. The Treatment of Purulent Pachymeningitis and Subdural Suppuration with Special Reference to Penicillin. *J. Neurol. Neurosurg. Psychiatry, 11*, 143, 1948.

Wilensky, A. D. Osteomyelitis of the Skull. *Arch. Surg., 27*, 83, 1933.

CHAPTER 4

CONCUSSION AND CONTUSION OF THE BRAIN AND THEIR SEQUELAE

SIR CHARLES SYMONDS

INTRODUCTION

It might appear from the title of this chapter that we were about to describe certain pathological states in the brain resulting from trauma, together with the appropriate symptoms of each, in the same way, for example, as we might describe those of epidural and subdural hemorrhage. Such expectations are not to be realized. Concussion and contusion are terms which are in general use for the description of certain groups of symptoms commonly observed after head injury, and attributed to the direct effects of the injury upon the brain. Of the pathology of these symptoms we know very little. The reasons for this defect are that the patients who present opportunity for clinical study usually recover with their lives, so that there is no opportunity for inspection of the brain; and those who die live for so short a time that there is little opportunity for the observation of symptoms.

The Facts of Morbid Anatomy

The pathology of brain injuries is considered fully in Chapter 2 of this volume. The approach to the clinical problems with which we are concerned, however, demands a brief review of what may be found either at autopsy or at operation.

In the fatal cases, with or without fracture of the skull, there is, as a rule, laceration of the leptomeninges with blood-stained fluid in the subdural and subarachnoid spaces. Associated with this, there is laceration of the superficial parts of the brain, especially in certain situations. These are at the site of the blow, if its incidence has been local; at the point of contrecoup; and at the temporal poles and undersurface of the frontal lobes. In the line of force of the injury there are hemorrhages in the brain substance, as also around the areas of superficial laceration or contusion. Surrounding the larger hemorrhages, there are petechial hemorrhages and areas in which the microscope shows the perivascular spaces to be distended with blood. Scattered hemorrhages of the smaller size may be found in other parts of the brain and brain stem. In addition to the swelling due to hemorrhage, there are areas of edema and, apart from hemorrhage and edema, there are foci in which direct injury to the neurons is apparent in the form of demyelinization and pathological alterations in the contour of the axis cylinders (Greenfield, 1938).

Occasionally, in patients who survive, we observe focal symptoms which are clean cut, for example, dysphasia, and are able in the same case to inspect the appropriate area of cortex in the course of an exploratory operation. We find that in such a case the cortex is swollen and hemorrhagic, sometimes torn. In proportion to the severity of the injury the patient may make a complete or partial recovery from his symptoms.

The Facts of Clinical Observation in Relation to Those of Morbid Anatomy

The clinical story in a fatal case of brain injury will almost invariably have been that of coma from the moment of the injury to that of death within a period of two or three days.

But there are patients who, after hovering on the brink of death, emerge from coma into stupor and so, gradually, through stages presently to be described, to recovery of consciousness, after which they may present a variety of symptoms — headache, inability to concentrate, and slowness in thinking, indicating some persistent damage to the intracranial contents. It is reasonable to assume in such instances lesions of the same kind that are found post mortem or at operation, and to seek in this assumption an explanation of the symptoms observed both during and after the period of unconsciousness.

We have noted for example that in the fatal cases laceration and contusion are most frequently observed at the frontal and temporal poles. These are parts of the brain which may be damaged without the development of any characteristic focal symptoms. We also know from our experience of other cerebral disease, that cortical damage, wherever it may be, if it is extensive enough, may interfere with cerebral function as a whole, and especially with its highest levels. It is at least possible that in patients who survive, damage of this type and distribution may play an important part in the causation of symptoms, from which ultimately recovery may be complete. We have on several occasions seen areas of old hemorrhagic softening at the frontal and temporal poles in the brain of a patient known to have had a severe head injury many years previously, and with a history of complete recovery.

If we follow the path indicated by these observations, it is a fairly easy journey by stages to the assumption that the patient who has been unconscious only for an hour or so, with no physical signs of focal injury, would show, if we could see his brain, lesions of a kind which might account both for the loss of consciousness and his subsequent complaints.

At about this point, however, the path begins to be less plain. Soon it divides and, either way, we are brought to a halt before an intriguing problem. On the one hand, there is that of the patient who is unconscious only for a few moments, or at most a few minutes, and, on the other hand, that of the patient who is never unconscious at all, but presents symptoms such as headache, giddiness, nervousness, difficulty in concentration, and so on, of the type with which we are also familiar as a sequel of more or less prolonged unconsciousness.

It will be profitable first to consider these two problems separately, and then, retracing our steps, to view them in joint perspective.

Symptoms of Brain Injury without Loss of Consciousness. Let us take first the case of the man who has suffered a head injury without loss of consciousness. It may be at once or after a day or two, he complains that he gets a headache when he exerts himself, or when he is tired or bothered: stooping makes him giddy; he does not sleep as well as he should; he has lost confidence and power of concentration. These symptoms, being purely subjective, were in the past commonly described as neurotic, without any clear implication of what that term should mean. In recent years, a clearer appreciation, on the one hand, of what is meant by a neurosis, and, on the other hand, of the clinical value of symptoms, has led to the conclusion that these patients are suffering from physical effects of the injury. Wilfred Trotter (1925, 1930, 1932) was among the first to put forward this view, and his designation of this clinical syndrome as that of a minor cerebral contusion has been widely accepted.

The Phenomenon of Immediate Loss of Consciousness Following Head Injury. The problem of pathology in the case of the patient who is unconscious only for a few minutes is one which has given rise to much thought and discussion, but has no generally accepted solution. The facts are that in the instant after the injury we may observe a complete paralysis of cerebral function. From this state there is recovery so rapid that we cannot interpret the clinical phenomena in

102

terms of any of the lesions which we have so far described, or, in fact, in terms of any lesion which we can visualize. Indeed, there are recorded cases in which death has occurred within a few minutes of the injury from failure of the respiratory center, and at autopsy no lesion has been visible. It has been argued that for this clinical phenomenon we must seek an explanation in terms of a pathology which is different, not only in degree, but in its essentials, from that which we have accepted for all the symptoms so far considered. It follows that if the latter are to be spoken of as the symptoms of cerebral contusion, the syndrome of immediate and transient loss of cerebral function should have a separate name, and it is with this especial meaning that the term concussion is often used with the distinct implication of a separate pathology. Trotter (1932), for example, suggests that concussion in this sense is the result of momentary cerebral anemia from compression or indentation of the skull.

Let us consider this argument from its inception. It is impossible to explain total or sub-total paralysis of cerebral function, with complete recovery in a few minutes, in terms of any lesions which we can visualize. But this is almost equally true if the process of recovery is somewhat slower. There are many cases in which, with the return of all consciousness after a lapse of several hours, recovery of cerebral function appears to be complete. It seems, indeed, beyond the limits of possibility to explain such an occurrence in terms of laceration, edema, hemorrhage, or direct injury to the neurons of a kind which would be visible under the microscope. The contrast between the severity of the disturbance of function on the one hand, and the rapidity and completeness of recovery on the other hand, is too great. But is it unreasonable to postulate direct injury to the neurons of a degree which may result in loss of function for a period of minutes, hours, or even days, without any coarse structural lesion — injury of a kind which is clinically effective but pathologically subliminal? There is abundant evidence in clinical neurology of a wide gap between the degree of injury required to abolish function, and that required to cause damage of the kind that we should necessarily expect to see under the microscope. One may take, for example, injury to a peripheral nerve from a blow, or from compression or stretching. From any of these causes function may be abolished for several days, yet be completely restored within a period which excludes the possibility of destruction and repair.

If the analogy be accepted, we are entitled to suggest that the instantaneous loss of cerebral function, so frequently observed after head injury, is the result of sudden direct damage, by stretching or compression, to the nerve cells or fibers in the brain. The depth of the initial disturbance and the rate of recovery may depend upon such factors as the situation and the number of neurons involved, and the severity of the injury. Such injury is compatible with complete recovery of function within a few minutes, at the end of several hours, and possibly after several days. It does not involve any coarse structural lesion. Structural damage to the meninges, blood vessels and neurons may occur at the same time, and may add to the clinical picture in various ways. It may delay recovery of consciousness as the result of increased intracranial pressure or subarachnoid hemorrhage; it may introduce symptoms resulting from gross focal lesions; it may give rise to sequelae, such as headache, giddiness, and nervousness; and it may result in a persistent defect of function at the higher levels from destruction of myelin and axis cylinders. The greater the severity of the initial direct and recoverable injury (as measured roughly by the duration of unconsciousness), the greater the probability of associated coarse damage.

If, as we have suggested, the immediate loss of consciousness following brain trauma depends upon a single type of injury, and the duration of unconsciousness is dependent largely upon the severity or extent of this injury, we might expect to discover in the clinical picture some unity irrespective of duration. This we believe exists. If we take first a case in which the duration of unconsciousness is a matter of a few hours, we shall observe a more or less regular sequence of clinical stages. In the first stage, if we are fortunate enough to see the patient very early, there is a complete paralysis of cerebral function which may extend for a moment to the vital centers. In the next stage, pulse and respiration having returned, the state is that of coma, flaccid paralysis, and abolition of reflex function. Reflex function rapidly returns and, following this, movement of a simple purposive type, such as withdrawal of a limb from a painful stimulus. At this stage the mental state is that of stupor. The patient may respond to a forcible command, but is otherwise unconscious of his surroundings. Following this, there is a stage in which voluntary movement and speech return, but without control or direction. The mental state is that of restless confusion, and the patient is generally resistive and often violent. Gradually, behavior becomes quieter and more controlled, and speech more coherent, but the state of mental confusion persists. The next stage is one of automatism, in which the patient will respond naturally to simple questions, and perform accustomed actions in an orderly and effective way. He is still, however, dazed and imperfectly aware of his surroundings, will repeatedly ask a question already answered, and afterwards has no memory of what occurred during this phase.

We submit that this same sequence of events is to be observed in a case in which the process of recovery occupies a period of several days, and again in a case in which recovery is complete within a few minutes. In the latter, of course, opportunity of close observation is scant, and when it is available, the march of events is so rapid that it is difficult to be sure of the sequence. We believe, however, that there is sufficient ground for concluding that there is a fundamental unity in the clinical picture. It is that of a generalized disturbance of cerebral function extending at first to the levels which are, physiologically speaking, the lowest — those which control vegetative function. There is a subsequent return of function, level by level, the highest functions being the last to recover. The process of recovery, whether rapid or slow, is always gradual. The case in which recovery is slow naturally affords most opportunity for detailed observation. It is, as it were, a slow-motion presentation of a sequence which may in other cases be so rapid that the eye can hardly follow it.

We have drawn attention (Symonds, 1935a) to the resemblance between the state of unconsciousness after head injury and that which follows an epileptic attack. In both there are to be observed variations in the depth and in the duration of the disturbance of function which may to some extent be independent of one another. A minimal epileptic attack may be followed by immediate return to full consciousness, or by a prolonged phase of postepileptic automatism. This is also true of the traumatic case. After a major epileptic attack, and more especially after a series of such attacks, the patient may pass through phases of coma, stupor, delirium, confusion and automatism, which again show a striking resemblance to the traumatic sequence. Between these two extremes it is easy to find other examples of similarity. In fact, there is hardly any variant of postepileptic disturbance of consciousness which may not sometimes be observed after head injury. Common to both also is a rapidity and completeness of recovery which is remarkable in relation to the severity of the initial disturbance. Whatever the pathology of traumatic unconsciousness, it would seem that physiologically speaking the disturbance may be of the same order as that which occurs in epilepsy.

We will now retrace our steps and review together the two problems which we have considered separately. We have observed that a man may suffer immediate unconsciousness as the result of injury, and recover completely within a few minutes. Not only is there complete recovery of conciousness. but in a great many cases, as soon as the highest levels of cerebral function have returned, there is complete recovery in every sense. Headache there may be for the rest of the day, but the next morning the patient awakes as well as ever. This may be true even when the duration of unconsciousness has been much longer. We have observed the case of a young man who was unconscious for two or three days, and had a complete amnesia of three weeks' duration, but at the end of that time claimed and appeared to be well in every way. On the other hand we have found that a man who has not been unconscious at all may suffer for a long time — and it may be in some degree for the rest of his life — from headache, giddiness, and minor mental disorder. The discrepancy is striking, and leads us to the conclusion that, as far as direct injury to the intracranial contents is concerned, there are two separable effects. One — that responsible for the immediate loss or disturbance of consciousness, whether brief or protracted — is an effect upon cerebral function as a whole. The other — responsible for a group of symptoms among which persistent headache is prominent — comprises the effects of injury upon various parts of the meninges, brain, brain stem, and possibly, as we shall see, the labyrinths. The two effects may be independent of one another. More often they are associated.

There is clearly an opportunity at this point for separate nomenclature. We might call the immediate loss of consciousness concussion, and extend this term to cover the whole period of confusion and amnesia, however long, describing all other symptoms under the heading of contusion. Thus we might speak of a patient as having been "concussed" for so many hours or days, and afterwards showing (or not showing) symptoms of contusion. This idea of concussion as a clinical effect of generalized direct injury to the nerve cells, which might last a long time, was in the past generally accepted and might well be revived. It is now supported by experimental observation in animals (Denny-Brown and Russell, 1941; Williams and Denny-Brown, 1944; Windle, Groat, and Fox, 1944; Groat and Simmons, 1950); by pathologic findings in humans (Strich, 1956); and by electroencephalographic records in man showing a generalized and

106

consistent disorder of rhythm which may persist for days or weeks (Williams, 1941 (a)).

Windle, Groat and Fox (1944), using the method described by Denny-Brown and Russell (1941) to produce experimental concussion in animals, found, as they did, that when the animal was sacrificed immediately afterwards there was no histological abnormality. But if there was a long enough delay between the concussion and the time the animal was killed, changes were to be seen in many of the nerve cells, which lost their Nissl granules, undergoing chromatolysis. This appeared to begin 14 hours after the injury, becoming clearly defined in two days, and proceeding to complete dissolution of Nissl substance in some cells between the sixth and eighth days. Carrying their experiments further they discovered that these changes in the nerve cells were for the most part reversible, but that a proportion of the affected cells in all regions studied underwent complete lysis. Groat and Simmons (1950) followed up this work by doing nerve cell counts in selected brain-stem areas of control guinea pigs, and guinea pigs in which concussion had been induced by a single blow to the head 13 months prior to sacrifice. A considerable cell deficit was disclosed in the injured animals. This work suggests a possible explanation of the punch-drunk syndrome, in which it may be supposed that repeated minor injury results in cumulative cell loss.

Strich (1956) has examined the brains of five patients who survived a closed head injury in a more or less decerebrate and extremely demented state for 5 to 15 months, being kept alive by skilful nursing care and artificial means of nutrition. Widespread, diffuse degeneration of the white matter, demonstrable by the Marchi method, was present in all these cases. There was no clinical or pathological evidence to indicate anoxia, edema, or vascular lesions as the basis of this degeneration, which the author suggests must be attributed to physical damage to nerve fibres at the time of the injury.

These studies support the view already expressed that what is generally called concussion might prove to be the clinical effect of generalized direct injury to the neurons of a kind that might last a long time. They further indicate that the effects of such injury are by no means all, or always, reversible, and may indeed lead to a fatal issue after several months. In the light of these observations there is now much to be said for the use of the term concussion in a pathological sense, indicating direct neuronal injury as opposed to contusion, with loss of consciousness as its immediate clinical effect. Transient loss of consciousness without aftermath should be regarded as the minimal effect of concussion, allowance being made in the terminology of head injuries for persistent, severe, and sometimes irreversible effects from the same kind of injury. We might thus speak of cases of slight, moderate, and severe concussion according to the degree and duration of the disturbance of consciousness, and acknowledge the occurrence of permanent sequelae. This appears to the writer a logical and inevitable step. The idea of concussion as an essentially benign type of injury must be abandoned.

It is obvious however that when confusion is prolonged, we cannot tell how far this may be due to a more severe degree of the initial generalized effect of the injury, or how far to such complicating factors as subarachnoid hemorrhage, laceration, contusion, edema, or increased intracranial pressure. The longer the duration of confusion, the greater is the probability that such complicating factors are present. It has been argued that concussion as a term of clinical usage should be reserved for traumatic disturbance of consciousness without residual symptoms on the assumption that the generalized disorder of cerebral function is invariably and completely reversible (Denny-Brown, 1945). Though it is by no means certain that the assumption is correct it is reasonable to suppose that a patient who has transient loss of consciousness from head injury without aftermath has suffered no more than concussion, and as a clinical event this is so common and so distinct that it is convenient to have a word for it. Concussion in this sense is established by tradition, and will probably be retained. *It is obviously a diagnosis which can only be made in retrospect, that is to say, when after a momentary loss of consciousness, sufficient time has elapsed to show that there are no sequelae.*

CLINICAL PICTURE

For the reasons already given we shall not attempt any formal distinction between cerebral concussion and contusion. We shall describe first the generalized effects of brain injury in which loss or disturbance of consciousness is the constant and most conspicuous feature; second, the syndromes attributable to local injury *(local contusion);* and third, the syndrome of traumatic headache, giddiness and nervous instability *(minor contusion syndrome).*

108

1. Generalized Effects of Brain Injury, with Loss or Disturbance of Consciousness

We had better perhaps begin with a statement of what is meant by unconsciousness. Russell (1932) holds that the state of full consciousness is that in which any occurrence in which the patient is actively or passively concerned makes an impression on the memory, and can be subsequently called to mind. Any state of consciousness less than this is to be regarded as a grade of unconsciousness. According to this view, any patient who has a posttraumatic amnesia must be deemed to have been unconscious for the duration of the amnesia, and the patient who has been more deeply unconscious cannot be said to have recovered consciousness until the function of recent memory has returned. This definition, as Russell points out, has the merit that the patient's subsequent memory of when he "woke up" or "came to" provides a not inaccurate indication of when consciousness returned. Mapother (1937) objects to this definition as too loose, and considers that the only practicable criterion of "recovery of consciousness" is awareness of external environment and accessibility. We shall adhere to Mapother's definition as being that which is generally accepted, but shall lay stress on the duration of the posttraumatic amnesia as indicating a general defect of cerebral function after consciousness has been regained.

In order to secure uniformity of case records during World War II, medical officers in the British Services were provided with brief definitions of unconsciousness and the different degrees of confusion which, if generally adopted, would simplify the classification of cases, though it would not replace accurate description of the symptoms observed (M.R.C. War Memorandum, 1941).

Loss of consciousness at the onset is the rule in all cases of severe head injury. There are, however, certain exceptions which are instructive. A glancing blow may fracture the skull without loss of consciousness. The same is true of a circumscribed injury from a hard and relatively sharp object, such as an angular projection on an automobile. In such a case there may be not only fracture of the skull, but penetration of the brain without unconsciousness. Again, fracture of the base of the skull may occasionally result from an injury, in which the line of force is in this plane, without loss of consciousness. High velocity missiles that penetrate the brain seldom cause loss of consciousness unless they are very large (Eden and Turner, 1941). On the other hand, widespread impact of the skull against a comparatively yielding

109

substance, as for example, a fall from a horse onto soft ground may result in unconsciousness without any visible injury to the head. Unconsciousness may also result, without direct injury to the head, from a fall from a height on to the feet or buttocks. It appears, therefore, that the type of injury which most readily causes unconsciousness is that which subjects the intracranial contents as a whole to sudden displacement.

The clinical picture when unconsciousness immediately follows the injury is subject to so much variation that we could not hope to present in detail a pattern which would fit more than a single case. We shall attempt to sketch, in broad outline, the main features of the syndrome as they appear in injuries of slight, moderate and severe degree. Such distinctions of degree are, of course, arbitrary. However, it seems worthwhile to consider the very mild and exceptionally severe injuries apart from the main body of cases, for at the two extremes the problems offered to the physician in relation to prognosis and treatment are so entirely different that they call for a separate approach.

A. *The Slight Degree of Injury.* In the least degree of injury there is no loss of consciousness at all. A familiar example is that of the football field. A player receives a blow on the head, and is dazed for a moment, but continues to take his part in the game in a manner which excites no comment, though it may be noticed that he is lacking in initiative in the face of any unusual situation. He may possibly in the interval ask another member of his side what is the score, and a moment later repeat the question. At a varying period of time after the injury he comes to himself with a complete amnesia, both for the blow and the subsequent events up to the moment of his recovery. Having regained orientation and the capacity for retaining the memory of current events, he will probably exhibit traces of defective inhibition at the highest levels of mental function. The expression of this will vary with the disposition of the individual. It usually takes the form of talkativeness and elation, but may be seen as irritability or moodiness. The variety is comparable with that seen as the result of alcoholic intoxication. The sufferer may or may not at one stage or another complain of headache. Occasionally other symptoms develop. Complete recovery is the rule within a few hours. The whole sequence of events is comparable with that which may occur after a minor epileptic attack. The outstanding clinical feature in this type of injury is the *traumatic automatism* with its corresponding *traumatic amnesia*.

In the next degree of injury the sufferer is for a few moments com-

110

pletely unconscious. This state is associated with flaccid paralysis and loss of reflex function. Consciousness is rapidly regained, and with it, reflex function and voluntary movement. At first the patient is confused. For a minute or two he is often restless and resistive. The confusion rapidly passes, and is succeeded by a phase of automatism. There is subsequently amnesia for the injury, and often for the events immediately preceding the injury (retrograde amnesia), and for a period following the injury which includes the phase of automatism. The whole sequence may be over in ten or 20 minutes. At some time or another during the stage of recovery vomiting is a common symptom. After he has recovered from the other symptoms, the patient will generally complain of headache, and will often for a short time show minor changes in his disposition of the type already described.

There is no doubt that most of the patients in this group completely recover within a period of 24 hours. A certain number, however, develop symptoms of the kind that we shall describe later — headache, giddiness, and nervous instability — and such development may be sometimes delayed for several days. As an occasional but rare occurrence one may see associated symptoms of focal brain injury.

B. *The Moderate Degree of Injury.* As our criterion for this degree of injury we may take, of course, in arbitrary fashion, failure to recover consciousness within five minutes of the injury, but with subsequent recovery of consciousness within two or three hours. The initial symptoms are the same as those described for a case of the mild degree. The state of coma, however, lasts longer, probably several minutes, and is followed by one of profound stupor in which, though purposive movements of the protective kind are possible, the patient is totally unaware of his environment and inaccessible. In this state he is at first mute, unresponsive to command, and inert. Later he begins to be restless and, while still mute and stuporous, may become resistive and violent. The first evidence of returning consciousness, as a rule, is a positive response to some simple command, such as, "Put out your tongue." Later he will occasionally reply to a question, such as, "What is your name?" though the basic state is that of restless confusion with an occasional relapse into stupor. During or after the period of unconsciousness there may be incontinence of urine, and vomiting. After recovery of consciousness the patient remains confused and may exhibit phases of delirium especially at night. In this state of *traumatic delirium* his behavior is unpredictable and often violent. He will frequently try to get out of bed, put on his clothes, or run out of the room, will

111

refuse his medicines, and will fight with those who try to control him. This state of confusion with delirium (sometimes known to surgeons as that of cerebral irritation) may be transient, lasting only an hour or two, or may persist for several days. So long as there is delirium there may be relapse into stupor from time to time. The delirious stage is followed by one of quiet and relatively well-mannered confusion *(traumatic confusional state)*, in which the patient is capable of conversation and to some extent biddable, but thought is incoherent, there is misinterpretation of the surroundings, and behavior may be impulsive and sometimes violent. In this state the patient may be able to feed himself and is no longer incontinent, but he may show no regard for decency. Speech, though coherent, shows evidence of the basic confusion of thought. This state of confusion, again, may pass rapidly or last for days. It is succeeded by that of automatism in which there is clear awareness of the environment with reasonable and adequate response to inner need and external stimulus. In this stage the general behavior shows little or no deviation from the normal. The mood is often elated with undue talkativeness. There is lack both of insight and judgment, and gross defect of memory for recent events, with consequent disorientation for time, place and person. Often there is a tendency to confabulate, such as is seen in Korsakoff's psychosis and, arising out of this, as Russell (1935) has pointed out, false accusations may be made in connection with the accident. Next comes recovery of the power to remember current events with correct orientation and insight into the nature of the illness, and with this the posttraumatic amnesia is at an end.

The whole sequence of events, so far described as following recovery of consciousness within a period of two hours, may be compressed into a few hours or may extend over several days, exceptionally several weeks. As a general rule, the longer the period of unconsciousness the longer is the duration of the subsequent stages up to the end of the state of automatism and the termination of the amnesia, but there are striking exceptions to this rule.

In the process of recovery there may be a halt at any one stage, and this may sometimes be of long duration. Moreover, from any particular stage there may at first be relapse. The last point may be of considerable clinical importance. A patient who has become sufficiently clear to answer a few simple questions may relapse into stupor so that for a time he cannot be roused. In such an instance the suspicion of compression from meningeal hemorrhage is justly raised. It will be found, however, that in the case of uncomplicated brain injury the setback

112

does not go very far. Stupor seldom becomes so profound that there is no response whatever to a shouted command. Subsequent developments are, of course, different in the two cases. In both there may be fluctuations in the state of consciousness, but in the uncomplicated brain injury the tendency is towards improvement, while in the case of compression it is in the opposite direction. As a rare occurrence one may encounter a delayed onset of unconsciousness without any subsequent evidence of compression. The victim of the accident may, for example, ask a bystander for help, or give his name and address to a policeman and subsequently lapse into stupor. In such cases the patient usually has no memory afterwards of what he has said or done in the relatively lucid interval. This phenomenon, being seldom observed, has been little investigated. It is difficult to explain, except on the assumption that the development in the interval of hemorrhage and edema has been sufficient to abolish a level of cerebral activity already damaged to the point of precarious function.

We have said enough to indicate that the clinical picture, so far as the mental state is concerned, is capable of great variety as the result of relapse and fluctuation in the process of recovery, and especially by reason of the variable duration of any one, or all, of its stages. All that is uniform is a more or less regular sequence in the return of cerebral function from the lowest levels towards the highest. It is this uniformity of stages and sequence, however, which is the essence of the picture.

During the phase of automatism there may be complaint from time to time of bodily symptoms, such as headache. The observer may, of course, remain ignorant of this if he relies upon his interrogation of the patient. We have on several occasions, having enquired of the patient, been told that he had had no headache, when the nurse has informed us that this has been a frequent though intermittent complaint. After the termination of the amnesia the mental state is seldom at first normal, though on account of defective insight, the patient may think it so. Defective inhibition with consequent overactivity and impulsiveness, emotional instability, and some defect or slowness of the intellectual functions, may persist for some time, though ultimate recovery is the rule.

We have so far been concerned mainly with those symptoms of the injury which are manifest in disorder of the mental function. In the way of abnormal physical signs on examination of the nervous system there is little to record. In the stage of coma the deep and superficial reflexes are at first absent. As they return the plantar responses are sometimes extensor. Sometimes an extensor response is present on one side only. Unless there is evidence in the form of hemiparesis of a severe focal lesion, both plantar responses are as a rule flexor by the time the patient has emerged from the state of traumatic confusion.

The temperature is at first subnormal, the pulse rapid and feeble, the respiration sometimes uneven and shallow. The respiration returns to normal within a few minutes. The temperature after a few hours rises. If the injury is relatively mild the rise of temperature is not much above 100°F (orally) and there is a slow irregular decline to normal within two or three days. In such a case the pulse rate rises and falls with the temperature. In cases of more severe injury (as a rule, therefore, associated with a longer duration of unconsciousness) the rise of temperature is higher and more prolonged. It seldom, however, rises above 102°F, or remains above normal for longer than a week. In such cases the pulse rate may again follow the temperature, but in a certain proportion it is abnormally slow. In this group, whether the pulse rate has been rapid or slow in the first few days, there is often a secondary bradycardia which may persist for a week or ten days.

Lumbar puncture reveals either an increased pressure or a blood-stained fluid, or both together in the majority of cases. Thus, in 49 estimations of pressure made in 40 cases Russell (1932a) found the pressure above 200 mm in 30. In only nine instances, however, was the reading above 300 mm. A comparision of the cerebrospinal fluid pressure with the mental state of the patient at the time of estimation showed no constant relationship. On twelve occasions the pressure was above 200 mm in cases in which consciousness had become clear (termination of traumatic amnesia), while on seven occasions in which the pressure was below 200 mm the patient was stuporous. It would appear from these observations, which have been amply confirmed by others, that, while the intracranial pressure is often raised in cases of head injury of the group under consideration, the rise is seldom very high as compared, for instance, with that which may be observed in a patient with a sub-tentorial tumor whose mental state is alert and wakeful. Further, there is no correlation between the degree of raised pressure and the mental state of the patient. The evidence, therefore, contradicts the assumption, at one time popular, that traumatic delirium and stupor might be simply explained in terms of increased intracranial pressure as the result of widespread cerebral edema. Nevertheless it seems fair to conclude that the increase of intracranial pressure so often present may play a part both in the causation of symptoms and in delaying their recovery. Whether the increased pressure

114

is due to brain swelling (as appears likely), to obstruction of the flow of cerebrospinal fluid towards the channels of absorption, or to disturbance of the mechanism regulating the balance of secretion and absorption, is at present a matter of conjecture.

A blood-stained fluid is found in a considerable proportion of cases indicating rupture of vessels in the leptomeninges or hemorrhage from the cortical vessels into the subarachnoid space. In many cases the amount of blood is trivial, but in a series of 200 cases of head injury (of which probably one third were of a milder degree than the group now under consideration) Russell (1932b) found on 32 occasions more than 1000 red blood corpuscles per cubic millimeter. All these patients, except one who was deeply comatose at the time of lumbar puncture, showed some rigidity of the neck muscles. Few patients with much blood in the fluid were conscious, and all those with a red cell count of over 100,000 per cubic millimeter were either stuporous or comatoe. Comparable observations have been recorded by Paterson (1943). Russell has argued with some reason that subarachnoid hemorrhage may be an important factor in causing the clinical symptoms, instancing the experimental work of Bagley (1928a, b, 1929) who produced unconsciousness and convulsions in dogs by subarachnoid injection of their own blood, and the stupor and delirium frequently observed in patients with subarachnoid hemorrhage from a leaking aneurysm. But, on the other hand, we must record the observation from time to time of a case in which traumatic stupor and delirium have coexisted with a cerebrospinal fluid containing nc trace of blood though examined within 48 hours of the injury. We must conclude, therefore, as in the case of increased intracranial pressure that subarachnoid hemorrhage cannot be held responsible in any important degree for the symptoms which we have described. It may add the signs of meningeal irritation and account in some measure for the delirium and fever of the early stages. With regard to the correlation established by Russell between the mental state and the amount of blood in the cerebrospinal fluid, we must observe that in cases of severe brain injury, laceration, not only of the meninges, but of the brain substance, is likely to occur, and it is at least as likely that the increased gravity of the mental symptoms is due to cortical laceration as to subarachnoid hemorrhage.

Russell (1932b) adds some important observations upon the rate of disappearance of blood from the cerebrospinal fluid after injury. The red cells begin to disappear rapidly from the first day after the accident, and at the end of four or five days the cerebrospinal fluid becomes clear and yellow-brown in color. It follows that the presence of many red cells in the cerebrospinal fluid after this lapse of time indicates continued or recurrent hemorrhage.

In a certain number of the cases in this group signs of local injury to the brain or cranial nerves will be observed. With the latter we are not concerned in this chapter. The signs of local brain injury will be considered in the following section.

After the general disturbance of cerebral function has subsided a large proportion of these patients will complain of headache, giddiness, and other symptoms of the kind to be described later. It is nevertheless remarkable that a patient may at the end of a traumatic amnesia, lasting several days, show no symptoms of this order.

C. *The Severe Degree of Injury.* In this group, comprising all cases in which there has been no recovery of consciousness within two or three hours of the accident, there is yet a considerable variety in the subsequent course of events. There is no doubt that many of these patients recover quite rapidly and are ready for convalescence in two or three weeks. They constitute the group, however, in which the patient is as a rule unconscious when first seen by the physician, whose primary concern will be not so much with the ultimate degree of recovery as with the chances of immediate survival. The mortality rate in these cases of severe head injury is generally estimated at about 20 per cent. Jefferson (1932) found it 23 per cent in a consecutive series of 1004 cases, Munro (1934) 17 per cent in a series of 1494. All observers agree that there is a rapid decline in the number of fatalities after the first 24 hours. Russell (1932a) found the mortality rate in patients who survived this period 8 per cent and Munro 7.2 per cent. After 48 hours Jefferson (1933) found it less than 1 per cent. These figures, which speak for themselves, indicate the general nature of the clinical problems to be faced in the early stages.

In the most severe cases there is evidence at first of surgical shock — subnormal temperature, a pale moist skin, and a weak rapid pulse. When this state persists and is associated with a persistent state of coma, with widely dilated pupils, sluggish corneal reflexes, cyanosis, stertorous respiration, and flaccid limbs, death usually follows within a few hours. In patients who survive this phase a careful study of the temperature chart on the one hand and the state of unconsciousness on the other offers the best guide to a true appreciation of the case (Rawling, 1927; Russell, 1932a; Woodhall, 1936; Davis, 1938). A persistently subnormal temperature with a rising pulse rate is of ill omen even though the patient is beginning to emerge from coma. So also is a steep rise of temperature and pulse rate especially if associated with rapid and uneven respiration. In many of the cases which end fatally the temperature continues to climb until the end reaching a height of 104 or 105°F.

In many cases the temperature having risen to 101 or 102°F, remains at about this level with a corresponding rise of pulse rate, and as a rule a quickened respiration. In these patients, improvement in the state of consciousness and a gradual fall in the temperature are indications of commencing recovery. A secondary sharp rise of temperature is often the prelude to a fatal issue. An estimation of the state of consciousness throughout is of the greatest importance. Once the patient has reached a stage at which he can be roused to answer questions it is certain that he will recover so far as the initial generalized brain injury is concerned, though he is, of course, still liable to such complications as meningitis, and extradural or subdural hemorrhage. In elderly people also the mortality from pneumonia is by no means negligible.

The subsequent course of events in patients who survive the first 48 hours is much the same as that already described in the preceding section though its march is often slower. The stage of stupor seldom lasts more than a day or two, but the traumatic delirium may continue for days or weeks, and the same is true of the subsequent stages of confusion and amnestic-automatism. This clinical syndrome or sequence, when it is prolonged, is commonly described as an acute traumatic psychosis, but we believe that it represents only a long-drawn-out example of what may occupy a day or two after an injury of moderate degree.

Recovery from the residual symptoms of general cerebral defect — slowness and difficulty in thought and memory, emotional instability, alterations in disposition, and impairment of judgment — is slower and less complete in this group than in the milder injuries. Improvement may continue slowly for a year or 18 months, but in many cases there are permanent sequelae of this kind.

Headache and giddiness are common complaints in the course of recovery, and the former symptom especially may persist indefinitely.

Symptoms and signs of focal brain injury are naturally more frequent in this group than in those previously described. It is, however, remarkable in what a small proportion of cases the effects of such injury, in so far as they can be estimated, are sufficiently severe or persistent to cause ultimate disability. The observation is one which lends support to the view that the symptoms of severe mental disorder in the early stages are due more to a generalized direct effect upon the neurons than local contusion and laceration.

Lumbar puncture in the most severe cases of this group is at first contraindicated. The less the patient is disturbed the better. When it is performed a blood-stained fluid is the rule. The pressure is sometimes raised, but may be within normal limits in a fatal case.

Postmortem examination in this group reveals as a rule the picture already described of widespread and scattered hemorrhage, with laceration of the meninges and cortex.

A detailed account of the syndrome of "blast concussion" and cerebral injuries due to explosion waves is available in an article by Cramer (*Surgery in World War II, Neurosurgery,* Vol. 1, P. 215-260, Office of the Surgeon General, Dept. of the Army, Washington, D. C., 1958). Various parts of the body including the abdomen, chest and nervous system may be injured as a result of a shock wave caused by a nearby explosion in the atmosphere or underwater. The cerebral manifestations include loss of consciousness, headache, tinnitus, tremor, and various psychiatric symptoms. Congestion and hemorrhages affecting the leptomeninges and brain have been found at necropsy. (Ed.)

Sequelae of the Generalized Effects of Brain Injury

Amnesia. As a permanent sequel of the injury there is loss of memory, which is almost always complete for the events immediately preceding the accident and for the accident itself (retrograde amnesia) and for a variable period after the accident (posttraumatic amnesia). The duration of the retrograde amnesia, after the patient has had full time to recover from the injury, is usually brief. Russell (1935) found that in 180 out of 200 cases it was not more than a few seconds or minutes. Of the remainder only four had a retrograde amnesia of longer than 24 hours, the longest period being seven days. The duration of the retrograde amnesia in his cases was by no means always proportional to that of the posttraumatic amnesia, but long periods of retrograde amnesia were more commonly present in cases with long posttraumatic amnesia. A long retrograde amnesia, therefore, appears generally to be evidence of severe or extensive brain injury.

As Russell (1935) has pointed out patients who remain for any length of time in the state of amnestic-automatism in the course of recovery from a severe injury, may at this stage have a much more extensive retrogradae amnesia. We have observed a case (Symmonds, 1937) in which on the thirtieth day after the injury the patient, who was aged 29, persisted in giving his age as 19, and attempted in a plausible way

118

to describe his surroundings in terms of the college where he had been at that age. In such cases the extent of the retrograde amnesia becomes shorter with the progress of recovery. Shrinkage of the retrograde amnesia may continue for some time after the patient has regained his orientation and memory for recent events, and may be taken as evidence of continued recovery of cerebral function. Observation of this point may, therefore, be of some clinical importance. A permanent retrograde amnesia longer than a few hours has in our experience always been associated with a story of severe injury, with a long posttraumatic amnesia, and with some permanent defect of mental function other than the amnesia, and the detailed observations of Russell and Nathan (1946) confirm this impression.

The duration of the posttraumatic amnesia is generally estimated by the patient's recollection of when he awoke to what was going on around him. The patient's statement needs critical examination before even a rough estimate of duration can be arrived at. It will generally be found that the end point is far from clear. Before — and sometimes several days before — the patient becomes continuously aware of his surroundings, some happening of emotional significance, such as a visit of a relative, may succeed in making a permanent impression. Often the return of continuous awareness and recollection is preceded by several isolated memories of this kind.

A statement of the duration of posttraumatic amnesia needs to be qualified, therefore, by explanation of the end point taken, whether that of the patient's first memory after the accident, or his recollection of the hour or day from which he preserves a continuous memory of his surroundings. Russell (1935) mentions a posttraumatic amnesia of eight weeks as the longest observed in his series of 200 cases. In some cases it may be longer. We have observed a young man with a post-traumatic amnesia of six months; he subsequently made a complete recovery so far as his capacity for work and social adjustment was concerned, though slight alterations in his disposition, and subjective difficulty of thought and recent memory, remained as permanent sequelae.

Permanent Defect of Mental Function. Whether persistent defect of mental function can result from generalized brain injury of the kind we have attributed to concussion is doubtful. When patients with residual defects are carefully examined, there is nearly always some evidence to be found of local contusion either in the history, the physical signs or the electroencephalogram. It is true that patients with prolonged disturbance of consciousness following head injury are more likely to show perma intellectual defect, but these are the cases in which there is most often

119

evidence of coarse lesions (Moore and Ruesch, 1944). There are, however, striking exceptions to these rules, — cases in which there has never been any clinical evidence of contusion (absence of focal signs, absence of blood in the cerebrospinal fluid, normal cerebrospinal fluid pressure, and absence of electroencephalographic evidence of focal injury), in which the disturbance of consciousness lasts for days or even weeks with no demonstrable residue of intellectual impairment or personality disorder. Denny-Brown (1945) concludes that such cases are probably examples of severe, uncomplicated concussion and that the persistent defects more commonly seen in patients who have had a long period of confusion and long posttraumatic amnesia, are due to associated cerebral contusion and laceration. According to this view permanent defect of mental function is not due to concussion and would more correctly be described under the heading of local cerebral contusion. In a sense, however, the symptom is an effect of generalized brain injury for it probably depends more upon the extent than the situation of the damage.

The fact of practical importance is that in patients who have emerged from prolonged confusion, residual intellectual impairment is common. Moore and Ruesch (1944) found gross intellectual defect at the end of six months in 31 per cent of a group of such cases. Ruesch (1944) found some measurable intellectual defect in about one-half of all patients suffering from head injury examined in the earlier stages, the functions primarily affected being speed, judgment, and ability to keep up a sustained effort. If the impairment were reversible its duration was usually less than three months. Even when there is no intellectual impairment demonstrable by formal tests it may be found when the patient attempts to resume his former occupation, his employers or associates observing slowness, faulty judgment, and undue liability to fatigue. The patient himself may be aware of these defects, which are then apt to provoke an anxiety state, but in some cases there is lack of insight. These defects of mental function are rarely such as to cause total disability for work. In a manual laborer they are of relatively small consequence, but they may so reduce the capacity of the intellectual worker that he is permanently unfit to return to his business or profession. Patients who before the injury have arrived at what may be called the presenile age, or are suffering from cerebral arteriosclerosis are especially apt to show gross and persistent intellectual impairment. They sometimes recover up to a point and relapse into progressive dementia.

Traumatic personality disorder cannot be measured, and its existence as a residual organic symptom apart from intellectual impairment has been the subject of debate. There is, however, no doubt about its occurrence in children in the form of behavior disorder, associated with deterioration, or failure of development of a moral sense (Strecker and Ebaugh, 1924; Beekman, 1928; Blau, 1936). The clinical picture resembles that seen not uncommonly after encephalitis lethargica and the outlook is unfavorable. In adults behavior disorder of a gross kind is rare, though explosive irritability may lead to acts of violence (Hooper et al, 1945). The relatives of patients who have apparently recovered from severe head injury and show no measurable intellectual defect will often give convincing descriptions of subtle changes in the personality not unlike those described after prefrontal leucotomy. Paterson (1944) has admirably summarized the emotional aspects of the posttraumatic personality, emphasizing that the majority of the posttraumatic emotional changes fall into two groups — excessive fear and anxiety on the one hand, and euphoria and aggression on the other. A study of the previous personality pattern is essential for an appreciation of the posttraumatic personality changes. Unlike the cognitive, these cannot yet be assessed in a test situation. Only careful observation over some period and comparison with the previous behavior can give a clue to the disorder. The relationship of such disorder to psychoneurosis following head injury has been clearly described by Kremer (1944) in the following words:

"Finally there is that group of patients who manifest the change by the production of what appear to be psychoneurotic symptoms. We know that diseases affecting the cerebrum such as encephalitis lethargica can produce a symptomatology indistinguishable from an affective disorder in the predisposed. A head injury may do exactly the same. If an individual will produce the same reaction to a head injury as he would to his girl friend throwing him over, or an attack of influenza, or breaking his leg, then the neurosis can only be posttraumatic in a chronological sense. If, however, the head injury changes a stable individual of stable stock into one who can no longer adjust himself to the stresses and strains of life, and to the stresses and strains produced by his own disabilities then I feel the neurosis is posttraumatic in an etiological sense and is therefore a true personality change. In most cases the problem is not at all simple or clear-cut and all too frequently the pathogenesis is mixed. My reason for raising this point is that I have frequently read as a comment on a case that the patient is suffering from a psychoneurotic reaction to his head injury, when a more correct interpretation would have been that because of his head injury the patient's personality is now such that he develops a psychoneurosis."

Epilepsy. Epilepsy as a late sequel of the type of brain injury under consideration deserves mention here, though it is more probably the result of local rather than generalized damage. (Chapter 17)

Headache and Giddiness. These symptoms, which have already been mentioned as a common but inconstant feature of the aftermath of generalized brain injury with loss of consciousness, will be described in detail later in this chapter. In general, their severity and duration are greatest in the cases of severe injury.

2. Syndromes Attributable to Local Brain Injury
(Local Cerebral Contusion)

The symptoms and signs of local injury occur most frequently in association with those of moderate or severe generalized brain injury, with loss of consciousness, but there are exceptions, of which certain aspects deserve preliminary consideration. We have previously observed that the type of accident most likely to cause a generalized disturbance of cerebral function is that in which the skull is subject to widespread impact. Local injury of the brain may occasionally result, with little or no disturbance of consciousness, as the result of a force whose distribution is sharply limited. This is most obvious when there is penetration of the skull by a sharp object, such as a spike, with laceration of the subjacent cortex, but it may sometimes happen without penetration of the skull or even without fracture, as the result of force which is at the same time severe and circumscribed. The tangential bullet wound offers an example, and a glancing blow from an automobile another. We have also observed a number of cases in which the impact of an object, heavy enough to possess momentum, but possessed of some resilience, upon the lateral aspect of the skull, has caused severe local injury with little generalized effect. We have, for example, seen a boy who was struck on the left temple by a cricket ball, was never completely unconscious, and continued to play in a state of automatism for an hour or two, with a subsequent posttraumatic amnesia for several hours. It was noticed by others at the end of the game that he was suffering from dysphasia, a state from which he gradually recovered in the course of two weeks.

In such an instance as that just related, the diagnosis of local contusion is easy enough. It is, of course, much more difficult in the case of a patient who is unconscious at the time of examination. Nevertheless, as Riddoch (1932) has insisted, careful neurologic examination will often reveal, even at this stage, the signs of focal damage. As the

122

patient emerges from unconsciousness and becomes accessible and co-operative, examination is easier, but the opportunity in the case of transient damage may have been lost.

We shall not attempt a complete description of the syndromes of local injury, but shall be content to indicate their main features.

Epileptic attacks, occurring within the first few hours of the injury, are probably always symptomatic of cortical contusion or laceration, though it is possible that they may sometimes be due to the irritation of subarachnoid hemorrhage from a meningeal tear without actual injury of the brain substance. The character of the fit will naturally vary with the situation of the lesion. These early attacks have a good prognosis (Wagstaffe, 1928; Ascroft, 1941).

Hemiplegia is sometimes seen in closed head injuries and is then probably due to traumatic thrombosis of the internal carotid or middle cerebral arteries (Cairns, 1942). Hemiparesis is not uncommon as the result of local contusion. If present, its degree together with the state of the reflexes should, of course, be noted clearly for a progressive hemiplegia is usually evidence of compression by epidural or subdural hemorrhage.

The establishment of sensory defect of cortical or subcortical type demands a cooperative patient. Possibly it is for this reason that such defect is seldom observed. In most cases the effects of local contusion are quick to recover, and may have done so before an adequate examination of sensory function is possible.

Defects in the visual fields, resulting from lesions of the optic radiations or occipital cortex, are not very uncommon.

Anosmia, which is of common occurrence with a fracture running through the cribriform plate, may also be symptomatic of contusion involving the olfactory lobes.

Visual agnosia in its different forms is an uncommon symptom in closed injuries. The same observation applies to motor and sensory apraxia. Symptoms of this order when they are associated with those of generalized brain injury cannot be distinguished until the patient has emerged from the state of confusion.

Aphasia may be suspected when in the course of recovery from unconsciousness the patient appears wakeful and alert yet unable to converse. The defect may, of course, be on the receptive or on the outgoing side, or involve both functions. Some degree of dysphasia is in our experience a relatively common symptom of local injury, possibly for the reason that damage to those areas of the cortex which are concerned with speech is more revealing in its effects than that which may exist elsewhere.

The question whether there is any clinical picture, which is characteristic of frontal lobe contusion, is one which has been much debated. Pfeiffer (1928) suggests that absence of spontaneity in movement and expression, amounting sometimes to a catatonic state, may be symptomatic of frontal lobe injury. Jefferson (1933) believes that many of the symptoms of severe mental disorder seen after head injury are due to contusion of the frontal lobes, and instances especially incontinence of urine persisting for several days after recovery of consciousness. We should hesitate to give symptoms of this kind any localizing value so long as they appear in the setting of mental disorder which we have considered as a general effect of brain injury, but we meet with cases from time to time in which, after the traumatic amnesia is at an end, apathy, indifference, lack of spontaneity, and occasional incontinence constitute a picture which is comparable with that seen often enough in instances of frontal lobe tumor, or after frontal lobectomy.

Another question which has been the subject of debate during recent years is whether contusion of the basal ganglia may give rise to the picture of traumatic parkinsonism. The argument for this possibility is that small hemorrhages in this situation are not infrequently observed in fatal cases, and that the parkinsonian syndrome may occasionally be observed in young persons with an antecedent history of severe head injury, and none of encephalitis lethargica. On the other hand, it must be admitted that in many cases, which are accepted as postencephalitic parkinsonism, there is no history of acute illness, that no case has been recorded with a convincing postmortem account of the traumatic lesion, and that the possibility of an occasional coincidence of past head injury and insidious encephalitis is considerable. The question has been reviewed by Weil and Oumansky (1937) with no satisfactory conclusion. We have observed a few cases in which the clinical evidence in favor of traumatic parkinsonism was convincing, the patient being known to be in good health before a severe head injury, after which unilateral symptoms of this type were apparent, and in one instance were progressive.

Syndromes attributable to injury of the structures in the floor of the third ventricle have perhaps not attracted as much attention as they deserve. Disturbance of the sleep function after head injury, apart from anxiety symptoms, is not uncommon. It may take the form of hypersomnia, insomnia, or disturbances of the rhythm of sleep of the kind observed after encephalitis lethargica. Many instances of narcolepsy

124

have been reported after head injury usually at a considerable interval after the accident. Diabetes insipidus is not very uncommon, the symptoms usually appearing immediately or within a day or two of the injury; it may be associated with other evidence of injury in this neighborhood (diplopia, visual field defect). Loss of sexual desire and potency, and amenorrhoea, may also occur as the result of damage in this region.

The clinical picture of pure cerebellar disorder from closed head injury is rare. Syndromes attributable to contusion of the brain stem (and possibly involving the cerebellum) are, however, not uncommon in closed head injuries. Duret (1920) drew attention to the fact that in fatal cases small hemorrhages were often found in relation to the walls of the ventricles, and especially the aqueduct of Sylvius and fourth ventricle. He suggested that this was due to distension of these cavities by displacement of cerebrospinal fluid at the moment of the injury. Whatever may be the exact cause, signs of midbrain contusion are, as Riddoch (1932) insists, not infrequent if looked for in the early stages of severe head injuries. The commonest evidence is in the pupils, which may show irregularity, inequality, eccentricity, and impairment of reflex reactions. If the patient is cooperative diplopia may be elicited, and we have drawn attention (Symonds, 1932) to the frequency with which this proves to be of nuclear type.

The other common sign of brain stem contusion is nystagmus, usually associated with the complaint of vertigo. Involvement of the cranial nerve nuclei in the pons and medulla, or of the long conducting tracts at this level, is rare, probably because any lesion large enough to produce such damage will usually have been fatal within the first few minutes. We have observed cases, however, in which such signs have been present and have in some degree remained permanent.

Ataxia and incoordination of the cerebellar type may, of course, be attributable to injury of the cerebellar type may, of course, be the brain stem. They are generally associated with nystagmus and vertigo.

Kremer et al (1947) have recorded nine cases of closed head injury with severe signs of midbrain damage. The dominant clinical signs were cerebellar and included severe dysarthria and disturbance of balance. The cerebellar signs were usually most pronounced on one side, and the limbs of the side showing the greater ataxia tended also to show increased tendon reflexes and parkinsonian tremor. In one case there was sensory loss suggesting injury to the medial fillet. Oculomotor and pupillary disturbances were present in most cases. In two instances, air encephalography disclosed a marked dilatation of the aqueduct of Sylvius.

Tangential injury of the vertex with depressed fracture may cause partial obliteration of the superior longitudinal sinus with a somewhat characteristic clinical picture. There is weakness of both lower limbs (one being usually affected more than the other) with bilateral extensor plantar responses, and, as shock passes off, spasticity and increase of the tendon jerks. When the patient is cooperative it is usually discovered that there is sensory defect of cortical type associated with the weakness, loss of postural sense being the most evident.

Headache, from the onset, or after recovery of consciousness, is a constant complaint in cases of local brain injury. It is usually referred to the site of the injury, and is of a throbbing, intermittent character, and increased by effort or change of posture. Giddiness on movement also is a frequent complaint. These two symptoms will be discussed in detail later.

Sequelae of Local Brain Injury

A distinction must be made at once between "penetrating" and "closed" injuries. In the former, not only is damage to the brain more severe and longer lasting, but there are all the sequelae of infection to be considered. Moreover, the risk of epilepsy as a sequel is far greater in the penetrating than in the closed injuries. In the closed injuries, local damage to the brain, so far as this is capable of assessment by means of physical examination, is usually quick to recover, and seldom results in permanent disability. How far the mental changes, already described as a sequel of generalized injury, may really be due to massive focal damage in silent areas, is a question which cannot at present be answered.

Dysphasia we have observed more often than any other symptom to persist in disabling degree. Slight degrees of motor or sensory defect are not uncommon, and may be a source of disability to the manual worker. Visual field defects from intracerebral injury show a capacity for recovery which is much greater than that observed when the optic chiasm is involved. Residual defect is seldom enough to be of serious importance. Diplopia and other symptoms of brain stem contusion may persist.

The residual effects of injury to the cranial nerves are dealt with in Chapter 5.

Epilepsy. Epileptic attacks in the early stages have already been

126

mentioned. More often there is a latent interval of several months before the first fit and the liability then as a rule persists. It has been observed that the incidence of traumatic epilepsy is not higher in patients with the longer posttraumatic amnesias, and this is consistent with the view that the responsible lesion is not a residue of concussion but an associated cerebral laceration or contusion (Denny-Brown, 1944). The incidence of epilepsy after head injuries seen in civilian practice is difficult to assess owing to the variety of the clinical material analysed in this respect. Schou (1933) found it 4.5 per cent in 200 cases of head injury reported to an insurance company, Russell (1932) reported 3.5 per cent in 200 consecutive cases of head injury admitted to hospital.

Cumulative Effects of Repeated Injury (Punch Drunk). (See also Chapter 16.) The effects of repeated minor injury are especially to be seen in professional pugilists who in the course of their trade are frequently knocked unconscious. Martland (1928) drew attention to a clinical syndrome indicating cumulative organic damage, which he had observed often enough in pugilists to support the ring-side diagnosis of "punch drunk" in such cases. His observations and conclusions have since been confirmed by others (Parker, 1934; Carroll, 1936; Ravina, 1937; Winterstein, 1937). The first symptoms observed are slowness and uncertainty of movement in the lower limbs, and unsteadiness in gait. The upper limbs may then be affected in the same way, one half of the body being usually earlier involved than the other. Involuntary movements of the type associated with disease of the basal ganglia may be observed. An extensor plantar response may occasionally be found. Some degree of dysarthria is common, and the mental state shows evidence of deterioration, especially affecting intelligence and recent memory. According to experienced observers the slighter degrees of this malady are by no means uncommon. The symptoms are permanent and may be progressive in some degree without further repetition of the injury.

Hydrocephalus. As a rare but important sequel of local injury, presumably involving the aqueduct of Sylvius, fourth ventricle, or basal meninges, hydrocephalic symptoms may develop. Usually these take the form of intermittent attacks of severe headache with drowsiness, and sometimes with vomiting. The acute symptoms last only a few hours but the headache may continue for several days. The history is usually that of severe generalized injury, with subsequent recovery, and between the attacks the patient is reasonably well. We have reported (Symonds, 1935b) an example of such a case in which the attacks continued at intervals of two or three months, six years after the accident. Moritz and Wartmann (1938) have reported four cases of progressive hydrocephalus following head injury with postmortem evidence of an obstructive leptomeningitis involving the roof of the fourth ventricle. The meningeal adhesions contained hemosiderin. In three of these cases the symptoms of hydrocephalus developed within four months of the injury. In the fourth there was an interval of several years. *

Headaches and Giddiness. These symptoms may in some cases persist after the signs of local brain injury have disappeared, and may remain as permanent, sometimes disabling, sequelae.

3. The Syndrome of Headache, Giddiness and Nervous Instability (Minor Contusion Syndrome)

It is not to be supposed that these symptoms necessarily occur together. The group is, however, a convenient one for descriptive purposes and this for several reasons. The first is that these three symptoms very often do occur together. The second is that they may occur with or without a history of unconsciousness, and that their severity and duration has no constant relationship to the degree and duration of unconsciousness if it has occurred. The syndrome, therefore, cannot be regarded merely as a sequel of the generalized effect of brain injury.

* Obliteration of the subarachnoid spaces as a result of organized blood may give rise to progressive hydrocephalus manifested by the signs and symptoms of increased intracranial pressure. Pneumoencephalography in such cases reveals dilatation of the ventricular system without visualization of the cortical subarachnoid spaces. In recent years cases of symptomatic occult hydrocephalus with normal cerebrospinal fluid pressure, some occurring as a consequence of severe head injury with subarachnoid hemorrhage, have been described (Adams, R. D., Fisher, C. M., Hakim, S., Ojemann, R. G., and Sweet, W. H. Symptomatic Occult Hydrocephalus with "Normal" Cerebrospinal Fluid Pressure. *N. Engl. J. Med.,* 273, 117, 1965; Adams, R. D. Further Observations on Normal Pressure Hydrocephalus. *Proc. Roy. Soc. Med.,* 59, 1135, 1966; Ojemann, R. G., Fisher, C. M., Adams, R. D., Sweet, W. H., and New, P. F. J. Further Experience with the Syndrome of "Normal" Pressure Hydrocephalus. *J. Neurosurg., 31,* 279, 1969). Dementia, psychomotor retardation, unsteadiness of gait and pyramidal signs are the usual clinical findings. Isotope cisternography is a useful diagnostic aid (James, A. E., Jr., DeLand, F. H., Hodges, F. J. III, and Wagner, H. N., Jr. Cerebrospinal Fluid (CSF) Scanning: Cisternography. *Am. J. Roentgenol. Rad. Therapy and Nuclear Med., 110,* 74, 1970). Treatment consists of a shunting operation to reduce the cerebrospinal fluid pressure. (Ed.)

The third is that these symptoms are not, as a rule, associated with any evidence of local brain injury.

These three symptom complexes comprise a group, therefore, whose association with the syndromes previously described is inconstant. As compared with such phenomena as unconsciousness, or focal symptoms, they are less significant. Therefore, they may reasonably be described together as the *minor symptoms of contusion*. The fact that they often occur, either single or in combination after slight injury, without either unconsciousness or focal symptoms, has led to their being described as the symptoms of minor contusion. This is, strictly speaking, inaccurate, for the symptoms in question, though they *may* occur after slight injury, are equally, if not more often, observed after severe injury.

Headache is by far the commonest and most important symptom. Giddiness is seldom complained of unless it is, or has been, associated with headache. The term nervous instability demands a word of explanation. We are in need of a separate terminology for those symptoms of minor mental disorder which appear to be especially associated with head injury. We have already discussed certain symptoms of mental disorder which may be observed as a sequel of the generalized effects of brain injury with loss of consciousness, and have called these traumatic intellectual impairment and personality disorders emphasizing in this connection the defects of memory, judgment and insight, which form a part of the clinical picture. The symptoms of mental disorder which we shall describe as belonging to the minor contusion syndrome doubtless have an organic basis, but are of a different degree. They are in the main symptoms of instability rather than loss of function, and they may occur, not only in the course of recovery from severe injury, but as the more immediate effect of slight injury without disturbance of consciousness. The term traumatic psychasthenia already suggested by Mapother (1937) in a wider sense might have filled the need indicated for description of these mental symptoms of minor degree, had not the word psychasthenia been used previously to designate compulsive and obsessional neuroses. Nervous instability as a heading admittedly lacks psychiatric precision, but in the sense proposed it appears preferable to any more formal label.

Having already emphasized the fact that minor symptoms of contusion are commonly observed in the course of recovery from moderate or severe brain injury with loss of consciousness, or in association with symptoms of focal contusion, we propose now to describe the evolution of the minor contusion symptoms as they appear after a brief loss of consciousness, or after a head injury with no loss of consciousness at all.

129

It is first to be remarked that the onset of any or all of these symptoms may be delayed. After a brief loss of consciousness, for example, the sufferer may appear to have completely recovered in a few hours, yet in the course of a few days may begin to complain of headache, giddiness, or undue fatigue of body and mind. Occasionally it may be a week or more after the accident before the patient seeks advice on account of such symptoms, and he may have continued at his full work during this time. The same may be true in the case of a man who has not lost consciousness at all, but has sustained a bruise or laceration of his scalp. This latent interval has often been attributed unjustly to the effects of a compensation neurosis, but it is in fact observed quite commonly in cases where no such possibility exists.

Headache. This, the commonest individual symptom resulting from head injury, displays many variations. Its distribution may be general or localized. If localized, it is often related to the site of the injury, which may be tender to pressure. The character of the headache is most frequently throbbing. Sometimes the pain is described as hammering. There may also be sharp stabs of pain. Sometimes there is a description of weight or pressure without or within the head. It is more usually intermittent than continuous. Often it takes the form of attacks which last from a few minutes to an hour or two. This type of headache is frequently precipitated by physical effort or movement, especially stooping, but may occur spontaneously. Attacks of headache may also be induced by noise, bright light, and mental effort or fatigue. The factors which precipitate, usually aggravate an existing headache. The pain is generally relieved in some degree by physical rest, and mental quiet. Posture sometimes has an effect which varies from one case to another. One patient may be more comfortable sitting, another lying. In the early stages the headache, if severe, may be accompanied by vomiting.

With appropriate treatment there is always a tendency to improvement, but relapse is very apt to occur as the result of premature exposure to physical or mental stress. Recovery under the most favorable conditions is often slow, and in some cases a persistent liability to headache remains as a sequel of the injury.

As a general rule traumatic headache is more severe and more persistent in the cases in which at the onset there has been profound and prolonged loss of consciousness.

So little is known of the mechanism of headaches in general that it is not surprising that we are at a loss for a complete explanation of those which are posttraumatic. The character of the severe throbbing, or sometimes bursting, headache, often complained of in the early stages, is suggestive of increased intracranial pressure. Russell (1932a) has recorded observations of the cerebrospinal fluid pressure in 30 cases in relation to the presence or absence of headache at the time of puncture. In 90 per cent of the cases in which the headache was severe the pressure was above 200 mm of water. But pressures above 200 mm of water were also recorded in 4 cases out of 6, in which there was no admission of headache at the time of puncture.

Encephalography in a certain number of cases has revealed a moderate degree of dilatation of the ventricular system (Bielschowsky, 1928; Friedman, 1932; Davies and Falconer, 1943) but there is no constant relation between this and a liability to headache.

Penfield and Norcross (1936) have shown that persistent localized headache, referred usually to the site of the injury and provoked by physical effort, may be due to adhesions between dura and arachnoid resulting from minute subdural hemorrhage.

Bremer et al (1932) regard vasomotor instability as an important cause of traumatic headache and instance the analogy of migraine.

It is probable that all these factors may play their part.

It is noteworthy that although headache is the commonest individual sequel of closed head injuries there are many patients who have no headache at all and among these are some of those with the most severe injuries as measured by the duration of the posttraumatic amnesia. This may mean that headache when it occurs is not an effect of the generalized or concussive injury but is due to associated contusion. Guttmann (1943) in a study of 158 cases of civilian head injury admitted to an accident ward found that less than half the patients complained of headache at any time after the accident, and only 20 per cent on discharge from hospital, though a follow-up showed that the percentage increased later. In most cases in which headache was complained of six months after the injury, he found psychological factors present in their causation. Brenner et al (1944) in a detailed study of 200 consecutive cases of head injury admitted to hospital found headache present in 69 per cent at some time. The complaint was present in 62 per cent of patients while in hospital, and in 41 per cent at or after discharge. In 32 per cent headache persisted for longer than two months after the injury. In this last group headache was characteristically associated with dizziness and nervous symptoms (fears, anxiety, fatigue, irritability and/or inability to concentrate), and psychological factors were frequently present in the etiology. Although the duration of posttraumatic amnesia when present was not related

131

to the incidence of headache, this symptom was significantly less frequent in those who had no initial disorder of consciousness.

Giddiness. The complaint of giddiness or dizziness is next to headache (with which it is usually associated) the most common symptom after head injury.

True spontaneous vertigo is rare and when it occurs is nearly always associated with clinical evidence, either of damage to the inner ear or eighth nerve, or a lesion of the brain stem (Symonds, 1942). The complaint of giddiness in relation to quick movement of the head, however, is not uncommon. It may be described as a sense of movement in surrounding objects, or of movement in the sufferer, or of unsteadiness as if he were about to fall. It may be provoked especially by movement in certain directions, for example, looking upwards, or turning to one side. It is of brief, often momentary, duration. Although objective evidence, such as nystagmus, or abnormality of posture, is usually lacking, this type of giddiness corresponds closely with that complained of in association with proved lesions of the labyrinth or its central connections in the nervous system. On clinical grounds, therefore, it is reasonable to suppose damage to these parts. The problem of localization has been investigated by otologists (Mygind, 1918; Linthicum and Rand, 1931; Barré and Greinier, 1932) with somewhat inconclusive results. Either over- or underexcitability may be found on testing vestibular function. There is seldom any evidence of cochlear damage. Portmann and Despons (1937) conclude that underexcitability is usually associated with some degree of deafness, and indicates a peripheral lesion. Overexcitability, which is more common, points to central damage. Sometimes this type of giddiness may be provoked, together with headache, by physical effort.

The work of Dix and Hallpike (1952) has led to the observation that the complaint of giddiness after head injury may not infrequently be due to damage of the otolith end organ. In such cases the complaint is of transient vertigo on changing the position of the head in relation to the direction of the force of gravity, as in looking up or down, rising from the horizontal to the erect posture, or vice versa, or turning over in bed. The diagnosis may be confirmed by the test for positional nystagmus. The patient should be sat on a couch and his head turned to one side. He should then be brought back into the supine posture with the head, supported by the examiner, hanging over the edge of the couch, while he looks at the examiner's finger. When the test is positive there is vertigo and nystagmus, often appearing after a delay of a few seconds, and transient though the posture is maintained. On sitting up transient vertigo and nystagmus often recur. The test should be applied with the head turned first to one side and then to the other. Gordon (1954) has emphasized the importance of performing this test in all cases in which there is complaint of posttraumatic giddiness, for it provides objective evidence of an organic basis.

Another type of traumatic giddiness is that in which there is no resemblance to true vertigo. The complaint refers to a general disturbance of the senses, including that of balance. Vision may be obscured for the moment, and the patient feels dazed. Such attacks may occur spontaneously, but are more often provoked by stooping, or rising suddenly from the horizontal to the erect posture.

Both varieties of giddiness need to be distinguished from minor epileptic attacks, which are not very rare in the phase of recovery from a severe injury with prolonged unconsciousness.

Complete recovery from traumatic giddiness is the rule, though in some cases it may be slow.

Friedman et al (1945) investigated the complaint of giddiness in 200 consecutive cases of head injury admitted to hospital and found it present in 51 per cent. It was always intermittent, of variable duration, frequency and severity, and the outstanding precipitating factor was change of posture. Its incidence was significantly higher in patients with a posttraumatic amnesia over 12 hours. At the same time psychological factors were prominent in patients who continued to complain of the symptom for longer than two months after the injury, and in this group there was a characteristic association of headache and nervous symptoms (fears, anxieties, fatigue, and irritability).

Nervous Instablity. Many of the patients who suffer from headache and giddiness complain also of symptoms which will be grouped under this heading. One of the most frequent is an undue liability to fatigue both mental and physical. There may also be intolerance of noise and light (apart from the aggravation of headache by these causes), insomnia, anxiety, and depression. The patient's spontaneous complaint is usually that of nervousness. Doubtless these symptoms are partly, often largely, due to psychogenic causes. They cannot, however, always be ascribed to the memory of the accident, for that is often blotted out by the retrograde amnesia; nor, as Russell (1932a) has pointed out, are they by any means confined to compensation cases. They are certainly to be observed most often in persons with a family and personal history containing evidence of neurotic liability, and are also dependent upon the degree of vexation and distress occasioned by the circumstances

133

arising out of the accident. They are more apt to occur in elderly and arteriosclerotic than in young and healthy persons.

The patients who exhibit these symptoms of minor posttraumatic mental disorder may present no measurable evidence of organic damage. Formal tests of memory, power of calculation, or reaction time may show no defect. It is difficult, however, for anyone who has studied a large number of these cases to escape the conclusion that the organic factor is present. Those in which there is no question of compensation provide the best point of departure. In this group it will be found that the young person of sound stock, whose previous history shows him to have stood up well to mental or physical stress, who is inured to risk of injury, and who is in a position to afford a period of disability without serious disadvantage, is least likely to develop symptoms of this kind. Nevertheless it is not uncommon for such a person to find himself intolerant of noise, indisposed for serious reading or card games, ready to rest after a single round of golf instead of his usual two, and unduly irritable under annoyance. The individual with a potential, or already evinced, disposition to depression, anxiety or insomnia, is likely to develop symptoms of this order in addition. If circumstances are such that disability involves loss of money or position, the symptoms are aggravated.

Our experience of the more severe effects of brain injury shows that the highest levels of cerebral function are the most vulnerable and the last to recover. Close observation of the symptoms which we have just described under the term nervous instability has convinced us that they are in part due to a disturbance of function at these levels, as a physical effect of the trauma. As a result the sufferer is not himself. His best qualities are in abeyance, revealing the second-best. He is slightly less of a man, and more of a child. Hence there is a tendency for his reactions to inner need or external stress to be inadequate or neurotic. The greater the stress, as in the case of a workman with dependants, and without reserves of capital, the greater the liability to neurosis.

When there is question of compensation, there is of course the additional element of motivation. Hysterical symptoms, such as pseudo-paralysis and tremors, are common, partly because the patient suffering from the effects of cerebral injury has nothing to show for his disability. The problem of assessing the organic element in these cases is one of great difficulty. It must be based upon a full knowledge of the family and personal history, together with an appreciation of the psychological situation arising out of the accident. The severity of the injury, as measured by the duration of the traumatic amnesia if present, or the presence in the early stages of signs of local brain injury, and associated symptoms such as headache and giddiness, must also be taken into account (Symonds, 1937b).

The immediate prognosis in severe injuries with loss of consciousness has already been discussed. Jefferson (1963) presented a graph of 152 fatal cases, showing that 91 deaths occurred during the first 24 hours, 18 in the second, 10 in the third, and 9 in the fourth 24-hour period. From this time onward to the end of the first fortnight, the mortality level is practically steady at two or three per diem. This series includes deaths from epidural and subdural hemorrhage and from meningitis. After this interval there is, of course, still some risk to life from subdural hematoma, and from infection in compound injuries or fractures communicating with the ear or nose, and, so long as a state of traumatic stupor persists, from exhaustion and pneumonia, especially in old persons. In the patients with severe injury who recover with their lives the next question which often presents is that of the prognosis with respect to their mental capacity. Recovery from stupor and confusion we may regard as certain, but we may expect when unconsciousness has been of long duration that after the traumatic amnesia is at an end, intellectual impairment and personality disorder will be in evidence. How severe these symptoms may be, and how long they may last, we cannot tell. There is no doubt, however, that improvement in this respect is slower and less certain of reaching the desired end with advancing age, and in a case of severe injury over the age of 60, the prospect of adequate mental restitution is doubtful. The younger folk, as a rule, do well, though at the other end of the scale one has to remember the risk of demoralization which is peculiar to children.

The rate of improvement after return of consciousness is usually rapid for the first week or two and subsequently slow. It may continue for at least a year.

As another aspect of serious mental disorder, we have to bear in mind psychoses of the affective or schizophrenic type precipitated by the injury.

The prognosis in cases of local contusion or laceration of the brain, so far as life is concerned, depends almost entirely upon the question of infection. In closed, or non-infected, injuries restoration of function is usually complete. It is rare to see persistent disability, for example, from hemiparesis. The fact is, doubtless, that patients with extensive contusion of one or other hemisphere die within the first few days. The ultimate outlook for patients with severe dysphasia, or brain stem lesions, is, as has been mentioned, not quite so hopeful as for the rest.

We have already noted the risk of epilepsy following local injury, especially if complicated by infection.

The prognosis for symptoms of the minor contusion syndrome is difficult to assess. Such symptoms appearing after severe injury with prolonged loss of consciousness are more likely to be persistent than when unconsciousness has been brief or is absent from the story, but this is no absolute rule.

Russell (1934a) in some valuable observations upon the after history of 200 patients admitted to hospital unconscious, or with a history of having been unconscious, found, as might have been expected, that the element of compensation neurosis was important. 139 of his patients were working men and women, of whom 27 were entitled to compensation. In this latter group 30 percent reported unfit for full work 18 months after the injury. In the remaining 112, with no claim for compensation, 83 per cent had returned to work within six months of the accident, and only 9 per cent reported unfit for full work 18 months after the accident. Russell's observations confirm also the impression that age is of importance in prognosis. In the group of non-compensation cases already referred to, 101 were under the age of 50: of these 88 had returned to full work within six months; 6 remained unfit after 18 months. Of the 11 patients over the age of 50, only 5 had returned to full work within six months; 5 remained unfit after 18 months.

Russell also contributed observations upon the duration of disability in relation to that of the traumatic amnesia, which may be summarized as showing that, for persons under the age of 40 with no factor of compensation, it is to be expected that, following a traumatic amnesia of less than one hour, 95 per cent will be fit for full work within two months of the accident. After a traumatic amnesia of 24 hours or more, 80 per cent will be fit for full work within six months of the injury. The return to work in Russell's patients did not, of course, imply complete freedom from symptoms. Of his total number of 200 patients, 120 still complained of symptoms two months after the accident, and of these 66 per cent continued to have symptoms at the end of 18 months. Headache was not only the commonest complaint, but the most persistent.

Following Russell others have made studies along the same lines. Guttmann (1943) in a series of 300 consecutive admissions of head injuries to a civilian hospital found that among the survivors the average working time lost by wage-earners was roughly eight weeks. For those with a posttraumatic amnesia (P.T.A.) of one hour or less it was four to five weeks; for a P.T.A. of one to 24 hours it was five to six weeks; and for a P.T.A. of one to seven days, nine weeks. In patients who stayed off work for an unusually long time he concluded that social and psychological factors were responsible rather than the physical effects of the accident.

Symonds and Russell (1943) in a study of service patients admitted to a military hospital for symptoms attributable to accidental head injuries divided their material into a group of 242 consecutive cases admitted in the acute stage, and another of 718 cases admitted in the later stages on account of delayed recovery. In the acute series five died and of the survivors 9 per cent were invalided and the remainder were returned to duty. Of these some relapsed and were invalided later so that the total invaliding rate was 20 per cent. They found as a general rule that as the duration of the P.T.A. lengthened the prognosis became worse, but that a third of the most severe cases (P.T.A. over seven days) returned to duty successfully and that at the other end of the scale of those with a P.T.A. of less than one hour 11 per cent were invalided. They concluded that their figures indicate both the value and the limitations of the duration of the P.T.A. as a criterion of prognosis. All that can be said for it is that it is the best single criterion at present available. Of those who returned to duty successfully 92 per cent did so in less than three months. In comparing the duration of incapacity with that in Guttmann's cases it must be remembered that service patients have to return to environmental conditions more severe than for civilians. In their 718 chronic cases Symonds and Russell found the invaliding rate 52 per cent. These were men admitted, as a rule from other hospitals, because of unsatisfactory progress and were therefore a selected group. In this group the duration of the P.T.A. had little relation to prognosis, indicating the presence of other factors. Predisposition to psychological breakdown as judged from the family and personal history obtained from the patient was assessed as positive or negative in all cases of both series and was found to be positive in 17 per cent of the former (acute) and 42 per cent of the latter (chronic). They concluded that predisposition in this sense was a factor in determining (1) the unsatisfactory progress of the chronic group on account of which they were selected for admission to the hospital and (2) the relatively bad prognosis for the chronic group as compared with the unselected acute group. Symonds and Russell point out however, that of their predisposed pa-

137

tients 33 per cent returned to duty successfully so that predisposition does not necessarily carry a bad prognosis. Kozol (1945, 1946) in a detailed analysis of the pre-traumatic personality in relation to the symptom pattern of posttraumatic disability has taken this point further and concludes from the study of civilian cases that there is little or no correlation between the pre-traumatic personality as assessed by a psychiatric inventory and the liability to development of posttraumatic mental symptoms. A patient with a pre-traumatic "neurotic" personality may be free from symptoms. A patient with a pre-traumatic "normal" personality may be crippled by mental symptoms. He concludes that this does not mean that the pre-traumatic personality may not play a large, or even the sole, part in the production of mental symptoms. It does mean that the development of posttraumatic mental symptoms may not generally be ascribed to the pre-traumatic personality. He stresses the fact that the development of psychoneurotic symptoms does not justify an assumption that such patients had pre-traumatic neurotic personalities, a point which is consistent with our view that in some cases psychoneurotic symptoms may be partly, or even largely, due to an alteration in the personality as the result of physical brain injury. He found a high correlation between the existence of persistent complicating psychological factors and the severity and persistence of psychiatric sequelae.

The greater importance attached to the pre-traumatic personality in prognosis by Symonds and Russell may possibly be explained by the nature of their material and a different method of assessing predisposition. Kozol (1946), concluding that the reasons that some patients did not exhibit sequelae were about as complex as the reasons that some did, observes that the patient who was altrocentric, rather than egocentric, social-minded and endowed with a high sense of responsibility, was most likely to escape substantial sequelae despite the fact that such a person might be heavily burdened with neurotic traits. Compensating personality traits of this kind in service patients during the war were perhaps weighed more heavily against an assessment of predisposition than they would be in civilians. Denny-Brown (1945), following up 200 patients admitted for head injury to a civilian hospital, found that the duration of disability was longest in two groups, those in whom there was evidence of coarse brain injury, and those in whom adverse environmental factors were present. In the former focal neurologic signs, focal or general electroencephalographic change and a prolonged P.T.A. appeared to be of greatest significance, and the presence of blood in the spinal fluid and fracture of the skull of less importance.

In the environmental group, anxiety derived from the injury, with special relation to problems of future occupation and compensation, was prominent. The symptoms associated with prolonged disability, whether the injury measured by the P.T.A. had been severe or mild, were predominantly those of anxiety.

For practical purposes it is of value to divide the patients into three groups: (1) those who are unconscious when first seen by the physician, (2) those who are reported to have been unconscious, and (3) those who have not lost consciousness.

1. The Patient Who Is Unconscious When First Examined

It is important in such cases to note, if possible before the patient is moved, whether there is any dangerous degree of bleeding from the scalp, and whether there is any evidence of gross injury of parts other than the head. Fracture-dislocation of the cervical spine is not infrequently associated with head injury. The unconscious patient should therefore be handled and moved with particular care to avoid undue movement of the head in relation to the spine.

The patient should be laid flat in the supine position with head a little rotated to one side. In case of vomiting, the rotation should be increased for the time being to prevent aspiration of vomitus.

Bleeding from the scalp if present should be controlled by a firm pad and bandage. Nothing will control severe hemorrhage except suture, and occasionally this may be necessary as a temporary measure while the patient is being removed to a hospital.

The presence and degree of surgical shock should be noted. A pallid, moist skin and rapid feeble pulse are immediate indications for measures to procure warmth. If shock be present, the less the patient is disturbed the better, but a rough examination should be made of the degree of unconsciousness, and a note should be made of the size and equality of the pupils.

If shock be absent, the tone of the limbs should be examined.

Whenever possible the patient should be moved to a hospital rather than his own home, both for the sake of more continuous observation, and in case of surgical emergency.

So long as there is evidence of shock the disturbance involved in taking x-rays of the skull should be avoided. X-rays are in fact of little value as a guide to treatment in this type of case, except when there is question of epidural hemorrhage, and as a general rule the procedure may well be postponed, as Munro (1934) suggests, until the second or third week after the accident. For the same reason, after the patient has been admitted to hospital, further examination should be postponed so long as there are symptoms of shock present.

As soon, however, as the patient is fit for the examination a note should be made of the state of consciousness. Can he reply to a simple question forcibly put, such as, "How are you?" or "What is your name?" Failing this, is he capable of performing simple movements to command, such as, "Open your eyes" or "Put out your tongue"? If he is unresponsive to these tests, will he withdraw a limb when pinched or turn his face away from the prick of a pin?

The pupils should be carefully examined and a note made of their size, and if there is any inequality.

A sufficient examination of the nervous system should be made to demonstrate the presence or absence of any difference in the power, tone and reflexes on the two sides of the body.

From this time onward, the nurse should be instructed to make a note two-hourly, not only of the pulse, temperature, and respiration, but of the state of consciousness, the size of the pupils, and any apparent defect in movement or power on the two sides of the body. These observations should be continued at the same frequency during the first 48 hours, and thereafter at four-hourly intervals until or unless consciousness has been regained. It is only by such means that the development of meningeal hemorrhage can be detected. In some cases the onset of compression by meningeal hemorrhage is associated with a rise of blood pressure. A similar rise however may be observed in the so-called reactionary phase of recovery from uncomplicated head injury, and there are cases of meningeal hemorrhage which show arterial hypotension throughout. Repeated blood pressure readings therefore are unnecessary.

In the case of profound stupor, spoon feeding may be inadequate, and is sometimes dangerous owing to an imperfect gag reflex. In either case feeding by nasal tube is indicated. The tube is best left in situ, the end being strapped to the forehead, so that small quantities of nutritious fluids with appropriate vitamin content can be given at frequent intervals.

The bladder should be watched for evidence of retention of urine, and should be catheterized if necessary.

The patient should during this phase be nursed in the lying posture

140

with a single pillow half on his side and should be turned from one side to the other at four-hourly intervals to avoid pulmonary edema. Penfield and Cone (1943) advise that he should be kept semi-prone and at times should be prone, with his head in a horseshoe head-rest to allow mucus to drain. In any case mucus should be aspirated when necessary and the mouth kept clean.

At the end of 36 hours if the patient has recovered from shock, but is still unconscious and quiet, lumbar puncture should be performed, as a diagnostic procedure to ascertain the cerebrospinal fluid pressure, and whether blood is present and if so to what extent. It has been the custom of many physicians and surgeons in the past to withdraw fluid if the pressure is high until a normal level is obtained and to repeat this procedure daily or at regular intervals on the ground that increased intracranial pressure is an important cause of symptoms. It is doubtful, however, how often this is the case and, as Penfield and Cone (1943) point out, if the intracranial pressure is high enough to cause brainstem compression from herniation of the temporal lobes into the incisura tentorii, or of the cerebellar tonsils into the foramen magnum, lumbar puncture is dangerous. As a therapeutic procedure it is probably better reserved for cases in which the level of consciousness and other symptoms make it certain that no dangerous degree of increased intracranial pressure exists, and the patient is complaining of severe headache. The effect of reducing the cerebrospinal fluid pressure to a normal level should then be observed and the procedure be repeated if beneficial, as in some cases it is. If the fluid is heavily blood-stained this is an additional argument for drainage as irritation of the meninges by blood appears in itself to be a cause of headache. With regard to the use of hypertonic solutions, whether intravenously or by the rectum, together with a limited fluid intake, this practice has now been abandoned in most clinics with a large experience of head injuries for theoretical as well as practical reasons. The former have been reviewed by Denny-Brown (1943), who concludes that there is no substance for the belief that the increased intracranial pressure is due to a generalized cerebral edema of the kind that would be relieved by such measures. Munro (1934) many years ago pointed out that the therapeutic brain shrinkage achieved by hypertonic solutions is only temporary and may be followed by a secondary wave of edema. Again, if there is meningeal hemorrhage it may be suddenly increased by shrinkage of the brain. Finally it has been the experience of many that stuporous patients after head injury may be actually short of body fluids and that their mental as well as their general condition will then improve with

141

an increased fluid intake (Denny-Brown, 1943; Penfield and Cone, 1943; Falconer, 1944, 1945). In this same connection, see Chapter 6.

The control of restlessness in the early stages should be achieved as far as possible by skilful nursing. Nevertheles sedatives are often required.* The most formidable problem is that of the confused and excited patient who will not take medicines by mouth. The balance of opinion is decidedly against the use of morphine because of its depressant effect on respiration. Falconer (1944, 1945) recommends that it should be given only if other sedatives fail and then in doses of 1/12 to 1/16 of a grain repeated as necessary. He has found these doses reasonably safe and efficacious. For the intravenous injection of sedatives the patient needs to be restrained, and the arm to be used splinted. Pentothal may then be given slowly until the required depth of narcosis is reached. Eden (1943) used intravenous paraldehyde for the same purpose in a dose of 3 cc. Once the patient has been quieted he can be kept quiet with paraldehyde given by rectum at well judged intervals, the dose recommended by Eden being 8 drams. For patients who can take drugs by mouth paraldehyde is best in 3 dram doses. Sodium amytal grains 3 to 6 is an alternative. It must however be emphasized that all narcotic drugs tend to produce confusion and should therefore be used as little as possible. Often the reason for giving them is to prevent the patient from disturbing others rather than for his own benefit, and when this is so and the delirious state is likely to be prolonged it is better that he should be transferred to a psychiatric clinic with nursing and other facilities better adapted to the care of the refractory patient.

In the later stages sedatives are better not given as a routine, but a moderate dose of amylobarbitone sodium during the day, and 1 or 2 tablets of Nitrazepam (Mogadon) at night time are sometimes needed for restlessness and insomnia.

For severe headache an occasional powder containing five grains each of aspirin and pyramidon and 1/6 grain of heroin hydrocloride is justifiable.**

After the patient has emerged from the state of traumatic confusion

*M. M. Peet has pointed out that a very full bladder especially in alcoholic patients may produce extreme restlessness and that catheterization may then allay the condition. (Ed.)

**We have found this prescription valuable. In countries where heroin is not procurable a quarter of a grain of morphine hydrochloride may be substituted or half a grain of codeine phosphate.

the line of treatment to be followed will depend upon the symptoms which he then presents. So long as there is complaint of headache or giddiness he will require such measure of physical rest and freedom from mental stimulus as appears necessary to give him the greatest degree of relief from these symptoms.

Mental inadequacy of major or minor degree will require appropriate measures of control and restraint. Nothing is more important in the later stages of treatment than a carefully graduated convalescence.

2. The Patient Who Is Reported to Have Been Unconscious

A note should be made at once of the reported duration of unconsciousness, and the patient's mental state when examined, whether clear or confused, correctly oriented or not, with normal or impaired capacity for the memory of current events. The state of the pupils should be observed and a routine neurologic examination made as soon as practicable. The patient is best admitted to hospital, and x-rays should be taken on admission. Subsequent treatment should follow the same lines as those advised for the patient who is unconscious when first examined.

The minimum period of strict rest in bed with freedom from mental stimulus in such a case should be 48 hours even though the unconsciousness has been of brief duration. After this period the patient, if symptom free, may be encouraged rapidly, but by carefully graduated steps, to submit himself to greater degrees of physical effort and mental stress. If at any stage symptoms, such as headache, giddiness, insomnia, or nervous instability, develop, the forward march must be retarded accordingly, the object being to gain relief of symptoms, but as soon as this has been obtained, to explore the possibilities of further progress. The patient who, after recovery of consciousness, from the first presents symptoms of this order should be kept at strict rest until there is a well marked improvement, after which his progress should be guided in the same way.

Lumbar puncture should be performed if headache is severe, and if the cerebrospinal fluid pressure is found high, the effect of reducing it by withdrawing fluid should be tried. If the procedure should be successful it may be repeated.

3. The Patient Who Has Never Been Unconscious

These cases will be treated on their own merits. It is unnecessary to assume that every scalp wound implies a probability of associated cerebral damage. The patient who presents the symptoms of such intracranial injury from the first will be treated accordingly on the lines already indicated. The possibility of a delayed onset, however, must be borne in mind. After any considerable impact upon the head, therefore, it is wise to prescribe a day's rest and thereafter, light occupation for a day or two, with a warning to the patient that should he develop any further symptoms, he ought to report them to the physician without delay. The treatment then will take the form of physical and mental rest.

We have already remarked upon the importance of a graduated convalescence. The ideal to be aimed at is that the patient should have mental and physical rest of a certain degree, until under such conditions he is symptom free – that he should then proceed to a stage of greater activity, and so on. The rate of progress is determined not by any rule, but by experiment in the individual case. One man may be fit to return to his normal way of living in a week or two after his injury. Another, after the same initial symptoms, may need a month or two before he is equally recovered. We believe that preconceived notions as to the duration of disability to be expected after injury of a particular degree are apt to result in unnecessarily prolonged invalidism. The patient who is symptom free should be encouraged to go ahead rapidly, but by gradual steps, which should be prescribed by the physician.

In practice, the ideal of obtaining freedom from symptoms before allowing an advance is often unattainable. Many patients after moderate or severe injuries never attain absolute freedom from symptoms. Few can afford to protract convalescence indefinitely in the hope of doing so. For most it would be harmful if they did. Hope deferred is a potent cause of neurotic invalidism. In our advice to the patient recovering from a head injury of this degree, we should be guided by these considerations, and try to strike a balance from the first. We had better warn him that recovery from the symptoms of cerebral contusion is often slow, but we may honestly assure him if he is under middle age that the risk of disability in any degree is extremely slight, even though he may be left with some relic of the injury, such as an increased liability to headache and fatigue. In the later stage of his convalescence – sometimes earlier – we may find it necessary to advise him to go forward despite symptoms, rather than await their complete disappearance.

The principles thus outlined have, we believe, now been generally applied to the convalescent treatment of patients with head injuries and the day is past when a fixed period of rest is prescribed for all patients with a specified degree of injury irrespective of their symptoms. While it is true that the duration of the posttraumatic amnesia, measuring the severity of concussion, is within limits a useful guide to the probable duration of incapacity in closed head injuries, it must be remembered that incapacity may also result from local injury with mild concussion, or in some cases with none. Table 1 compiled by Symonds and Russell (1943) relates the duration of incapacity to that of posttraumatic amnesia in a consecutive series of 167 service personnel admitted to hospital immediately after the injury, and treated by the methods which have been described, who were returned to military duties and proved by

TABLE 1

Duration of Treatment in Acute Cases with a Satisfactory Follow-Up Report after Return to Duty

MONTHS FROM INJURY TO DISCHARGE TO DUTY	DURATION OF POSTTRAUMATIC AMNESIA					
	Nil	Under 1 hour	1-24 hours	1-7 days	Over 7 days	Total
Under ½	4	4	—	—	—	8
Over ½	7	20	10	1	—	38
1 - 2	7	19	23	15	1	65
2 - 3	6	13	12	5	7	43
3 - 4	—	2	3	1	1	7
4 - 5	—	—	2	2	1	5
5 - 6	—	—	—	—	1	1
Over 6	—	—	—	—	—	—
	24	58	50	24	11	167

follow-up reports not to have relapsed. From this table it will be seen that it cannot be accepted as a fixed rule either that the patient with a brief P.T.A. will need a short period of treatment, or that the patient with a long P.T.A. will need prolonged treatment. It is true that if the P.T.A. has been less than one hour there is a much greater chance that the patient will be fit for duty in quite a short time than if it has lasted for several days. Thus comparing the figures for a P.T.A. of less than one hour with those for a P.T.A. of one to seven days we find that 41 per cent of those in the former group returned to duty in less than a month as compared with 4 per cent of the latter. But there is no such striking correlation between the longer periods of incapacity and duration of P.T.A. for if we compare the same two groups in this respect we find that of the patients with a P.T.A. of less than one hour 26 per cent were still incapacitated at the end of two months as compared with 33.3 per cent of those with a P.T.A. of one to seven days. The duration of treatment, including convalescence, therefore must be decided not by any fixed rule but by the symptoms of the individual patient and their response to treatment.

Russell and McArdle (1946) have drawn attention to the part played for good or ill by the patient's relatives in convalescence, emphasizing their importance as allies of the physician in dispelling anxiety and building up that sense of personal and social security which is especially helpful for this particular class of invalid in preventing the development of psychoneurotic symptoms.

BIBLIOGRAPHY

Ascroft, P. B. Traumatic Epilepsy after Gunshot Wounds of the Head. *Br. Med. J.*, *1*, 739, 1941.

Bagley, C., Jr. Blood in the Cerebrospinal Fluid. *Arch. Surg.*, *17*, 18, 1928.

Bagley, C., Jr. Blood in the Cerebrospinal Fluid. *Arch. Surg.*, *17*, 39, 1928.

Bagley, C., Jr. The Grouping and Treatment of Acute Cerebral Traumas. *Arch. Surg.*, *18*, 1078, 1929.

Barré, J. A. and Greiner, G. Les Troubles Vestibulaires chez les Traumatisés Craniens (Etude basé sur 100 cas personnels). *Rev. d'Oto-Neuro-Ophtalmol.*, Paris, *10*, 633, 1932.

Beekman, F. Head Injuries in Children. *Ann. Surg.*, *87*, 355, 1928.

Bielschowsky, P. Störungen des Liquorsystems bei Schädeltraumen. *Zeit. f. d. ges. Neur. u. Psych.*, Berlin *117*, 55, 1928.

Blau, A. Mental Changes Following Head Trauma in Children. *Arch. Neurol. Psychiat.*, *35*, 723, 1936.

Bremer, F., Coppez, H., Hicguet, G., and Martin, P. Le Syndrome Commotionnel Tardif dans les Traumatismes Fermés du Crane. *Rev. d'Oto-Neuro-Ophtalmol.*, Paris, *10*, 161, 1932.

Brenner, C., Friedman, A. P., Merritt, H. H., and Denny-Brown, D. Posttraumatic Headache. *J. Neurosurg.*, *1*, 379, 1944.

Cairns, H. The Vascular Aspects of Head Injuries. *Lisboa Medica*, *19*, 375, 1942.

Cairns, H. Rehabilitation after Injuries to the Central Nervous System. *Proc. R. Soc. Med.*, *35*, 299, 1942.

Carroll, E. J., Jr., Punch Drunk. *Am. J. Med. Sci.*, *191*, 706, 1936.

Davies, H. and Falconer, M. Ventricular Changes after Closed Head Injury. *J. Neurol.*, *6*, 52, 1943.

Davis, B. F. Physiologic Indications in the Treatment of Brain Injuries. *Am. J. Surg.*, *39*, 512, 1938.

Denny-Brown, D. Cerebral Concussion. *Physiol. Rev.* *25*, 296, 1945.

Denny-Brown, D. Intellectual Deterioration Resulting from Head Injury. *Res. Publ. Assoc. Nerv. Ment. Dis.*, *24*, 467, 1945.

Denny-Brown, D. The Clinical Aspects of Traumatic Epilepsy. *Am. J. Psychiatry*, *100*, 585, 1944.

Denny-Brown, D. Disability Arising from Closed Head Injury. *J.A.M.A.*, *127*, 429, 1945.

Denny-Brown, D. The Principles of Treatment of Closed Head Injury. *Bull. N.Y. Acad. Med.*, *19*, 3, 1943.

Denny-Brown, D. and Russell, W. Experimental Cerebral Concussion. *Brain*, *64*, 93, 1941.

Dix, M. R. and Hallpike, C. S. The Pathology, Symptomatology and Diagnosis of Certain Common Disorders of the Vestibular System. *Proc. R. Soc. Med.*, *45*, 341, 1952.

Duret, H. *Traumatismes Cranio-Cérébraux*. Paris: 1920.

Eden, K. and Aldren Turner, J. W. Loss of Consciousness in Different Types of Head Injury. *Proc. R. Soc. Med.*, *34*, 685, 1941.

Eden, K. Mobile Neurosurgery in Warfare. *Lancet*, *2*, 689, 1943.

Falconer, M. The Management of Closed Head Injuries. *N. Z. Med. J.*, *43*, 274, 1944, and *44*, 15, 1945.

Friedman, A. P., Brenner, C., and Denny-Brown, D. Post-traumatic Vertigo and Dizziness. *J. Neurosurg.*, *2*, 36, 1945.

Friedman, E. D., Head Injuries: Effects and Their Appraisal. III. Encephalographic Observations. *Arch. Neurol. Psychiat.*, *27*, 791, 1932.

Gordon, N. Post-traumatic Vertigo with Special Reference to Positional Nystagmus. *Lancet*, *1*, 1216, 1954.

Greenfield, J. G. Some Observations on Cerebral Injuries. *Proc. R. Soc. Med.*, London, *32*, 43, 1938.

Groat, R. A., and Simmons, J. Q. Loss of Nerve Cells in Experimental Concussion. *J. Neuropathol. Exp. Neurol.*, *9*, 150, 1950.

Guttmann, E. Postcontusional Headache. *Lancet*, *1*, 10, 1943.

Guttmann, E. The Prognosis in Civilian Head Injuries. *Br. Med. J.*, *1*, 94, 1943.

Helsmoortel, J., Jr., Bauwens, L., and Van Bogaert, L. Le Syndrome Résiduel des Traumatismes Cranio-Cérébraux Fermes. Etude de 43 observations au point de vue Labyrinthique, Ophtalmologique et Neuro-Psychiatrique. *Rev. d'Oto-Neuro-Ophtalmol.*, Paris, *10*, 581, 1932.

Hooper K. S., McGregor, J. M., and Nathan, P. W. Explosive Rage Following Head Injury. *J. Mental Sci.*, *91*, 458, 1945.

Jefferson, G. Discussion of the Diagnosis and Treatment of Acute Head Injuries. *Proc. R. Soc. Med.*, London, *25*, 742, 1932.

147

Jefferson, G. Remarks on the Treatment of Acute Head Injuries. *Br. Med. J.*, 2, 807, 1933.

Kozol, H. Pre-traumatic Personality and Psychiatric Sequelae of Head Injury. *Arch. Neurol. Psychiat.*, 53, 358, 1945 and 56, 245, 1946.

Kremer, M., Post-traumatic Personality Change. *Proc. R. Soc. Med.*, 37, 564, 1944.

Kremer, M., Russell, W. R., and Smyth, G. E. A Mid-Brain Syndrome Following Head Injury. *J. Neurol. Neurosurg. and Psychiatry*, 10, 49, 1947.

Linthicum, F. H. and Rand, C. W. Neuro-Otological Observations in Concussion of the Brain. *Arch. Otolaryngol.*, 13, 785, 1931.

Mapother, E. Mental Symptoms Associated with Head Injury: The Psychiatric Aspect. *Br. Med. J.*, 2, 1055, 1937.

Martland, H. S. Punch Drunk. *J.A.M.A.*, 91, 1103, 1928.

Medical Research Council War Memorandum No. 4. *A Glossary of Psychological Terms Commonly Used in Cases of Head Injury.* London: H. M. Stationery Office.

Moore, B. E. and Reusch, J. Prolonged Disturbances of Consciousness Following Head Injury. *New Engl. J. Med.*, 230, 445, 1944.

Moritz, A. R. and Wartman, W. B. Post-traumatic Internal Hydrocephalus. *Am. J. Med. Sci.*, 195, 65, 1938.

Munro, D. The Diagnosis, Treatment and Immediate Prognosis of Cerebral Trauma. *New Engl. J. Med.*, 210, 287, 1934.

Mygind, S. H. Traumatic Vestibular Diseases. *Acta Otolaryngol.*, 1, 515, 1918-1919.

Parker, H. L. Traumatic Encephalopathy ('Punch Drunk') of Professional Pugilists. *J. Neurol. & Psychopath.*, 15, 20, 1934.

Paterson, A. Disorders of Personality after Head Injury. *Proc. Soc. Med.*, 37, 556, 1944.

Paterson, J. H. Some Observations on the Cerebrospinal Fluid in Closed Head Injuries. *J. Neurol.*, 6, 87, 1943.

Penfield, W. and Cone, W. Elementary Principles of the Treatment of Head Injuries. *Can. Med. Assn. J.*, 48, 99, 1943.

Penfield, W. and Norcross, N. C. Subdural Traction and Post-traumatic Headache. Study of Pathology and Therapeusis. *Arch. Neurol. Psychiat.*, 36, 75, 1936.

Pfeiffer, B. Die Psychischen Störungen nach Hirnverletzungen. *Bumke Handb. der Geisteskrankheiten.* Berlin, 7: Teil 3, 415, 1928.

Portmann, G. and Despons, J. A Propos des troubles vestibulaires dans le syndrome post-commotionnel. *Rev. de Laryngol.*, 58, 585, 1937.

Ravina, A. L'encéphalite Traumatique ou 'Punch Drunk.' *Presse Med.*, 45, 1362, 1937.

Rawling, L. B. Head Injuries. *Postgrad. Med. J.*, London, 2, 113, 1927.

Reusch, J. Intellectual Impairment in Head Injuries. *Am. J. Psychiatry*, 100, 480, 1944.

Riddoch, G. Discussion of the Diagnosis and Treatment of Acute Head Injuries. *Proc. R. Soc. Med.*, London, 25, 735, 1932.

Russell, W. R. Cerebral Involvement in Head Injury. *Brain*, 55, 549, 1932.

Russell, W. R. Discussion of the Diagnosis and Treatment of Acute Head Injuries. *Proc. R. Soc., Med.* London, 25, 751, 1932.

Russell, W. R. The After-effects of Head Injury. *Trans. Med. Chir. Soc.*, Edinburgh, *113*, 129, 1933-1934.

Russell, W. R. Discussion on Intracranial Pressure: Its Clinical and Pathological Importance. *Proc. R. Soc. Med.*, London, *27*, 832, 1934.

Russell, W. R. Amnesia Following Head Injuries. *Lancet*, 762, Oct. 5, 1935.

Russell, W. R. and McArdle, M. J. Convalescence after Head Injuries. Advice for the Patient's Relations. *Practitioner*, *156*, 370, 1946.

Russell, W. R. and Nathan, P. W. Traumatic Amnesia. *Brain*, *69*, 280, 1946.

Schou, H. I. Trauma Capitis and Epilepsy. *Acta. Psych. et Neurol.*, *8*, 75, 1933.

Strecker, E. A. and Ebaugh, F. G. Essentials of Neuro-psychiatric Sequelae of Cerebral Trauma in Children. *Arch. Neurol. Psychiat.*, *12*, 443, 1924.

Strich, S. J. Diffuse Degeneration of the Cerebral White Matter in Severe Dementia Following Head Injury. *J. Neurol. Neurosurg. Psychiatry*, *19*, 163, 1956.

Symonds, C. P. The Effects of Injury upon the Brain. *Lancet*, 820, Apr. 16, 1932.

Symonds, C. P. Disturbance of Cerebral Function in Concussion. *Lancet*, 486, Mar. 2, 1935.

Symonds, C. P. The Effects of Head Injury Remaining after One Year. *Rapports, VIIme Congres International des Accidents et des Maladies du Travail*, Brussels, *2*, 11, 1935.

Symonds, C. P. Traumatic Epilepsy. *Lancet*, 1217, Nov., 30, 1935.

Symonds, C. P. Prognosis in Cerebral Concussion and Contusion. *Lancet*, 854, Apr. 11, 1936.

Symonds, C. P. Mental Disorder Following Head Injury. *Proc. R. Soc. Med.*, London, *30*, 1081, 1937.

Symonds, C. P. Assessment of Symptoms Following Head Injury. *Guy's Hosp. Gaz.*, *51*, 461, 1937.

Symonds, C. P. Differential Diagnosis and Treatment of Post-Contusional States. *Proc. R. Soc. Med.*, *35*, 601, 1942.

Symonds, C. P. and Jefferson, G. The Treatment of Head Injuries. *Br. Med. J.*, 677, Oct. 12, 1935.

Symonds, C. P. and Russell, W. R. Accidental Head Injuries: Prognosis in Service Patients. *Lancet*, *1*, 7, 1943.

Trotter, W. An Address on the Management of Head Injuries. *Lancet*, 953, Nov. 7, 1925.

Trotter, W. An Address on the Evolution of the Surgery of Head Injuries. *Lancet*, 169, Jan. 25, 1930.

Trotter, W. Injuries of the Skull and Brain. In *Choyce's System of Surgery*. London: Cassell & Co., 3, 358, 1932.

Turner, W. A. Epilepsy and Gunshot Wounds of the Head. *J. Neur. & Psychopathol.*, *3*, 309, 1922.

Wagstaffe, W. W. The Incidence of Traumatic Epilepsy after Gunshot Wound of the Head. *Lancet*, 861, Oct. 27, 1928.

Weil, M. and Oumansky, V. Parkinsonisme Traumatique. *Rev. Neurol.*, Paris, *67*, 489, 1937.

Williams, D. The Electroencephalogram in Acute Head Injuries. *J. Neurol. and Psychiat.*, *4*, 107, 1941.

Williams, D. and Denny-Brown, D. Cerebral Electrical Changes in Experimental Concussion. *Brain*, *64*, 223, 1941.

Windle, W. F., Groat, R. A., and Fox, C. A. Experimental Structural Alterations

149

in the Brain During and after Concussion. *Surg. Gynec. Obstet.*, 79, 561, 1944.

Winterstein, C. E. Head Injuries Attributable to Boxing. *Lancet*, 719. Sept. 18, 1937.

Woodhall, B. Acute Cerebral Injuries. Analysis of Temperature, Pulse and Respiration Curves. *Arch. Surg.*, 33, 560, 1936.

ADDENDUM (Ed.)

The thesis that diffuse injury to neurons provides the structural basis for concussion was further elaborated by Symonds in 1962. He reiterated his belief that "the term concussion should not be confined to cases in which there is immediate loss of consciousness with rapid and complete recovery but should include the many cases in which the initial symptoms are the same but with subsequent long continued disturbance of consciousness, often followed by residual symptoms." He further stated that "The effects of the trauma may or may not be reversible. In the most severe degree of concussion, there is widespread irreparable damage. In the slightest degree there may be rapid and complete recovery of cerebral function, but this does not necessarily exclude the possibility that a small number of neurons may have perished — a number so small as to be negligible at the time, but leaving the brain more susceptible as a whole to the effects of further damage of the same kind." Russell (1959) expressed similar views regarding the physical basis of concussion. Additional pathologic data in support of this concept were provided by Strich (1961), Nevin (1967), Peerless and Rewcastle (1967), and Oppenheimer (1968). Supplementing her original report, Strich described widespread degenerative changes in the white matter of the cerebrum and brain stem following injury in an additional 15 cases. Evidence of damage to nerve fibers was observed by Nevin in 29 of 40 cases of fatal head trauma. Peerless and Rewcastle found microscopic evidence of axonal and small vessel injury localized to the basal and midsagittal areas of the diencephalon and mesencephalon in 37 cases of head trauma, the survival period ranging from a few hours to 243 days. Oppenheimer examined the brains of 59 patients with head injuries who had survived at least 15 hours and found aggregates of microglial cells in about three-quarters of them.

Considerable evidence exists to substantiate the belief that wakefulness is dependent on normal activity of the brain-stem reticular formation and that the alteration of consciousness associated with concussion is related to dysfunction of this system. As indicated by Lindsley (1960), "Wakefulness is maintained by excitation of the reticular formation and the ascending reticular activating system through collaterals from all sensory pathways, by corticofugal impulses originating in various regions of the cortex, and by humoral factors which affect particularly the rostral portions of the reticular formation. Increased activity of the ascending reticular activating system through any of these sources of excitation acts upon the cortex by changing the pattern of its electrical activity from the slow waves and spindle bursts of sleep, or the alpha waves of relaxed wakefulness, to a pattern of low-voltage fast waves commonly referred to as 'activation.' Electrocortical activation is accompanied by behavioral arousal and by alertness and attention." The function of the reticular activating system following trauma was investigated by Foltz and Schmidt (1956). They found that the sensory evoked potentials in the reticular formation of the monkey were abolished during coma resulting from concussion, whereas the evoked potentials in the medial lemniscus remained unchanged. Earlier, French and Magoun (1952) had demonstrated that destructive lesions in the central cephalic brain stem of monkeys resulted in a state of chronic unresponsiveness, whereas stimulation of this region produced a change in the direction of arousal of the dormant animal and altered the pattern of electrocortical activity accordingly. Gurdjian et al (1958, 1966) observed neuronal damage in the brain stem and reticular formation, as well as in the medial temporal lobes and posterior thalamus following experimental concussion in the dog. Friede (1961) found chromatolysis and loss of nerve cells in the reticular formation, lateral vestibular nucleus, red nucleus and, less often, in other nuclei of the brain stem following experimental concussion in cats, produced by stretching of the cervical cord at the craniovertebral junction. The cellular changes in the brain stem were interpreted as secondary phenomena, consequent upon damage to large fibers in the ventral tracts of the cord at the odontoid level. Cytologic alterations in the brain stem after experimental concussion had previously been reported by Windle, Groat, and Fox (1944); Groat, Windle, and Magoun (1945); and Groat and Simmons (1950). Recently, however, Ommaya (1966) and Unterharnscheidt and Sellier (1966) failed to confirm these findings (see also Unterharnscheidt, 1970). Apropos of these experimental observations, it should be recalled that, in 1944, Jefferson had arrived at essentially similar conclusions on the basis of clinical and pathological evidence, and attributed traumatic stupor to lesions of the brain stem and hypothalamus. While the activity of the reticular formation appears to play a fundamental role in regulating the level of consciousness, undoubtedly it does so in collaboration with other parts of the brain, especially the thalamus and cerebral cortex (Brodal, 1969). The literature on the reticular formation is extensive; for a more detailed account of this subject, and of the physiology of contusion, the reader is referred to the publications of French (1958), Magoun (1936), Pearce (1964), Ward (1966), and Brodal (1969).

The facts concerning consciousness and brain-stem function are not to be taken as an indication that concussion is essentially due to brain stem involvement. As indicated by Russell (1959), "The brain stem and cerebral hemispheres are so intricately interdependent that widespread trauma to the hemispheres is just as likely to inactivate the brain stem temporarily as the brain stem is to inactivate the hemispheres; and as the traumatic oscillations are likely to be more extensive at the cortex and subcortical white matter than the brain stem, it seems likely that the neuronal damage in the hemispheres is usually responsible for the clinical concussion."

A study by Zangwill (1961) revealed that even in cases of mild concussion "retrograde amnesia is at first considerably longer than is commonly supposed," often lasting days, weeks or even months. Within a few days it diminishes markedly and by the time of discharge its duration almost always is reduced to a few seconds. Although the general trend is for memory of more remote events to return first, "very seldom did memories appear to return in strict chronologic order. Islands of memory emerged in sporadic fashion and gradually became linked in chronologic sequence. Indeed memories dating from shortly before the accident were often available when memory for the preceding hours or days was still grossly defective." Zangwill further found that after complete recovery a patchy amnesia for remote events well outside the accepted scope of the retrograde amnesia was often demonstrable. In cases of severe head trauma the residual memory defect may involve events which occurred long before the accident.

A discussion of traumatic amnesia was included in a paper on disorders of memory by Symonds (1966). Attention was again drawn to the fact that amnesia may follow slight degrees of trauma unaccompanied by any appreciable clouding of consciousness. In considering the localization and pathogenesis of the lesions responsible for memory disorder in cases of closed head injury, the uniformity of the clinical symptoms led Symonds to postulate widespread commotion rather than focal damage. It was suggested that the amnesic syndrome is caused by damage to activating structures situated mainly in the hippocampal system (temporal lobes, mammillary bodies, and parts of the thalamus) responsible for counterbalancing a natural bias towards forgetting.

Extracts from the publications of Russell and his associates dealing with head trauma, and specifically traumatic amnesia, have been compiled together with a commentary in a recent monograph (The Traumatic Amnesias, 1971). The material is presented in an exemplary manner.

The basis of the post-concussional syndrome remains a matter of dispute. The argument in favor of psychologic factors has been supported by Miller (1961, 1966), whose observations led him to express skepticism regarding the importance of cellular damage. He found that the severity and duration of post-concussional symptoms were inversely related to the severity of the injury, and that recovery as a rule was contingent upon the settlement of compensation claims. While cognizant of the diversity of opinion concerning its etiology, Friedman (1969) is nevertheless of the opinion that, "The posttraumatic syndrome in which headache plays a prominent part has no pathological counterpart, and is most frequently associated with minor head injuries with or without concussion, rather than with major trauma." He considers persistent posttraumatic headache to be functional in origin in the vast majority of cases, and believes that compensation is a significant factor in some instances.

Commenting on Miller's views, Russell (1966) questioned the validity of conclusions drawn from a study of cases examined partly for compensation purposes, and Zangwill (1966) indicated that results of his psychological studies appeared to favor an organic basis for the post-concussional syndrome. Taylor (1967) also believes that such symptoms are the result of physical factors. Lesions in the brain-stem nuclei and white matter, disorders of vestibular function, alterations of capillary permeability, slowing of cerebral blood flow (Taylor and Bell, 1966; Taylor, 1969) and metabolic abnormalities are held responsible for concussional sequelae.

No abnormality of cerebral blood flow was found by Skinhøj (1966) in patients with the post-concussion syndrome studied about a year after injury; however, a significant reduction of cerebral blood flow was observed in patients with cerebral contusions or lacerations. (Also of interest in this connection are the observations of Salmon and Timperman (1971). Using intracarotid Xenon 133, they found a reduction of cortical blood flow through the gray matter in cases of severe posttraumatic encephalopathy. The blood flow through the white matter of severely demented patients studied several years after trauma was increased).

It has also been suggested that involvement of cervical structures may play a part in the genesis of the posttraumatic syndrome (Jacobson, 1969; Ishii, 1969).

Probably both organic and psychologic factors play a role to varying degrees in any particular case. While admitting that the symptoms of the post-concussional syndrome are of a psychologic nature, Symonds (1962) further stated that "This does not mean that they have no physical basis, but it does mean that they are related to all those qualities which constitute the patient's personality, and to his whole attitude of mind. Prominent in this will be his attitude towards his illness, its causes and prospects, and the question of compensation if it exists." The problems posed by the post-concussional syndrome are well summarized in an editorial published in 1967 in the *British Medical Journal.*

Positional nystagmus of the benign paroxysmal variety was found in 15 per cent of cases of post-concussional vertigo (Harrison, 1956). The recovery period in such cases was appreciably longer than in those in which it was not observed.

A high incidence (91 per cent) of vestibular symptoms was reported by Toglia (1969) following closed head injury and so-called whiplash injury of the neck. He proposed the following classification of labyrinthine damage:

1. Labyrinthine concussion characterized by a resolution of symptoms in a few weeks.

2. Paroxysmal positional vertigo.

3. Labyrinthine contusion, in which the inner ear is irreversibly damaged and symptoms subside gradually, though not necessarily completely.

The end results of a series of 500 cases of head injury, consisting of 170 children and 330 adults, were reported by Rowbotham (1964). The overall mortality was 9.2 per cent, the figures for children and adults being 4.7 per cent and 11.5 per cent respectively. Neurologic sequelae were more frequent among adults, and included the following (adults): visual impairment (9 cases); unilateral deafness (6); hemiparesis (5); epilepsy (5); anosmia (4); diabetes insipidus (2); dysphasia (2); and pulsating exophthalmos (1). Five patients, two of whom had previously exhibited psychiatric symptoms, were listed as

154

psychotic, and an equal number as psychoneurotic. Personality changes were of frequent occurrence among the children.

The long-term prognosis of severe head injuries among civilians is indicated in a study of 100 such cases, referred for medicolegal assessment, by Miller and Stern (1965). The follow-up period varied from 3 to 40 years, the average being 11 years. Initially, the patients were not examined immediately following trauma but after periods varying from 3 months to 14 years (average 3 years). Ninety-two survivors were available for reexamination. About half the cases suffered closed injuries, and the average duration of the P.T.A. was 13 days. Twenty-one of 25 patients with pareses recovered, as did also two with dysphasia. By and large, patients with involvement of the first, second, fifth (sensory) and eighth cranial nerves at the time of the initial examination failed to improve. Psychiatric symptoms persisted in 16 patients, the diagnosis being dementia in 10 and psychoneurosis in 4. Convulsions developed in 19, usually within 2 years of injury. Ten of 85 adults were totally disabled from an occupational standpoint and 72 were fully employed, 45 at their usual jobs.

A reduction in the mortality rate of closed head injuries over a 20-year period, from 9 per cent in 1948 to 3.5 per cent in 1966, was reported by Lewin (1967). It is generally recognized that most patients with mild or moderately severe head trauma recover completely or to a satisfactory degree. According to Lewin (1967) some 80 per cent of patients who survive more severe trauma (P.T.A. over 24 hours) eventually are able to resume their former work. The remaining 20 per cent, however, are left with a major disability. Lewin (1965) also reported that of some 130 patients unconscious for a month or longer following injury, two-thirds survived, of whom three-quarters eventually made a reasonably adequate socioeconomic adjustment despite some degree of mental or physical disability.

The prognosis and course of 44 patients with prolonged traumatic unconsciousness was investigated by Van der Zwan (1969). Coma had lasted at least three weeks in each instance. Thirty-five patients survived, of whom 27 were examined two years or more following injury. A third or more complained of headache, forgetfulness, loss of interest and initiative, difficulty in concentration and word finding, emotional lability, and a change in their sleep pattern; ten complained of neurasthenic symptoms. Function of the oculomotor, facial, or acoustic nerve was defective in one-third to one-half the cases; the optic and olfactory nerves were each affected in five cases. Coordination was disturbed in over one-third of patients and five were hemiparetic. Fits occurred in four. Psychologic and intellectual disturbances were frequent. Memory was defective in 20 and the ability to deal with abstractions impaired in 19. "In all patients, more or less, there was marked slowness in thinking, action and speech." Seven patients were invalids unable to earn a living independently.

Memory, intellect, and personality may suffer as a consequence of head trauma, the resultant psychiatric disability in some instances proving a serious handicap. Among 3552 cases of cerebral trauma sustained during the war years in Finland, a posttraumatic Korsakoff syndrome was observed in 29 (Hillbom and Jarho, 1969). Fifty-eight per cent of the cases had suffered closed head injuries. The authors suggest that the lesions responsible for the memory disturbances are bilateral, affecting the limbic system and its frontal lobe connections.

A series of 1168 adult patients with closed head injuries was studied by Ota (1969) during both initial and chronic stages. Generalized disorders of intellectual function occurred in 22 cases (1.9 per cent), character changes in 68 (5.8 per cent), neurotic manifestations in 255 (21.8 per cent), and psychotic states in 52, 20 of which were classified as organic. The incidence of epilepsy was 3.3 per cent.

Carlsson et al (1968) found that the capacity for mental restitution following closed head trauma was appreciably influenced by the age of the patient and the duration of coma. The chances of restitution decreased sharply after the age of 50. Prolonged coma had a similar deleterious effect after the age of 20.

Based on a study of 305 cases of acute head trauma in children up to the age of 14 years, about half of whom had lost consciousness, Hjern and Nylander (1964) concluded that neurologic sequelae were infrequent and that there was little risk of occurrence of psychiatric symptoms following slight injury per se. Mental sequelae, as a rule, appeared in children whose home environment was unstable or who had previously shown evidence of psychiatric disorder.

The effects of head trauma in a series of 105 children were examined by Black et al (1969). Almost two-thirds had been rendered comatose and over half sustained a fracture. Although 44 per cent suffered some sort of neurologic dysfunction following injury, the ultimate residual deficit, with few exceptions, was generally minor in degree. Compared with adults, the predominant posttraumatic symptoms in children were of a behavioral nature. Sixty-nine per cent of those free of symptoms prior to injury remained asymptomatic thereafter, 9 per cent developed headache, and 22 per cent behavioral manifestations. The four most common problems were hyperkinesis, temper outbursts, impaired attention, and headache; discipline and eating problems, hypokinesis, and disturbances of sleep occurred less often. The incidence of headache rose with age and was more prevalent in girls. Behavioral disturbance, particularly hyperkinesis, appeared more frequently in boys.

Posttraumatic epilepsy is dealt with elsewhere in this volume, and will be considered only briefly at this point. Summarizing a discussion on posttraumatic epilepsy in 1969, Caveness stated, "It is evident that some of the men who have fits as a result of trauma have but a single attack. Others have a few, or several, attacks and then no more. And still others have frequent attacks that, even though they may begin early, persist throughout the remainder of their lives." Virtually all observers are in agreement that the risk of posttraumatic epilepsy is much less after closed head injury than following penetrating wounds. Fits occur in about 5· per cent of cases of blunt injury, whereas their incidence following dural penetration is in the neighborhood of 40 per cent. The study of Jennett (1962) would indicate that the risk of epilepsy following blunt trauma is "about 1 per cent for all injuries uncomplicated by early epilepsy, hematoma, or depressed fracture even when the P.T.A. is of more than 24 hours' duration." Even in cases in which the dura remains intact, seizures are much more common after missile injuries. According to Jennett (1969, 1969) epilepsy after closed head trauma occurs much more frequently during the first week after injury (early epilepsy) than in any of the subsequent seven weeks. Localized focal motor fits were observed to occur commonly during the first week but infrequently in the next seven weeks; temporal lobe epilepsy did not appear during the first week but occurred often during the course of the next seven weeks. Fits within the first week of injury occurred in 3.9 per cent of 821 cases analyzed by Jennett and Lewin (1960). Seizures occurred more commonly in children under five years of age and in cases in which the P.T.A. was over 24 hours. Late epilepsy occurred in over 25 per cent of patients with early epilepsy; fits recurred in over 70 per cent of those in whom they first appeared after the first week. While depressed fracture and prolonged P.T.A. (more than 24 hours) alone increase the likelihood of late epilepsy, their occurrence in combination is associated with an appreciably higher incidence of epilepsy (Jennett, 1965, 1969). The frequency of late fits is also greater in patients with depressed fracture in whom the dura has been penetrated or who manifest early epilepsy. Late epilepsy developed in 28.5 per cent of cases with intracranial hematoma. Somewhat more than half the patients with late epilepsy experience their first seizure within a year following injury (Jennett 1962, 1965); in over 25 per cent of cases the onset of fits is delayed beyond the fourth year.

Courjon (1969) found that the incidence of late epilepsy in closed trauma was 2 per cent. It was higher in patients with early fits (13 per cent), in those in whom an intracranial hematoma had been evacuated, and in those in whom localized spikes or waves of ictal discharges were observed in the electroencephalogram at an early stage (15 per cent).

A tendency towards cessation of attacks is evident in an appreciable number of posttraumatic epileptics (Caveness, 1969; Courjon, 1969).

BIBLIOGRAPHY

Black, P., Jeffries, J. J., Blumer, D., Wellner, A., and Walker, A. E. The Posttraumatic Syndrome in Children. In A. E. Walker, W. F. Caveness, and M. Critchley (Eds.), *The Late Effects of Head Injury*. Springfield, Ill.: Charles C Thomas, 1969. Pp. 142-194.

Brodal, A. The Reticular Formation. In *Neurological Anatomy in Relation to Clinical Medicine*. 2nd ed. New York: Oxford, 1969. P. 807.

Carlsson, C. A., von Essen, C., and Löfgren, J. Factors Affecting the Clinical Course of Patients with Severe Head Injuries. Part 1: Influence of Biological Factors. Part 2: Significance of Posttraumatic Coma. *J. Neurosurg.*, 29, 242, 1968.

Caveness, W. F. Posttraumatic Epilepsy: Critique. In A. E. Walker, W. F. Caveness, and M. Critchley (Eds.), *The Late Effects of Head Injury*. Springfield, Ill.: Charles C Thomas, 1969. P. 560.

Chason, J. L., Hardy, W. G., Webster, J. E., and Gurdjian, E. S. Alterations in Cell Structure of the Brain Associated with Experimental Concussion. *J. Neurosurg.*, 15, 135, 1958.

Courjon, J. A. Posttraumatic Epilepsy in Electroclinical Practice. In A. E. Walker, W. F. Caveness, and M. Critchley (Eds.), *The Late Effects of Head Injury*. Springfield, Ill.: Charles C Thomas, 1969. Pp. 215-227.

Foltz, E. L. and Schmidt, R. P. The Role of the Reticular Formation in the Coma of Head Injury. *J. Neurosurg.*, 13, 145, 1956.

French, J. D. The Reticular Formation. *J. Neurosurg.*, 15, 97, 1958.

French, J. D. and Magoun, H. W. Effects of Chronic Lesions in Central Cephalic Brain Stem of Monkeys. *Arch. Meurol. & Psychiat.*, 68, 591. 1952.

French, J. D., von Amerongen, F. K., and Magoun, H. W. An Activating System in Brain Stem of Monkey. *Arch. Neurol. & Psychiat.*, 68, 577, 1952.

Friedman, A. P. The So-called Posttraumatic Headache. In A. E. Walker, W. F. Caveness, and M. Critchley (Eds.), *The Late Effects of Head Injury*. Springfield, Ill.: Charles C Thomas, 1969. Pp. 55-71.

Friede, R. L. Experimental Acceleration Concussion. *Arch. Neurol.*, 4, 449, 1961.

Groat, R. A., Windle, W. F., and Magoun, H. W. Functional and Structural

Changes in the Monkey's Brain During and After Concussion. *J. Neurosurg.,* 2, 26, 1945.

Gurdjian, E. S., Lissner, H. R., Hodgson, V. R., and Patrick, L. M. Mechanism of Head Injury. P. 112-128 in *Clin. Neurosurg.,* Vol. 12. Baltimore: Williams and Wilkins, 1966. P. 419.

Harrison, M. S. Notes on the Clinical Features and Pathology of Post-concussional Vertigo, with Special Reference to Positional Nystagmus. *Brain,* 79, 474, 1956.

Hillbom, E., and Jarho, L. Posttraumatic Korsakoff Syndrome. In A. E. Walker, W. F. Caveness and M. Critchley (Eds.), *The Late Effects of Head Injury.* Springfield, Ill.: Charles C Thomas, 1969. Pp. 98-109.

Hjern, B. and Nylander, I. Acute Head Injuries in Children. *Acta Paediatrica, Supplement 152,* 1964. P. 1-37.

Ishii, S. Significance of Soft Tissue Neck Injuries in the Posttraumatic Syndrome. In A. E. Walker, W. F. Caveness, and M. Critchley (Eds.), *The Late Effects of Head Injury.* Springfield, Ill.: Charles C Thomas, 1969. Pp. 123-134.

Jacobson, S. A. Mechanism of the Sequelae of Minor Craniocervical Trauma. In A. E. Walker, W. F. Caveness, and M. Critchley (Eds.), *The Late Effects of Head Injury.* Springfield, Ill.: Charles C Thomas, 1969. Pp. 35-45.

Jefferson, G. The Nature of Concussion. *Br. Med. J., 1,* 1, 1944.

Jennett, W. B. *Epilepsy after Blunt Head Injuries.* Springfield, Ill.: Charles C Thomas, 1962. P. 150.

Jennett, W. B. Predicting Epilepsy after Blunt Head Injury. *Br. Med. J., 1,* 1215, 1965.

Jennett, W. B. Epilepsy after Blunt (Nonmissile) Head Injuries. In A. E. Walker, W. F. Caveness and M. Critchley (Eds.), *The Late Effects of Head Injury.* Springfield, Ill.: Charles C Thomas, 1969. Pp. 201-214.

Jennett, W. B. Early Traumatic Epilepsy. Definition and Identity. *Lancet, 1,* 1023, 1969.

Jennett, W. B., and Lewin, W. Traumatic Epilepsy after Closed Head Injuries. *J. Neurol. Neurosurg. Psychiatry, 23,* 295, 1960.

Lewin, W. Observations on Prolonged Unconsciousness after Head Injury. In J. N. Cummings and M. Kremer (Eds.), *Biochemical Aspects of Neurological Disorders,* 2nd series. Oxford, 1965. Pp. 182-198.

Lewin, W. Severe Head Injuries. *Proc. R. Soc. Med., 60,* 1208, 1967.

Lindsley, D. B. Attention, Consciousness, Sleep and Wakefulness. In H. W. Magoun (Ed.), *Handbook of Physiology.* Section 1. *Neurophysiology.* Vol. *III.* Washington, D. C.: American Physiological Association, 1960. Pp. 1553-1593.

Magoun, H. W. *The Waking Brain,* 2nd ed. Springfield, Ill.: Charles C Thomas, 1963. P. 188.

Miller, H. Accident Neurosis. *Br. Med. J., 2,* 919, 992, 1961.

Miller, H. Mental After-Effects of Head Injury. *Proc. R. Soc. Med., 59,* 257, 1966.

Miller, H., and Stern, G. The Long-Term Prognosis of Severe Head Injury.

Ommaya, A. K. Experimental Head Injury. In W. F. Caveness and A. E. Walker *Lancet, 1,* 225, 1965.

Nevin, N. C. Neuropathological Changes in the White Matter Following Head Injury. *J. Neuropathol. Exp. Neurol., 26,* 77, 1967.

159

(Eds.), *Head Injury.* Conference Proceedings. Philadelphia: J. B. Lippincott Co., 1966. Pp. 260-275.

Oppenheimer, D. R. Microscopic Lesions in the Brain Following Head Injury. *J. Neurol. Neurosurg. Psychiatry, 31,* 299, 1968.

Ota, Y. Psychiatric Studies on Civilian Head Injuries. In A. E. Walker, W. F. Caveness, and M. Critchley (Eds.), *The Late Effects of Head Injury.* Springfield, Ill.: Charles C Thomas, 1969. Pp. 110-119.

Pearce, G. W. The Reticular System with Reference to Head Injuries. In G. F. Rowbotham, *Acute Injuries of the Head.* 4th ed. Baltimore: Williams and Wilkins, 1964. P. 584.

Peerless, S. J. and Rewcastle, N. B. Shear Injuries of the Brain. *Can. Med. Assn. J., 96,* 577, 1967.

Post-Concussional Syndrome. *Br. Med. J. 3,* 61, 1967.

Rowbotham, G. F. *Acute Injuries of the Head.* 4th ed. Baltimore: Williams and Wilkins, 1964. P. 584.

Russell, W. R. *Brain. Memory Learning.* London: Oxford, 1959. P. 140.

Russell, W. R. Comments. Mental Sequelae of Head Injury. *Proc. R. Soc. Med., 59,* 266, 1966.

Russell, W. R. *The Traumatic Amnesias.* London: Oxford, 1971.

Salmon, J. H. and Timperman, A. L. Cerebral Blood Flow in Posttraumatic Encephalopathy. *Neurology, 21,* 33, 1971.

Skinøj, E. Determination of Cerebral Blood Flow in Man. In W. F. Caveness and A. E. Walker (Eds.), *Head Injury.* Conference Proceedings. Philadelphia: J. B. Lippincott Co., 1966. Pp. 431-438.

Strich, S. J. Shearing of Nerve Fibers as a Cause of Brain Damage due to Head Injury. A Pathological Study of Twenty Cases. *Lancet, 2,* 443, 1961.

Symonds, C. Concussion and Its Sequelae. *Lancet, 1,* 1, 1962.

Symonds, C. Disorders of Memory. *Brain, 89,* 625, 1966.

Taylor, A. R. Post-concussional Sequelae. *Br. Med. J., 3,* 67, 1967.

Taylor, A. R. The Cerebral Circulatory Disturbance Associated with the Late Effects of Head Injury. In A. E. Walker, W. F. Caveness and M. Critchley (Eds.), *The Late Effects of Head Injury.* Springfield, Ill.: Charles C Thomas, 1969. Pp. 46-54.

Taylor, A. R. and Bell, T. K. Slowing of Cerebral Circulation after Concussional Head Injury. *Lancet, 2,* 178, 1966.

Toglia, J. U. Dizziness after Whiplash Injury of the Neck and Closed Injury: Electronystagmographic Correlations. In A. E. Walker, W. F. Caveness and M. Critchley (Eds.), *The Late Effects of Head Injury.* Springfield, Ill.: Charles C Thomas, 1969. Pp. 72-83.

Unterharnscheidt, F. J. Discussion, Mechanisms of Head Injury. In E. S. Gurdjian, W. A. Lange, L. M. Patrick, and L. M. Thomas (Eds.), *Impact Injury and Crash Protection.* Springfield, Ill.: Charles C Thomas, 1970. Pp. 43-62.

Unterharnscheidt, F. and Sellier, K. Mechanics and Pathomorphology of Closed Brain Injuries. In W. F. Caveness and A. E. Walker (Eds.), *Head Injury.* Conference Proceedings. Philadelphia: J. B. Lippincott Co., 1966. Pp. 321-341.

Van der Zwan, A. Late Results from Prolonged Traumatic Unconsciousness. In A. E. Walker, W. F. Caveness, and M. Critchley (Eds.), *The Late Effects of Head Injury.* Springfield, Ill.: Charles C Thomas, 1969. Pp. 138-141.

Ward, A. A., Jr. The Physiology of Concussion. In W. F. Caveness and A. E. Walker (Eds.), *Head Injury*. Conference Proceedings. Philadelphia: J. B. Lippincott Co., 1966. Pp. 203-208.

Zangwill, O. L. Psychological Studies of Amnesic States. *Proc. Third World Congr. Psychiat.*, Montreal (1961), 3, 219, 1963.

Zangwill, O. L. Comments. Mental Sequelae of Head Injury. *Proc. R. Soc. Med.*, 59, 266, 1966.

Chapter 5

INJURY TO CRANIAL NERVES AND OPTIC CHIASM

W. BRYAN JENNETT, M.D., F.R.C.S.

Cranial nerve injury usually occurs at some point on the intracranial course of the nerves along the skull base but may involve central connections in the brain stem or the extracranial course in the orbit or face. The importance of recognizing this last group is that the neurological deficits to which these lesions give rise may be erroneously regarded as prima facie evidence of brain injury, whereas they may occur with injuries that are confined to the face or orbit. Intracranial involvement of the central nervous system may result from the initial injury, from subsequent local swelling, or from such specific complications as tentorial herniation secondary to intracranial hematoma or brain swelling.

Missile injuries can obviously produce any cranial nerve palsy, according to the track involved, and no specific patterns emerge. The following account applies to non-missile (blunt) head injuries.

Olfactory Nerve

Some 7 to 10 percent of most large series of injuries have anosmia, at least temporarily (Leigh, 1943; Hughes, 1964; Sumner, 1964). This may result from major injuries associated with anterior fossa fractures, which grossly damage the olfactory nerves; but half the cases of anosmia follow injuries associated with less than an hour's posttraumatic amnesia and, among these mild injuries, occipital blows that produce a contrecoup effect are quite common. In one series over a third of patients having anosmia soon after injury recovered, usually within three months; but when the posttraumatic amnesia exceeded 24 hours the anosmia almost always persisted (Sumner, 1964). Recovery usually occurred within three months and was complete; but late recoveries were recorded even after years; and some patients suffered parosmia, a distortion of normal olfactory sensation.

Anosmia may rightly form the basis of a claim for damages both because of the loss of pleasure and on account of the danger of failing to recognize potential hazards such as leaking domestic gas or the smell of burning; in certain occupations the loss may be a serious disability. For these reasons, and the fact that permanent anosmia may follow quite mild injury, the testing of the sense of smell assumes great importance. An investigation has shown that several of the traditional test odors are inconsistently recognized by normal subjects (Sumner, 1962); the most reliable are coffee, benzaldehyde (almond), tar, and oil of lemon. Loss of taste is frequently complained of, and anosmic patients certainly lose much of the flavor of food; but testing will show trigeminal taste intact, that is, salt and vinegar; and pungent odors such as ammonia are still appreciated.

Optic Nerve and Chiasm

The commonest site of injury involving the optic nerve seems to be the optic canal. The mechanism may be vascular rather than compressive because an inferior altitudinal hemianopia is usual, similar to that often produced by vascular disease. A fracture into the canal is rarely seen; sometimes the head injury has been quite mild with no loss of consciousness, especially in children. Loss of vision occurs immediately and, if this is complete, loss of light reflex also; within three weeks pallor of the disc may be obvious. A more anteriorly placed lesion (in the orbit) may be associated with thread-like fundal vessels, again suggesting a vascular component. When the chiasm is involved bitemporal hemianopia is common, or one blind eye and temporal hemianopia in the other; there may be CSF rhinorrhea (via sphenoidal sinus) and pituitary insufficiency may declare itself due to damage to the gland or stalk. Chiasmal lesions are occasionally delayed in onset, and only in such circumstances is exploration justified. The more anterior lesions are maximal at onset, and if recovery is to occur it begins in a few days; even a little recovery within 48 hours justifies an optimistic outlook. *

Oculomotor Nerves

These nerves are involved in some 5 percent of injuries. Orbital injuries may damage nerves and muscles, whilst mechanical displace-

---

* The optic nerves, chiasm, proximal optic tracts, and posterior half of the eyes of 84 patients with closed head injuries were examined at necropsy by Crompton (*Brain*, 93, 785, 1970). Mainly shearing lesions and ischemic necrosis of the optic nerves and chiasm were found. (Eds.)

ment of the globe due to fracture of the orbital walls may cause diplopia without there being any disorder of eye movements. All three nerves may be involved in fractures of the superior orbital fissure, or in lesions of the cavernous sinus (carotico-cavernous fistula). Brain-stem lesions cause complex disorders of conjugate movement, gaze palsies, or convergent spasm; these may occur in isolation after relatively mild injuries and hysteria may be suspected, so bizarre are the movements, but they usually disappear within a few weeks as a rule (Jefferson, 1961). Loss of upward gaze alone, associated with a mild degree of ptosis, results from pressure on the tectal plate of a bilateral posterior tentorial hernia, commonly due to chronic subdural hematoma; that part of the third nerve nucleus which controls upward movement is most dorsally placed in the midbrain.

More often a unilateral tentorial hernia, due to a rapidly developing extradural or acute subdural hematoma, damages one third nerve trunk and, at postmortem examination, distortion of the nerve and hemorrhage into it may be seen. This accounts for the dilated pupil so characteristic of rapid compression; since the patient is usually in coma by this time the other functions of the third nerve cannot be tested but, if prompt surgical evacuation of the clot leads to recovery of consciousness, ptosis and limited upward and inward movement of that eye may become obvious, even after the pupil has returned to normal. Occasionally the movement fails to recover completely, diplopia is a continuing complaint, and a muscle operation may eventually be required. Isolated third nerve lesions also occur from orbital fissure injuries, and recovery is common. If a third nerve lesion is detected soon after injury it should be recorded to avoid its being misinterpreted later as evidence of developing compression and tentorial herniation.

The sixth nerve alone may be affected by petrous fractures which may also cause facial paralysis. Bilateral sixth nerve palsies may develop due to raised intracranial pressure from various complications.

Nystagmus is usually the result of vestibular damage but may occur with cerebellar or brain-stem injury.

Trigeminal Nerve

Infraorbital sensory loss is common in maxillary fractures, due to involvement of the fifth (trigeminal) nerve in the floor of the orbit; less often the supraorbital nerve is affected. Only occasionally does a petrous fracture or carotico-cavernous fistula involve the fibers intra-

164

cranially, and then facial pain or dysesthesia may result as well as sensory loss.

Facial Nerve

Petrous fractures, manifested frequently by bleeding from the ear or by post-auricular ecchymosis (Battle's sign) are quite often associated with facial palsy; but in 40 percent of palsies no fracture can be identified. In 10 percent the palsy is delayed in onset by a few days, usually in patients with severe head injury and fracture. Occasionally the delayed development of paralysis indicates the onset of otitis media or even meningitis, but more often is due to edema. Steroids have been shown to reduce the incidence of delayed palsies if given soon after injury when a petrous fracture is found (Potter, 1967). Almost all patients with delayed palsy recover, as do most of those with immediate palsy and no special measures are called for. Facial paralysis may result from extracranial damage caused by lacerations in the parotid region or fracture of the neck of the mandible, and the outlook is then less favorable as the branches involved may have been completely severed.

Acoustic Nerve

This is probably the most commonly damaged nerve of all, figures of over 8 percent being quoted. However, there are difficulties in distinguishing between nerve damage and direct injury to the end organs (cochlea and ossicles and the vestibular apparatus) which appear to suffer some degree of damage even in quite mild concussions. An investigation of a large series of patients still complaining of vertigo from several weeks to several months after injury, and in whom conventional neurologic examination revealed no abnormality, has shown clear evidence of vestibular and cochlear damage in over 50 percent (Toglia, 1969). This finding suggests that the persisting dizziness and hyperacusis so commonly complained of after mild injuries has an organic basis. Such damage may be revealed only by formal neuro-otological testing which includes inducing nystagmus by change of position and by caloric stimulation; both the effect of these maneuvres and the analysis of the nystagmus is more easily measured by electro-nystagmography which also enables nystagmus to be recorded with the eyes closed or in a darkened room with fixation abolished.

165

Most of the patients with obvious deafness have middle-ear damage, with hemotympanum; the deafness may recover as blood is absorbed. However, one in four has associated facial palsy, and one in five CSF otorrhea. Gross inner-ear damage is less common, and is often associated with middle-ear involvement also; the fracture line in such instances is often continued down from the vault. Once the stage of bleeding and CSF leakage is over, it may be possible to distinguish between conductive deafness due to middle-ear damage, and nerve deafness due to inner-ear damage; the sound of a tuning fork on the forehead is localized to the ear affected by conductive deafness, but is heard in the normal ear if there is nerve involvement. Pure tone audiometry will establish the extent of the deafness, and may indicate whether damage is conductive, in the end organ, or in the central nervous connection.

Glossopharyngeal, Vagus, Accessory, and Hypoglossal Nerves

These four cranial nerves are almost never involved in blunt injuries. Those cases reported are either freak penetrations by sharp objects or missile injuries, and no consistent pattern emerges.

REFERENCES

Hughes, B. In G. F. Rowbotham, *Acute Injuries of the Head*. 4th ed. Edinburgh: Livingstone, 1964.

Jefferson, A. Ocular Complications of Head Injuries. *Trans. Ophthal. Soc. U. K.*, *81*, 595, 1961.

Leigh, A. D. Defects of Smell after Head Injury. *Lancet*, *1*, 438, 1943.

Potter, J. M. Prevention of Delayed Tramautic Facial Palsy. *Br. Med. J.*, *4*, 464, 1967.

Sumner, D. Testing the Sense of Smell. *Lancet*, *2*, 896, 1962.

Sumner, D. Post-traumatic Anosmia. *Brain*, *87*, 107, 1964.

Toglia, J. U. Dizziness after Whiplash Injury of the Neck and Closed Head Injury. In E. A. Walker, W. F. Caveness, and M. Critchley (Eds.), *The Late Effects of Head Injury*. Springfield, Ill.: Charles C Thomas, 1969. Pp. 72-83.

CHAPTER 6

EFFECTS OF HEAD INJURY ON METABOLISM AND OTHER ORGAN SYSTEMS

ROBERT L. McLAURIN, M. D.

AND

LIONEL R. KING, M. D.

Injury to the brain cannot be treated as an isolated event but must be considered in its proper physiological setting. Since management of most head injuries is non-surgical, it follows that appropriate treatment consists mainly of establishing and supporting the optimum milieu to promote recovery of the damaged brain. It is essential, therefore, that the secondary effects of the injury on other organ and metabolic systems be recognized. The following discussion summarizes the present knowledge regarding such secondary effects and includes recommendations for recognition and treatment.

During the past three decades a considerable body of information has been developed defining the metabolic and physiologic sequelae of acute trauma. In many respects the effects of head injury are similar to those that occur after other bodily trauma but may differ only in degree. However, certain effects of craniocerebral trauma appear to be unique (e.g., pituitary damage) and these areas need further exploration.

SYSTEMIC METABOLISM

Fluid and Electrolytes

Awareness of the normal responses of water and electrolyte metabolism following head injury is essential for at least two reasons: it allows the physician to maintain an internal milieu which is most consistent with recovery of the injured brain, and it permits recognition of excessive metabolic response which may simulate posttraumatic hematoma or may compound the neural damage. This section will summarize briefly the present knowledge of metabolic responses and then describe the pathophysiology and manifestations of excessive reactions.

167

Water retention for a variable number of days is a normal metabolic sequel to bodily trauma as well as to head injury. The retention results primarily from release of antidiuretic hormone from the hypothalamico-hypophyseal system. LeQuesne (1955), one of the early investigators of water and salt metabolism after bodily trauma, noted that primary water retention was the most consistent metabolic event. The period of water retention is characterized by low urine output, high specific gravity, and high urine electrolyte concentration. The volume of urine output during this retention period, therefore, is not an index of the adequacy of hydration. The water retention may be considered to be "inappropriate" since it is not a response to osmotic or volume receptors and may lead to hypotonicity of the body fluids. In most instances the retention is of no clinical significance and gradually recedes during the first three to four days after head injury. A definite temporal relationship has been noted between the period of water retention and that of sodium retention althougth the two responses are probably not etiologically related (King et al, 1965).

Sodium retention, a normal response after bodily trauma, has also been found to occur after craniocerebral injury. The mechanism by which this occurs involves stimulation of the hypothalamus which leads to release of ACTH and consequent aldosterone secretion. The period of sodium retention is variable and appears to be related directly to the severity of the head injury. Retention has been arbitrarily defined as excretion of less than 50 percent of the administered sodium. Using this criterion, the retention period is usually between two and four days with a mean of about three days. It is, therefore, usually concomitant with water retention despite the completely separate endocrine pathways of control. The severity of retention as well as its duration is subject to variation — patterns of progressively increasing retention have been observed in some patients while maximum initial retention followed by abrupt cessation has been noted in others. It has been postulated that sodium retention following head injury is actually a combination of two separate mechanisms, an initial one involving renal hemodynamics and a later adrenal response. The variability of pattern may, therefore, reflect different combinations of these mechanisms.

Although there seems to be a relationship between general severity of head trauma and sodium retention, there is no agreement about a relationship to the location of injury. Although Sweet et al (1948) attributed disturbances of salt metabolism to frontal lobe damage, this has not been found by other observers. Experimentally, however, the hypothalamus, the brain stem, the caudal diencephalon, and the sub-

168

commissural organ have been implicated in salt metabolism (Gilbert and Glaser, 1961).

A consistent observation after head injury is lack of correlation between serum sodium and the occurrence of sodium retention. Despite active retention, the serum sodium is usually found to be 130-135 mEq/L during the first few days after injury. The mechanism of the mild hyponatremia may be due to shift of sodium into cells, relatively excessive water retention, variations of sodium deposits in bone, or a combination of these factors. Whatever the mechanism, it is noteworthy that mild posttraumatic hyponatremia is not indicative of depletion of body sodium and a need for more vigorous sodium administration.

The principal hazard of posttraumatic metabolic responses is the occasional occurrence of an excessive reaction which may result in profound metabolic and intracranial imbalance. One such reaction was originally termed the "cerebral salt wasting syndrome" (Peters et al, 1950). It is characterized by excessive sodium excretion and hyponatremia. The basic defect, however, is in water balance rather than salt metabolism. Hypotonicity of the body fluids occurs as a consequence of the administration of excessive amounts of hypotonic fluids or of a sustained ("inappropriate") release of ADH. This prolonged release may result from the original intracranial trauma accompanied by an accentuated response secondary to mechanical positive pressure respiration. The result of hypotonicity is frank water intoxication if it occurs sufficiently rapidly. This may be characterized by changes in consciousness, proceeding to delirium and coma with convulsions, elevation of CSF pressure, and decreased frequency and voltage of EEG activity. The symptoms may be indistinguishable from those of posttraumatic hematoma. It is imperative that water intoxication be prevented or promptly treated. Prevention can be achieved easily by administration of salt to the daily intravenous fluid allotment while treatment includes water deprivation and/or administration of hypertonic saline.

The opposite metabolic excess is "cerebral salt retention", or "neurogenic hypernatremia" (Higgins et al, 1951) characterized by hypernatremia and hyponatruria. Again the basic defect is referable to water metabolism and involves dehydration. Such dehydration may result from diabetes insipidus, decrease of thirst due to clouding of consciousness or disturbed osmoreceptors, inadequate fluid administration, or prolonged use of urea or high-protein feeding. The effects of hypertonicity, like those of hypotonicity, may present as neurologic symptoms. Awareness of this syndrome leads to prevention through adequate water intake or to early recognition and correction.

Potassium deficits immediately after head injury have been minimal provided there was no extrarenal loss. This may be due to the contribution of a negative nitrogen balance to potassium input (3 mEq potassium per gram of nitrogen lost). Calcium, phosphorus, and magnesium balances have received little attention in head injury patients. We found the losses of these minerals to be minimal and of no consequence unless the total nutritional input of the patient was solely intravenous fluids for long periods of time.

Nitrogen and Calories

Increased nitrogen loss has been recognized for several decades as an essential part of the metabolic response to trauma. Physical inactivity and inadequate nutritional intake in the immediate posttrauma period as well as age, sex, and previous nutritional state of the patient make varying contributions. Increased catabolism from hormones released by the neuroendocrine response to trauma are important although this same response includes anabolic hormones as well. Currently the major source of nitrogen loss is thought to be skeletal muscle protein, and not liver, plasma protein, or autolysis of damaged tissue as previously believed.

Clinical observations in general trauma suggest that the degree of nitrogen loss relates to the degree of trauma. Such a relationship has not been demonstrated in craniocerebral trauma but this may reflect difficulty in defining grades of damage in head-injured patients.

In balance studies carried out in this clinic the range of nitrogen loss was quite wide, 4.6 to 26.5 grams a day (29 to 160 grams protein) with an average loss of 10.6 grams/day (66 grams protein) for periods up to 10 days which is about the same as that incurred following general body trauma (McLaurin, 1966 a). Although damage to a specific area of the brain could not be correlated with the magnitude of nitrogen loss, there was an indication that intracranial surgery for removal of hematomas or severely damaged brain tissue caused a reduction in urinary nitrogen loss. This would suggest that a continuing stressful stimulus was removed and the convalescence of the patient hastened.

There is evidence that nitrogen utilization rate is not diminished after trauma, but that nitrogen utilization becomes inefficient because of inadequate caloric intake (*Nutr. Rev.*, 24, 193, 1966). Our studies and others suggest that 250-300 calories per gram nitrogen with a nitrogen intake of 10-15 grams/day (62 to 92 grams protein) should keep the majority of patients in nitrogen equilibrium. This should be easy enough to achieve with current techniques of intravenous hyperalimentation or with tube feedings in suitable patients. High protein, high caloric intake in some patients may precipitate hyperglycemia or azotemia if attention is not directed to fluid balance and insulin requirements (McLaurin, 1966 b).

Following the first few days of observation and treatment of intracranial complication, adequate nutrition of the head-injured patient becomes of primary importance. We were able to correlate nitrogen loss with the length of hospitalization. This may merely indicate muscle loss due to hemiparesis and inactivity as well as the difficulty of maintaining nutrition in a semi-comatose or uncooperative patient who is likely to develop secondary complications of pneumonia, genitourinary tract infections, and gastroenteric bleeding.

In the early post-injury period attention should be directed to prevention and treatment of respiratory complications (vide infra) and fluid and electrolyte problems. Our clinical estimations for minimum daily maintenance in an adult patient who does not have any extrarenal losses are: water 2000-2500 cc, sodium 80-100 mEq, and potassium 30-40 mEq. In a patient who was adequately nourished previous to injury, a short period of caloric and nitrogen deficit is not detrimental. After the first few days, especially in the severely injured, 10-12 grams of nitrogen (62-75 grams of protein) and 2800 calories should be added to the daily regimen. In the late convalescent phase caloric requirements can be reduced to 150 cal/gram nitrogen.

Neuroendocrine and Intermediary Metabolism

Clinical evidence of dysfuntion of the hypothalamus or pituitary gland following head injury is unusual aside from diabetes insipidus. Although isolated case reports of hypothalamic obesity, hypercholesterolemia, persistent hyperosmolarity, and hypopituitarism do appear periodically, the overall incidence is minimal in view of the large number of head injuries that occur. There is ample autopsy evidence, however, that pituitary damage following fatal head injury is quite common (Kornblum and Fisher, 1969). Whether survivors have no damage or subclinical damage is conjectural.

The effect of hypothalamic-pituitary injury on endocrine changes which have been demonstrated to occur following general body trauma is unknown. Evidence for increased activity of antidiuretic hormone, cortisol, aldosterone, catecholamines, growth hormone, and prolactin has been accumulated. The stimulus for release of most of these hormones

171

is mediated via the hypothalamus. In spite of the fact that secretion of FSH and LH appear to be inhibited, and TSH secretion seems to be unchanged, the testes and thyroid glands as well as the pituitary and adrenal glands can be shown to increase in weight following injury (Chatterjee et al, 1970). Whether this endocrine response would be exaggerated following injury to the head or whether it would be hindered cannot be answered at this time because of paucity of data. Theoretically, head injury with its damage to the higher regulatory centers should exhibit unique disturbances in intermediary metabolism and the hormones which affect it. We have not been able to demonstrate this except possibly with growth hormone which appears to have a paradoxical response to glucose loading after head injury (Knowles).

In a study of plasma cortisol levels after head injury, it was found that these levels were much higher than those reported in elective surgery, remained elevated for several days after injury, and were still elevated as long as four months later in patients with neurological deficits and extracranial complications (King et al, 1970). The persisting high levels may contribute to the marked catabolic response seen after some head injuries. The circadian rhythm of cortisol secretion was abolished post-injury and frequently was not yet present even when normal plasma levels had been attained. Finer regulation of ACTH release may be at fault for long periods after a head-injured patient has apparently returned to his previous level of function. In two separate series of head-injured patients who presented no evidence of endocrine dysfunction to ordinary clinical examination, about one-third demonstrated poor ACTH response to administration of Metapyrone. These patients had been unconscious for a longer period of time than those who gave a normal response. In addition, some of those with limited ACTH reserve had no suppression of their basal ACTH secretion when given dexamethasone (McCarthy et al, 1964; Rinne, 1966).

Acute effects of head injury on intermediary metabolism have not been studied extensively. Transient glucose intolerance was found to be present immediately post-injury in monkeys receiving a standardized head injury (Lewis et al, 1969). The degree of intolerance could not be related to the degree of injury as measured by clinical observation. Glucose tolerance had returned to pretrauma levels by the third post-injury day.

In patients with varying degrees of head injury studied three to five days after trauma and serially thereafter, it was demonstrated that glucose intolerance as estimated by glucose disappearance rate from blood was present in all patients but the degree of glucose intolerance could not be correlated with the degree of injury. Glucose tolerance did improve, however, as the injury became more remote in time. The fasting blood sugar level and mean post-loading blood glucose level were statistically higher in those with more severe grades of trauma. Plasma immunoreactive insulin was higher, both fasting and post-glucose loading, in patients with mild trauma only. Those with more severe grades of trauma had lower fasting levels of immunoreactive insulin and decreased response to glucose loading. As the patient progressed in time from the injury, the post-glucose plasma insulin levels became more normal. The changes in carbohydrate metabolism seem to relate more to trauma than to head injury per se (King et al, 1971).

Free fatty acid mobilization is an integral part of the neuroendocrine response to trauma as well as other forms of stress. Although this phenomenon has been studied following experimental trauma, a recent review of the literature failed to uncover studies of free fatty acid response in human accident victims (Warner, 1969). Lipid metabolism will undoubtedly be disturbed following head injury, but its exact characterization awaits further study. One important aspect of fatty acid mobilization during stress is the tendency for fatty acids to cause intravascular thrombosis. Recent studies have shown that patients with severe brain trauma manifest hypercoagulable blood to a greater degree than patients with multiple injuries exclusive of central nervous system involvement (Attar et al, 1969).

Acid-Base Balance

Different types of acid-base disturbances have been observed in patients who had sustained general bodily trauma. In a series of general surgery patients, 64 percent were found to have an alkalosis in the postoperative period (Lyons and Moore, 1966). The majority of these patients were being mechanically ventilated; transfusion alkalosis, hypoxia, and endogenous adrenal steroid effects were thought to be factors as well. In a large group of severely wounded combat casualties, metabolic acidosis was present in those with hypotension (Collins et al, 1970). The degree of acidosis correlated well with the degree of hypotension. Those with injuries to the extremities had hyperventilation to the extent that respiratory alkalosis was present in 34 percent.

Cook et al (1961) in an early survey of head-injured patients found no survivors among those with acid-base disturbances. The overwhelming majority had respiratory acidosis or a mixed metabolic and respiratory acidosis. In a later report from the same clinic 75 percent of patients with severe head injury had respiratory alkalosis (Huang et al, 1963). The difference in the incidence of respiratory alkalosis in the two studies may relate to the fact that in the later study tracheostomy was done frequently and more attention paid to tracheobronchial toilet. In these patients, survival time depended not only on degree of acid-base imbalance but also on degree of oxygen saturation and magnitude of abnormalities of ventilation.

Our experience with severe head injuries indicates that soon after injury most patients have an arterial pH that is normal or slightly acidotic. Usually within the first 24 hours a respiratory alkalosis develops. Soon after injury urinary excretion of hydrogen ion is elevated, but then progressively decreases due to a decrease in both titratable acidity and urinary ammonia with an increase in urinary bicarbonate. This suggests that early after injury a mixed respiratory alkalosis and metabolic acidosis are present and that with supportive therapy (fluids and correction of hypoxia) the metabolic acidosis may remit and the respiratory alkalosis be "unmasked."

Brain-injured patients usually have a decrease in cerebrospinal fluid pCO_2, pH and bicarbonate ion concentration with an increase in CSF lactate and pyruvate concentration (Zupping, 1970). These changes are consistent with a metabolic acidosis in the CSF, which seems to be severe soon after injury and gradually returns to normal over a period of days, especially in those who recover. The severity of the CSF metabolic acidosis relates to the severity of the head injury and seems dependent on the amount of lactate produced by the injured and hypoxic brain tissue. It has been suggested that the level of CSF lactate can be used as a measure of gross brain damage because those patients with a concentration in excess of 3 mM/liter (27 mg%) usually do not survive (Kurze et al, 1966). The CSF lactate correlates poorly with the arterial lactate. There is, however, an excellent inverse correlation between the elevation of CSF lactate and the depression of CSF bicarbonate ion (Katsurada et al, 1969). The latter is easier to determine and could be used to judge severity of injury in place of lactate.

RESPIRATORY SYSTEM

During the past decade considerable progress has been made in understanding respiratory pathophysiology and the management of ventilatory problems following head injury. It is essential that the principles of respiratory abnormalities be understood since they not only constitute the most common cause of death in patients who survive

174

48 hours after injury but they also lead to a compounding of the cerebral damage as a result of hypoxia. It is appropriate, therefore that, pulmonary insufficiency after head injury be considered in a discussion of metabolic disturbances.

Certain patterns of ventilation have been defined in relation to specific areas of damage to the central nervous system (Plum and Posner, 1966). One type of respiratory pattern commonly seen after head injury is central neurogenic hyperventilation, in which the damage is apparently at the pontine level. This hyperventilation leads to hypocarbia and is not altered by exposure to 100 percent oxygen, indicating that hypoxemia is not responsible for the hyperventilation. Cheyne-Stokes respiration, characterized by regular alternating periods of hyper- and hypoventilation, results from increased sensitivity of the respiratory mechanism to hypercarbia and the occurrence of post-hyperventilation apnea. This pattern of respiration is not commonly seen after acute head injury but is presumed to result from bilateral supramedullary brain injury. A third pattern of respiration which may occur after trauma is an "ataxic" respiratory effort characterized by irregular rate, rhythm, and volume. It is due to damage to the medullary respiratory centers, is associated with hypoxemia, and is an ominous prognostic sign.

In experimental animals, uncomplicated cerebral concussion produces transient apnea but no other respiratory abnormalities occur. In addition, there is no significant change in blood and CSF pH, pCO_2, and pO_2. It was postulated (Grubb et al, 1970) that any further ventilatory or acid-base changes are due to secondary effects arising from pulmonary complications or the epiphenomena of head injury which result in increased intracranial pressure. Increased intracranial pressure alone, however, produces neither transient apnea nor the prolonged hyperventilation seen clinically (Moody et al, 1969).

Head injury, like other trauma, leads to an initial period of hyperventilation, which is to be distinguished from the very rapid shallow respiration that results from specific local brain-stem damage (Moore et al, 1969). This early hyperventilation results in hypocarbia and mild respiratory alkalosis. It is characterized by high tidal volumes, some increased respiratory rate, and true alveolar hyperventilation.

Despite the existence of hypocarbia during this initial hyperventilation, hypoxemia is nearly always present to some degree. The hypoxemia results from impaired ventilation-perfusion relationships. These ventilation-perfusion abnormalities are associated with increased physiologic dead-space and increased physiologic shunting (increased alveolar-arterial oxygen tension difference). Aspiration of gastric contents, which may occur routinely early after head injury, may contribute to the increased alveolar-arterial gradient. Thus, the existence of impaired ventilation-perfusion relationships will preclude normal oxygenation regardless of the drive which leads to hyperventilation. Although correction of hypoxemia does not correct the ventilatory pattern, it still must be the objective of pulmonary care.

The importance of prevention or correction of hypoxemia is apparent, since it may contribute further damage to the brain which has already been compromised by mechanical impact. The need to correct hypocarbia and alkalosis, however, remains debatable. While hypocarbia is useful as an adjunct to intracranial surgery because it decreases brain volume by vasoconstriction, it is not certain whether the cerebral vessels are responsive to CO_2 changes following trauma and whether vasoconstriction is advisable. In this connection, it is noteworthy that hypocarbia and alkalosis may be responsible for alterations of cerebral function seen in traumatized patients without head injury. Some of these cerebral effects may be the result of a shift of the oxyhemoglobin dissociation curve toward the left as pH rises. This leads to a higher oxygen saturation in the venous blood and, if oxygenation is borderline, the net effect may be a degree of cerebral hypoxia. Vasospasm resulting from hypocarbia will accentuate the condition.

Following the stage of hyperventilation, hypocarbia, and alkalosis the patient usually demonstrates progressive pulmonary insufficiency, if he remains unconscious, and unless vigorous respiratory support is rendered. This stage is characterized by an increasing alveolar-arterial gradient and the need for administration of greater concentrations of oxygen. As respiration is either assisted or controlled by mechanical devices, hypocarbia usually persists but alkalosis may be supplanted by metabolic acid-base imbalance. The pulmonary insufficiency results from a combination of factors, including aspiration pneumonitis, bacterial pneumonia, pulmonary emboli, pulmonary edema, and possible chest trauma. Management during this phase requires frequent cleansing of the upper respiratory passage, use of endotracheal intubation or tracheostomy, careful avoidance of bacterial contamination of the tracheobronchial tree, and judicious use of oxygen and mechanical respiratory support. The toxicity of 100 percent oxygen is now clearly recognized. Because arterial blood gases do not reflect the cerebral environment as accurately as do the CSF gases, it may, in the future, be advisable to adjust ventilator therapy on the CSF pH and pCO_2 (Gordon and Rossanda, 1968).

Pertinent to a discussion of ventilation control by mechanical respirators is a consideration of the related factor of "inappropriate secretion of antidiuretic hormone." It has been noted that a significant number of patients on prolonged mechanical ventilation show evidence of water retention (Sladen et al, 1968). The pathophysiology of this phenomenon is presumed to involve a decrease of pulmonary blood volume and left atrial pressure due to the positive pressure respiration. Decrease of afferent impulses from the stretch receptors of these structures leads to increased output of ADH and consequent water retention. This, in turn, may contribute to hypotonicity of body fluids and to the resulting cerebral swelling. In addition, the excess water contributes to pulmonary failure by addition of extravascular pulmonary water and increasing alveolar-arterial oxygen gradient.

The syndrome of water retention can best be detected by frequent weighing of the patient and careful assessment of fluid balance. In calculating fluid intake it must be remembered that the nebulizer may contribute as much as 500 ml per day. Moreover, it is expected that a patient with little or no caloric intake should lose about 400 grams per day and that failure to lose this amount means water retention.

CARDIOVASCULAR SYSTEM

The effects of brain stimulation on cardiovascular function have been generally acknowledge for some time. The occurrence of cardiovascular changes in the head-injured patient and the application of therapeutic regimens based on this knowledge, have not been as widely recognized. Abnormalities in the electrocardiogram described in intracranial disease are large T waves, prominent U waves and prolonged QT or QU intervals (Abildskov, 1970). The T waves may have normal or abnormal polarity. These changes are due to direct effect of altered autonomic tone on functional alteration of ventricular recovery time. In one series (Millar and Abildskov, 1968) a high incidence of notched T waves was found suggesting asymmetric alteration of sympathetic tone resulting in two populations of ventricular recovery times. Increased height of P wave has also been described (Hersch, 1961). Arrhythmias include sinus arrhythmias with wandering pacemaker, atrial fibrillation, and ventricular tachycardia. Whether myocardial damage contributes to the EKG changes is not settled (vide infra) although the frequency of EKG change exceeds that of myocardial damage. These persistent EKG changes are quite different from the transient changes described

177

immediately after experimental concussion, i.e., bradycardia, shortened Q-Tc, and S-T segment elevation (Fernando et al, 1969).

Pathological changes in the myocardium have been described (Connor, 1968) in patients with intracranial disease. This was originally noted in subarachnoid hemorrhage although it has been described to a lesser extent in head injury. Focal myocytolysis was found at autopsy in 2 percent of those dying from head injury. A milder form of myocardial damage, fuchsinophilic degeneration, was described in 6 percent of head-injured patients in another series (Connor, 1970). Survival in these patients was less (2.8 days) than in those dying with focal myocytolysis (6 days). Myocardial damage varying from hyalinization of cytoplasm with loss of striations to widespread areas of myocardial degeneration and necrosis has been produced in mice by intracranial injection of whole blood. Histochemical staining showed depletion of succinic and B-hydroxybutyric dehydrogenase activity in the myofibers (Burch et al, 1967).

Functional myocardial changes described in patients with head injury (Brown et al, 1967) included increased heart rate and stroke index, reduced stroke work, and central venous pressure lower than in healthy controls. Cardiac index, arterial pressure, peripheral resistance, and central blood volume were not different from control subjects. Intracranial pressure was correlated positively with cardiac output and inversely with total peripheral resistance. When these studies were repeated following recovery, the changes had returned to normal suggesting a functional insufficiency of the ventricles immediately after head injury. Two patients with severe hypotension, normal blood volumes, but a decrease in cardiac index, central blood volume and heart rate had restoration of values to normal with sympathomimetic amines, suggesting a decrease in ventricular contractility due to the absence of endogenous sympathetic neural stimuli.

Pulmonary edema has been reported in 11-28 percent of patients with intracranial disease of all types but in almost 100 percent of battle casualties with head injury. Severe CNS stimulation sets off a massive autonomic discharge which has the following hemodynamic consequences: a) systemic vasoconstriction with increased peripheral resistance causing large amounts of blood to be shifted into the pulmonary vascular bed, and b) loss of ventricular compliance. Experimentally, in animals, as intracranial pressure is elevated there is an increase in venous return and in cardiac output leading to moderate rises in systemic and pulmonary vascular pressures. Peripheral resistance, however, may fall. Further stress causes total peripheral resistance to rise so that diastolic pressure must be maintained at higher levels to perfuse the brain. In about 20 percent of animals extreme elevations in total peripheral resistance (greater than 11,000 dyne-sec/cm 5) caused a decrease in cardiac output with distention of the left atrium and pulmonary edema (Simmons et al, 1969).

Other effects may contribute to the pulmonary edema: increased arteriovenous shunting in the lung (with arterial hypoxemia) and in the periphery (with increased venous constriction and increased volume return to the heart of acidotic blood). Persistent strong autonomic discharge results in failure of the heart to relax in diastole and hence emia all act to produce pulmonary edema (Simmons et al, 1969).

Cardiovascular complications can best be prevented by a comprehensive approach. Attention to pulmonary ventilation will reduce hyit cannot accommodate the increased venous return causing a further rise in left atrial and left centricular pressure. Thus, increased venous return, massive peripheral vasoconstriction, and loss of left ventricular compliance in combination with systemic acidosis and arterial hypoxpoxia. Because both pulmonary edema and pulmonary shunting with arterial hypoxemia relate to marked increases in intracranial pressure, therapy directed to this point should obviate these complications. In addition, the effects of autonomic discharge can be reduced by alpha-adrenergic blocking agents or bilateral stellate ganglion block (Ducker et al, 1969). Use of cardiac monitoring for detection of cardiac arrhythmias may eventually be routine in the immediate post-injury period.

GASTROINTESTINAL TRACT

The relationship between intracranial disease and gastric ulceration has been recognized for nearly two centuries. John Hunter, in 1772, reported observations on two patients who had sustained craniocerebral trauma and who at autopsy had ulceration and perforation of the gastric wall. It is noteworthy, however, that in both instances the patient died very shortly after the head injury, whereas subsequent experience has shown that the clinical evidence of ulceration rarely occurs before three days post-injury. The relationship was subsequently supported by several writers and the role of the vagus nerve was defined. Cushing, for whom the ulceration has been named, stimulated modern investigation by his lucid description of the syndrome (1932) and his suggestion that the lesion developed as a result of diencephalic activity. Since then numerous investigators have confirmed the role of autonomic impulses arising in the hypothalamus.

179

The clinical setting for gastric ulceration and hemorrhage is a patient who has sustained severe injury resulting in signs of brain-stem damage. Watts and Clark (1969) have shown that the incidence of gastric bleeding is much higher in those individuals who have posttraumatic decerebrate rigidity. The role of intracranial hypertension has not been established and it seems likely that increased pressure is neither necessary nor contributory per se. The existence of ulceration and bleeding is recognized by blood-stained or "coffee-ground" vomitus or gastric aspirate. Severe hematemesis may occur and occasionally the first clue to gastric bleeding is the onset of oligemic shock. This is particularly apt to occur in the pediatric age group. Bleeding seldom occurs before the third post-injury day or after the first week.

Watts and Clark (1969) have demonstrated the existence of gastric hyperacidity after severe head injury. The greatest secretion of acid occurred in decerebrate comatose patients. The same authors also noted a direct relationship between gastric hemorrhage and hyperacidity. Factors other than acid secretion may also play a role in the development of ulceration; gastric blood flow, cellular populations, and mucus formation may all be contributory. Leonard (1967) demonstrated that hypothalamic lesions affect each of these factors. Moreover, the hypothalamic stimulus also activates the anterior hypophysis which in turn leads to increased adrenal steroid output. This may be compounded by efforts to control cerebral edema through the use of glucocorticoids which enhance ulcer formation. Finally, increased output of catecholamines occurs after head injury and has been implicated in experimental ulcerogenesis.

Management of gastric ulceration begins with attempts at prevention. Aspiration of gastric secretion after head injury serves two purposes: prevention of aspiration pneumonitis and decrease of hyperacidity. Watts and Clark (1969) have recommended that gastric acidity be monitored in the comatose patient after head injury and that anticholinergic agents be employed if the acidity increases to pathologic levels. In this clinic, antacids and anticholinergic drugs have been used in any comatose patient who is receiving glucocorticoids. The hazard of imposing a metabolic alkalosis in a patient whose acid-base balance may already have been altered by respiratory abnormalities must be kept in mind whenever continuous gastric aspiration is employed.

REFERENCES

Abildskov, J. A. Electrocardiographic Wave Form and the Nervous System. (Editorial) *Circulation*, *41*, 371, 1970.

Anonymous. Reduction of Nitrogen Deficits in Surgical Patients Maintained by Intravenous Alimentation. *Nutr. Rev.*, *24*, 193, 1966.

Attar, S., Boyd, D., Layne, E., McLaughlin, J., Mansberger, A. R., and Cowley, R. A. Alterations in Coagulation and Fibrinolytic Mechanisms in Acute Trauma. *J. Trauma*, *9*, 939, 1969.

Brown, R. S., Mohr, P. A., Carey, J. S., and Shoemaker, W. C. Cardiovascular Changes after Craniocerebral Injury and Increased Intracranial Pressure. *Surg. Gynec. Obstet.*, *125*, 1205, 1967.

Burch, G. E., Sun, S. C., Colcolough, H. L., DePasquale, N. P., and Sobal, R. S. Acute Myocardial Lesions Following Experimentally-induced Intracranial Hemorrhage in Mice: A Histological and Histochemical Study. *Arch. Pathol.*, *84*, 517, 1967.

Chatterjee, S., Prasad, G. C., and Udupa, K. N. Changes in Endocrine Gland during Fracture Repair and Effect of their Ablation. *J. Trauma*, *10*, 890, 1970.

Collins, J. A., Simmons, R. L., James, P. M., Bredenberg, C. E., Anderson, R. W., and Heisterkamp, C. A. The Acid-free Status of Seriously Wounded Combat Casualties. I. Before Treatment. *Ann. Surg.*, *171*, 595, 1970.

Connor, R. C. R. Heart Damage Associated with Intracranial Lesions. *Br. Med. J.*, *3*, 29, 1968.

Connor, R. C. R. Fuchsinophilic Degeneration of Myocardium in Patients with Intracranial Lesions. *Br. Heart J.*, *32*, 81, 1970.

Cook, A. W., Browder, E. J., and Lyons, H. A. Alterations in Acid-base Equilibrium in Craniocerebral Trauma. *J. Neurosurg.*, *18*, 366, 1961.

Cushing, H. Peptic Ulcers and the Interbrain. *Surg. Gynec. Obstet.*, *55*, 1, 1932.

Ducker, T. B., Simmons, R. L., and Martin, A. M., Jr. Pulmonary Edema as a Complication of Intracranial Disease. *Am. J. Dis. Child.*, *118*, 638, 1969.

Fernando, O. U., Mariano, G. T., Jr., Gurdjian, E. S., and Hodgson, V. R. Electrocardiographic Patterns in Experimental Cerebral Concussion. *J. Neurosurg.*, *31*, 34, 1969.

Gilbert, G. J. and Glaser, G. H. On the Nervous System Integration of Water and Salt Metabolism. *Arch. Neurol.*, *5*, 179, 1961.

Gordon, E. and Rossanda, M. The Importance of the Cerebrospinal Fluid Acid-base Status in the Treatment of Unconscious Patients with Brain Lesions. *Acta Anaesthesiol. Scand.*, *12*, 51, 1968.

Grubb, R. L., Jr., Naumann, R. A., and Ommaya, A. K. Respiration and the Cerebrospinal Fluid in Experimental Cerebral Concussion. *J. Neurosurg.*, *32*, 320, 1970.

Hersch, C. Electrocardiographic Changes in Head Injuries. *Circulation*, *23*, 853, 1961.

Higgins, G., Lewin, W., O'Brien, J. R. P., and Taylor, W. H. Metabolic Disorders in Head Injury. *Lancet*, *1*, 1295, 1951.

181

Huang, C. T., Cook, A. W., and Lyons, H. A. Severe Craniocerebral Trauma and Respiratory Abnormalities. *Arch. Neurol.*, 9, 113, 1963.

Hunter, J. On the Digestion of the Stomach after Death. *Philosoph. Tr.*, 62, 447, 1772. (Cited by Leonard.)

Katsurada, K., Sugemoto, T., and Onji, Y. Significance of Cerebrospinal Fluid Bicarbonate Ions in the Management of Patients with Cerebral Injury. *J. Trauma*, 9, 799, 1969.

King, L. R., Knowles, H. C., Jr., McLaurin, R. L., and Lewis, H. P. Glucose Tolerance and Plasma Insulin in Cranial Trauma. *Ann. Surg.*, 173, 337, 1971.

King, L. R., McLaurin, R. L., and Knowles, H. C., Jr. The Balances of Water, Sodium, Potassium, and Nitrogen in Cranial Surgery and Trauma Estimated by Computer Analysis. *Surg. Gynec. Obstet.*, 120, 761, 1965.

King, L. R., McLaurin, R. L., Lewis, H. P., and Knowles, H. C., Jr., Plasma Cortisol Levels after Head Injury. *Ann. Surg.*, 172, 975, 1970.

Knowles, H. C., Jr. Personal communication.

Kornblum, R. N. and Fisher, R. S. Pituitary Lesions in Craniocerebral Injuries. *Arch. Pathol.*, 88, 242, 1969.

Kurze, T., Tranquada, R. E., and Benedict, K. Spinal Fluid Lactic Acid Levels in Acute Cerebral Injury. Pp. 254-259. In W. F. Caveness and A. E Walker (Eds.), *Head Injury.* Philadelphia: J. B. Lippincott Co., 1966. P. 589.

Leonard, A. S. Neuroendocrine Influences on Gastric Secretory Factors and Ulcer Formation. Pp. 133-163. In E. Bajusz. *An Introduction to Clinical Neuroendocrinology.* Basel/New York: S. Karger, 1967. P. 573.

LeQuesne, L. P. *Fluid Balance in Surgical Practice,* (1st ed.). Chicago: The Year Book Publishers, Inc., 1955.

Lewis, H. P., King, L. R., Ramirez, R., Brielmaier, J., and McLaurin, R. L. Glucose Intolerance in Monkeys Following Head Injury. *Ann. Surg.*, 170, 1025, 1969.

Lyons, J. H., Jr., and Moore, F. D. Posttraumatic Alkaloses: Incidence and Pathophysiology of Alkalosis in Surgery. *Surgery,* 60, 93, 1966.

McCarthy, C. F., Wills, M. R., Keane, P. M., Gough, K. R., and Read, A. E. The SU-4885 (Methopyrapone) Response after Head Injury. *J. Clin. Endocr. Metab.*, 24, 121, 1964.

McLaurin, R. L. Some Metabolic Aspects of Head Injury. Pp. 142-157 in W. F. Caveness and A. E. Walker (Eds.), *Head Injury.* Philadelphia: J. B. Lippincott Co., 1966a. P. 589.

McLaurin, R. L. Metabolic Changes Accompanying Head Injury. *Clin. Neurosurg.*, 12, 143, 1966b.

Millar, K., and Abildskov, J. A. Notched T Waves in Young Persons with Central Nervous System Lesions. *Circulation,* 37, 597, 1968.

Moody, R. A., Ruamsuke, S., and Mullan, S. Experimental Effects of Acutely Increased Intracranial Pressure on Respiration and Blood Gases. *J. Neurosurg.*, 30, 482, 1969.

Moore, F. D., Lyons, J. H., Jr., Pierce, E. C., Jr., Morgan, A. P. Jr., Drinker, P. A., MacArthur, J. D., and Dammin, G. J. *Posttraumatic Pulmonary Insufficiency.* Philadelphia: W. B. Saunders Co., 1969. P. 234.

Peters, J. P., Welt, L. G., Sims, E. A. H., Orloff, J., and Needham, J. A. A Salt-wasting Syndrome Associated with Cerebral Disease. *Trans. Assoc. Am. Physicians,* 63, 57, 1950.

Plum, F., and Posner, J. B. *Diagnosis of Stupor and Coma*. Philadelphia: F. A. Davis Co., 1966. P. 197.

Rinne, U. K. Corticotrophin Secretion in Patients with Head Injuries Examined by the Metopirone Test. *Psychiatr. Neurol., 152,* 145, 1966.

Simmons, R. L., Martin, A. M., Heisterkamp, C. A. III, and Ducker, T. B. Respiratory Insufficiency in Combat Casualties: II. Pulmonary Edema Following Head Injury. *Ann. Surg., 170,* 39, 1969.

Sladen, A., Laver, M. B., and Pontoppidan, H. Pulmonary Complications and Water Retention in Prolonged Mechanical Ventilation. *New Engl. J. Med., 279,* 448, 1968.

Sweet, W. H., Cotzias, G. C., Seed, J., and Yakovlev, P. Gastrointestinal Hemorrhages, Hyperglycemia, Azotemia, Hyperchloremia, and Hypernatremia Following Lesions of the Frontal Lobe in Man. *Proc. Assoc. Res. Nerv. & Ment. Dis., 27,* 795, 1948.

Warner, W. A. Release of Free Fatty Acids Following Trauma. *J. Trauma, 9,* 692, 1969.

Watts, C. and Clark, K. Gastric Acidity in the Comatose Patient. *J. Neurosurg., 30,* 107, 1969.

Zupping, R. Cerebral Acid-base and Gas Metabolism in Brain Injury. *J. Neurosurg., 33,* 498, 1970.

CHAPTER 7

THE DIAGNOSIS AND TREATMENT OF UNCOMPLICATED HEAD TRAUMA

HARRY A. KAPLAN, M. D.

High speed travel on overcrowded highways and the congested personnel traffic of urban areas have resulted in an ever-increasing number of injuries. Casualties are usually transported by ambulance to nearby regional hospitals, some of which are large municipal or community institutions with adequate personnel and equipment for handling all types of injuries. A large number are taken to smaller hospitals without facilities for the comprehensive care of the severely injured. It is true that the majority of patients with head injuries do not require the services of a specialist; however about 12 to 15 percent do and it is important that such cases be recognized and appropriate treatment initiated as early as possible. In smaller community hospitals the initial evaluation of the majority of patients with head injury is usually made by general practitioners. Neurologists and/or neurosurgeons may serve these institutions on a consultant basis. A single visit by a neurosurgeon may be adequate if all that is needed is assurance that the patient does not require special care. In some cases, however, hour-to-hour or day-to-day observation may be essential in order not to overlook a complication such as an intracranial hematoma requiring early surgical treatment. Seldom in the smaller hospital without a neurosurgical service is a neurosurgeon available for repeated appraisal of the patient's condition. The facilities, including the necessary personnel, for proper execution of a cranial operation may not be at hand. Moreover, severely injured patients are subject to a multitude of complications for which a variety of laboratory studies are required, as well as the services of diverse specialists. Consequently, unless the hospital accepting the responsibility for the treatment of such cases is geared for total intensive care, patients with major injuries should be transferred to a facility that can cope with all the problems that may be encountered.

184

From an embryologic viewpoint the brain may be divided into five components, each having certain specific functions (Kaplan, 1966). Beginning rostrally and proceeding in a caudal direction, these components are: telencephalon, diencephalon, mesencephalon, metencephalon and myelencephalon. The most rostral component, the telencephalon, is composed of the cerebral cortex and underlying white matter, the olfactory lobe, and basal ganglia. The next segment, the diencephalon, comprises all the thalamic structures. Continuing caudally, the mesencephalon or midbrain consists of the dorsal corpora quadrigemina, a central tegmental portion and the cerebral peduncles. The metencephalon includes the cerebellum and pons. The most caudal segment is the myelencephalon or medulla oblongata.

The cerebral cortex is concerned with functions of the highest order, including vision, sensation, motor performance, speech, and intellectual activity. Depending on the region affected, focal traumatic lesions, occurring as a consequence of penetrating wounds of the head, for example, may produce varying degrees of motor or sensory deficits or disturbances referable to the speech mechanism. Injuries involving the tegmentum of the diencephalo-mesencephalic area may result in alteration of the state of awareness depending on the severity and extent of the damage. Oculomotor and pupillary changes also may occur as a consequence of midbrain injury. In some patients, damage to the midbrain may produce a state of decerebrate rigidity characterized by opisthotonus, extension of the extremities, and pronation of the hands; this posture may be augmented by sensory stimulation. Trauma to metencephalic structures is associated with disturbances of coordination and cranial nerve palsies. Injuries affecting the medulla and/or the upper cervical spinal cord, with or without concomitant cervical spine fracture, may lead to sudden death. Compression of the medulla by downward displacement (herniation) of the cerebellum, often associated with marked cerebral edema, may give rise to gasping respiration, a most ominous sign.

In determining the extent of brain damage following a blow to the head, consideration should be given primarily to the probable mechanism of injury and the clinical findings. The outstanding abnormal clinical feature in a closed head injury is the alteration of the conscious state. The phenomenon of loss of awareness following a head injury with recovery in a matter of seconds is generally referred to as cerebral concussion. Controversy still exists regarding the pathophysiology of this transitory loss of consciousness (Courville, 1953; Symonds, 1962; Taylor, 1967). Many investigators believe that morphological changes in the cerebral cells account for this altered state. In the boxing arena, it is well known that a fighter dazed by one blow to the head may be alerted by a second, less forceful blow to the same site. Professional pugilists will, therefore, throw the second punch to the abdomen in order to cause the dazed boxer to lower his guard. Then the opponent delivers the solid knockout punch to the head. This common practice of boxers who are aware of the effect of a glancing blow in alerting a dazed opponent, would suggest that a pathophysiological state develops which may be almost immediately reversible and, therefore, is not due to a morphological alteration of the cerebral cells.

Patients who have sustained a closed head injury and a disturbance in the state of awareness lasting for hours, days or weeks, as a rule exhibit changes in the brain differing from those attributed to cerebral concussion. In such cases of prolonged unconsciousness, one usually finds evidence of cerebral contusion, i.e., bruising and hemorrhagic extravasation. Patients dying as a result of head injury and who have been in coma from the moment of injury, often have contusions of the base of the frontal and rostro-mesial aspects of the temporal lobes on one or both sides of the brain. The close location of these lesions to the "seat of alertness" in the diencephalo-mesencephalic region strongly suggests concomitant involvement of structures in this area either directly or as a result of vascular changes.

Intracranial hemorrhage is a complication that may influence the state of awareness. The classical clinical syndrome of extradural hemorrhage following a blow to the head, sequentially consists of immediate loss of awareness, recovery of consciousness (lucid interval) followed by a relatively rapid dilatation of the pupil on the side of the lesion, stupor progressing to coma, hemiplegia, decerebration and, finally, death, if treatment is withheld. However, many patients with epidural clots and associated contusions at the base of the brain do not exhibit a lucid interval. The same sequence of events, extended over a longer period, may be observed with subdural hemorrhage. Deepening stupor may also be caused by intracerebral hemorrhage. It must be borne in mind that intracranial bleeding may occur concomitantly at different sites, both intra- and extracerebral. In cases which present the classic syndrome of an epidural hematoma, the immediate loss of awareness following the blow should be regarded as cerebral concussion. The lucid interval represents the time it takes the enlarging blood mass to compress the brain, and cause focal vascular insufficiency and edema.

186

The subsequent depression of consciousness, pupillary dilatation, and hemiparesis result from midbrain compression by uncal herniation secondary to the swollen hemisphere underlying the clot. Further compression is usually associated with severe hypoxia and/or hemorrhage in the midbrain causing a decerebrate state.

Increased intracranial pressure per se is not acceptable as an explanation of the abnormal neurological features, including unconsciousness, and the changes that may be observed in the vital signs of patients having sustained a head injury. The concept of increased intracranial pressure as the major causative factor for these abnormalities was initiated by the work of Kocher (1901) and Cushing (1901) shortly after the turn of the present century. These investigators based their conclusions on observations made in animals after applying varying degrees of pressure to the surface of the uninjured brain. In most instances of closed head injury in man, the major factor that accounts for alteration of the state of consciousness and of the vital signs is related to immediate or delayed injury to cell groups in the rostral brain stem (Aronson and Kaplan, 1957). Intracranial blood clots, whether extra- or intracerebral, produce increasing regional edema of the adjacent white matter and secondary compression ventro-medially, resulting in clinical features indicative of upper brain stem compression. Browder and Meyers (1938) found that a rising intracranial pressure altered the systemic blood pressure, pulse, and respiratory rate and state of consciousness only slightly until the cerebrospinal fluid pressure approached the diastolic blood pressure. A manometric estimation of intracranial pressure at the lumbar site may be extrapolated as a crude measure of the extent of the intracranial lesion and resulting edema. Removal of a part of the intracranial bulk of cerebral tissue and/or cerebrospinal fluid may, in some instances, allow an increase in cerebral blood flow with resultant improvement in the clinical state.

EXAMINATION

Physical Findings

To avoid overlooking associated injuries, often of a serious nature, which may escape a cursory scrutiny, it is of the utmost importance that the patient who has suffered head trauma be subjected to a thorough, meticulous examination, one including a detailed history and a complete investigation of his general physical and neurological status. All parts of the body must be examined and all observations carefully recorded.

Completeness aids immeasurably in the immediate assessment of the patient's problems and, in the event of multiple injuries, in deciding the order of therapeutic priority.

Surface injuries of the scalp, face and neck should be carefully examined. The significance of swellings, especially those of the upper eyelids and of the mastoid region, and of cutaneous abrasions must be determined. Bilateral orbital ecchymoses involving the upper lids and ecchymoses behind the ear are highly suggestive of basilar skull fracture. Bleeding from the nose or ears may indicate a basilar fracture but may also result from local trauma. Careful inspection of all scalp lacerations is to be made with particular reference to contour and continuity of the underlying skull. Employing sterile technique, the physician should explore the laceration digitally and view and palpate the underlying structure. Attempts should be made to estimate the site of maximal impact to the head, especially when several contusions and/or lacerations of the scalp are present. Such information is particularly useful whenever the subsequent course of events points to the likelihood of an extradural hematoma; the hematoma frequently is located directly beneath the site of maximal impact. Swelling of the scalp may assume a doughnut-like contour, especially in children, suggesting a depressed fracture of the skull. An x-ray examination with special views of the head should be made to verify such a diagnosis. A large boggy swelling of the scalp, especially in young children, occurring in conjuction with a pallid skin (anemia) and a fast pulse indicates a probable extradural hematoma (Ingraham et al, 1949). Hooper (1954) has reported the frequent association of extradural hematoma of the posterior fossa with trauma involving the back of the head, the site of injury being indicated by a local contusion or laceration. A boggy swelling of the entire scalp, particularly over the vertex in young children, suggests a fracture with disruption of the dura and arachnoid and seepage of cerebrospinal fluid. Thin bloody fluid escaping from the nose (rhinorrhea) or from the external auditory canal (otorrhea) indicates a compound fracture of the frontal fossa or of the petrosal portion of the temporal bone respectively.

Proptosis may be caused by a retrobulbar hemorrhage or a carotid-cavernous fistula. Auscultation of the head, routinely performed, may reveal a bruit and thereby establish the diagnosis of a fistulous communication.

The size of the pupils should be measured in millimeters and their reaction to light recorded. Every effort should be made to visualize the optic fundi. One must be mindful of the fact that pupillary changes may be the result of direct injury of the eye, as well as trauma involving the optic or oculomotor nerves. Mydriatics should not be used lest important pupillary changes that may occur at a later date be obscured. Testing of the corneal reflex may aid in the estimation of the patient's conscious level, as well as in determining the function of the fifth and seventh cranial nerves. Any asymmetry of the face should be noted. Vigorous movement of the neck is to be avoided. This admonition applies especially to stuporous patients with abrasions of the forehead; not infrequently, it is later found that such patients have sustained both cerebral trauma and fracture of the cervical spine.

One next proceeds to examine the trunk and limbs. All bony elements including the clavicles, ribs, pelvis, spine, and those of the limbs are carefully palpated. Ecchymoses in the suprapubic or perineal regions may be indicative of a pelvic fracture. The chest and abdomen must be examined for possible visceral injury or hemorrhage — lesions frequently responsible for surgical shock.

If the patient is unable to void, a catheter should be inserted into the bladder and the urinary output measured. Hematuria signifies trauma involving some portion of the urinary tract. Rectal examination may disclose the presence of fresh blood or, rarely, palpable evidence of extraperitoneal hemorrhage. The posture of the limbs and mobility of the joints should be noted. One must also be on the lookout for circulatory or peripheral nerve injury which is not infrequently found in association with fracture of a long bone.

Having completed the general physical examination and determined the nature of the injuries sustained, one's attention should be directed to the abnormal features signifying dysfunction of the brain. A rapid, but systematic, neurologic examination should be performed. The completeness of the neurologic examination depends on the conscious state of the patient. An estimate of the posttraumatic state of awareness is readily made by interrogating the patient with regard to the accident. If memory is intact concerning the accident and the subsequent course of events, and the patient fully oriented, then it would appear that transitory unconsciousness had not been sustained. On the other hand, although oriented and aware of his surroundings, if the patient nevertheless has no recollection of the accident and the immediate sequence of events thereafter (anterograde amnesia), loss of consciousness at the time of injury or shortly thereafter must have occurred. Most patients who have had significant cerebral dysfunction following a craniocerebral injury may, for a time, be unable to recall major hap-

189

penings that transpired hours, days or even months prior to injury (retrograde amnesia).

Patients with evidence of head trauma, lying motionless, with flaccid limbs, and wholly unresponsive to all forms of noxious stimuli, have obviously suffered a severe brain injury. Others completely out of contact with their surroundings and alternately stuporous and restless likewise have probably sustained serious brain damage. The examiner's diagnostic acumen is put to the test in the evaluation of these clinical states whenever there are associated injuries. Especially when there are multiple fractures, the patient's state of confusion and drowsiness may in part be due to such factors as shock and/or fat emboli. When a history is unavailable and there is little or no external evidence of head injury, as in the case of an unconscious patient found on the street, one must consider in the differential diagnosis the many causes of coma other than cerebral trauma, including alcohol, diabetes, epilepsy, uremia, drug intoxication, and cerebrovascular and infectious disease.

Flaccidity of the extremities with varying degrees of paralysis may be caused by injury to brain, spinal cord, or peripheral nerves. Cerebral injury usually produces paresis of one or both extremities on the side opposite the lesion. Intracranial blood clots, however, may produce paretic extremities on the same side as the hemorrhage. A quantitative determination of motor function may be difficult in uncooperative or stuporous patients. Spontaneous movements of the face and limbs should be observed as well as the responses to noxious stimuli. Facial paralysis may be revealed by an asymmetric grimace induced by supraorbital pressure. Reflex activity should be tested, with particular attention to the plantar responses. Quadriplegia or paraplegia as a rule signifies a spinal cord lesion. Even in a drowsy or mildly stuporous patient, some evaluation of the response to a pinprick can be made, thus furnishing a crude estimate of impairment of sensory and motor function and the location of the lesion.

Speech, cranial nerve function, especially ocular motility, coordination, and gait should also be tested whenever the patient's state of consciousness and cooperation permit.

Continued observation and repeated examinations at frequent intervals are essential to the recognition of an epidural hemorrhage at an early stage. The possible occurrence of this complication must be borne in mind in every case of head injury. It is lethal unless diagnosed and treated before it has caused irreparable damage to the brain stem.

Vital Signs

The respiratory rate, blood pressure, pulse and temperature are regularly recorded. Abnormalities of thoracic movements, as well as any changes in the depth and rate of respiration, should be noted. Irregular respiration with periods of apnea is, at times, observed in patients with extradural or subdural hematoma in the posterior cranial fossa. Cheyne-Stokes breathing occurs commonly in those with severe craniocerebral trauma and is, in part, due to an alternating action of oxygen and carbon dioxide on the respiratory center. Involvement of the diencephalo-mesencephalic regions may be associated with rapid labored breathing affecting inspiration and expiration equally, so-called central hyperventilation. Damage to the hindbrain may give rise to a gasping type of respiration, frequently terminal.

The complexity of problems related to multiple injuries renders interpretation of the vascular response most difficult. This is not intended to imply that a careful record of these parameters is not important. Changes in blood pressure and pulse rate may represent an early signal that all is not well and should initiate an immediate reexamination and reassessment of the patient's problem. A slow or rapid pulse early in the course of the illness may not of itself be of diagnostic value; however, a rising blood pressure and slowing of the pulse sometime later may indicate the development of an intracranial clot of significance. A progressive drop in blood pressure and an increase in pulse rate are indicative of impending shock, in which case immediate reexamination for determination of the causative factor is imperative.

In cases of mild head injury the temperature is not significantly elevated. Hyperthermia associated with a rapid pulse and respiratory rate occurs following severe trauma and is of ominous significance. A secondary rise in temperature usually signifies an infectious complication.

ANCILLARY AIDS

Routine laboratory studies should include a complete blood count and urinalysis, blood sugar, blood urea nitrogen and electrolyte determinations, serology, blood typing, and prothrombin time. Further laboratory tests are performed according to clinical indications. Should the possibility of a drug overdose be entertained, appropriate tests should be made.

Radiography

Roentgenograms of the head should include the following views: anteroposterior, posteroanterior, occipital (Towne) and right and left lateral. While of no direct help in determining the extent of cerebral damage, plain skull roentgenograms may provide a considerable amount of information. They may reveal the site and type of a fracture, the position of the pineal gland relative to the midline and the presence of a foreign body or of air within the cranial cavity. The finding of a fracture across the grooves of the middle meningeal vessels should alert one to the possibility of an extradural hematoma.

A roentgenogram of the chest taken at the same time as the skull films provides a base line for subsequent comparison, should the occasion arise.

Since a fracture of the cervical spine is not an infrequent accompaniment of head trauma, it is advisable to obtain cervical spine roentgenograms in all stuporous patients suspected of having sustained craniocerebral trauma.

More definitive diagnostic roentgenography involves the use of contrast media. Pneumoencephalography and cerebral angiography provide the only means of definitely diagnosing an intracranial blood clot. Arteriography is the definitive procedure of choice in this respect and has virtually replaced pneumoencephalography in the study of head trauma in the acute and chronic stages.

Spinal Puncture

Lumbar puncture is of relatively little value as a diagnostic aid following trauma. A spinal tap performed shortly after a head injury is useful primarily for medicolegal reasons or for the purpose of deciding what disposition to make of some patients on a busy hospital service. An alert, oriented patient relatively free of complaints, with a clear cerebrospinal fluid, may be allowed to leave the hospital the day following injury, while one with a bloody cerebrospinal fluid should be held for further observation. Increased intracranial pressure may not register on a manometer attached to a needle inserted into the lumbar thecal sac because of obstruction of the subarachnoid space at the level of the foramen magnum as a result of cerebellar herniation. Lumbar puncture may indeed be hazardous under such circumstances. It is also well known that a spinal puncture performed shortly after a severe head injury may reveal clear cerebrospinal fluid; several hours may be required for blood to reach the lumbar subarachnoid space. In cases of suspected meningitis or brain abscess, examination of the cerebrospinal fluid is obviously of great importance.

Electroencephalography

Electroencephalography may be of some help in selected instances of craniocerebral trauma. This examination may be performed without disturbing a severely injured patient. The degree and location of the brain damage determine the type of electrical activity. Localized damage to the cerebral cortex will produce a focal abnormality in the EEG, while a brain stem injury may produce bilateral changes. A patient with a surface clot compressing the brain and underlying cerebral edema may show a low voltage, slower frequency, and washed-out appearance of the brain waves on the side of the lesion (Kaplan, 1956). Because of the relatively abnormal basic patterns of some individuals, serial records become necessary if the EEG is to be used as an indicator of brain injury.

Brain Scan

The uptake of radioactive material about an area of traumatized tissue may be increased, thereby providing evidence of focal brain injury. The scan may become positive only about four to six days after trauma. In cases of subdural hematoma an area of increased radioactive uptake in a crescentic distribution may be observed directly over the brain in the anteroposterior projection. Care must be taken not to misinterpret the increased uptake by extracranially injured tissue for brain damage.

Echoencephalography

By comparing ultrasound reflections from each side of the head, a shift of the midline may be revealed. Such displacement would suggest the presence of an intracranial mass. Because of its simplicity, and its safety and rapidity of performance, echoencephalography is a useful method of studying patients suspected of harboring an intracranial mass lesion. It is not an infallible guide, however, and failure to demonstrate a midline shift does not necessarily exclude the presence of a hematoma. Experience with the technique is required to avoid misinterpretation of extraneous echoes.

While the brain scan, echoencephalogram, and electroencephalogram may provide useful data, in the final analysis the diagnosis of an intracranial blood clot can only be definitely established preoperatively on the basis of the cerebral angiogram. This statement is not meant to imply that angiography must invariably be performed preoperatively in all cases of suspected intracranial hemorrhage. Surgical treatment is urgently required in cases of epidural bleeding and to delay operation in a critically ill patient for the purpose of performing an angiogram is unjustified.

TREATMENT

A person found lying in the street, especially one in profound stupor, should be carefully placed on his side with his face slightly turned towards the ground to allow drainage by gravity of oronasal secretions. Keeping in mind the possibility of an associated fracture of the cervical spine, the head and neck should be maintained in normal alignment with the rest of the vertebral column. Any obvious fractures of the extremities should be splinted and bleeding areas controlled by pressure dressings. For transportation to a hospital without risking cord damage in the event a vertebral fracture has been incurred, adequate help is required to lift the patient onto a firm stretcher so as to avoid flexion or extension of the spine. Apparatus should be available in the ambulance for maintaining an open airway and assisting respiration if necessary. Upon arrival at the hospital, the patient is transferred to a portable bed. He is examined completely, and appropriate studies, including x-rays, are performed. Disposition of the patient is made at this time. If conscious and cooperative, he may be sent home or, alternatively, detained for a short period for observation. If drowsy or stuporous, he is hospitalized and, if critically ill, admitted to an intensive care unit. In a large municipal hospital where many head-injured patients are received, those who appear only slightly injured and who are under the influence of alcohol are kept under observation in a special, short-term holding ward for a period of 12 hours. Appropriate care is provided for patients with multiple injuries.

The majority of patients with closed head trauma admitted to a hospital do not require intensive medical treatment. Those who are drowsy or mildly confused are kept under observation for periods of one to two weeks; vital signs are monitored. In most cases only symptomatic treatment and general nursing care are required. A relatively small number will develop evidence of an epidural blood clot soon after trauma, others of a subdural hematoma usually at a later stage. Both, particularly the former, demand early recognition and prompt surgical management.

Patients who are in deep stupor or coma from the time of injury present a more complex problem. Such patients have obviously suffered extensive brain damage associated in some cases with intracranial hemorrhage of surgical significance. The diagnosis of an intracranial hematoma in a comatose patient may be exceedingly difficult. If there is reason to suspect an epidural clot in a critically ill patient, one should immediately proceed with exploratory trephination. Otherwise, bilateral angiography should be considered (1) in patients with a demonstrable focal neurologic deficit, (2) whenever stupor deepens, and (3) in the event improvement in the state of consciousness is not evident after a period of 48 hours. The treatment of the comatose patient with a complicating intracranial hematoma postoperatively is similar to that of the patient without an associated clot.

The various items to be considered in the treatment of the severely head injured patient are the following: circulatory support, respiratory care and assistance, treatment of cerebral edema and hyperpyrexia, correction of metabolic abnormalities, and general medical care.

Circulatory Support

Shock is a rare occurrence in patients having sustained a head injury alone. More often, in those with moderate to severe injury of the brain, the blood pressure is slightly elevated and the pulse slowed. The occurrence of shock should prompt a search for an associated injury, usually one involving the chest, abdomen, pelvis or extremities. Prolonged bleeding from an extensive scalp laceration may occasionally lead to shock. Appropriate therapeutic measures must be promptly initiated. Monitoring the central venous pressure provides a guideline to intravenous fluid replacement.

Respiratory Care and Assistance

Respiratory insufficiency produces injurious effects by raising the intracranial pressure (cerebral vasodilatation) and by inducing hypoxia. Elevation of the intracranial pressure may compromise the cerebral circulation.

195

To maintain a clear airway the naso-oro-pharynx and tracheobronchial tree should be kept free of secretions by frequent suction, using a plastic catheter. If necessary, an endotracheal tube may be inserted. This may be left in place for 48 to 72 hours. If an artificial airway is required for longer periods, a tracheostomy should be done. It should be understood that a tracheostomy is not a wholly innocuous procedure. Complications such as misplacement, blockage by secretion, ulceration, infection, hemorrhage, emphysema, and pneumothorax occur not infrequently. The tracheostomy tube should be cuffed to prevent aspiration of secretions; a low pressure cuff or one permitting a minimum leak is desirable. Periodic deflation, immediately preceded by aspiration of secretions, must be performed at one- to two-hour intervals. The care of the tracheostomy wound and tube must be meticulous. Gentle, frequent suction through a sterile catheter should be carried out to maintain an open airway at all times. Just before suctioning the inspired oxygen concentration should be increased. Daily cultures should be taken from the indwelling tracheostomy tube and, when indicated, appropriate antibiotic therapy instituted. The inner tracheostomy tube should be frequently removed and thoroughly cleansed. Mechanical ventilation may be required to assist inadequate spontaneous respiration. Blood gas analysis should be freely utilized to assess pulmonary function and the efficacy of therapy.

At times, it is difficult to differentiate between agitation due to a brain injury and that caused by hypoxia. The supply of oxygen to the brain depends on the hemoglobin concentration of the blood, the degree of oxygen saturation, and the adequacy of cerebral blood flow. Hypoxia, regardless of cause, requires the administration of oxygen. However provided, the oxygen should always be humidified. If the patient has a clear airway and is breathing well spontaneously, the oxygen may be passed through a nebulizing type of humidifier into a face mask. If the oxygen is to reach the lungs through a naso-tracheal tube or through a tracheostomy tube, it should be delivered through a high humidity generator such as an ultrasonic or heat nebulizer. The advice of a specialist in the field of inhalation therapy should be available, whenever necessary.

Cerebral Edema

The intracranial pressure is a measure of the extent of cerebral damage and associated edema. Edema may be of varying severity and is accentuated by hypoxia and cerebral ischemia. It may be sufficiently extensive and pronounced to act as an expanding lesion, causing brain stem compression and ultimately death. Hyperosmolar solutions such as urea and mannitol may be employed in an attempt to control the edema and intracranial hypertension, provided the presence of a significant intracranial clot has been excluded. Unfortunately the effects of such hypertonic solutions are only transient and repeated administration produces deleterious fluid and electrolyte disturbances. Moreover, a secondary rise in intracranial pressure (rebound phenomenon) may occur thereafter. The danger attending the use of hypertonic solutions in the treatment of brain injuries and the varied response of the cerebrospinal fluid pressure were pointed out many years ago by Browder (1930).

There is evidence to indicate that the adrenal corticosteroids may be useful in the treatment of posttraumatic edema. Dexamethasone is most commonly prescribed, an initial dose of 10 mg being administered intravenously, followed by 4 mg intramuscularly at 6-hour intervals. The dosage is gradually reduced over a period of a week.

Another method currently being attempted to reduce intracranial pressure following injury involves the use of hyperventilation to induce hypocapnia. Its effect appears to be longer lasting (Paulson, 1972).

While on theoretic grounds hypothermia should be especially beneficial in the treatment of head trauma, this expectation has not been borne out in actual practice. To date, the results of hyperbaric oxygen therapy have not been impressive.

Temperature Control

Hyperpyrexia is a common occurrence in patients with severe head injury, probably as a result of hypothalamic involvement. It is a life-threatening complication which must be promptly treated. Irreversible damage to the central nervous system may follow sustained elevation of temperature in a patient who is hypoxic. A rectal temperature of 102 to 103 degrees F may be arbitrarily taken as an indication to institute antithermic measures. All covering should be removed, and the patient sponged with cold water. A damp sheet may be placed over the patient and an electric fan brought into play. Ice packs, colonic irrigation with cold water, and the use of cooling (hypothermia) blankets may be required. To reduce heat production, shivering should be prevented with chlorpromazine.

The metabolic response to head injury is similar in many respects to that following body trauma elsewhere (McLaurin, 1966). Sodium and water are retained for several days and a mild hyponatremia develops. The nitrogen loss may be appreciable. Potassium balance, however, remains unaffected.

Dehydration may occur as a result of various factors and leads to hypertonicity and hypernatremia. It may be caused by an inadequate fluid intake, fever, excessive use of hypertonic solutions and diabetes insipidus. A primary neurogenic disturbance due to brain damage has also been suggested (primary cerebral salt retention). Excessive secretion of antidiuretic hormone, on the other hand, causes water retention and hyponatremia. Recognition and correction of these fluid and electrolyte disturbances is important because of their potential threat to life and because they may produce profound neurologic and mental changes. The treatment of dehydration consists of the administration of water and correction of the underlying causative mechanism. In cases of inappropriate secretion of antidiuretic hormone, the therapy of choice is water restriction; should evidence of water intoxication appear (coma, convulsions), hypertonic saline administered intravenously is effective in restoring normal osmolality and reversing the neurologic disturbances.

Comatose patients are maintained initially on intravenous fluids (1500-2500 cc daily), usually only for a few days. Frequent determinations of the blood and urinary electrolytes and a record of the urinary output provide useful guides to therapy. Acid-base imbalances, which may occur as a consequence of respiratory disturbances, are revealed by measuring the blood pH, and pCO_2 and CO_2 content. Respiratory acidosis is indicative of inadequate ventilation. Improved ventilation decreases acidosis and hypercapnia and enhances oxygenation. Severe respiratory alkalosis due to sustained hyperventilation may necessitate the cautious use of drugs to depress the activity of the respiratory center.

If after 48 hours the patient remains unable to ingest food, he must be fed by means of a soft, flexible nasogastric tube. Starting with about 50 cc water per hour, the quantity of fluid and its caloric content are increased so that within a few days a total of about 2500-3000 cc of liquid providing about 2500 calories is being administered each day (200-250 cc every 2 hours). Aspiration of the gastric contents should be performed before each feeding to minimize the likelihood of gastric reflux and aspiration. Patients who remain in coma for prolonged periods almost invariably lose weight despite a high protein intake.

Spinal Puncture

Spinal puncture, with drainage of cerebrospinal fluid for therapeutic purposes, is mentioned only to be condemned. Its beneficial effect, if any, in cases of head trauma is transient at best. Moreover, it is fraught with danger, sudden death having been known to occur as a consequence of herniation.

General Medical Care

Comatose patients must be kept on their side or semiprone, preferably with the head slightly elevated and their position changed every two hours. The semiprone position is especially useful in maintaining a satisfactory airway and — by facilitating drainage — avoiding aspiration. The extremities should be put through a full range of motion at all joints whenever the patient is turned. In cases of prolonged coma, splints may be required to prevent contractures. The skin should be kept clean and dry and the bedsheets free of wrinkles. Beds should be provided with padded siderails to avoid injury to restless patients. Restraints should be kept to a minimum; whenever they are needed, they must be judiciously applied so as not to cause vascular or peripheral nerve damage. At times sedatives are required to control severe agitation. Paraldehyde, chlorpromazine, diazepam or a barbiturate may be administered in small doses. The use of sedatives at an early stage following injury, when the clinical course of the patient is of vital importance and must not be obscured, is obviously inadvisable. Morphine, because of its depressant action on respiration and consciousness, is best avoided at all times. Convulsions are treated with phenobarbital, diphenylhydantoin or Valium.

Patients not fully alert are usually incontinent of urine. To avoid a continually wet bed and maceration of the skin, urine is collected by means of a condom catheter in the male and an indwelling Foley catheter in women. The use of a catheter also provides a means of measuring urinary output.

Stool softeners such as Colace followed by suppositories may be effective in relieving constipation. Otherwise, an enema may be administered every few days. The presence of a fecal impaction should be determined by rectal examination.

The dentures of comatose patients should be removed and the lips and mouth lubricated to prevent drying of the mucous membranes. Careful attention must be paid to the state of oral hygiene.

In the event the eyes do not close adequately and spontaneous blinking does not occur, the instillation of methylcellulose affords protection to the cornea. It may be necessary to close the eyes of a comatose or stuporous patient with a facial paralysis by means of adhesive tape applied to the eyelids or by suturing the eyelids.

PROGNOSIS

Survival following head trauma depends on: (1) the severity of the brain injury, (2) the astuteness of the physician in recognizing and treating complications, particularly those of a life-threatening nature such as intracranial bleeding, before an irreparable state is reached, and (3) the ability of the physician and hospital personnel to effectively handle the many problems presented by the seriously injured patient.

The state of consciousness of the patient is the most important single factor in estimating the chances of recovery from injury to the brain. Yet, the duration of the state of impaired awareness is not necessarily an index of the ultimate outcome of the patient. Some patients have been unresponsive for prolonged periods, even weeks to months, and seemingly have made a reasonably good recovery (Kaplan, 1965). Permanent sequelae in those who have sustained a serious head injury may be mental or physical, or both, and may be of a degree that precludes resumption of former occupation and social activities.

From a large series of head-injured patients, 96 cases were studied intensively by the author from the time of entry into the hospital through autopsy. Severe damage to the postero-inferior frontal and antero-mesial temporal regions was found in those surviving for only one to three days. Those surviving longer than four days had either moderate bilateral or unilateral damage to these areas. Those who died within the first three days and who had no injury to the base of the temporal and frontal lobes were found to have other lesions such as clots, brain stem hemorrhages, cerebellar contusions and cervical spinal cord injuries. Brain stem hemorrhage was found in 50 percent of the group of patients who expired within 24 hours; this type of lesion was not present in patients who lived longer than two weeks.

In attempting to correlate respiratory alterations with observations at necropsy it was found that gasping respirations usually occurred in association with severe injury of the base of the brain or with large intracranial clots. In such cases, cerebellar herniation with medullary compression was present. Patients with mild to moderate damage of the base of the brain, who survived from 24 hours to 48 hours, usually had labored respirations affecting both inspiration and expiration. A rapidly changing respiratory pattern was observed in many patients dying within four days; the breathing of four patients who died within 24 hours after head injury was normal on admission but soon became labored and gasping. This appeared to be related as much to poor respiratory care as to the basic brain damage.

The effects of brain injury on the circulatory system were less prominent. Evidence of shock was not often found in patients with head injury alone and occurred only in those who expired within a few minutes after admission to the hospital. The circulation was frequently maintained for relatively long periods after cessation of spontaneous respiration. A slow pulse, i.e., below 60 per minute, was not found in any patient surviving over four days.

Laboratory data and information obtained from ancillary diagnostic procedures performed shortly after admission to the hospital were of relatively little value in prognosis.

REFERENCES

Aronson, S. M. and Kaplan, H. A. Pathogenesis of Cerebral Lesions Resulting from Contact Trauma to the Head. *Bull. N. Y. Acad. Med.*, *33*, 450-454, 1957.

Browder, E. J. Dangers in the Use of Hypertonic Solutions in the Treatment of Brain Injuries. *Am. J. Surg.*, *8*, 1213-1217, 1930.

Browder, E. J. and Meyers, R. Behavior of the Systemic Blood Pressure, Pulse Rate and Spinal Fluid Pressure Associated with Acute Changes in Intracranial Pressure Artificially Produced. *Arch. Surg.*, *36*, 1-19, 1938.

Courville, C. B. *Commotio Cerebri*. Los Angeles, Calif.: San Lucas Press, 1953, pp. 63-80.

Cushing, H. Concerning a Definite Regulatory Mechanism of the Vasomotor Center Which Controls Blood Pressure During Cerebral Compression. *Bull. Johns Hopkins Hosp.*, *12*, 290-292, 1901.

Hooper, R. S. Extradural Hemorrhages of the Posterior Fossa. *Br. J. Surg.*, *42*, 19-26, 1954.

Ingraham, F. D., Campbell, J. B., and Cohen, J. Extradural Hematoma in Infancy and Childhood, *J.A.M.A.*, *40*, 1010-1013, 1949.

Kaplan, H. A. Chronic Residua of Head Trauma. *Clin. Neurosurg.*, *12*, 266-276, 1965.

Kaplan, H. A. Basic Aspects of the Brain and the EEG. *Am. J. EEG. Tech.*, *6*, 55-61, 1966.

Kaplan, H. A., Huber, W., and Browder, E. J. Electroencephalogram in Subdural Hematoma. *J. Neuropath. Exper. Neurol.*, *15*, 65-78, 1956.

Kocher, T. Hirnerschütterung, hirndruck und chirurgische eingriffe bei hirnerkrankungen. In: *Nothnagel, H., Specielle Pathologie und Therapie.* Vienna: A. Hölder, 1910. Vienna, Vol. IX, Part III: 1-457.

McLaurin, R. L. Some Metabolic Aspects of Head Injury. In W. F. Caveness, and A. E. Walker (Eds.). *Head Injury.* Conference Proceedings. Philadelphia: J. B. Lippincott Co., 1966. Pp. 142-157.

Paulson, O. B. Intracranial Hypertension. *Anesthesiology*, *36*, 1-3, 1972.

Symonds, C. Concussion and its Sequelae. *Lancet*, *1*, 1-5, 1962.

Taylor, A. R. Post-concussional Sequelae. *Brit. Med. J.*, *3*, 67-71, 1967.

The author wishes to express his gratitude to Dr. Jefferson Browder for reviewing the chapter and offering many helpful suggestions.

Chapter 8

TRAUMATIC INTRACRANIAL HEMORRHAGE

E. S. GURDJIAN, M. D.

AND

L. M. THOMAS, M. D.

Traumatic intracranial hemorrhage may be extradural (epidural), subdural, subarachnoid, or intracerebral in location. A condition closely linked with subdural hematoma is subdural accumulation of cerebrospinal fluid. Intracerebral hemorrhage may be massive or petechial. In this chapter, we are concerned primarily with massive epidural, subdural, intracerebral, and intracerebellar hematomas. Detailed discussion of these various types of hemorrhage follows.

EXTRADURAL HEMORRHAGE

Extradural hemorrhage, or a collection of blood between the skull and dura, is a complication that occurs in about 1 to 3.1 percent of patients with cranial injuries (Munro, 1938; Voris, 1947; Echlin, 1949). In our series of 647 cases of skull fracture, there were seven instances of middle meningeal hemorrhage. An extradural hemorrhage may result from a rupture of the middle meningeal artery and veins, the dural sinuses (sagittal and lateral sinus), or the diploic or emissary vessels. A middle meningeal hemorrhage is the commonest source of an extradural hematoma. Dural sinus injury with resultant extradural hemorrhage is not frequently seen, and diploic and emissary vein bleeding rarely produces a lesion of surgical significance.

Middle Meningeal Hemorrhage

Middle meningeal hemorrhage is un uncommon complication of head injury. In the absence of associated traumatic intracranial lesions prompt treatment of this condition is frequently gratifying. A hematoma of

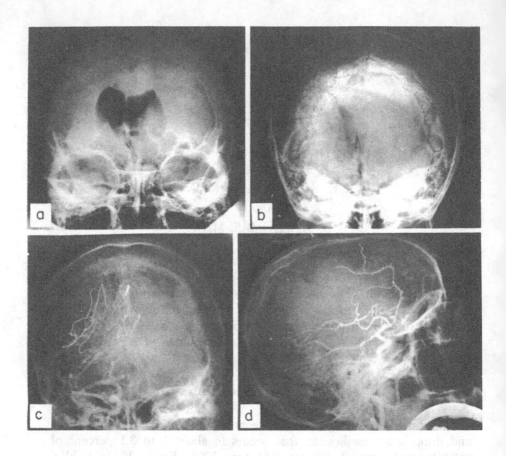

Fig. 1. a, Encephalogram in a patient with a left parietal epidural hematoma. b, Encephalogram with left temporal hematoma. c—d, Angiogram with parietal epidural hematoma.

middle meningeal origin is almost always unilateral. The classic clinical syndrome is that of a short period of unconsciousness initially followed by a lucid interval, after which consciousness again deteriorates and focal signs appear. This sequence of events has been known to occur in association with middle meningeal hemorrhage for almost 100 years.

204

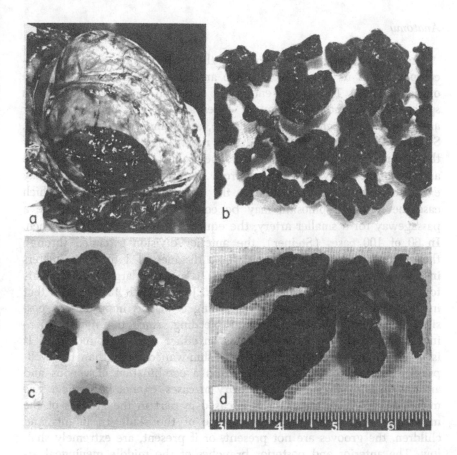

Fig. 2.   a, The usual position of an epidural hematoma seen in the autopsy room. b, 100 gm. epidural clot removed at operation. c, 30 gm. epidural clot with depressed fracture. d, Epidural clot removed 31 days after injury. No membrane was seen surrounding the clot.

However, there may be many variations of this pattern owing to associated intracranial damage or differences of individual response. Other intracranial mass lesions may give rise to a clinical picture similar to that of middle meningeal hemorrhage.

205

Anatomy

The middle meningeal artery and the two or three veins that accompany it in its intracranial course are the chief source of this type of hemorrhage. The artery enters the cranium through the foramen spinosum in about 57 percent of cases and divides into an anterior and posterior branch near the foramen, according to Plummer (1896). Steiner (1894) stated that the artery runs along the greater wing of the sphenoid for 1 to 5 centimeters before its division. At times, the anterior branch may be given off from the ophthalmic artery and may enter the cranial cavity through the supraorbital fissure, in which case the foramen spinosum may be completely absent, or may be a passageway for a smaller artery, the equivalent of the posterior branch. In 60 of 100 cases (Steiner), the anterior division extended through the greater wing of the sphenoid for a distance of 1 to 3 centimeters in a bony canal. The anterior division is usually larger and appears to be the continuation of the main trunk. Jones (1911, 1912) states that in the majority of cases, venous bleeding is just as important or possibly more important than arterial bleeding, since the middle meningeal artery has two or more veins on either side, surrounding it. It is much easier to tear or damage the thin-walled veins than the well-protected artery (Jones). That there is a combination of venous and arterial bleeding in the great majority of cases, cannot be denied. The meningeal artery in the adult is encased in part in the grooves of the meningeal vessels on the inner surface of the skull. In infants and children, the grooves are not present, or if present, are extremely shallow. The anterior and posterior branches of the middle meningeal artery supply the greatest extent of the dura in the middle two-thirds of the cranium.

Small, interconnecting vessels between the dura and the diploic channels of the skull also may be torn as the dura is dissected off the skull by epidural bleeding. These are mostly venous channels. Undoubtedly, bleeding from this source is a contributing factor in the formation of the clot.

Pathology

Middle meningeal hemorrhage results from a laceration of the artery and the veins when a fracture crosses a groove in which they lie. Starting with a small amount of hemorrhage initially, separation of the dura from the bone is begun and increases as the hematoma enlarges, owing to continued bleeding not only from the meningeal vessels, but also from the connecting veins between the diploë and the dura. In the great majority of cases, there is a linear fracture, but depressed fractures may also be associated with middle meningeal hemorrhage. In our experience, seven instances of middle meningeal bleeding were associated with depressed fractures. Penetrating wounds have also been known to cause middle meningeal hemorrhage (Guthrie, 1842).

The clot is often a discus-like mass, varying in weight in the fresh state from 25 to 100 grams. In postmortem examinations, Vance (1926) reported a middle meningeal clot of 300 grams, and Moody (1920) one of 246 grams. The clot usually is found in the temporoparietal region, as first noted by Kroenlein (1885). Frontotemporal and parieto-occipital sites are next in frequency. Frontal extradural clots have been described and we have had one example in this location. McKenzie (1938) emphasized that the clot in the parietotemporal region may extend posteriorly over the cerebellar lobe and should be looked for in that location, in some cases.

Occasionally, an extradural clot may occur without a fracture. Bell (1816) has shown, experimentally, that a separation of dura from bone may occur from blunt impact without an associated fracture.

The size of the clot is not always directly proportional to the severity of the symptoms. In some cases, a small clot may be associated with early signs of compression, and cause death. In others, a large clot may be present and be tolerated for several days or even weeks. Jacobson (1885), Moody (1920), and Vance (1926) have described such cases. In our own series, we operated on one patient 31 days after injury. The clot of this patient contained portions that were "liver-like" in consistency and surrounded by liquid. Rowbotham and Whalley (1952) reported a case operated upon 27 days after injury. They found a membrane surrounding the clot much like a subdural hematoma, with dark watery fluid in the center. The indication for operation was the appearance of papilledema. Air study and exploration revealed the lesion.

Associated damage to other parts of the brain may be present. Bloody cerebrospinal fluid is commonly found in patients with extradural hematoma. Bruises and lacerations of the temporal and frontal poles of the hemispheres may occur. The coexistence of massive intratemporal hemorrhages with extradural hematomas was described by Moody (1920). Pringle (1938) has seen subdural hemorrhages in association with extradural hematomas. In our own group (56 cases), there were three patients with subdural accumulation of cerebrospinal fluid, nine

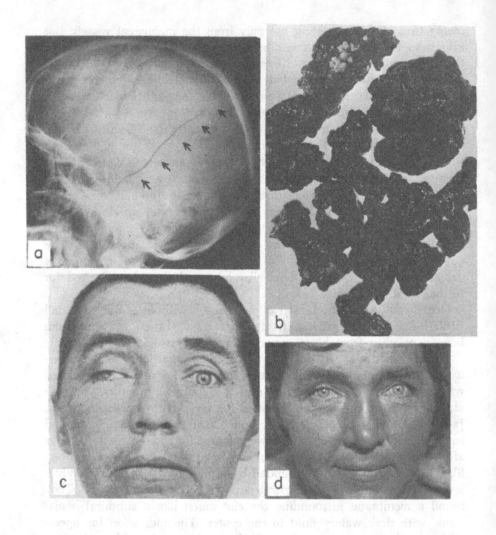

FIG. 3.   a, Typical fracture with epidural hematoma. b, 65 gm. clot removed in the same case. c—d, Third nerve paralysis associated with temporal epidural hematoma with recovery.

with subdural hemorrhages and four with massive temporosphenoidal hemorrhages.

Extradural middle meningeal hemorrhage is almost always unilateral, but a bilateral lesion was present in one of the earliest cases recorded in the literature. Hill operated upon the patient in 1750. First one side was explored with removal of the clot and then the other, three days later. The patient recovered and was well 20 years later. Bilateral lesions have been reported by Pringle (1938), Roy (1884), Wiesmann (1885), Browder and Turney (1942), Munro and Maltby (1941), and MacCarty, Horning, and Weaver (1948). Two instances occurred in our own group of cases.

Etiology

Extradural hematoma of middle meningeal origin is essentially a disease of young adult life. Formerly it was thought that in infancy this complication was rare. The study of Campbell and Cohen (1951) showed that such hematomas may occur during infancy and childhood. They reported 15 cases of middle meningeal hemorrhage under the age of two and a similar number between the ages of two and twelve. Hematomas of this type in infancy have been reported from time to time. Wakely and Lyle included in their (1934) paper the case of a patient 14 months of age, who fell from a first-story window to the pavement, a distance of 18 feet. The child was unconscious ten hours later. No physical findings were reported, but a left temporo-parietal extradural clot was removed at operation. Recovery followed. Goode (1936) reported the case of an infant 13 months of age who fell from its mother's arms, a distance of four feet, and struck its head. Two hours later the child was unconscious. There were twitchings of the left side of the face and arm, and eventually of the leg. Later, the patient became paralyzed on that side and the eyes turned to the right. The child was operated upon and a large extradural clot removed from the right temporoparietal region. A three and one-half year old child who fell from a swing and died within 12 hours was found at postmortem examination to have a right middle meningeal hemorrhage together with a fracture (Jacobson, 1885). The relative infrequency of this condition during infancy may be attributed to the greater degree of adherence of the dura to bone and to the lack of vascular depressions in the bone in the form of meningeal grooves or canals. After the age of ten, it occurs more frequently, but it is typically encountered in adult life. Included in our data is the record of a three-month-old infant with an epidural hematoma that was operated upon with a good result. We have had a total of 13 cases under the age of 12 years.

Middle meningeal hemorrhage in the newborn is rare. Various reviews on birth injuries do not discuss the subject of hemorrhage into the extradural space. Ballance (1919) described a case of extradural hemorrhage of middle meningeal origin at birth, due to a depressed fracture of the left frontoparietal area. There were no localizing signs and operation on the twelfth day was followed by recovery. The clot was in part liquid. Lefkowitz (1936) described a patient with extradural hemorrhage of middle meningeal origin due to a birth injury. The baby was delivered by version and extraction. At birth, the infant did not breathe spontaneously and was cyanotic. There was no fracture of the skull, but a fracture of the right humerus was noted. The spinal fluid was bloody and there were generalized convulsions two days after birth. On the fourth day, there were twitchings of the left side of the face. On the sixth day, the temperature rose to 105 degrees and the patient died. At autopsy, a discus-shaped extradural mass was found in the right temporoparietal region. There was a small amount of subarachnoid hemorrhage in the right Sylvian fissure, and a small subdural clot along the tentorium cerebelli. No fracture of the skull was found.

An extradural hematoma most commonly occurs after a fall or a direct blow to the head. Low velocity impacts are the usual cause of this type of hemorrhage. Penetrating wounds, such as those caused by a poker, spade, or brick, have resulted in an extradural hemorrhage, according to Jacobson (1885). Impacts received in fighting and in automobile accidents, as well as gunshot and shell wounds, have been known to produce this lesion. Bicycle accidents have been found to result in a higher incidence of middle meningeal hemorrhage than other causes, an observation borne out by our autopsy material. Simple and open depressed fractures may be associated with this condition.

Symptoms and Signs

State of Consciousness. In patients with an extradural hematoma of middle meningeal origin, the state of consciousness may vary. 1) There may be an initial short period of unconsciousness, followed by a lucid interval before a secondary period of unconsciousness supervenes; 2) there may be no initial coma following the blow, but impairment of consciousness may occur minutes, hours, or days later; 3) there may be no loss of consciousness at any time, the clinical manifestations consisting of headache, drowsiness, and such focal signs as weakness or paralysis of one-half of the body; 4) disorientation, semi-coma, and a fairly normal mental state may alternate over a period of days; 5) coma persisting from the time of injury may become more profound. Alcoholism may obscure a lucid interval. It is obvious that a lucid interval, which has been emphasized as a characteristic feature of this condition, does not occur in every instance but, when present, it is of great diagnostic significance. It must be stressed that a lucid interval is not pathognomonic of middle meningeal hemorrhage. The length of the lucid interval may vary from 15 minutes to many days. Moody (1920) recorded a lucid interval of 30 days and Gurdjian (1958) one of 31 days. Rowbotham and Whalley (1952), and King and Chambers (1952) also reported cases of 27 and 30 days' duration, respectively. In Jacobson's series (1885), 32 of 63 cases had a definite lucid interval. In Kennedy and Wortis's group (1931), 15 of 17 patients had a lucid interval. McKenzie (1938) described a group of 20 patients, only one of whom was unconscious throughout the entire clinical course. Jacobson aptly commented that the lucid interval may not be evident for several reasons: (1) because of its brevity, it is overlooked; (2) because of alcoholic intoxication; and, finally, (3) because of associated brain damage.

At the present time, when deceleration impacts incurred in automobile accidents are common, associated brain damage often occurs. Under these circumstances, a lucid interval may not be observed, contrary to what occurred before the era of fast transportation. Deepening of the initial state of unconsciousness is a frequent pattern. In our series, one patient had a short period of unconsciousness following the accident after which he regained full consciousness. Beginning a week after the accident, the patient complained of headache. Examination disclosed swelling of the left optic disc together with a slight right lower facial weakness and a right Babinski sign. A 67-gram extradural hemorrhage of middle meningeal origin was removed on the thirteenth day. In this case, there was an associated subdural hemorrhage. Another patient exhibited disorientation alternating with periods of unconsciousness over a four-week period. He developed weakness of the right half of the body and an operation was performed on the thirty-first day. A large extradural clot on the left side with liquid and solid components was removed, followed by recovery.

In our group of patients a lucid interval occurred in 25 of the 56 cases. In 18 instances the patients were unconscious throughout their clinical course. There was a short period of unconsciousness after the trauma, following which full consciousness was regained in two cases; in 11 cases, drowsiness and disorientation were the features observed throughout the entire period before operation.

It must be emphasized that changes in the state of consciousness are important in the diagnosis of middle meningeal hemorrhage. A lucid interval may occur, but more frequently, unconsciousness that is present from the start becomes deeper. It should also be pointed out that a patient with a large extradural hemorrhage may remain conscious for several days. Careful observation and repeated examinations are essential to establish the diagnosis in each individual case.

Ocular Manifestations. Hutchinson (1867) first called attention to the presence of a dilated pupil on the same side in cases of extradural hemorrhage. He attributed the pupillary change to a partial involvement of the third cranial nerve, resulting from pressure of the clot against the nerve at the superior orbital fissure. The pupillary fibers appear to be more sensitive to injury as they course along the superior aspect of the nerve. Woodhall, Devine, and Hart (1941), and McKenzie (1938) suggested that uncal herniation through the incisura may be the cause of the third-nerve involvement. The possibility that increased intracranial pressure from a mass lesion may compress the third nerve between the superior cerebellar and the posterior cerebral arteries as it passes between them, was suggested by Cushing (1910). Sunderland and Bradley (1953), in a well-documented paper, stated that third-nerve paralysis in middle meningeal hemorrhage is always caused by uncal herniation and resultant distortion of the third nerve on the same side as the lesion. They noted initial constriction of the pupil, followed by dilatation. If the pressure continues unbated, the third nerve on the opposite side also becomes involved and both pupils eventually becomes dilated and fixed. In instances in which the oculomotor nerve is not involved, there may be more room for expansion, or the pressure may be produced more slowly.

A dilated pupil on the side of the clot is an important sign, and, in our group of cases, this was observed on the side of the lesion in 34 out of 56. A constricted pupil on the same side as the hemorrhage is noted occasionally. This was observed in four patients in our series. Kennedy and Wortis (1931) found that it was present in four of 17 cases. The pupils were equal in 18 patients in our group. When the pupils are equal in size, the hemorrhage may be in a parietooccipital position, while a dilated pupil on the side of the lesion often indicates that there may be a hematoma in the temporal area extending toward the base. This was noted by Hutchinson many years ago (1867).

Complete third-nerve paralysis as a complication of middle meningeal hemorrhage has been described by Kroenlein (1885) who also reported a case with a sixth-nerve paralysis associated with a parietooccipital extradural hematoma. There have been six instances in our own material of unilateral complete third-nerve paralysis. The fourth nerve was thought to be involved in one case with oculomotor dysfunction, and the sixth nerve in another. In one case there was a divergent squint. Recovery of function has occurred in every instance of survival, including the pupillary reaction to light which, in our experience, has been the last to recover. The presence of a third-nerve paralysis on one side with contralateral weakness or paralysis, simulates the midbrain syndrome described by Weber. Such an alternating oculomotor paralysis is also seen with middle meningeal hemorrhage, and in some patients with a subdural hemorrhage (Fig. 3 c, d).

Changes in the fundi may occur in middle meningeal hemorrhage. There were six instances of choked disc in our series and 11 of engorgement of the veins. In a group of 20 cases, McKenzie (1938) observed choked discs in one, and slight or questionable choking in five.

Focal Signs. Many authors have described typical focal signs in extradural hemorrhage – dilatation of the pupil on the side of the lesion, and weakness or paralysis of the opposite half of the body. In Jacobson's series of 63 cases, paralytic or paretic phenomena were absent in only two instances. In our own group, 47 of 56 patients showed focal signs. At times, there may be an ipsilateral paralysis, as occurred in three cases. This may result from uncal herniation on the side of the lesion causing compression of the brain stem against the contralateral border of the incisura, and resulting in a weakness or paralysis on the same side as the hematoma.

Generalized rigidity of the body has been described as an accompaniment of middle meningeal hemorrhage. This was reported many years ago by Jacobson (1885) and by Wiesmann (1885), and subsequently reemphasized by Jefferson (1921). The body may become uniformly rigid. Flexion and extension of body parts are not possible. It is a decerebrate or decorticate state without opisthotonos. Such generalized rigidity is undoubtedly due to severely increased intracranial pressure resulting from the rapid formation of a mass in the cranial cavity and uncal herniation. Bilateral pyramidal tract signs may occur at a late stage. Uncal herniation with brain stem involvement may result in secondary hemorrhages from anoxic compression and increased capillary permeability, causing death. Jacobson thought that in a unilateral lesion the pressure on the affected side may cause paralysis of the opposite half of the body, and if the pressure is sufficiently severe, there may be implication of the cortex on the opposite side which produces, in addition, a weakness or paralysis on the same side as the lesion, thereby resulting in bilateral involvement. A more reasonable explanation is that the ipsilateral signs are due to uncal herniation

213

causing displacement of the brain stem against the opposite margin of the tentorium and compression of the contralateral pyramidal tract. Multiple foci of brain damage may also account for bilateral pyramidal tract signs. Rarely, bilateral middle meningeal hemorrhage may be responsible for signs referable to both sides.

Occasionally, there may be no localizing signs. In our own group, two patients had clots in the frontal region, and two had posterior parietal and occipital hematomas without evidence of localization. Localizing signs may be absent, either because the clot is situated over a "silent" area of the cortex, or because the hemorrhage, being one of slow seepage, permits the brain to accommodate itself to the enlarging mass.

Convulsions have been observed repeatedly in patients with epidural hematoma. Goode (1936), Relton and Haslam (1894), Kroenlein (1885), Stewart (1921), Wakely and Lyle (1934), Wiesmann (1885), and others have discussed this symptom. Usually, the convulsions are generalized although jacksonian fits may also occur. Kennedy and Wortis (1931) reported five instances of convulsions, two of the jacksonian type, in 17 patients. In a rapidly deteriorating patient, a decerebrate state may develop.

Sensory deficits have been described by Wiesmann. Unilateral impairment of sensation was noted in seven out of 225 patients with middle meningeal hemorrhage. Aphasia, both motor and sensory, has occurred in association with left-sided lesions. In some cases, it may not be recognized until after removal of the clot. Catatonia was noted in one case in our group. This patient was also aphasic. The hematoma was located in the left temporoparietal region.

Posturing, such as lying with the face toward the side of the lesion, was observed by Wiesmann in three cases. Conjugate deviation of the eyes to the side of the lesion in early cases is fairly common, and has been described by Stewart.

Appearance of the Scalp. Before roentgenograms were available, middle meningeal hemorrhage was diagnosed on the basis of the appearance of the scalp, as well as the above mentioned clinical phenomena. A "puffy" swelling of the scalp in the temporoparietal region, a dilated pupil and paralysis of the opposite half of the body were considered indicative of extradural hemorrhage. The "puffy" swelling on the side of the fracture may be caused by leakage of the clot from within the cranial cavity into the extracranial tissues.

The possibility of an epidural hemorrhage should be considered in cases of open fracture of the skull and of penetrating wounds caused by bullets, knives, or shell fragments occurring in association with some of the above mentioned signs of compression.

Roentgen Findings. The roentgen examination is valuable and should precede operative intervention. A linear fracture is almost always seen in patients with middle meningeal hemorrhage. The fracture usually crosses the middle meningeal groove or grooves. In some cases, there may be a depression in the parietotemporal region. This occurred in seven instances of our group of 56. The disclosure of a shifted pineal gland is important, being indicative of lateralization. In our autopsied cases, there was one bilateral frontal hematoma, unassociated with a fracture. We have seen, associated with extensive epidural hematomas, examples of fractures of seemingly insignificant size in the vicinity of the temporal fossa which could not have been diagnosed by roentgen studies. Consequently, the absence of a demonstrable fracture does not exclude the possibility of an epidural hematoma.

In the infant, the presence of a diastatic fracture of the lambdoid suture should suggest the possibility of an epidural hematoma of lateral sinus or diploic origin.

The pulse may be slow, full, and bounding in character at an early stage. A "pressure pulse" has been emphasized by the older writers such as Jacobson and Kroenlein. Characteristically, the pulse rate is between 40 and 55 early in the course of the disease, but in the untreated patient, the rate increases until the pulse becomes rapid and thready.

Respirations have been described as being slow and deep and, in the later stages, stertorous and Cheyne-Stokes in type. Eventually, hyperpnea, associated with a rapid pulse and pulmonary edema, occurs.

The temperature in the uncomplicated case of middle meningeal hemorrhage is usually only slightly elevated, but it may increase to higher levels in the untreated patient. Temperatures of 99 to 101° F are usually seen early in the course of the condition.

The blood pressure is of little value in establishing a diagnosis of increased intracranial pressure in the great majority of cases. Occasionally however, the pressure may rise and be accompanied by other signs of compression.

Spinal Fluid Findings. In most cases of present-day middle meningeal hemorrhage, there is associated subarachnoid bleeding. Hence, the presence of bloody cerebrospinal fluid is not incompatible with an extradural hematoma. Kennedy and Wortis (1931) noted bloody cerebrospinal fluid in 11 of 15 cases and McKenzie (1938) in 9 of 14.

In our group, there were 25 patients who had blood in the cerebrospinal fluid out of a total of 28 in whom spinal puncture was performed. The spinal fluid pressure in usually high, although it may be rather low in some instances. The highest pressure in our series was 650 mm of water. In one case, it was only 45 mm of water after a previous puncture the day before had shown a pressure of 135 mm. In McKenzie's series the pressure of the cerebrospinal fluid varied between 75 and 300 mm of water. A normal or subnormal cerebrospinal fluid pressure does not exclude an extensive extradural clot. In such a case, one should be guided by the general condition of the patient, and if there is evidence of deterioration, operative intervention may be urgent.

Diagnosis

In a typical case, the diagnosis of a middle meningeal hemorrhage offers little difficulty. A lucid interval associated with a dilated pupil on one side, and weakness or paralysis of the opposite half of the body, is a syndrome highly suggestive of middle meningeal hemorrhage. That other lesions, such as subdural hematoma, intracerebral hematoma and, at times, subarachnoid hemorrhage with localized swelling of the brain, also may result in a similar syndrome, is unquestioned. In the majority of patients with extradural hematoma, associated damage to other parts of the brain often complicates the picture so that diagnosis without further investigation may be difficult.

One receives some help from roentgen studies of the skull, particularly as to the presence of a linear fracture crossing the middle meningeal groove or grooves, or of a depression in the parietotemporal region (Fig. 3a). The presence of a shifted pineal may lead to a correct diagnosis.

Angiography and echoencephalography are the most useful diagnostic aids. Electroencephalography is of little help in acute cases but may aid in localization or lateralization in patients with a more protracted course. Pneumoencephalography may also be helpful in patients with a more chronic course and may provide diagnostic information in cases of posterior fossa masses (Fig. 1a, b).

Bilateral carotid angiography has been the most reliable diagnostic procedure in our hands. It is quickly carried out — preferably under local anesthesia. Typical angiographic patterns (Fig. 1c, d) are readily recognized and provide a guide to the proper placement of trephine and craniotomy openings. Although an epidural hematoma over the convexity may present an angiographic picture similar to that of subdural hematoma, the confusion is of no practical importance since treatment of the two conditions is similar.

Echoencephalography, in skilled hands, may demonstrate a midline shift and can thus serve as a screening test for the presence of mass lesions. It must be emphasized, however, that progressive deterioration or the onset of focal signs demands angiographic evaluation, a negative echoencephalogram notwithstanding.

In an occasional case of head trauma, there may be an associated injury to the neck resulting in thrombosis of the cervical internal carotid artery and manifested by contralateral hemiplegia. Lemmen and Schneider (1952) noted such a lesion in two patients. Angiography in the presence of such a complication is, of course, diagnostic, and would obviate the necessity for intracranial exploration. By this diagnostic method one may also identify other vascular lesions simulating the syndrome of an epidural hematoma.

Treatment and Surgical Considerations

The importance of early surgical treatment of epidural hematoma of middle meningeal origin has long been recognized. Kroenlein (1885), Plummer (1896), Auvray (1913), Steiner (1894), and others worked out the exact localization of the various branches of the middle meningeal artery to permit accurate trephination. Cushing (1912) stated that the usual hematoma of middle meningeal origin may be exposed by a subtemporal decompression. This is still the method of choice with many present-day surgeons. A low osteoplastic flap was suggested by Krause many years ago for the removal of convexity hematomas.

If an angiogram or an air study has been done, the exact location of the clot may be determined and the appropriate exposure performed. When the hematoma is near the base, a subtemporal decompression will be adequate in the great majority of cases. With a hematoma of the convexity extending toward the occipital or the frontal areas, a bone flap would be more desirable. In those instances in which no diagnostic studies have been done, the use of openings in the skull along the fracture site is proper. However, the so-called "woodpecker" surgery sooner or later may lead to serious difficulty. A burr opening may be a centimeter or two from the border of a mass which is eventually exposed at autopsy, much to the chagrin of the surgeon.

Common carotid and external carotid artery ligation in cases of middle meningeal hemorrhage was practiced in the latter part of the

19th century. Jacobson (1885) advised against such procedures but suggested that the external carotid artery be used if ligation is decided upon. Thorman, quoted by Wiesmann (1885), is thought to have done the first extracranial middle meningeal ligation in 1828. Verbruggen (1937) described a case in which external carotid ligation was necessary to stop the extradural bleeding. Raney, Raney, and Peterson (1953) suggested ligation of the external carotid artery in patients with extradural hematoma as a temporizing operation until more adequate surgical facilities are available to permit definitive surgery. We have not practiced ligation of the external carotid artery in any of our cases.

The technical aspects of subtemporal decompression for a middle meningeal hematoma are shown in Figure 4. In b_1, b_2, b_3 a subtemporal decompression is outlined. In b_2 the fracture site is located; a burr opening is made near the fracture site exposing the hematoma. The opening in the skull is enlarged to the size of a silver dollar or more, and bleeding vessels are either coagulated or ligated with silk as shown in b_3. The clot is removed piecemeal or by suction. The dura may be opened to determine whether or not there is an associated subdural accumulation of cerebrospinal fluid or blood. It is extremely important to control all bleeding and, for this purpose, attaching the dural margins to extracranial structures by means of sutures is very useful. An actively bleeding middle meningeal artery is seen infrequently; it has usually thrombosed before operation. In an occasional case, the epidural space may have to be packed. The pack may be removed 24 hours later. Occasionally an intracerebral hematoma may be present, usually in the temporal lobe on the same side as the lesion. If this is suspected on the basis of the angiogram, needling the brain with a cannula or more extensive exploration of the temporal lobe should be carried out after removal of the epidural collection. Small amounts of Gelfoam may be used for hemostasis; as much as possible of the Gelfoam should be removed before closure.

In Figure 4 c the management of a frontal epidural hematoma by a bone flap is shown. After the clot is removed, bleeding points on the dura are either coagulated or ligated with silk or silver clips; the dura is opened so as not to overlook such other lesions as a collection of cerebrospinal fluid or a hematoma, the presence of the latter being suggested by a tense bluish dura. After complete hemostasis, dural margins are sutured to pericranium or temporal muscle and the wound closed in layers. In many instances, it may be desirable to completely detach the bone flap from temporal muscle in order to assure hemostasis

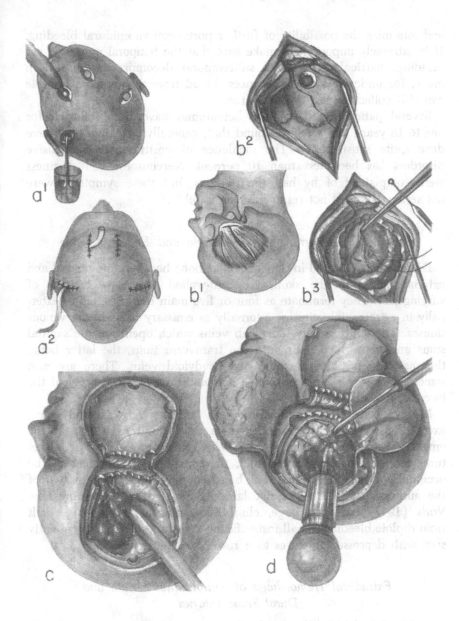

Fig. 4. a¹—a², multiple burr openings for drainage of a liquid subdural hematoma or subdural accumulation of CSF. b¹—b³, removal of epidural hematoma through a subtemporal approach. Bleeding vessels may be ligated, coagulated, or dural bleeding may be controlled by tenting the dura. c, epidural hematoma outside the confines of the temporal muscle; removed by bone flap. d, solid acute subdural hematoma removed by a bone flap.

and minimize the possibility of further postoperative epidural bleeding. It is extremely important to make sure that the temporal muscle is not bleeding, particularly when a subtemporal decompression has been made, for under these circumstances, blood from the temporal muscle can still collect in the epidural area.

Several patients with epidural hematomas have been followed for one to 18 years, and we have found that, generally speaking, they have done quite satisfactorily. The incidence of posttraumatic convulsive disorders has been less than 10 percent. Nervousness and dizziness were complained of by half the patients, but these symptoms were not serious and did not result in any disability.

Extradural Hemorrhage from Diploic and Emissary Veins

Diploic veins, located in the cancellous bone between the internal and external tables of the skull, are thin-walled, irregular channels of varying size. They terminate as four or five main branches, either externally in extracranial veins, or internally as emissary veins in the venous sinuses. There are usually four such veins which open into the sagittal sinus and two which drain into the transverse sinus, the latter being the mastoid emissary, and the post-condyloid veins. There are also some emissary veins in the midline occipital area in the vicinity of the torcular Herophili.

Massive hemorrhage from diploic and emissary veins is rarely seen, except, possibly, in the posterior fossa as a result of a tear of the emissary vein in the torcular area. With comminuted, depressed fractures in the region of the mastoid, there may be involvement of the occipital emissary vein. Epidural bleeding may ensue, but in two of the authors' cases this was not large enough to cause compression. Voris (1947) has seen large, clinically significant hematomas result from diploic bleeding. Small insignificant extradural clots are frequently seen with depressed fractures as a result of diploic bleeding.

Extradural Hemorrhage of Dural Sinus Origin and Dural Sinus Injuries

The two important dural sinuses that may be associated with extradural hemorrhage are the lateral and sagittal sinuses. A tear of the sinuses or of vessels in an extradural location leading into the sinuses may result in extensive hemorrhage in the epidural space. Parietal and occipital emissary veins and midline occipital venous connections

220

may be torn without necessarily involving the dural sinus per se, and may result in extensive extradural collections. Many examples of extradural posterior fossa hematomas have been described in the papers of Anderson (1949), Bacon (1949), Gordy (1948), Beller and Peyser (1952), Turnbull (1944), Campbell and Cohen (1951), Guthkelch (1949), Munro and Maltby (1941), Grant and Austin (1949), Munslow (1951), Kessler (1942), Schneider et al (1951), Hooper (1954), and others. The reviews of Campbell, Whitfield, and Greenwood (1953), and of Beller and Peyser (1952) are especially instructive.

Pathology

The superior longitudinal sinus is more frequently involved than the lateral sinus. Most commonly, injury to the superior longitudinal sinus is caused by a closed or compound fracture producing a depression at the midline. Because of the low venous pressure, there may be little bleeding from the sinus until the fragments of bone are removed at operation. The literature contains many examples of fatal hemorrhage from a lacerated superior longitudinal or lateral sinus during the operative removal of depressed fragments of bone and foreign bodies. Air embolism also may complicate extensive tears of the venous sinuses during repair. Bergmann (1904), Doench (1933), and others have discussed air embolism, and the latter described a case in which death followed immediately after air entered a torn sinus which was exposed for but a moment. A peculiar "suction noise" due to air aspiration within the sinus preceded the patient's last gasp.

Extradural hematomas, particularly in the posterior fossa, may be associated with a linear fracture of the occipital bone. Whenever a fracture of the occipital area is associated with a progressive clinical deficit, an extradural mass should be suspected, and a trephine exploration of the area should be carried out. A low venous pressure, 5 to 9 mm of mercury, may cause a slow hemorrhage with delayed signs of compression, such as occurred in the case described by Coleman and Thompson (1941). More commonly, an extradural hematoma in the posterior fossa may result from a perforating wound of the skull and sinus. This occurred in one of our cases.

Extradural hematomas that result from involvement of the superior longitudinal sinus may simulate middle meningeal hemorrhage. There may be a lucid interval and, with the escape of blood laterally, the cortex may be compressed first on one and then on the opposite side. Wharton (1901) described a case of a sagittal sinus extradural

221

hematoma which extended over the right hemisphere. There was a lucid interval and, along with increasing drowsiness, the patient developed a paralysis of the left half of the body. A middle meningeal hemorrhage was diagnosed, but in the absence of a hematoma in the right temporal area, Wharton followed the fracture line upward by extending his incision; near the midline he uncovered a four ounce clot. There was profuse bleeding from the sagittal sinus. The patient's wound was packed and he eventually recovered.

The syndrome of the superior longitudinal sinus described by Holmes and Sargent (1915), and Levi-Valensi and Ezes (1930) may be seen in patients with extradural hematomas from superior longitudinal sinus injuries. In one of our cases with an avulsion type of injury at the midline, there was a huge epidural hematoma with bilateral pyramidal tract signs. In another case, there was rigidity of both lower limbs and of the left upper limb, with bilateral pyramidal tract signs due to a perforating wound (ice-pick injury) of the superior longitudinal sinus. This caused not only an extensive extradural hemorrhage, but also a hemorrhage within the dura compressing the interhemispheric region.

Symptoms and Signs of Lateral Sinus and Sagittal Sinus Hemorrhage

In the presence of uncomplicated hemorrhage from either one of these sinuses, a dynamic syndrome results, with the patient becoming increasingly more stuporous as a result of the hematoma forming in the epidural area, either over the convexity or in the posterior fossa on one or the other side. When a patient with no localizing signs is found to have a fracture, whether it be in the occipital area or in the interparietal region, exploration in the vicinity of the fracture is indicated in the face of increasing deterioration of the state of consciousness. When definite localizing signs appear, angiography may be valuable.

In the case of superior sagittal sinus injury with bleeding, unilateral or bilateral symptoms and signs may develop. If the lesion remains confined mainly to the midline, both motor cortices may eventually be involved. If, on the other hand, the hemorrhage extends to one or the other side, the signs and symptoms may simulate those of middle meningeal hemorrhage, and unilateral manifestations develop. Associated injuries to other parts of the brain, as well as a lesion within the dura, such as a subdural or intracerebral hematoma, may complicate the picture and give rise to confusing neurologic findings.

In the case of lateral sinus bleeding uncomplicated by other injuries to the brain, increasing stupor and eventually hypotonia of the extremities may develop, as first described by McKenzie (1938) and also observed in the case of Coleman and Thompson (1941). If such a patient also has a linear or a comminuted or depressed fracture of the occipital squama, operative intervention is mandatory. The case of Coleman and Thompson is interesting, since the patient was not unconscious immediately following an impact to the occiput caused by a fall from a moving truck. There was a small hematoma of the scalp. Twenty-four hours later, the patient developed headache, drowsiness, and vomiting. Neurologic examination disclosed no abnormality and the patient was again sent home. The following night, he returned to the hospital in a drowsy state, complaining of headache and, in another 12 hours, developed nuchal rigidity, generalized hypotonia, and arreflexia. The roentgen study showed a midline occipital fracture extending into the foramen magnum. The patient slept on his right side and, whenever his position was changed, he would invariably resume lying on that side. At operation, a large hematoma was found in the posterior fossa, mostly to the right of the midline. The bleeding was thought to arise from the torcular Herophili; probably there was a tear of connecting veins between the torcular and extracranial structures. The patient made a complete recovery; the reflexes and muscle tone were regained before he was discharged from the hospital.

A posterior fossa extradural hemorrhage may, therefore, be associated with increasing drowsiness, unconsciousness, and hypotonia and arreflexia on the same side as the lesion. However, the review of Campbell, Whitfield, and Greenwood (1953) indicates that a majority of patients with such lesions do not conform to a typical clinical pattern and that the diagnosis depends upon judicious evaluation of the evidence (e.g., occipital trauma, increasing stupor) combined with a high index of suspicion.

Dural sinus injuries are frequently caused by tears or punctures occurring in association with depressed fractures. In our group of depressed fractures, 14 instances of dural sinus injury of one variety or another were found.

In a paper on venous sinus injuries incurred in the Korean War, Meirowsky (1953) discussed the management of 112 cases, seven with multiple wounds. There were 124 sinus wounds in the 112 patients; the mortality was 11.6 percent. Meirowsky suggested removal of the thrombus from a transected vessel in order to prevent infection. He pointed out that continued liquefaction of brain tissue following operation in many cases of trauma involving the midportion of the sagittal sinus and occasionally of the posterior segment of the sinus may necessitate a secondary resection of necrotic and infarcted cerebrum four to seven days after the initial procedure. Fatal air embolism is a possibility to keep in mind when dealing with venous sinus tears. One should never explore the area of laceration in a venous sinus without first exposing a wide area surrounding the lesion.

Angiography. Angiographic studies using delayed or serial techniques will demonstrate the draining veins and sinuses, thus permitting accurate preoperative evaluation. Rarely, it may be necessary to inject contrast material directly into the superior sagittal sinus.

Treatment and Surgical Considerations

In dural sinus injuries, three important types of lesions may be encountered: (1) extradural bleeding; (2) subdural bleeding alone or in association with extradural hemorrhage; and (3) torn sinus which either bleeds externally or is kept from bleeding by the pressure of the surrounding tissues, depressed fragments, and foreign matter; with the low venous pressure, hemostasis by these means is possible.

The management of extradural bleeding caused by dural sinus injury is essentially the same as for that of middle meningeal origin. Bleeding points are controlled with the electrocautery, silver clips, or Gelfoam as indicated. The sagittal sinus may be ligated in the anterior half of its extent but should not be ligated when found torn in the posterior half of its course. The lateral sinus, if necessary, may be doubly ligated on either side without serious complications, except, possibly, edema of the optic discs which eventually resolves. A small discrete tear in a sinus may be repaired by suture. One may be able to apply a piece of muscle over the opening in the sinus and fix the muscle in position with a suture passed from the dura of one side to that of the other. Several sutures may be necessary to obtain complete hemostasis.

The management of an epidural hematoma in the posterior fossa is shown in Figure 5b. Usually a unilateral exposure on the side of the fracture in the occipital bone is adequate. A paramedian incision is made in the back of the head and neck, as shown in Figure 5 b$_1$, and the exposed bone trephined. After removal of the blood clot from the epidural space, the dura may be opened, keeping in mind the possibility of an associated subdural or intracerebellar hematoma. The dura is

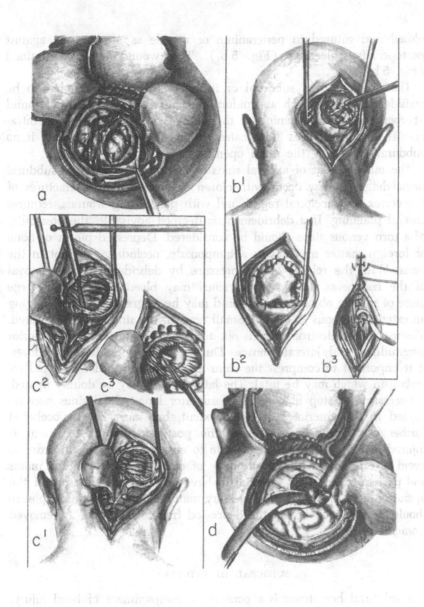

Fig. 5. a, chronic subdural hematoma removed by bone flap. b¹—b³, posterior fossa epidural hematoma removed through large burr opening. b², demonstrates tenting of dura after removal of clot. c¹—c³, excision of intracerebellar hematoma through a unilateral suboccipital approach. d, intracerebral hematoma removed through a transcortical incision after a bone flap.

closed and sutured to pericranium or muscle as a safeguard against postoperative bleeding (Fig. 5 b₂). The wound may be drained (Fig. 5 b₃).

The presence of a subdural or intracerebral mass lesion has to be considered, even though an epidural hematoma may have been found at operation. Thus, opening of the dura and inspection of the intracranial dural structures is indicated. If one is satisfied that there is no subdural collection, the dural opening is then tightly closed.

The management of a dural sinus tear without epidural or subdural hemorrhage, as may occur with closed or open depressed fractures of the vertex and occipital region and with penetrating wounds, requires careful planning. If a debridement is deemed advisable, the possibility of a torn venous sinus should be considered. Depressed pieces of bone or foreign matter may act as a tamponade, occluding the rent in the sinus. With the release of the pressure by debridement and removal of the fragments, the lacerated sinus may bleed profusely. A large piece of muscle obtained beforehand may be of great value in plugging an extensive venous laceration. Small tears in the sinus may be sutured. The use of the electrocautery is not advisable in injuries of the superior longitudinal and lateral sinuses. During these operative procedures, it is important to compress the sinus at all times in order to avoid air embolism which may be fatal. The lateral sinus may be doubly ligated, if necessary, to stop bleeding. The superior longitudinal sinus may be ligated in the anterior half of its extent, but must not be occluded further posteriorly. In the event the posterior half of the sinus is injured, every effort should be made to ensure its patency in order to avoid interference with the drainage of cortical veins from the motor and parietal areas. It is essential to have an adequate exposure of the operative field to permit the necessary manipulations. Such an exposure should be provided before the depressed fragment of bone is removed from the sinus.

SUBDURAL HEMATOMA

A subdural hematoma is a common accompaniment of head injury. Varying amounts of blood in the subdural area were present in a little over 20 percent of 151 consecutively autopsied cases of head injury. Small bilateral subdural collections were noted in four cases. There was one subdural hematoma of "surgical" size over the cerebellar hemisphere. The incidence of subdural accumulation of blood among surviving patients is probably not as high although Munro (1938) stated that in his series of cases there was an average of 20 percent with subdural hematoma, including both surviving and non-surviving patients. Subdural hematomas may be classified into three groups on the basis of the rapidity of the clinical course and the time of onset of symptoms and signs: (1) acute; (2) subacute; and (3) chronic. The group termed *acute* includes cases in which symptoms and signs appear almost immediately following trauma, requiring intervention in three days or less. Those in the *subacute* group are patients who may be symptomatic from the very beginning, yet tend to show improvement for several days until about a week to eight days after the injury, when they deteriorate, making surgical intervention necessary in three to 14 days. The *chronic* group consists of cases that are over two weeks old. This classification is rather arbitrary. In general, it indicates that if bleeding is sufficiently severe to cause symptoms almost immediately, we are dealing with an acute process, whereas if the hemorrhage is less pronounced and/or is tolerated by the host for a week or so, it falls into the subacute category. The chronic group includes patients who have severe associated brain injury, and may, therefore, be quite ill from the beginning, tending to improve for several weeks, until symptoms resulting from expansion of the chronic subdural hematoma appear. Also designated as cases of chronic subdural hematoma are patients whose initial hemorrhage is unassociated with brain injury, and who are quite comfortable for several weeks, until signs of compression supervene. The division of subdural hematomas into acute, subacute, and chronic forms is of prognostic value.

Browder (1943), Voris (1941), and Echlin (1949) have emphasized that the earlier intervention is necessary in patients with a subdural hematoma, the higher the mortality. In our series of 1285 cases of craniocerebral injuries, there were 61 patients with subdural hematoma. The mortality was highest in those requiring operation within 24 hours and decreased as the time interval between injury and operation rose. Of 16 patients operated upon within 24 hours, 14 died (87 percent mortality); of 6 who required operation between 24 and 72 hours following trauma, 3 died (50 percent mortality); there were 4 fatalities among 18 operated upon 3 to 15 days after injury (22 percent mortality). The operative mortality of chronic subdural hematoma is 10 to 15 percent.

In the following sections the three forms of subdural hematoma will be described separately, although it is admitted that the pathological process is the same in all. The differences arise from the size of the clot, the degree of tolerance by the host, and the extent of associated brain damage.

Acute Subdural Hemorrhage

Acute subdural hemorrhage may be unilateral or bilateral and it may be located in any area within the cranial cavity. Usually it occurs in the frontotemporoparietal area. (Fig. 6)

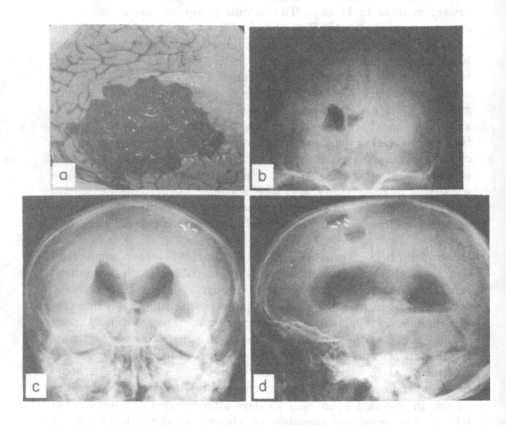

FIG. 6. a, Acute subdural hematoma seen in autopsy room. b, Encephalogram in acute subdural hematoma. Left ventricle compressed, no subarachnoid air over left side. c—d, Ventriculogram in a patient with interhemispheric acute subdural hematoma.

228

Pathology

Subdural hematomas may result from tears of connecting veins between the surface of the brain and the dural sinuses, such as those along the sagittal sinus and those at the base and at the temporofrontal junction, which empty into the sphenoparietal sinus. The latter, Browder feels, is a site of predilection for some of the acute subdural hemorrhages. Other connecting veins extend from the surface of the temporal lobe to the lateral sinus or to the superior petrosal sinus. A subdural collection may also result from contusions of the brain surface with a tear of venous and arterial channels, usually the former; arterial channels may also be torn with extensive hemorrhage. In open injuries, a tear of the surface vessels may be associated with a subdural hemorrhage, or an extensive intracerebral hematoma may point to the surface of the brain through a dehiscence in brain tissue. Intracerebral hematomas in the path of penetrating wounds may enter the subdural space as a result of the egress of blood through the track. Subdural hemorrhage also may result from tears of venous sinuses, usually as a consequence of penetrating wounds or birth injuries. Large collections of blood may accumulate in unusual locations, such as the anterior or middle fossae, over the optic chiasm, between the hemispheres above the corpus callosum, and over the occipital lobes or cerebellar hemispheres, unilaterally or bilaterally.

The subdural collections are of varying size. In some instances the clot may weigh as much as 300 grams, or even more. The usual collections encountered, particularly in the operating room, vary between 30 and 150 grams. The collection may be solid in the beginning and become liquefied over a period of several days. According to Browder, the longer the interval after injury, the greater the likelihood of a more solid clot at the time of exploration. Combinations of solid and liquid clot are frequently seen in acute subdural hematomas. One may find that in the frontoparietal area the clot is liquid, whereas in the temporal region it is more solid in consistency. The most common location of the clot is the frontoparietotemporal area.

Associated damage elsewhere in the cranial cavity is frequently seen. Contusions and tears of the brain surface may be present. Petechial hemorrhages, large intracerebral clots, and subarachnoid hemorrhages are frequently coexistent. A skull fracture may or may not be present. Among 151 autopsied cases, there were 22 with "surgical" subdural clots of 30 grams or more; 7 were associated with a fracture on the same side, and 8 with one on the opposite side; there was no fracture in the remaining 7 cases. It is evident, therefore, that in more than half of the cases there was either no fracture, or else the fracture was contralateral to the hematoma.

A frontotemporoparietal localization of an acute subdural hematoma may be explained on the basis of the anatomic relations of the brain and skull in this region. The frontal and temporal lobes are snugly fitted against the anterior fossa, the sharp edge of the lesser wing of the sphenoid, and the middle fossa. The connecting veins from the surface of the brain that enter the anterior two-thirds of the sagittal sinus, and other connecting veins from the temporal lobe and the temporofrontal junction that empty into the sphenoparietal sinus, may be found torn at autopsy (Leary, 1934). Bleeding from these vessels would tend to collect in the frontoparietotemporal region. With mass movements of the brain, tears of these connecting veins through rotational acceleration may result in extensive bleeding into the subdural space. In the more posterior portions, such as in the occipital area, the relationships are not comparable and, consequently, large collections do not usually occur in these regions. Contusions of the frontotemporal junction, the frontal base, and pole may be associated with subdural collections over the frontal and temporal regions.

Subdural hematomas are unusual in the posterior fossa. They may be produced by penetrating wounds in this area. Posterior fossa subdural hemorrhage extending to the base of the brain and also over the cerebellar lobes may occur as a consequence of tears of the vein of Galen in association with birth injuries. Such subdural collections may also result from tears of the lateral sinuses and of the cerebellar veins emptying into the venous sinuses. A few such examples were described by Meirowsky. Coblenz (1940) found an encysted form of subdural hematoma in the posterior fossa in a two-week-old infant, comparable to a subacute or chronic subdural hematoma over the cerebral hemispheres. Depressed fractures in the occipital area may be associated with a posterior fossa subdural hemorrhage produced by a tear of the lateral or sigmoid sinus or of a tributary vein.

Etiology

Acute subdural hemorrhage usually occurs as a result of trauma, although occasionally it may be associated with rupture of an intracranial aneurysm or arteriovenous malformation, bleeding within a brain tumor or abscess, or with a blood dyscrasia. In the non-traumatic cases the clinical presentation is characterized by a sudden increase in signs and symptoms accompanied by bloody cerebrospinal fluid. Trauma of any variety may result in a subdural hemorrhage. Penetrating injuries, including bullet, shrapnel, and stab wounds, may at times be associated with subdural hemorrhage. Open fractures of the skull involving the dural sinuses may produce this type of lesion. In one of our cases an ice-pick wound of the superior sagittal sinus was associated with an extensive interhemispheric subdural hematoma. Penetrating wounds of the lateral, sagittal, cavernous, petrosal, and sphenoparietal sinuses may result in extensive subdural collections.

During infancy and childhood subdural hematomas are much more common than other forms of hemorrhage within the cranial cavity. The papers of Luys (1898), Alpers (1943), Wharton (1901), Peet and Kahn (1932), Ingraham and Matson (1944) and others that discuss injuries of early life describe many examples of subdural hematoma resulting from trauma at birth. Distortion of the head with tears of dural sinuses may result in extensive subdural collections. The most common causes of subdural hemorrhage in infants and children are falls and automobile accidents. Subdural hemorrhage from traction and tear of connecting veins following evacuation of large collections of fluid in hydrocephalic infants has been reported (Davidoff and Feiring, 1953).

Symptoms and Signs

State of Consciousness. In the acute variety of subdural hematoma, which implies that the patient has a severe degree of bleeding or that the clot occurs in association with extensive brain damage, the patient is usually unconscious from the beginning. At times, even in this group, a lucid interval may be seen. In our series, 20 of 65 patients with acute subdural hematoma had a lucid interval. More commonly, the patients may appear to be in fair condition at first, and then show a deterioration of consciousness in a matter of hours. Unconsciousness deepens, or the patient may show some degree of stabilization for the first several days. Progressive impairment of consciousness occurred in 32 of our 65 patients. In the acute type of subdural hematoma, one is dealing with a critical condition in which deterioration may be rapid, with the outcome decided in a few days.

Ocular Manifestations. These include inequality of pupils, extraocular paralyses, and retinal abnormalities. Inequality of pupils is not as common in the subdural group as it is in cases of epidural hematoma. A dilated pupil on the side of the lesion is seen in about half of the cases, but the dilatation is less marked than in epidural hematomas, and may vary from day to day. A constricted pupil on the side of the lesion is also seen occasionally.

In Browder's series (1943) of 289 cases of all types, the pupils were found to be unequal in 46 percent. In 29 percent, the larger pupil was on the side opposite that of the subdural collection. In only 11 percent was there a widely dilated pupil on the same side as the lesion. In 17 of our 65 cases, a dilated pupil on the side of the lesion with contralateral weakness or paralysis was found; 35 of the 65 patients had a dilated pupil on one side. A widely dilated pupil is most probably the result of paralysis of pupilloconstrictor fibers due to uncal distortion and third-nerve compression at the incisural gap. With sufficient compression, the third nerve may be completely paralyzed, even on both sides.

A third-nerve paralysis is seen infrequently, except in those patients who have a widely dilated pupil. Oculomotor involvement may not only result from compression of the temporal lobe against the brain stem, but also from impingement on the nerve by the posterior cerebral artery, this too as a consequence of distortion of the brain stem brought about by transtentorial herniation. In the subacute and chronic varieties, complete third-nerve paralysis is seen more frequently. Sixth-nerve paralysis is probably due to distortion of the nerve resulting from increased intracranial pressure, and its presence Usually does not lateralize the lesion.

The fundi in patients with acute subdural hemorrhage may show evidence of engorgement of retinal veins. In other cases, there may be hemorrhages in the retina. This is seen more frequently in children and infants and is undoubtedly the result of the initial impact and its indirect effect upon the retina. Such hemorrhages, due to the blow, may also rarely occur in the adult. Occasionally, a choked disc is noted.

Focal Signs. Focal signs are extremely common in acute subdural hematoma. They were present in about 60 percent of the cases in Browder's series. Weakness of one-half of the body and evidence of pyramidal tract involvement were noted in 29 of 65 patients (45 percent) in our group with acute subdural hematoma. Echlin (1949) reported an incidence of 45 percent of pyramidal tract signs in patients with acute subdural hematoma.

Weakness or paralysis on the same side as the hematoma was seen in 22 percent of Browder's entire series, and we also have encountered

232

many examples of this seeming paradox (15 percent). Uncal herniation with compression of the brain stem by the incisural edge of the opposite side is most probably the cause of the ipsilateral weakness or paralysis in such cases.

Decerebrate states may develop in a rapidly forming subdural hematoma. In our group of cases, jacksonian convulsions were noted in nine patients and generalized convulsions in seven.

One should look carefully for localizing signs in an unconscious patient. A Babinski toe reflex is a dependable sign. Occasionally, one may find a difference in the tendon reflexes on one side as compared with the other. Loss of the abdominal reflexes, usually on the side opposite the hematoma, may be demonstrable. Observation of the patient for several minutes may show that only one-half of the body is under volitional control. A painful stimulus, such as pinching the toe or the trapezial border in the neck, may reveal evidence of weakness of one-half of the body. Facial paresis may also become evident.

In some patients with left cerebral involvement, the extremities may be in a catatonic-like state. Obviously, these patients are too ill, in the great majority of instances, to complain of or to be tested for visual, speech, sensory, and other disturbances, ordinarily readily demonstrable in the conscious individual.

Pulse, Respiration, Temperature, and Blood Pressure. In general, the pulse and respiration may be somewhat slower than normal, but this is not seen as often in acute subdural hemorrhage as in epidural hematoma. Because of the associated damage to other parts of the brain and body, a fast and thready pulse is much more commonly noted early in a majority of these patients. Only occasionally may the blood pressure rise due to the increase in intracranial pressure. The temperature in many of these patients is somewhat higher than in epidural hematomas; levels of 101 to 103°F are common. Respiration soon becomes hyperpneic and, in some instances, stertorous and Cheyne-Stokes in type.

Spinal Fluid Findings. The spinal fluid is frequently bloody in patients with acute subdural hematoma. The amount of blood in the cerebrospinal fluid does not indicate the extent of the subdural hemorrhage, being indicative only of the degree of subarachnoid bleeding. The red color of the cerebrospinal fluid deepens as more spinal fluid is allowed to escape. This indicates that a greater concentration of blood is present higher up in the cerebrospinal fluid system. The spinal fluid pressure is usually high (300 to 450 mm of water) but may also be low. A very bloody spinal fluid under a low pressure (hypotension of the cerebrospinal fluid) is a serious prognostic sign. A normal or subnormal cerebrospinal fluid pressure does not rule out the presence of a massive subdural hematoma on one or both sides.

Diagnosis

The diagnosis of an acute subdural hemorrhage is difficult at times because of the associated injury to the brain. Increasing deterioration of consciousness and the appearance of hemiparesis or hemiplegia are the important manifestations. These are indications for further diagnostic (and therapeutic) measures. In patients who have no localizing signs and who remain unconscious for two or more days without showing definite improvement, diagnostic studies to exclude the presence of an acute subdural hematoma are indicated. Electroencephalography, air studies, echoencephalography, angiography, as well as exploratory trephination, may be employed.

Electroencephalography is not always helpful in diagnosing acute subdural hematoma. In many instances, in the first 48 hours after injury, the electroencephalogram does not lateralize the lesion. If lateralization is demonstrable, it is usually on the basis of suppression of electrical activity on the side of the lesion. In view of the usual brain-stem involvement in many patients with closed head injuries, the electrical pacesetting mechanism may be impaired with bilateral dysrhythmias resulting. In others, a low voltage record is found and is not diagnostic.

Exploratory trephination may be worthwhile. Frontoparietal openings 3.5 cm on either side of the midline at or near the coronal suture may show the presence of a subdural hematoma on one or the other side.

Echoencephalography, a technique used to demonstrate a midline shift, provides a useful means of screening patients suspected of harboring intracranial mass lesions but does not substitute for angiography in cases in which the diagnosis remains in doubt or in which deterioration clearly occurs.

Carotid angiography is the diagnostic method of choice in our opinion. Bilateral studies should be made, utilizing oblique views as indicated to locate anterior and posterior lesions. Intracerebral as well as extracerebral masses are delineated by angiography. In the absence of angiographically demonstrated lesions, conservative treatment may be continued. It should be borne in mind, however, that normal carotid angiography does not rule out a posterior fossa hematoma. This possibility must not be overlooked and diagnostic exploration must be carried out if indications for it exist.

234

Treatment and Surgical Considerations

As has been pointed out, the earlier one has to intervene surgically in the presence of an acute subdural hemorrhage, the poorer the prognosis. Browder (1943), Voris (1947), and Echlin (1949) have all made this observation. For instance, in Browder's series, 51 of a total of 227 surgically treated cases were operated upon within 24 hours with a resultant mortality of 82 percent. Of those operated upon between 1 and 7 days, the mortality was 48 percent. The mortality of patients operated upon between 7 and 14 days was 25 percent, and of those upon whom surgery was performed between 14 and 21 days, 21 percent. When the operation was performed after a period of 4 weeks, the mortality was 11 percent.

After a mass has been identified in the subdural space, the type of operation employed will depend somewhat on whether one is dealing with a liquid or solid clot. A liquid clot can be effectively drained through burr openings and the subdural area irrigated with saline introduced through a suitable rubber catheter (Fig. 4 a). On the other hand, if the clot is solid, as occurs soon after trauma, then a small bone flap is turned and the blood clot carefully evacuated (Fig. 4 d). In our experience, more than half of the cases have had a liquid clot.

Usually the wound is drained as shown in Figure 4 a$_2$. The subdural and epidural spaces may be drained in the event a bone flap has been turned. These drains may be removed in 24 to 36 hours.

The brain surface is easily bruised, particularly in the infant. Sudden changes in intracranial pressure may cause the brain to herniate through the burr opening with resultant injury. Consequently, when the presence of a subdural hematoma has been established by the opening in the skull, gentle pressure with a blunt instrument covered with cottonoid may permit escape of more blood. A cottonoid moistened with saline may be applied to absorb fluid from the subdural space which may then be aspirated with the suction unit.

Prognosis

The prognosis in cases of acute subdural hemorrhage is usually poor. Of the surviving patients, many have a protracted convalescence. Some of those with associated cerebral contusions – which occur commonly in the more severe cases – may later develop convulsions. Acute psychotic manifestations and disorientation for varying periods of time

235

are frequent. Personality deficits may be noted after an otherwise relatively good recovery. Severe injuries may cause persistent, disabling neurologic deficits. Adult patients do not improve as rapidly or as completely as those under the age of 17. In the latter group, the extent of recovery may be considerable, with relatively few or no remaining neurologic deficits.

Subacute Subdural Hematoma

When the hemorrhage into the subdural area is not large, and the spatial relations are not immediately jeopardized by the presence of the clot, the patient may carry on for several days without improvement. Before evidence of irreversible deterioration in the patient's condition develops, exploration for a subdural hematoma should be carried out. The results in this group of patients are much better than in those who come to operation within the first 72 hours. Those who are explored four to 15 days after injury belong in the class of subacute subdural hematoma.

Pathology

The origin of the hemorrhage in patients with acute subdural hemorrhage has been discussed. Concerning the subacute form, there is frequently an admixture of blood and cerebrospinal fluid and consequently the subdural collection is more liquid in the majority of cases.

Signs, Sympts, and Diagnosis

Persistent unconsciousness or drowsiness with disorientation three to 15 days after injury characterizes this class of patients. Thereafter further deterioration occurs. If, at the same time, inequality of the pupils and signs of weakness or paralysis of one half of the body develop, then te possibility of subdural hemorrhage must be considered, and the diagnosis established by exploration, angiography, or ventriculography. Jacksonian and/or generalized convulsions, may occur. Electroencephalography may reveal evidence of a localized lesion, and x-rays a shifted pineal. Arteriography is the diagnostic method of choice.

In our series, 44 cases of subacute subdural hematoma have been

236

analyzed. The majority were between the ages of 30 and 50. A lucid interval occurred in 29 patients; hemiparesis or hemiplegia was present in 19, and a dilated pupil in 10; a dilated pupil with contralateral paralysis was seen in 4; convulsions occurred in 13 (jacksonian in 5 and generalized in 8). The hematoma was bilateral in 6 instances. It was liquid in 26, solid in 6, and mixed in 12. Associated clots were epidural in one instance and intracerebral in another. The paralysis was on the same side as the clot in 4 patients. In the preoperative evaluation of the patient, angiography was of great help and 21 of the cases were so studied. The mortality in this group, operated upon between the third and the fifteenth day after injury, was 22 percent, much lower than in the acute variety.

Treatment and Surgical Considerations

Surgical treatment for subacute subdural hematoma is more successful than it is in cases of acute subdural hemorrhage. It is usually preceded by diagnostic procedures for confirmation of the lesion. The management of such cases should include the following steps: (1) careful neurologic evaluation to establish the need for intervention; (2) roentgen studies to show whether there is a shifted pineal or a fracture and its location; (3) angiography to delineate the site of the lesion; and (4) burr openings, usually two in number, to identify the type of clot and a small osteoplastic flap for its evacuation, if needed.

In our series of 44 cases, the operations were either multiple trephine openings with drainage of the fluid collection, a subtemporal decompression with a trephine opening for counterdrainage, or an osteoplastic craniotomy. Bone flaps were used in five patients, subtemporal decompression and burr holes in six, and multiple trephine openings in 33.

Angiography is especially valuable in diagnosis because of the possibility that it may disclose a coexisting intracerebral clot. Since an intracerebral clot with rupture of the overlying cortex may be associated with a subdural hematoma, and since the finding of a small amount of subdural hemorrhage may be mistakenly considered an adequate explanation of the clinical picture, the realization on the part of the surgeon that the angiogram shows more than a small surface subdural hematoma may prevent him from falling into the pitfall of overlooking an intracerebral collection of blood (Fig. 10 a, b, c, d). Evacuation of the intracerebral hematoma may be lifesaving.

Historical Note

Chronic subdural hematoma was recognized by Wepfer in 1657 and Morgagni in 1747, both of whom described the occurrence of blood cysts under the dura. Houssard (1817) thought that a subdural hema-

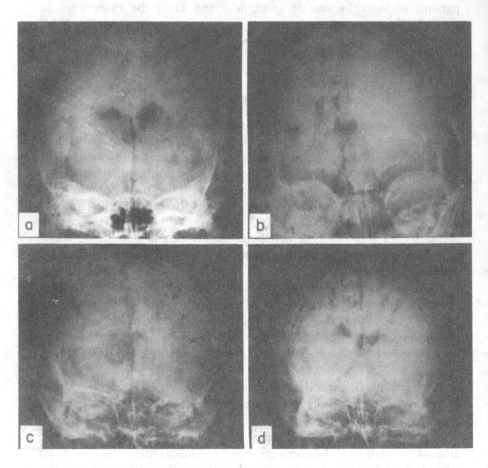

Fig. 7. a, Air study with right chronic subdural hematoma; b, With left chronic subdural hematoma; c—d, Bilateral chronic subdural hematoma.

toma was of inflammatory origin. In 1857, Virchow published his important studies ascribing the condition to an inflammation of the dura. According to Virchow, inflammation of the dura results in the deposition of fibrin which becomes vascularized and organized, forming a membrane. Rupture of blood vessels within the membrane is the

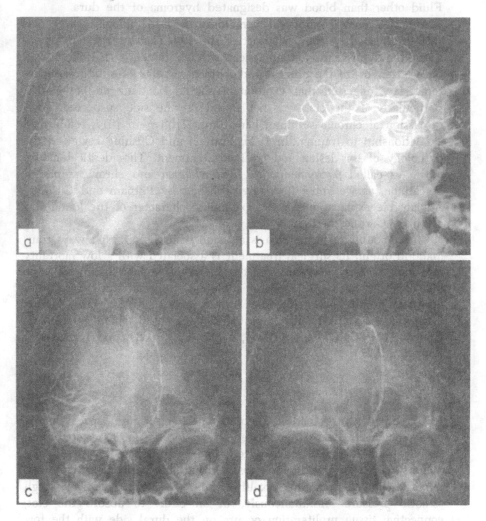

Fig. 8. a—b, Angiogram in right chronic subdural hematoma. c, Right angiogram and, d, left angiogram in right chronic subdural hematoma.

239

source of the hemorrhages. The term *pachymeningitis interna chronica* was applied to the fibrinous exudate which became organized. If extravasation was a prominent feature of the tissue, it was called *pachymeningitis hemorrhagica*. The expression hematoma of the dura was used to refer to the collection of blood in the subdural space. Fluid other than blood was designated hygroma of the dura.

Although chronic subdural hematoma as a pathologic entity was well established by the early part of the 19th century, the fear of entering the dural membrane influenced surgical thinking. In 1905, Bowen drew attention to the clinical and surgical aspects of subdural hematoma. He suggested that exploration should be done on both sides, particularly if the clot was not found on the side suspected. In a discussion of chronic subdural hematoma, Trotter, in 1914, established a relationship to trauma. In 1925, Putnam and Cushing reviewed the pathology of this lesion and outlined treatment. The identical nature of the so-called *pachymeningitis hemorrhagica* and chronic subdural hematoma, as we know it, was established by Putnam and Cushing. A plausible explanation for the expanding character of the lesion was given by Gardner in 1932.

Chronic subdural hematoma is a lesion which is almost always traumatic in origin. Its surgical treatment is associated with a low mortality rate and recovery may be expected in most patients. In view of the difficulties involved in diagnosing some cases, special studies are often necessary despite the likelihood of a high percentage of negative results Furlow (1936), Groff and Grant (1942), King and Chambers (1952), Browder (1943), Oldberg (1945), McKenzie (1938), and Horrax and Poppen (1937).

Pathology

If a quantity of blood accumulates in the subdural space that is not sufficient to cause immediate effects and is not associated with serious brain injury, it may be tolerated by the host for weeks and months with few or no symptoms. During this period, the clot may undergo liquefaction, the resulting fluid having a relatively high osmotic pressure. Simultaneously, in an effort to absorb the clot, connective tissue proliferation occurs on the dural side with the formation of a membrane. The arachnoid membrane having little or no blood supply, does not contribute to the attempt at absorption. Since the arachnoid is a semipermeable membrane, the clot tends to grow larger as cerebrospinal and other tissue fluids are drawn into the clot.

240

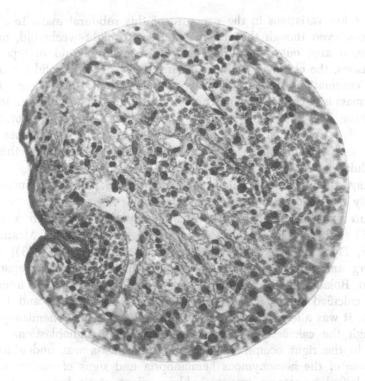

Fig. 9. Microscopic appearance of subdural membrane surrounding hematoma. One can see sinusoidal type of blood channels easy to tear causing repeated hemorrhages.

The size of the mass may also increase as a result of hemorrhage from the proliferating connective tissue membrane on the dural side of the clot (Fig. 9). At the borders of the mass, the proliferation continues until a very thin layer is formed on the inner (arachnoid) side of the mass. Eventually, such a mass causes headache, personality disorders and drowsiness. Later, neurologic deficits and evidence of increased intracranial pressure may develop.

Such a clot may occur on one or both sides of the brain. Although it usually is situated over the frontotemporoparietal area, it lies closer to the parietal region and midline. In this respect, it differs from the acute subdural hematoma, the solid component of which especially occupies more of the temporal region.

241

There are variations in the structure of this subdural mass. In some instances, even though the clot may be six to eight weeks old, there is little, if any, outer membrane and it is mainly liquid in type. In other cases, the clot may be liver-like in consistency and solid throughout. Combinations of solid and liquid components also occur. This entire mass is enclosed in an outer thick membrane and a very thin inner membrane. The liquid portion of the mass becomes lighter in color, and eventually it may be straw-colored. It has been stated that at times the cystic mass contains clear fluid. We have seen no examples of this in the adult.

Rarely, the mass may calcify or partly ossify. Many instances of partially calcified subdural hematoma have been reported in the literature. Chusid and DeGutierrez-Mahoney discussed such a case in 1953. Others include those reported by Critchley and Meadows (1933), Dyke and Davidoff (1938), Boyd and Merrill (1943), and Mosberg and Smith (1952). One of the earliest cases was reported by von Rokitansky in the middle of the 19th century. Of interest is the calcified subdural hematoma reported by MacLean and Levy (1955). It was a left-sided lesion with a left homonymous hemianopsia. Although the calcified mass was removed, later a glioblastoma was found in the right occipital lobe. The tumor mass was undoubtedly the cause of the homonymous hemianopsia and signs of compression. The calcified hematoma was probably a silent, static lesion.

Among others, Bassett and Lemmen (1952) reported several cases of subdural hematoma caused by bleeding from an intracranial aneurysm. After removal of a subdural hematoma, if the brain is still quite suffused with blood and under considerable pressure, the possibility of an associated intracerebral clot or a ruptured aneurysm should be considered. The importance of angiography in such cases is obvious. A subdural hematoma may also be caused by bleeding from an underlying tumor. In one of our cases, both a subdural hematoma and a subdural abscess were found. Subdural hematoma may occur in patients with cerebrovascular accidents.

The *age* of a chronic subdural hematoma is difficult to estimate except in a general way. Munro (1938) suggested that one be guided by the microscopic appearance of the hematoma wall and the protein content of the fluid in the cystic mass. The membrane of the hematoma on the dural side may form in about 15 days, though usually it takes 21 days or longer. Some attempts at fibroblastic proliferation occur as early as a few hours after the clot has formed. The thickness of the membrane increases after two or three weeks, but not in a manner that could suggest its exact age. Obviously calcification in the membrane of the hematoma implies that the lesion is several years old.

The protein content of the cystic portion of the hematoma increases up to 21 days according to Munro, then diminishes due to the effects of dilution. Unfortunately, this method of evaluating the age of the hematoma is also deceptive.

Etiology

In the adult, minor trauma may be the cause of a chronic subdural hematoma. Fights, falls — particularly in alcoholics — auto accidents, severe jolts of the head such as occasionally occur upon entering a car, may be responsible factors. Sometimes indirect injury to the head may produce a subdural hematoma. The trauma may be more severe. In our group of 114 cases, 33 were found to have a skull fracture in association with a chronic subdural hematoma. In Poppen's series (1955), a skull fracture was present in 8 out of a total of 119 cases.

By far the greatest number of our patients with chronic subdural hematoma were men, the proportion of males to females being almost 6:1. Most were between the ages of 20 and 60. In the older age group, between 60 and 80, we had 17 cases. One patient, aged 84, lived for another three years in good health after removal of the hematoma.

In a number of cases no definite history of injury was elicited. This may be due to the fact that the blow sustained may have been forgotten, or that the injury may have appeared insignificant. At any rate, 15 percent of the patients denied a history of trauma.

In the infant and young child, the picture is essentially the same as in the adult. Usually following a birth or postpartum injury, fall, or other accident, a subdural hemorrhage may form which may be well tolerated for some time because of the ease with which the skull can be deformed and enlarge at this early age. Such a child may appear hydrocephalic, except that his general demeanor is more nearly normal and he is more responsive to his environment. There may be a "cracked pot" resonance on skull percussion. The head does not enlarge to the extreme degree observed in the hydrocephalic child. A membrane that is thicker on the dural side and thinner on the arachnoid side, is present, and may contain large quantities of straw-colored fluid. While a liquid clot in an adult is effectively drained through one or two openings in the subdural space, in an infant a liquid clot surrounded by a membrane is often not cured by repeated drainage. (See also Chapter 15). A more lasting effect is obtained when a large

243

portion of the membrane, or as much of it as possible, is removed along with the contents of the cyst (Peet and Kahn, 1932).

Davidoff and Dyke (1938) have described a juvenile relapsing type of chronic subdural hematoma. In patients in whom a subdural hematoma resulted from an injury sustained during childhood or infancy, elevation of the sphenoid ridge and of the superior orbital plate and ridge develops, with deepening, widening, and lengthening of the middle fossa, hypertrophy of the frontal and ethmoidal sinuses, and thickening of the skull on the side of the lesion. These changes in the skull are the result of localized increased intracranial pressure followed by localized diminished pressure subsequent to absorption of the fluid content of the hematoma. A second injury at a later date is responsible for recurrence of hemorrhage into the original subdural hematoma, causing a reappearance of symptoms. Davidoff and Epstein (1955) described several examples of this type. Such a possibility should be considered in patients who have an asymmetric skull structure affecting the frontotemporal region.

Davidoff and Feiring (1953) reported the occurrence of chronic subdural hematoma in surgically treated hydrocephalus.

Symptoms and Signs

State of Consciousness. Except in those cases that are associated with a severe head injury, the state of consciousness is usually nearly normal up to the time of hospital admission. Patients who have sustained severe head trauma usually continue to improve following the initial period of impaired consciousness. After three to four weeks, headache reappears and the patient's state of consciousness deteriorates. The most common symptom in those who have not suffered a severe head injury is headache. Personality and other mental changes are common and in some instances a diagnosis of mental illness may be made. Chronic subdural hematoma is not a rare finding at necropsy in patients who have been confined to mental institutions. As knowledge concerning the causes of mental disease has increased and the necessity of appropriate diagnostic studies has become more widely recognized, this occurs much less often today than formerly.

Ocular Manifestations. Among our 114 patients, a dilated pupil on the side of the lesion was noted in 22. Dilatation of the pupil on the opposite side was seen in seven, and the pupils were equal in 85. Third-nerve paralysis was present in nine instances. There was one example of bilateral third-nerve paralysis shown by the presence of bilateral ptosis. The pupils were slightly dilated in this case. Papilledema was present in 27 cases.

Pupillary inequality may be due to cortical involvement or third-nerve injury. Compression of area 8 may result in constriction of the pupil followed by dilatation. Third-nerve involvement causes a marked dilatation of the pupil. Oculomotor paralysis in chronic subdural hematoma is produced by transtentorial *uncal* herniation compressing and distorting the brain stem.

Headache. In patients with chronic subdural hematoma, headache is quite common. Headaches were localized to the site of the lesion in 49 of our cases and generalized in 39. In the remaining patients, headache was not a symptom. Occasionally, the headache may be on the side opposite to that of the lesion. It is subject to considerable variation. For instance, following a lumbar puncture, it may disappear for a week or ten days and then reappear.

Focal Signs. These are frequently, though not invariably, present. A large subdural hematoma may compress the posterior cerebral artery through uncal herniation with resultant infarction affecting the occipital pole. Contralateral homonymous hemianopsia may thus be produced. Unilateral headache, weakness of the opposite half of the body, inequality of pupils, and a partial or complete third-nerve paralysis are present in some cases. Contralateral weakness or paralysis occurs in about 35 percent of patients. In about 10 percent of cases, the weakness or paralysis may be on the same side as the hematoma. Again, uncal herniation with compression of the brain stem by the margin of the incisura on the opposite side is the cause of the paradoxical finding of ipsilateral weakness or paralysis.

Pulse, Respiration, Temperature, and Blood Pressure. Alterations in vital signs in cases of chronic subdural hematoma are of little diagnostic significance until advanced cerebral compression has occurred. Then bradycardia may be observed, usually accompanied by headache and stupor. Slowing of the respiratory rate and an increase in blood pressure are infrequently seen.

Spinal Fluid Findings. Studies were made in 85 of our 114 cases. The spinal fluid was clear in 24, and bloody or xanthochromic in 61 cases. The pressure was over 300 mm of water in 51 instances, between 200 and 300 mm in 16, and between 100 and 200 mm in 11. The total protein was moderately elevated (50 to 100 mg%) in a little more than half of the cases.

Roentgen examination of the skull may show displacement of the pineal gland. This shift was diagnostic of the lesion in 22 of our 114 cases. Poppen (1955) observed a pineal shift in 40 out of a total of 119 patients with subdural hematoma. Usually, fractures are of the the linear type. In our group, 31 patients had linear fractures of the skull. In the series reported by Poppen, fractures of the skull were present in only eight patients out of 119. Unusual roentgen findings include erosion or thinning of the skull over the site of the hematoma. Asymmetrical development of the skull, anteriorly, may suggest a relapsing juvenile form of chronic subdural hematoma. Calcification occurs in some hematomas and may be visible in the roentgenogram over the cortex and adjacent to the inner table.

Side Involved. The hematoma was on the left side in 55 of our cases, on the right in 46, and bilateral in 12. The fact that the lesion is not infrequently bilateral makes it necessary to explore both sides at operation, unless adequate bilateral angiograms have been obtained. If bilateral hematomas are present, one is somewhat larger than the other, and consequently, a shift toward the side of the smaller one may give the false impression that only a unilateral lesion exists.

Diagnosis

The diagnosis of chronic subdural hematoma is not difficult if the lesion is suspected. In a general hospital service, it may be revealed during the course of investigation of a case of supposedly "cerebrovascular disease" or "tumor." Electroencephalography is of lateralizing value in approximately 50 percent of cases; as a means of providing localization it is much less accurate (Whelan et al, 1956). Echoencephalography may also lateralize the lesion. Radioisotope brain scanning provides a highly accurate method of diagnosis. Angiography remains the most reliable diagnostic procedure and may be performed with relative safety even in elderly patients and those in poor condition. Air study may uncover clots in unusual locations and seems to be better tolerated by these patients than by those with brain tumor (Martin et al, 1953), (Figs. 7, 8).

Treatment and Surgical Considerations

A chronic subdural hematoma may be evacuated by means of burr openings if the clot is mostly liquid (Jones, 1911 and 1912). If the clot is mainly solid, a small bone flap may be turned, one which adequately exposes and permits removal of the lesion. *Bilateral explorations* are indicated in all instances of suspected subdural hematoma, even though a lesion may have been found on the side initially explored, unless adequate bilateral angiograms have been done. In Figure 5 a, a solid subdural hematoma is shown being removed through a bone flap.

Occasionally a subdural hematoma may be found in the posterior fossa. In such a case, exploration of the posterior fossa may be done through either a unilateral (Fig. 5 c) or bilateral approach. In instances in which the authors have used the unilateral approach, a fracture line pointed the way to the lesion.

Following the removal of a large subdural hematoma over the hemisphere, the brain may fail to expand and fill the space occupied by the clot, remaining, instead, depressed and well away from the dura. Under these circumstances, we prefer to leave a rubber catheter connected to a sterile drainage system. Others have suggested the intraventricular or lumbar subarachnoid injection of saline (LaLonde and Gardner, 1948).

Prognosis

The treatment of a chronic subdural hematoma is successful in about 90 percent of cases. After removal of the clot, recovery may be rapid. The mental state returns to normal and, as a rule, patients are able to resume their usual type of work. Posttraumatic development of epilepsy is uncommon. We have encountered it in less than 10 percent of cases. Posttraumatic syndromes are also uncommon. In patients with associated brain injury, the prognosis may be less favorable, depending upon the severity of the cerebral trauma.

Follow-up Studies

Follow-up studies were done on 46 of the patients in our group. In the 7 who had acute subdural hematomas, the results of treatment have been poor in 6 and good in one. The outcome in 12 who had subacute subdural hematomas was good in 6, fair in 4, and poor in 2. A good result was achieved in 17 cases of chronic subdural hematoma; the outcome was fair in 8 and poor in 2. There were 5 instances of posttraumatic epilepsy in the entire group, 2 having had chronic hematomas, 2 subacute clots, and one an acute lesion. One patient with a chronic hematoma committed suicide nine months after injury and another was hospitalized in a mental institution; the head injury in the latter case was thought to be of importance in producing the mental abnormality. Patients wth slight deficits referable to speech or memory

247

or with minor alterations of behavior, none sufficiently serious to cause disability, were listed as having had fair results. A few patients in the group categorized as having good results complained of nervousness, occasional headache, and dizziness. Intellectual impairment, memory disturbances, nervousness, dizziness, easy fatigability, abnormal behavior, and crying spells were common sequelae in patients with acute subdural hematoma. There was a tendency for some of these patients to improve slowly and a few were fairly well rehabilitated after a few years.

It may be concluded that the outcome in patients with subdural hematoma is fairly good in those with the chronic variety and quite poor in those with the acute type, and that a good recovery may be expected in about half of those with subacute clots. Serious posttraumatic sequelae may occur even in cases of chronic subdural hematoma.

SUBDURAL COLLECTION OF CEREBROSPINAL FLUID (HYDROMA)

Pott (1819) reported finding subdural collections of clear or yellowish cerebrospinal fluid in some cases of head injury. Mayo described this condition in 1896 and Payr in 1916. It has since been the subject of a number of reports – Naffziger, (1924), Cohen and Elsberg (1927), Wycis (1945), Love (1937), McConnell (1941), and Abbott, Due, and Nosik (1943). Under the heading of Subdural Fluid Complicating Bacterial Meningitis, post-inflammatory collections of fluid in the infant have been described by McKay, Ingraham, and Matson (1953).

These collections of cerebrospinal fluid may not be surrounded by a membrane. Our own experience includes 47 such cases treated surgically. This condition was seldom recognized preoperatively, the diagnosis being made at the operating table.

Mechanism

Traumatic subdural accumulation of cerebrospinal fluid may result from a tear of the arachnoid membrane with escape of cerebrospinal fluid producing a loculated collection in the subdural space and localized pressure against the brain. The presence of small amounts of blood in the extra-arachnoid space may increase the osmotic pressure causing cerebrospinal and tissue fluids to enter the subdural space, thereby further increasing the volume of fluid in this region. Contusion and tears of the brain may lead to an accumulation of fluid in the adjacent subdural area through a similar mechanism. Coughing and sneezing

248

have been thought to cause tears of the arachnoid membrane in non-traumatic cases. Finally, certain inflammatory diseases involving the pia-arachnoid may result in collections of fluid in the subdural space, e.g., subdural effusions following meningitis (McKay, Ingraham, and Matson, 1953). In infants and children particularly, external hydrocephalus as a part of a congenital abnormality of the brain with agenesis may be mistaken for a subdural accumulation of cerebrospinal fluid.

Signs and Symptoms

The signs and symptoms of the subdural accumulation of cerebrospinal fluid are similar to those of a subdural hematoma which this condition mimics. The preoperative diagnosis, in many instances, is subdural hematoma, the nature of the lesion being established only at operation.

In our series of 47 cases, a lucid interval was noted in 12. Weakness or paralysis of one half of the body was observed in seven instances. Generalized and jacksonian seizures occurred in six cases. This condition was usually, but not always, unilateral. Skull fracture was present in about one-third of the cases. It must be remembered that a subdural accumulation of cerebrospinal fluid may coexist with a subdural or an epidural hematoma. This was true in three of our patients with epidural hematoma.

Diagnostic Tests

Diagnostic tests, including ventriculography and arteriography, are helpful. Angiography may show a unilateral or bilateral collection. A burr opening and incision of the dura reveals the lesion. In an infant, a subdural tap may be diagnostic and the injection of small amounts of air may show the extent of involvement. In three-fourths of the cases, the cerebrospinal fluid is bloody though the pressure is not particularly high, usually under 300 mm of water. In some of our cases, air accumulated in the subdural space following the evacuation of a large subdural collection of cerebrospinal fluid.

Treatment

Treatment involves drainage by means of burr holes on one or both sides, depending on the angiographic findings. On opening the dura, fluid, which is xanthochromic, straw-colored, or colorless in appearance, usually escapes under pressure. After enlarging the dural opening, one may be able to evacuate more subdural fluid by carefully depressing, with a blunt instrument, a cottonoid placed over the surface of the brain. The fluid tends to force the brain into the dural opening, and by carefully displacing the brain, additional large quantities of fluid may be drained. The introduction of a small piece of cottonoid immediately under the dura permits absorption of the cerebrospinal fluid which may then escape or be aspirated, allowing the brain to recede.

Although the operative procedure is simple and the fluid may be removed easily, the mortality in patients with this complication is still quite high (30 percent), undoubtedly due to associated intracranial damage. The possibility of another lesion such as an epidural or subdural hematoma occurring in association with a hydroma, should be given consideration.

INTRACEREBRAL AND INTRACEREBELLAR HEMATOMA

Intracerebral hemorrhage is less common than subdural hematoma, but more frequent than epidural bleeding. During a two-year period at the Detroit Receiving Hospital, 36 cases were operated upon for intracerebral hematoma out of a total of 950 cases of head injury (3.8 percent). During this time there were also, in the same hospital, 48 cases of depressed fracture, 7 patients with epidural and 61 with subdural hematomas. A large number of intracerebral hematomas was reported by Browder and Turney (1942). Echlin (1949) stated that intracerebral hematomas occur in about 1 percent of severe head injuries.

Mechanism of Production

The mechanism of production of intracerebral hematomas is mainly through mass movements resulting either in deep contusions of the brain, as may occur in the frontal and temporal regions, or tears of blood vessels which result in a hemorrhage within the brain substance. Deep contusions that produce softening and necrosis of brain with hemorrhage are the most common cause. Usually, when such a mass is removed, a large cavity is left in the brain, and this may eventually fill with cerebrospinal fluid or become connected with the ventricular system, resulting in porencephaly. The majority of such hematomas are

250

in the frontal and temporal regions. In our series, all except three were in these locations; three involved the parietooccipital area. The temporal and frontal lobes are the sites of predilection because of the mass movements of the brain and the shearing effects of the lesser wing of the sphenoid and the roof of the orbit on these areas. Occasionally, a vessel in the substance of the brain may be torn, resulting in a large hematoma, but this does not happen often. At times, the hemorrhage may be bilateral. One of our cases that came to autopsy had bilateral intracerebral hematomas in the temporal lobes.

Signs and Symptoms

The signs and symptoms of an intracerebral hematoma depend upon the location of the lesion. When it occurs in the temporal lobe, particularly on the left side, there may be a disturbance of speech associated with weakness of the right upper limb and the right side of the face. The neurologic deficit may increase with the development of stupor and eventual coma. Other patients may be comatose from the outset and exhibit weakness or paralysis of one-half of the body. Diagnostic studies are valuable in locating the clot.

In our series of patients, there were 6 females and 30 males. One patient complained of contralateral and 10 of generalized headache. There was a lucid interval in 15. The left side was involved in 20 and the right in 16 cases. Among the 36 cases, there were 7 with a central facial weakness, 20 with a contralateral hemiparesis, and 2 with an ipsilateral hemiparesis. In 22 of the 36 cases skull fracture was present on the same side as the hematoma in all but two. Generalized convulsions occurred in only one case. Focal signs were present in 22 out of the 36, and a pineal shift was found in 2 instances. Anisocoria was not as common as in subdural and epidural hematomas. The pupil was slightly dilated, or constricted, on the side of the lesion. Papilledema was noted in 7 cases. The cerebrospinal fluid was bloody in 21 and xanthochromic in 7; it was clear in 1 case. The cerebrospinal fluid pressure was frequently high. It was above 500 mm of water in 5 patients, and above 300 in an additional 7; in 6 cases it measured between 200 and 300 mm and in 3 between 100 and 200 mm.

Diagnosis

The diagnosis of an intracerebral hematoma is best confirmed by angiography. Air studies may be used in some instances. Browder

251

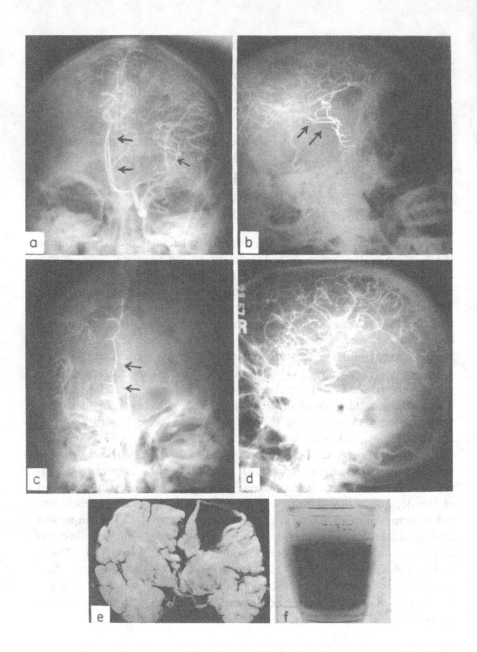

Fɪɢ. 10. a—d, Bilateral carotid angiography in a patient with left temporo-parietal intracerebral hematoma. e, Parietal intracerebral hematoma seen in another case in the autopsy room. f, Hematoma removed from patient whose angiograms are above.

(1943) has stated that exploration without any preliminary diagnostic studies is the best method of management. We believe that angiography is of inestimable value since the great majority of these clots occur in the frontal and temporal portions of the brain where delineation of abnormalities of the vascular pattern is readily demonstrated by this type of investigation.

Trauma involving the posterior fossa may be associated with intracerebellar hemorrhage (two cases in our series). It may be worthwhile to recount the case of a 27-year-old woman injured ten days prior to hospitalization. There was no history of unconsciousness at the time of the accident. She entered the hospital in a disturbed, drowsy state, that had developed three days earlier and had progressed. Roentgen examination of the skull showed no fracture. There were no localizing signs suggesting a mass lesion. She had mild nuchal rigidity and a slight fever, and was thought to have meningitis. Lumbar puncture revealed 40 red cells and 75 white cells, mostly lymphocytes, suggesting encephalitis. During the following day, her condition deteriorated and she died within a matter of minutes. At autopsy, she was found to have a right intracerebellar clot, partly solid and partly liquid, about the size of a hen's egg. Undoubtedly the clinical course in this case is best explained on the basis of increased intracranial pressure.

In war injuries, such lesions in the cerebellum are revealed by the presence of shell fragments and location of the cutaneous wound. An illustrative case was described by Webster, Schneider, and Lofstrom (1948). Their patient was in a manic state, vomiting, and complaining of severe headache. He had an insignificant appearing wound of the neck to the left of the midline. There was horizontal nystagmus on left lateral gaze, and incoordination was noted in the left upper and lower extremities. Roentgenologic examination revealed a comminuted fracture of the occipital bone to the left of the midline. Operation was performed through a curved incision to expose the left suboccipital region. A perforation into the posterior fossa was exposed and cerebellar tissue extruded through this opening. After opening the dura, there was a sudden extrusion of clots and dark blood, approximately 40 cc in amount. Following this, the herniating cerebellum receded and brain pulsations were observed. After thorough debridement, the wound was closed without drainage. Healing was by primary intention in spite of the fact that nine days had elapsed between the time of injury and operation. Two years later the patient was "getting along just fine.... I still don't have good use of my left hand."

Schneider, Kahn, and Crosby (1951) have suggested that such lesions in the cerebellum may be suspected on the basis of the lines of force involved in the head injury, one clue being the presence of an occipital fracture or of a contusion or laceration of the scalp in this region.

Hematomas of the cerebellum may, at times, pursue a subacute or chronic course. We have had a patient with a huge cystic mass in the right cerebellar lobe operated upon two and one-half months after injury. The cystic cavity contained straw-colored fluid. Microscopically, the cyst wall showed old hemorrhage. It was our impression that the lesion was originally an intracerebellar clot which had undergone absorption. The residual cystic mass compressed the cerebrospinal fluid pathways, causing increased intracranial pressure manifested by choked discs and severe headache. This posterior fossa lesion was diagnosed by ventriculography. The diagnosis of a subacute or chronic intracerebellar hematoma is difficult and fraught with uncertainty, since in many instances a hemorrhage into a preexisting tumor mass may behave essentially in the same manner. It is, therefore, not always possible to be absolutely sure of this diagnosis, unless the patient makes a sustained recovery, or the tissues available for microscopic study show unmistakable evidence of old hemorrhage.*

Treatment and Surgical Considerations

The treatment of intracerebral hematoma is operative removal of the clot. In the majority of our cases, the removal of the clot is effected through a large trephine opening (about 5 to 7 cm in diameter) over the suspected area; in a few, a bone flap is turned. A brain cannula is introduced permitting blood and softened brain to escape. In some instances, we have obtained as much as 2.5 ounces of old blood and debris by this technique. Following removal of the clot, the cavity is repeatedly irrigated with saline until clear fluid is obtained. In some cases the clot may be uncapped and aspirated under direct vision. Browder feels that a bone flap is preferable in the management of intracerebral hematomas. The surgical treatment of an intracerebral hematoma by means of a bone flap is shown in Fig. 5 d.

An example of an intracerebellar hematoma is seen in Fig. 5 c. Although these hematomas are rare, their removal may be followed by

* Four cases of traumatic intracerebellar hematoma occurring in association with contralateral supratentorial hemorrhage and contusion were reported by Schneider, Lemmen, and Bagchi (*J. Neurosurg.*, *10*, 122: 1953). (Ed.)

spectacular results. In Fig. 5 c, a right intracerebellar hematoma is exposed and excised after uncapping and entering the cavity containing the clot.

Prognosis

The prognosis for recovery of normal function in patients with intracerebral hematoma who survive is poor. The level of mentation is impaired and many patients have personality disorders for many months after injury. Epilepsy is a definite threat, but it does not occur as frequently as in open wounds. In our small group, it has occurred in about one-fifth of the cases.

CEREBROSPINAL FLUID PROTEIN IN VARIOUS HEMATOMAS. XANTHOCHROMIA

The normal protein content of the lumbar cerebrospinal fluid ranges from a low of about 20 mgm% to a high of about 45 mgm%. The presence of red blood cells increases the amount of protein roughly 1 mgm% per 1000 red blood cells per cu. mm. The increase of protein, however, does not depend upon the red blood cell count in the cerebrospinal fluid alone but occurs as a result of other factors as well. The highest levels are reached when there is loculation or blockage of the subarachnoid space, whatever the cause. An inflammatory reaction involving the pia-arachnoid also causes an increase of the cerebrospinal fluid protein content. Increase of cerebrospinal fluid protein may be seen in any of the intracranial hematomas and has little diagnostic significance per se.

In some cases of chronic subdural hematoma, there may be a moderate increase of the spinal fluid protein, up to between 80 and 100 mgm%. The protein elevation in intracerebral hematoma depends upon the proximity of the lesion to the subarachnoid space or ventricle and the amount of leakage of blood into the cerebrospinal fluid.

Yellow (xanthochromic) spinal fluid may be seen in any of the intracranial hematomas, as well as in other conditions, especially those associated with loculation of part of the subarachnoid space. It is almost always associated with an increase of the cerebrospinal fluid protein content.

Xanthochromia occurring in association with fresh blood in the subarachnoid space is evidence of preexisting hemorrhage, i.e., bleeding which has occurred some hours or days earlier. In the absence of recurrent bleeding, xanthochromia usually disappears in two to three weeks.

255

Postoperative bleeding is a complication to be recognized and treated with dispatch. Early reexploration is essential if irreparable damage due to uncal herniation and brain-stem compression are to be avoided. Among the signs and symptoms suggesting reaccumulation of blood are increasing stupor and focal findings not previously present. It is important to watch for such evidence as the development of a third-nerve paralysis combined with increasing weakness of one half of the body, and unilateral dilatation of the pupil in a patient who is stuporous or becoming lethargic. The pulse rate and the blood pressure should be recorded every half hour in the immediate postoperative period since a change in the direction of a bradycardia or an increase in blood pressure in a patient who is becoming more stuporous is very suggestive of postoperative bleeding.

Occasionally a patient in whom a subdural hematoma has been evacuated satisfactorily may relapse into a deepening stupor. Reexploration at the site of the hematoma may be negative but investigation farther posteriorly on the opposite side may reveal a clot previously overlooked.

We make it a practice to do a bilateral carotid angiogram before reexploration in patients in whom postoperative bleeding is suspected. A collection of blood on one or both sides may thus be outlined.

THE DIFFERENTIAL DIAGNOSIS OF INTRACRANIAL HEMATOMAS

The diagnosis of intracranial hematoma may be relatively easy or very difficult. Much depends upon the availability of an accurate history concerning the head injury and the symptoms immediately following. In a large city hospital to which many patients are brought in varying states of coma, and with external evidences of head injury, the differential diagnosis may be almost impossible on purely clinical grounds. This may be due not only to the lack of an adequate history but also to the presence of other diseases and, not infrequently, acute alcoholism or other intoxication. In such cases, spinal fluid examination, including a pressure determination, and x-rays of the skull may be helpful, the latter in regard to the presence of fracture and/or displacement of the pineal gland. Subsequent observation of the vital signs, and particularly the "curve" of unconsciousness (i.e., whether it is increasing, diminishing, or subject to unusual fluctuations) is important. Unilateral weakness may be of considerable significance. If it is increasing, a carotid arteriogram or multiple bilateral exploratory burr holes may be urgently required.

Fewer intracranial hematomas have been overlooked in recent years owing to the tendency to study or explore suspected cases sooner. Admittedly, not a few hematoma suspects turn out to be suffering from other conditions.

Given a typical history and clinical course, it is not difficult to make a diagnosis of epidural or subdural hematoma. In the former, an initial, often brief loss of consciousness follows a blow on the side of the head. Improvement sets in, with perhaps some headache and dizziness (the lucid interval), to be followed in hours or a day by the onset of deepening coma, usually with hemiplegia opposite the site of the blow. The demonstration of a fracture of the frontotemporal or temporoparietal skull on the injured side practically confirms the diagnosis. There are deviations from this "textbook" picture, such as the absence of the lucid interval and/or the slower development of signs over days rather than hours. In the case of subdural hematoma (subacute or chronic type), the clinical picture may simulate a brain tumor. Actually, the enlarging blood clots, though not neoplastic, act as expanding "tumors." The history — often of a mild head injury in the months preceding the onset — may be helpful, as may be the marked fluctuations of consciousness, progressive development of hemiplegia, and the displacement of a pineal gland as shown in the roentgenogram. The presence of xanthochromic cerebrospinal fluid, irrespective of its pressure, with some increase in the protein content, provides confirmatory evidence. A carotid arteriogram or pneumoencephalogram reveals the presence of a mass. Burr holes give the final answer by exposing a telltale, plum-colored dura overlying the hematoma. In the case of subdural hydroma, puncture of the normal-appearing dura reveals large quantities of clear or pale yellow fluid. Not infrequently signs of midbrain pathology complicate the picture, displacement of the temporal lobe resulting in transtentorial herniation and compression of the upper brain stem. The same displacement (uncal herniation) may impair the circulation of the posterior cerebral artery and produce a contralateral homonymous hemianopsia.

The intracerebral (or subcortical) hematomas may also simulate brain tumor. It may also be impossible to distinguish them on clinical grounds from a subdural hematoma. As for the rarer intracerebellar hematomas, Gurdjian and Webster (1958) emphasize the diagnostic importance of a perforation or a linear fracture in the occipital bone (overlying the cerebellum) in a patient who is "markedly disturbed and whose condition is deteriorating."

Not only tumor but such other conditions as brain abscess and hypertensive vascular lesions have also been erroneously diagnosed, especially when the clinical presentation was compatible with these entities and a history of head injury was not forthcoming. Conversely, other disorders manifested by coma have been encountered instead of hematoma when the clinical history and findings appeared to implicate head trauma. Burr holes in such obscure cases are quite justified as diagnostic tests to rule out the possibility of *associated* intracranial hematoma.

Cerebral edema occurs in association with cerebral contusion and/or hemorrhage, and also about areas of acute encephalomalacia. At times it may develop in the absence of such lesions and is believed by some to be due to vasomotor paralysis. This causes stasis in the cerebral venous channels and leads to a rise of cerebrospinal fluid pressure. Increased capillary permeability and tissue anoxia, and changes in the osmotic pressure of the affected tissues probably also play a part in producing edema. Fortunately, these cases are relatively rare. The patients are apt to be stuporous or even deeply unconscious and there is little or no improvement; there may be focal signs at times which suggest cerebral contusion, but this condition is not always present. The optic discs may show some swelling. The pineal gland may be displaced and angiography is likely to show displacement of vascular channels. The swollen brain may exert pressure on blood vessels, the posterior cerebral artery, for example, in the course of uncal herniation; rarely, the internal carotid artery is compressed. This clinical picture is practically indistinguishable from that of an expanding blood clot. The urgency of the condition may call for trephination and, if no clot is found, a right subtemporal decompression may have to be performed in an attempt to offset the increasing intracranial pressure. Dehydrating measures may have to be employed.*

Cerebral fat embolism may occur in cases of trauma involving long bones, especially of the lower limbs, and/or fat-containing tissues. Associated head injury may mislead the examiner into an erroneous diagnosis of an intracranial hematoma.

Symptoms of fat embolism appear after a latent period of variable length. The pulmonary manifestations include cough, chest pain,

*Hypothermia, the administration of steroids, and the use of controlled respiration with positive-negative pressures have also been suggested. The value of such measures, however, has not been clearly demonstrated. (Ed.)

cyanosis, increased respiratory rate, and rales. Headache, mental symptoms, convulsions, focal signs, and deepening coma reflect cerebral involvement. Cutaneous petechiae sometimes appear on the chest, extremities, and conjunctivae, and are of diagnostic significance. Fat droplets may be demonstrable in the sputum and/or urine.**

Gurdjian and Webster (1958) make reference to the appearance of hemorrhages and white patches of exudate in the retinae and emphasize the disappearance of old lesions coincident with the appearance of new ones. Papilledema has also been described.

Metabolic Disturbances. Various metabolic disturbances may occur following head trauma. Higgins, Lewin, O'Brien, and Taylor were among the first to study these metabolic disorders. In 1951 they reported six cases of fatal head injury with hyperchloremia and hypochloruria. In a subsequent article (1954), the metabolic effects observed in 76 patients unconscious for more than 12 hours following injury were presented. In 8 of these cases no abnormalities were found, and in another 50 the metabolic alterations, including proteinuria, hyperglycemia, renal glycosuria, elevation of blood urea, and diminution of plasma protein, were of transient duration. Major disorders consisting of hyperchloremia and hypochloruria (nine cases), hypochloremia and hyperchloruria (five cases), water deprivation, respiratory alkalosis, and renal uremia occurred in 18. Patients with hyperchloremia who expired had demonstrable injury to the undersurface of the frontal lobes.

Electrolyte disturbances may cause coma after a posttraumatic lucid interval, the resultant clinical picture being indistinguishable from that of a hematoma. This problem arose in a patient with hyponatremia and hypochloremia following head injury reported by Fagin, Mehan, and Gass (1958):

A girl of 17 was thrown out of a car when it collided with another vehicle. She was rendered unconscious. An x-ray of the skull showed a long, linear fracture of the left temporoparietal area. She improved progressively and in three days was able to converse normally; on the fourth day she was ambulatory, and her behavior and conversation rational. However, one week after the accident she became drowsy, soon exhibited spastic movements of the limbs, and became profoundly stuporous. The suspicion of an intracranial hematoma arose, but carotid angiography failed to substantiate this diagnosis. On the eighth day, she was in deep coma with irregular respirations. Examination revealed generalized mild

*Decreased arterial PO_2, and elevation of serum lipase are frequently found in cases of fat embolism. An electrocardiogram and chest x-ray may also be helpful in the diagnosis of this condition. (Ed.)

rigidity, intermittent right carpal spasm, overactive lower limb reflexes and a bilateral Babinski sign. Blood chemical studies were as follows: serum sodium 106 mEq/L (normal 137 to 147 mEq), serum chloride 88.7 mEq/L (normal 100 to 110 mEq), and the serum calcium, 4.28 mEq/L (normal 4.5 to 5.5 mEq). The serum potassium, carbon dioxide combining power, and blood sugar were normal.

Correction of the electrolyte imbalance brought about dramatic improvement by the next afternoon, and the patient recovered.

The metabolic disorders in head injury are discussed at length in Chapter 6.

LATE APOPLEXY

This rare condition was brought to the fore by Bollinger in 1891. It comes on days, weeks, months, or even later, following head injury in individuals in whom cerebral arteriosclerosis is supposedly not present. According to Gurdjian and Webster (1958), it is usually unrelated to the injury. In many of the cases arteriography has shown the presence of a thrombotic lesion, which of course raises a question as to the relationship between the trauma and thrombosis. If the vascular lesion occurs several weeks or months after the injury, there is no relationship, particularly if the injury was of minor degree. Sometimes the patient may have symptoms in the "free interval," and there may be suggestive focal signs with much fluctuation in symptoms before the final episode, be it thrombosis or hemorrhage.

A paralytic state appearing soon after head injury due to thrombosis of the internal carotid artery or other major vessel may result from contusion of the intima brought on by hyperextension, kinking, or the trauma of the deformation caused by the blow. In such a case, the thrombosis becomes complete and appropiate focal signs appear in a matter of several hours to a day or two.

Occasionally a hemorrhage may result from rupture of vessels crossing a cystic area caused by a previous injury. Such a cyst may contain clear or yellow fluid traversed by bands of tissue. Blood vessels present in these bands may rupture, producing a so-called "late apoplexy." The authors have seen such a hemorrhage occur in a porencephalic cavity associated with birth injury, after the patient had reached the age of sixteen years.

Cerebral arteriosclerosis is difficult to rule out as a basic cause, even in young subjects. Small areas of softening dependent upon secondary changes in vessels with alterations in local tension, as described by

260

Bollinger, are of very doubtful traumatic origin, nor is there general agreement with Marburg and Helfand's (1939) traumatic vasopathy, i.e., traumatic damage to vessel walls which may progress to a point of rupture with resulting hemorrhage.

BIBLIOGRAPHY

Abbott, W. D., Due, F. O., and Nosik, W. A. Subdural Hematoma and Effusion as a Result of Blast Injuries. *J.A.M.A.*, *121*, 664, 1943.

Alpers, B. J. Cerebral Birth Injuries, In S. Brock (Ed.), *Injuries of the Skull, Brain and Spinal Cord*, 2nd ed. Baltimore: Williams and Wilkins, 1943. Pp. 208-210.

Anderson, F. M. Extradural Cerebellar Hemorrhage; Review of Subject and Report of Case. *J. Neurosurg.*, *6*, 191, 1949.

Auvray, M. Traitement des Plaies des Sinus Veineux du Crane. *Arch. Gen. de Chir.*, *9*, 257, 1913.

Bacon, A. Cerebellar Extradural Hematoma. Report of a Case. *J. Neurosurg.*, *6*, 78, 1949.

Ballanace, C. A. *Surgery of the Temporal Bone*. London: Macmillan & Co., 1919.

Bassett, R. C. and Lemmen, L. J. Subdural Hematoma Associated with Bleeding Intracranial Aneurysm. *J. Neurosurg.*, *9*, 443, 1952.

Bell, Sir C. *Surgical Observations*. London: Longman, 1816.

Beller, A. J. and Peyser, E. Extradural Cerebellar Hematoma. Report of Three Cases. *J. Neurosurg.*, *9*, 291, 1952.

Bergmann, E. von. Surgery of the Head. In von Bergmann, E., von Bruns, P., and von Mikulicz, J. A. *System of Practical Surgery*, *1*, 17. New York and Philadelphia: Lea Bros. and Co., 1904.

Bollinger, O. Über traumatische Spätapoplexie. Ein Beitrag zur Lehre von der Gehirnerschütterung. *Internat. Beiträge zur wiss. Med.* (Festschrift Rud. Virchow), *2*, 459, 1891.

Bowen, W. H. Traumatic Subdural Hemorrhage. *Guy's Hosp. Rep.*, *59*, 21, 1905.

Boyd, D. A., Jr. and Merrill, P. Calcified Subdural Hematoma. *J. Nerv. Ment. Dis.*, *98*, 609, 1943.

Browder, J. A Résume of the Principal Diagnostic Features of Subdural Hematoma. *Bull. N. Y. Acad. Med.*, *19*, 168, 1943.

Browder, J. and Turney, M. F. Intracerebral Hemorrhage of Traumatic Origin. Origin. *N. Y. State J. Med.*, *42*, 2230, 1942.

Campbell, E., Whitfield, R., and Greenwood, R. Extradural Hematomas of the Posterior Fossa. *Ann. Surg.*, *138*, 509, 1953.

Campbell, J. A. and Campbell, R. L. Angiographic Diagnosis of Traumatic Head and Neck Lesions. *J.A.M.A.*, *175*, 761, 1961.

Campbell, J. B. and Cohen, J. Epidural Hemorrhage and the Skull of Children. *Surg., Gynec. Obstet.*, *92*, 257, 1951.

Chusid, J. G. and De Gutierrez-Mahoney, C. G. Ossifying Subdural Hematoma. *J. Neurosurg.*, 10, 430, 1953.

261

Secondary Hydrocephalus. *Surgery, 8,* 771, 1940.

Cohen, I. and Elsberg, C. A. Chronic Subdural Accumulations of Cerebrospinal Fluid after Cranial Trauma; Report of Case. *Arch. Neurol. Psychiat., 18,* 709, 1927.

Coleman, C. C. and Thomson, J. L. Extradural Hemorrhage in the Posterior Fossa. *Surgery, 10,* 985, 1941.

Critchley, M. and Meadows, S. P. Calcified Subdural Hematoma. *Proc. R. Soc. Med., 26,* 306, 1933.

Cushing, H. Strangulation of the Nervi Abducens by Lateral Branches of the Basilar Artery in Cases of Brain Tumor. *Brain, 33,* 204, 1910.

Cushing, H. Surgery of the Head. In W. W. Keen, *Surgery.* Philadelphia: W. B. Saunders, 1916. Pp. 17-276.

Davidoff, L. M. and Dyke, C. G. Relapsing Juvenile Chronic Subdural Hematoma. *Bull. Neur. Inst., New York, 7,* 95, 1938.

Davidoff, L. M. and Epstein, B. S. The Abnormal Pneumoencephalogram, 2nd ed. Philadelphia: Lea & Febiger, 1955.

Davidoff, L. M. and Feiring, E. H. Subdural Hematoma Occurring in Surgically Treated Hydrocephalic Children. *J. Neurosurg., 10,* 557, 1953.

Doench, H. O. Luftembolie bei Verletzung des Sinus Longitudinalis. *Zentralbl. f. Chir., 60,* 486, 1933.

Dyke, C. G. and Davidoff, L. M. Chronic Subdural Hematoma; Roentgenographic and Pneumoencephalographic Study. *Bull. Neur. Inst., New York, 7,* 112, 1938.

Echlin, F. Traumatic Subdural Hematoma — Acute, Subacute and Chronic; Analysis of 70 Operated Cases. *J. Neurosurg., 6,* 294, 1949.

Fagin, I. D., Mehan, D. J., and Gass, H. H. Hyponatremia and Hypochloremia as a Complication of Head Injury; Report of a Case Simulating Intracranial Hematoma. *Arch. Neurol. Psychiat., 80,* 562, 1958.

Ford, L. E. and McLaurin, R. L. Mechanisms of Extradural Hematomas. *J. Neurosurg., 20,* 760, 1963.

Freytag, E. Autopsy Findings in Head Injuries from Blunt Forces. *Arch. Pathol., 75,* 74, 1963.

Furlow, L. T. Chronic Subdural Hematoma. *Arch. Surg., 32,* 688, 1936.

Gardner, W. J. Traumatic Subdural Hematoma with Particular Reference to the Latent Interval. *Arch. Neurol. Psychiat., 27,* 847, 1932.

Goode, A. F. Extradural Haemorrhage in Child of 13 Months. *Lancet, 1,* 779, 1936.

Gordy, P. D. Extradural Hemorrhage of the Anterior and Posterior Fossae. *J. Neurosurg., 5,* 294, 1948.

Grant, F. C. and Austin, G. M. Evacuation of Traumatic Extradural Hemorrhage from the Posterior Fossa. *Ann. Surg., 130,* 963, 1949.

Groff, R. A. and Grant, F. C. Chronic Subdural Hematoma; Collective Review. *Int. Abstr. Surg., 74,* 9, 1942.

Gurdjian, E. S. and Webster, J. E. Extradural Hemorrhage. *Int. Abstr. Surg., 75,* 206, 1942.

Gurdjian, E. S. and Webster, J. E. *Operative Neurosurgery.* Baltimore: Williams and Wilkins, 1952.

Gurdjian, E. S. and Webster, J. E. *Head Injuries, Mechanisms, Diagnosis and*

Management. Boston: Little, Brown y Co., 1958.

Gurdjian, E. S. and Thomas, L. M. Surgical Management of the Patient with Head Injury. *Clinical Neurosurgery, 12.* Baltimore: Williams and Wilkins, 1966. Pp. 56-74.

Guthkelch, A. N. Extradural Hemorrhage as a Cause of Cortical Blindness. *J. Neurosurg.,* 6, 180, 1949,

Guthrie, G. J. *Injuries of the Head Affecting the Brain.* London: J. Churchill, 1842.

Higgins, G., Lewin, W., O'Brien, J. R. P., and Taylor, W. H. Metabolic Disorders in Head Injury. Hyperchloraemia and Hypochloruria. *Lancet, 1,* 1295, 1951.

Higgins, G., Lewin, W., O'Brien, J. R. P., and Taylor, W. H. Metabolic Disorders in Head Injury; Survey of 76 Consecutive Cases. *Lancet, 1,* 61, 1954.

Hill, J. *Cases in Surgery.* Edinburgh: R. Baldwin, 1772.

Holmes, G. and Sargent, P. Injuries of the Superior Longitudinal Sinus. *Br. Med. J., 2,* 493, 1915.

Hooper, R. S. Extradural Hemorrhages of the Posterior Fossa. *Br. J. Surg., 42,* 19, 1954.

Hooper, R. Head Injuries in Childhood. *The Australian and N.Z. J. Surg.,* 32, 11, 1962.

Horrax, G. and Poppen, J. L. The Frequency, Recognition and Treatment of Chronic Subdural Hematomas. *New Engl. J. Med.,* 216, 381, 1937.

Houssard, M. Observation d'un Kyste Considerable, Developé dans la Cavité de l'arachnoide chez un Sujet qui a Succombé avec les Symptomes d'une Apoplexie Sanguine. *Biblioth. méd.,* 55, 67, Paris, 1817.

Hutchinson, J. Lectures of Compression of Brain. *Clinical Lectures and Reports. London Hosp., 4,* 29, 1867.

Ingraham, F. D. and Matson, D. D. Subdural Hematoma in Infancy. *J. Pediatr.,* 24, 1, 1944.

Jacobson, W. H. A. Middle Meningeal Hemorrhage. *Guy's Hospital Rep., 28,* 147, 1885.

Jefferson, G. Bilateral Rigidity in Middle Meningeal Hemorrhage. *Br. Med. J., 2,* 683, 1921.

Jones, F. W. On the Grooves upon the Ossa Parietalia Commonly Said to be Caused by the Arteria Meningia Media. *J. Anat. and Physiol., 46,* 228, 1911.

Jones, F. W. The Vascular Lesions in Some Cases of Middle Meningeal Hemorrhage. *Lancet, 2,* 7, 1912.

Kennedy, F. and Wortis, S. B. Modern Treatment of Increased Intracranial Pressure. *J.A.M.A., 96,* 1284, 1931.

Kessler, F. K. Cerebellar Extradural Hematoma. *J. Neurol. Psychiat.,* 5, 96, 1942.

King, A. B. and Chambers, J. W. Delayed Onset of Symptoms Due to Extradural Hematomas. *Surgery, 31,* 839, 1952.

Krause, F. *Surgery of the Brain and Spinal Cord, Based on Personal Experiences, vol. 1.* Tr. by H. Haubold. New York: Rebman, 1909-1912.

Kroenlin. Über die Trepanation bei Blutungen aus der A. Meningea Media und geschlossener Schädelkapsel. *Deutsche Ztschr. f. Chir.,* 23, 209, 1885.

LaLonde, A. A. and Gardner, W. J. Chronic Subdural Hematoma. Expansion of Compressed Cerebral Hemisphere and Relief of Hypotension by Spinal

Injection of Physiologic Saline Solution. *New Engl. J. Med., 239,* 493, 1948.

Leary, T. Subdural Hemorrhages. *J.A.M.A., 103,* 897, 1934.

Lefkowitz, L. L. Extradural Hemorrhage as Result of Birth Trauma. *Arch. Pediatr., 53,* 404, 1936.

Lemmen, L. J. and Schneider, R. C. Extradural Hematomas of the Posterior Fossa. *J. Neurosurg., 9,* 245, 1952.

Levi-Valensi, A. and Ezes. Paraplégie corticale traumatique. Observation anatomoclinique. *Encéphale, 25,* 667, 1930.

Levy, L. L., Segerberg, L. H., Schmidt, R. P., Turrell, R. C., and Roseman, E. The Electroencephalogram in Subdural Hematoma. *J. Neurosurg., 9,* 588, 1952.

Love, J. G. Bilateral Chronic Subdural Hygroma. *J. Nerv. Ment. Dis., 85,* 161, 1937.

Luys, G. Fracture du Crane; Rupture du Sinus Lateral. *Bull. Soc. Anat. de Par., 73,* 450, 1898.

Luys, G. Les Blessures des Sinus de la Dure-mére. *Presse méd., 9,* 278, 1901.

MacCarty, C. S., Horning, E. D., and Weaver, E. N. Bilateral Extradural Hematoma, *J. Neurosurg., 5,* 88, 1948.

MacLean, J. A. and Levy, L. F. Calcified Subdural Hematoma. *Neurology, 5,* 520, 1955.

McConnell, A. A. Traumatic Subdural Effusions. *J. Neurol., Neurosurg. Psychiatry, 4,* 237, 1941.

McKay, R. J., Jr., Ingraham, F. D., and Matson, D. D. Subdural Fluid Complicating Bacterial Meningitis. *J.A.M.A., 152,* 387, 1953.

McKenzie, K. G. Extradural Haemorrhage. *Br. J. Surg., 26,* 346, 1938.

Marburg, O., and Helfand, M. *Injuries of the Nervous System.* New York: Veritas Press, 1939.

Martin, F. A., Webster, J. E., and Gurdjian, E. S. The Relative Accuracy of Electroencephalography, Air Studies and Angiography in a Series of Two Hundred Mass Lesions. *J. Neurosurg., 10,* 397, 1953.

Mayo, C. H. Brain Cyst with Recovery. *N. Y. Med. J., 59,* 434, 1896.

McLaurin, R. L. and Ford, L. E. Extradural Hematoma. Statistical Survey of Forty-Seven Cases. *J. Neurosurg., 21,* 364, 1964.

McLaurin, R. L. and Tutor, F. T. Acute Subdural Hematoma. Review of Ninety Cases. *J. Neurosurg., 18,* 61, 1961.

Meirowsky, A. M. Wounds of Dural Sinuses. *J. Neurosurg., 10,* 496, 1953.

Moody, W. B. Traumatic Fractures of the Cranial Bones; Clinical Considerations, with Especial Reference to Extradural Hemorrhage. *J.A.M.A., 74,* 511, 1920.

Morgagni, J. B. De Sedibus et Causis Morborum. Liv. 1, Epist. 3, Art. 1, Louvain, 1767.

Mosberg. W. H., Jr. and Smith, G. W. Calcified Solid Subdural Hematoma. Review of Literature and Report of an Unusual Case. *J. Nerv. Ment. Dis., 115,* 163, 1952.

Munro, D. *Cranio-cerebral Injuries: Their Diagnosis and Treatment.* New York: Oxford Univ. Press, 1938.

Munro, D. Cerebral Subdural Hematomas; a Study of Three Hundred and Ten Verified Cases. *New Engl. J. Med., 227,* 87, 1942.

Munro, D. and Maltby, G. L. Extradural Hemorrhage; A Study of Forty-Four Cases. *Ann. Surg., 113*, 192, 1941.

Munslow, R. A. Extradural Cerebellar Hematomas; Report of Two Cases. *J. Neurosurg., 8* 542, 1951.

Naffziger, H. C. Subdural Fluid Accumulations Following Head Injury. *J.A.M.A., 82*, 1751, 1924.

Oldberg, E. Subdural Hematoma. *Med. Clin. North Am., 29*, 62, 1945.

Payr, E. "Meningitis serosa" bei und nach Schädelverletzungen (Traumatica). *Med. Klin., 12*, 841, 1916.

Peet, M. M. and Kahn, E. A. Subdural Hematoma in Infants. *J.A.M.A., 98*, 1851, 1932.

Plummer, S. C. Research on the Surgical Anatomy of the Middle Meningeal Artery. *Ann. Surg., 23*, 540, 1896.

Poppen, J. L. Chronic Subdural Hematomas. *Geriatrics, 10*, 49, 1955.

Pott, Sir P. The Chirurgical Works of Percivall Pott, by Sir James Earle. 2 vols. Philadelphia: J. Webster, 1819.

Pringle, J. H. Traumatic Meningeal Hemorrhage with Review of 71 Cases. *Edinburgh Med. J., 45*, 741, 1938.

Putnam, T. J. and Cushing, H. Chronic Subdural Hematoma; Its Pathology, Its Relation to Pachymeningitis Hemorrhagica and Its Surgical Treatment. *Arch. Surg., 11*, 329, 1925.

Raney, R. B., Raney, A. A. and Peterson, E. W. Emergency Care of Suspected Middle Meningeal Hemorrhage; Technical Suggestions for the General Surgeon. *J.A.M.A., 153*, 1434, 1953.

Relton, B. and Haslam, W. F. Case of Hemorrhage from a Branch of the Middle Meningeal Artery. *Lancet, 1*, 469, 1894.

von Rokitansky, C. *Handbuch der pathologischen Anatomie.* Vol. 2, 717. Vienna: Br\umüller u. Seidel, 1844.

Rowbotham, G. F. and Whalley, N. Prolonged Compression of Brain Resulting from Extradural Haemorrhage. *J. Neurol., Neurosurg. Psychiatry, 15*, 64, 1952.

Roy, G. C. Fracture of Skull; Extensive Extravasation of Blood on Dura Mater, Producing Compression of Brain; Trephining; Partial Relief of Symptoms; Death. *Lancet, 2*, 319, 1884.

Schneider, R. C., Kahn, E. A., and Crosby, E. C. Extradural Hematoma of the Posterior Fossa. *Neurology, 1*, 386, 1951.

Smith, G. W., Mosberg, W. H., Pfeil, E. T., and Oster, R. H. The Electroencephalogram in Subdural Hematoma; with Review of the Literature and Presentation of Seven Cases. *J. Neurosurg., 7*, 207, 1950.

Solomon, N. H. Subepicranial Hydroma (False Meningocele). *N. Y. State J. Med., 49*, 1324, 1949.

Steiner, R. Zur chirurgischen Anatomie der Arteria Meningea Media. *Arch. f. klin. Chir., 48*, 101, Berlin, 1894.

Stewart, J. W. Fractures of Skull, Diagnostic and Prognostic Features. *J.A.M.A., 77*, 2030, 1921.

Sunderland, S. and Bradley, K. C. Disturbances of Oculomotor Function Accompanying Extradural Haemorrhage. *J. Neurol., Neurosurg. Psychiatry, 16*, 35, 1953.

Thorman, W. quoted by P. Wiesmann.

265

Trotter, W. Chronic Subdural Hemorrhage of Traumatic Origin and Its Relation to Pachymeningitis Hemorrhagica Interna. *Br. J. Surg.*, 2, 271, 1914.

Turnbull, F. Extradural Cerebellar Hematoma; A Case Report. *J. Neurosurg.*, 1, 321, 1944.

Vance, B. M. Fractures of the Skull; Complications and Causes of Death (A Review of 512 Necropsies and of 61 Cases Studied Clinically). *Arch. Surg.*, 14, 1023, 1926.

Vance, B. M. The Significance of Fat Embolism. *Arch. Surg.*, 23, 426, 1931.

Vance, B. M. Ruptures of Surface Blood Vessels on Cerebral Hemispheres as a Cause of Subdural Hemorrhage. *Arch. Surg.*, 61, 992, 1950.

Verbruggen, A. Extradural Hemorrhage. *Am. J. Surg.*, 37, 275, 1937.

Virchow, R. Haematoma Durae Matris. *Vërhandl. d. phys.-med. Gesellsch.*, 7, 134, Würzburg, 1857.

Voris, H. C. The Diagnosis and Treatment of Subdural Hematomas. *Surgery*, 10, 447, 1941.

Voris, H. C. The Diagnosis and Treatment of Extradural Hematomas. *Surgery*, 10, *Surg.*, 10 655, 1947.

Wakely, C. P. G. and Lyle, T. K. Problem of Extradural Hemorrhage; Report of 14 Cases. *Ann. Surg.*, 100, 39, 1934.

Webster, J. E., Schneider, R. C., and Lofstrom, J. E. Observation on Early Type of Brain Abscess Following Penetrating Wounds of the Brain. *J. Neurosurg.*, 3, 7, 1946.

Webster, J. E., Schneider, R. C., and Lofstrom, J. E. Observations upon Patients with Penetrating Wounds Involving the Cerebellum. *Ann. Surg.*, 127, 327, 1948.

Wepfer, J. J. Observationes Anatomicae ex Cadaveribus Eorum, quos Susptulit Apoplexia. Amsterdam, 1681. P. 5.

Wharton, H. R. Wounds of the Venous Sinuses of the Brain. An Analysis of Seventy Cases. *Ann. Surg.*, 34, 81, 1901.

Whelan, J. L., Haddad, B. F., Webster, J. E., and Gurdjian, E. S. Electroencephalographic Findings in Subdural Hematoma. A Report of 18 Cases. *Grace Hosp. Bull.*, 34, 11, 1956.

White, R. J., Verdura, J., and Locke, G. E. Emergency Cerebral Arteriography in Acute Head Injury. Presented at the annual meeting of the American College of Angiology, June, 1964, Las Vegas, Nevada.

Wiesmann, P. Über die modernen Indikationen zur Trepanation mit besonderer Berücksichtigung der Blutungen aus der Arteria Meningea Media. *Deutsche Ztschr. f. Chir.*, 21, 1, 1885, 22, 52, 1885.

Woodhall, B,. Devine, J. W., Jr., and Hart, D. Homolateral Dilation of Pupil, Homolateral Paresis and Bilateral Muscular Rigidity in Diagnosis of Extradural Hemorrhage. *Surg., Gynec. Obstet.*, 72, 391, 1941.

Wycis, H. T. Subdural Hygroma. A Report of 7 Cases. *J. Neurosurg.*, 2, 340, 1945.

BILBLOGRAPHY ON "LATE APOPLEXY"

Bollinger, O. Über traumatische Spätapoplexie. Ein Beitrag zur Lehre von der Gehirnerschütterung. *Internat. Beiträge zur wiss. Med.* (Festschrift Rud. Virchow), 2, 459, 1891.

Courville, C. B., and Blomquist, O. A. Traumatic Intracerebral Hemorrhage, with Particular Reference to its Pathogenesis and its Relation to "Delayed Traumatic Apoplexy." *Arch. Surg., 41,* 1, 1940.

DeJong, R. N. Delayed Traumatic Intracerebral Hemorrhage. *Arch. Neur. Psych., 48,* 257, 1942.

Doughty, R. G. Post-Traumatic Delayed Intracerebral Hemorrhage. *South. Med. J.,* 31, 254, 1938.

Friedman, E. D. Intracerebral Hemorrhage of Traumatic Origin. In S. Brock (Ed.), *Injuries of the Brain and Spinal Cord,* 3rd ed. (Chap. 6). Baltimore: Williams and Wilkins, 1949.

Harbitz, F. Traumatic Hemorrhage of the Brain: Late Post-Traumatic Hemorrhage. Norsk Mag. f. Laegevidensk, *92,* 501, 1931.

Harbitz, F. Traumatic Late Hemorrhages in Brain and Meninges and Their Significance in Accident Insurance; Addendum: Significance of Traumas in Development of Vascular Diseases. *Norsk Mag. f. Laegevidensk., 25,* 715, 1945.

Langerhans, R. Die Traumatische Spätapoplexie. Berlin: Hirschwald, 1903.

Marburg, O. Zur Frage der Hemorrhagia Cerebri bei jüngeren Menschen und deren differentieller Diagnose. *Deutsche Ztschr. f. Nervenh., 105,* 22, 1928.

Naffziger, H. C., and Jones, O. W. Late Traumatic Apoplexy. *Calif. and West. Med., 29,* 361, 1928.

ADDENDUM

(By the Editor)

Echoencephalography, radioactive brain scanning, and contrast radiologic examination, particularly arteriography, have been utilized extensively as diagnostic adjuncts in cases of suspected hemorrhage following head trauma. Employing pulsed ultrasound and recording the echoes reflected from within the cranium, echoencephalography provides a rapid, simple, and safe means of determining whether midline structures have been displaced. With experience, an accuracy of about 95 percent may be attained. Errors in interpretation and the fact that the diencephalic midline determined by this technique may not be shifted by lesions in front of or behind this level, or on both sides, limit its usefulness. For these reasons, a negative echoencephalogram does not necessarily exclude a hematoma and, depending on the clinical evidence, further investigation may be indicated. Nevertheless it remains a useful screening procedure.

Brain scans in cases of subdural hematoma usually disclose a "hot vascular rim" in the prone or supine position. False positive scans may, however, be encountered, as, for example, in patients with ecchymoses involving the soft tissues.

267

The advantages and wide sphere of applicability of angiography in the diagnosis and localization of intracranial hemorrhage are well reconized. Although this procedure has been utilized most frequently in cases of suspected subdural hematoma, it has also proved exceedingly valuable in demonstrating extradural hematomas in aberrant locations. Intracerebral clots also lend themselves to angiographic diagnosis though they may not be readily distinguishable from localized areas of edema.

Angiography has largely supplanted pneumoencephalography as a diagnostic procedure during the acute phase of head trauma. At times, however, as in cases of suspected posterior fossa hematoma, pneumoencephalography may be preferable.

It should be stressed that whenever an extradural hemorrhage is under consideration, special investigations must not be allowed to interfere with surgical treatment since the mortality rises sharply with delay (Hooper, 1969). In the event operation fails to disclose the lesion, angiography or air study must then be performed for purposes of localization.

For a detailed account of the radiologic aspects of head injury, including traumatic intracranial hemorrhage, the reader is referred to Chapter 10. (See also Schechter, 1966; Schechter and Zingesser, 1969).

Several important contributions dealing with extradural hemorrhage have appeared in recent years. Observations on a series of 83 cases were reported by Hooper (1959). In this series the highest incidence occurred during the third decade of life; only 2 of the 21 children under 15 years of age were less than 2 years old; the incidence during childhood was greatest at 8 years of age. Traffic accidents accounted for 39 percent of cases, falls were responsible for 36 percent, and 16 percent resulted from blows. By and large, the injuries were relatively mild. In a large proportion of cases, the abrasion or hematoma of the scalp, indicative of the site of impact, was situated directly over the extradural clot. This relationship occurred more commonly than one between the fracture line and hematoma. Injuries of the side of the head were associated with supratentorial clots, while the less common posterior fossa hemorrhages were caused by trauma involving the occipital region. In 34 of the cases, the hemorrhage was of arterial origin in 15; in 5 it arose from both artery and vein, and in 8 it resulted from tears of dural venous sinuses; the site of origin was not clear in the remaining 6 cases. The clinical picture developed most rapidly in cases in which the bleeding was arterial in origin. The pattern of the clinical presentation varied depending on the degree of initial injury and depth of coma, the site of trauma, the location and rapidity of formation of the clot, and the presence or absence of associated intradural lesions. Thus, in 8 cases, following an initial period of unconsciousness, operative treatment was instituted before deterioration occurred; 37 patients exhibited the classic clinical picture — a "lucid" interval after a period of initial unconsciousness, followed by stupor and, eventually, coma; transitory impairment of consciousness followed by progressive deterioration occurred in 15 cases; and in 16 the trend was one of progressively deepening coma. The middle fossa was the most common site of hemorrhage (54 cases). Evidence of trauma to the lateral aspect of the head was almost invariably discernible. Although the clinical picture varied, symptoms developed more rapidly when the clot was in this location than when it was situated elsewhere. Operation was required within 12 hours in 64 percent of the cases in this group. Contralateral signs appeared in 50 percent, and an ipsilateral dilated pupil in a slightly higher proportion. There was a coexisting intradural hemorrhage in 40 percent. The overall mortality was 25 percent. In 15 patients the extradural hematoma was located in the anterior fossa, trauma having been sustained in the lateral frontal region. Consciousness deteriorated gradually, and pupillary inequality was commonly observed; pyramidal signs were not marked. The average interval between injury and operation was 38 hours. The mortality in this group was 20 percent. A hematoma developed in the parasagittal region in five cases and in each instance there was some evidence of local trauma. The rapidity of development of the clinical picture varied. Pyramidal signs and pupillary inequality were present in four of the five cases, all of which survived. In nine cases the hematoma involved the posterior fossa and, in all but one, a fracture line crossing a venous sinus was present. The clinical presentation unfolded at a varying pace. In the acute form, loss of consciousness, pupillary dilatation, and signs of medullary compression developed rapidly. Headache, vomiting, nuchal rigidity, cerebellar and cranial nerve dysfunction, and retention of consciousness characterized the more chronic variety. Four of these nine patients died. There were 19 deaths (23 percent) in the entire series of 83 patients, one having succumbed prior to operation. In 25 percent of cases there was an associated intradural lesion, either a subdural or intracerebral hemorrhage or both; the mortality rate of this group was about four times greater (48 percent) than that of patients without coexisting intradural clots (12.5 percent). The mortality was higher in patients over 60 years of age. The major factor influencing mortality was the state of consciousness. The importance of early diagnosis and treatment and of intradural inspection at the time of operation was emphasized.

McKissock et al (1960 b) reported their experience with 125 cases of extradural hematoma. Exclusive of children, males predominated. In this series, as in Hooper's, the clinical course varied, with the syndrome characterized by a lucid interval occurring in only 27 percent of cases. Ten patients remained conscious throughout the entire course of their illness; in 17 cases there was no initial loss of consciousness, but coma subsequently supervened (this group included the greatest number of the very young); 35 patients were initially unconscious, but thereafter remained quite alert up to the time of operation; 33 patients exhibited a lucid interval; the remaining 30 patients were comatose from the time of injury until operation was performed. In all, consciousness was affected in 90 percent. Evidence of trauma to the scalp, usually over the site of the hematoma, was noted in the majority of cases. Pupillary abnormalities, most commonly a dilated ipsilateral pupil (63 cases), occurred in 74 patients. Four patients with bilateral dilated and fixed pupils survived. Weakness of the limbs or pyramidal signs were observed in 85 cases; in 4 patients in whom the course of events was one of slow progression, over a period of more than 7 days, the paresis was on the side of the lesion. Bradycardia (pulse rate below 60) was recorded in 57 cases. Signs of blood loss were evident in four patients, all infants. Roentgenograms available in 96 cases disclosed a fracture in 82 and suture diastasis in 3; over half the patients without a demonstrable fracture were less than 15 years of age. Ventriculography performed in 26 cases demonstrated the lesion in each instance. The location of the hematoma was as follows: temporal 100 cases, frontal 9, parietal or parietooccipital 11, posterior fossa 5. Three patients had bilateral clots. Coexisting subdural hematomas were present in 12 cases, ipsilateral in 8, contralateral in 2, and bilateral in 2. In two patients the extradural hematoma was associated with an intracerebral hemorrhage within the temporal lobe. At operation the bleeding site was identified in 43 cases and proved to be the middle meningeal artery in 35, the superior sagittal sinus in 2, the lateral sinus in 3, and the diplöe in 3. The surgical mortality (116 cases) was 23 percent. The lesion was not found at operation in 7 cases, and in 3 coexisting lethal lesions were overlooked; the surgical procedure was inadequate in 2 cases. Of the 91 survivors, 63 recovered fully, 8 remain totally disabled for physical or mental reasons, 16 are partially disabled and 4 have epilepsy. There were 27 children in this series under the age of 15 years, of whom 18 (67 percent) did not lose consciousness initially though 16 were comatose at the time of operation. X-rays of the skull did not demonstrate a fracture or suture diastasis in 21 percent. Whereas 58 percent of the adults were operated upon within 24 hours of injury, the comparable figure for children was 37 percent. Only two children died (7 percent mortality). Factors affecting prognosis included the level of consciousness, the age of the patient, and the rate of evolution of the clinical picture. No patient under seven years of age died, while no one over 60 survived.

A study of 167 cases of extradural hematoma was presented by Gallagher and Browder (1968). A fracture was demonstrated in 91 percent of cases by x-rays or at operation or necropsy. Clinical information of a nature to permit analysis was available in 106 instances. Three variations of the clinical syndrome could be distinguished. Little or no associated brain damage was suffered by 65 patients (61 percent) and these exhibited the classic sequence of events terminating in coma, ipsilateral pupillary dilatation, contralateral paralysis, bradycardia, and decerebration and death if unrelieved. A moderate degree of brain trauma was sustained by 19 patients (18 percent) whose clinical course differed from the previous group essentially only in that the duration of the initial state of impaired consciousness was more prolonged. Injury to the brain was severe in 22 patients (21 percent), being manifested by profound coma throughout their clinical course. Most injuries occurred as a result of a fall. The youngest patient was three years of age, the oldest 75, bearing out the impression that extradural hemorrhage may occur at any age though rarely at the extremes of life. Males predominated, there being only 11 females in the series. In about one-third of the cases the trauma appeared to be relatively insignificant; in 35 cases the accident was not followed by loss of consciousness. A lucid interval was recorded in 72 percent of those in whom an adequate history was available. A dilated pupil on the side of the hematoma developed in 94 patients; in 12 it appeared on the opposite side. Contralateral hemiparesis was apparent in 112 patients (67 percent); ipsilateral weakness was noted in two, both with extensive bilateral cerebral lacerations; most of the remaining cases exhibited decerebrate rigidity or flaccidity. Signs of decerebration developed in 72 cases (43 percent) and bradycardia appeared in 86 (about 50 percent). Lumbar puncture done in 113 cases revealed a normal pressure in 30 percent, a moderate increase in 33 percent and pronounced elevation in 37 percent. Operation was performed on 122 patients of whom 48 died, a surgical mortality of 40 percent; only 3 of 36 children expired following surgery. The surgical mortality was directly related to the level of consciousness at the time of operation;

decerebration affected the prognosis adversely. In the vast majority of cases (120), the hematoma was temporal in location, though frequently extending into adjacent areas; in 8 it was situated in the frontal region and in 35 its location was parietooccipital; there were 2 bilateral hematomas. Postmortem examination in 88 cases disclosed associated contusions of the frontal or temporal lobes in 41, lacerations often combined with subdural or intracerebral clots in 37, and hemorrhages in the brain stem or cerebellum in 16. In the surgical material, contusion of the cortex beneath the hematoma was frequently observed and in 8 instances (one contralateral) there was an associated subdural hemorrhage. In only a few cases did the extradural hematoma arise from a source other than the middle meningeal vessels. The method of surgical treatment depended on the clinical condition of the individual patient. In 41 cases the clot was evacuated through a subtemporal craniectomy while in 81 a bone flap was utilized.

The report of Jamieson and Yelland (1968) is also based on a series of 167 cases of extradural hematoma. The overall mortality was 16 percent, there having been a decline from 27 percent in the first 60 cases to 8 percent in the last 60. While most of these cases involved young adults, mostly males, the ages of the patients varied from nine months to 84 years. Traffic accidents accounted for almost half of the injuries. The hematoma was situated over the lateral convexity in 70 percent of cases; other locations included the anterior cranial fossa, floor of the middle fossa, occipital region, posterior fossa and, in a few instances, the vertex. Five patients had bilateral clots. The mortality was highest in posterior fossa lesions. Only one child out of a total of 22 under the age of 10 years succumbed. Concomitant subdural or intracerebral hematomas or cerebral lacerations were present in 47 percent and these cases were associated with a mortality rate four times greater than that of extradural hematoma alone. Only 20 of the 167 patients exhibited the syndrome characterized by a lucid interval; 38 remained unconscious and 41 were conscious throughout their clinical course; 91 were initially unconscious and 93 unconscious at the time of surgery. The level of consciousness when operated upon was distinctly related to the mortality rate. Abnormality of one pupil occurred in about one-third of cases and the incidence of hemiparesis was about the same. More than half the patients conscious at the time of operation manifested headache, irritability, and bradycardia. In patients with unilateral pupillary dilatation the mortality rate was 17 percent; when both pupils were dilated, the mortality was 47 percent, and when decerebration occurred, the figure rose to 78 percent. The textbook sequence of initial concussion followed by lucidity and then unconsciousness, together with pupillary dilatation, circulatory disturbance, and hemiplegia was observed in only four of the 167 patients. The evolution of the clinical picture varied in time from less than one hour to 14 days; it was slowest when the hematoma involved the frontal region. Over half the cases were operated upon within 24 hours. The mortality rate was highest in cases in which the clinical picture developed most rapidly. In almost all cases the operative procedure utilized to evacuate the hematoma was a local craniectomy. These authors emphasized that an alteration in the state of consciousness is the most important single sign of a developing extradural hematoma. They further indicated that the most useful of all investigations is an exploratory burr hole at the site of trauma to the head, and that, in most instances, neuroradiologic study is not warranted in view of the resultant delay in diagnosis and treatment.

Data on 21 cases of extradural hemorrhage in children are included in Mealey's monograph on pediatric head injuries (1968). Only two patients were less than four years of age. The hematoma was located in the temporoparietal area in 13 cases; the parietooccipital region was involved in four, the anterior fossa in three and the posterior fossa in one. The classic clinical picture was not observed in any of the cases. Four patients rendered unconscious initially continued to deteriorate; six never lost consciousness throughout their clinical course; while 11, who were not unconscious immediately following the injury, deteriorated subsequently. The usual phenomena associated with temporal lobe herniation were observed, including unilateral or bilateral dilated and/or fixed pupils, contralateral hemiparesis, decerebrate rigidity, and flaccid quadriplegia. Papilledema developed in patients with a protracted course. The overall mortality rate was 25 percent, being highest in patients operated upon within 12 hours (45 percent). Although acknowledging the usefulness of angiography in the management of extradural hematoma, Mealey emphasized that its use in any particular case is contingent upon the patient's condition and the urgency of the need for surgical intervention. With regard to extradural hematoma of the posterior fossa, he indicated that the operative indications are "mainly clinical, based on a smoldering course after occipital trauma severe enough to cause fracture or diastasis of the posterior cranial fossa."

The section on extradural hematoma in Matson's textbook (1969) is based on an experience with 44 patients under the age of 12. In almost half of the cases, the condition occurred during the first two years of life. Roentgenograms performed in 36 cases disclosed a fracture or diastasis of a suture in 26. Initial loss of consciousness was uncommon, occurring only in 11 patients. Evidence of trauma to the scalp was usually present. Aside from deterioration of consciousness, the most significant clinical feature was the appearance of lateralizing neurologic signs — contralateral weakness and ipsilateral pupillary dilatation. In about 30 percent of cases, several days elapsed before this sequence of events developed. Deterioration occurred rapidly in 26 cases operated upon within 12 hours of hospitalization. In infants, bleeding into the epidural space often resulted in anemia and a shock-like state. The source of the bleeding was the middle meningeal artery or one of its branches in about 60 percent of cases and a venous sinus in 20 percent. Evacuation of the clot was performed by means of a craniectomy in the temporal region. In young children, the clot was often relatively circumscribed, being limited to the middle fossa inferiorly or posteriorly, presumably because of the firm attachment of the dura to suture lines at this age. Four patients died; 30 of the survivors recovered completely.

The observations reported by Mealey (1960), Hawkes and Ogle (1962), and McLaurin and Ford (1964) are essentially similar to those already noted. Four cases of extradural hematoma at the vertex revealed by angiography were reported by Alexander (1961) and a single case each by Stevenson et al (1964) and Columella et al (1968). In each instance a fracture was present near the vertex and in four of the cases papilledema developed. In most cases the evolution of the clinical picture was relatively slow.

There are five main causes of death following operation for extradural hematoma (Hooper, 1969): delay in operation; circulatory collapse during operation; failure to remove the hematoma completely; recurrence; and failure to recognize and treat associated subdural or intracerebral clots.

With regard to the actual operative procedure, an exploratory burr hole is usually made in the temporal region and enlarged sufficiently to permit evacuation of the clot and to control bleeding. If exploration at this site fails to reveal a hematoma, additional burr holes are made in the parietal, parietooccipital, and frontal regions (Mealey, 1968; Hooper, 1969). Depending on the operative findings and the clinical situation, exploratory burr holes on the opposite side or over the cerebellum may be indicated. Following removal of the extradural clot, the subdural space should be inspected. In the event the hematoma has been definitively localized preoperatively, formal craniotomy is

274

probably the procedure of choice unless the more expeditious craniectomy is dictated by the patient's condition.

In view of the importance of careful observation for evidence of impending complications, particularly intracranial bleeding, in all cases of head trauma, the use of monitoring techniques comparable to those employed in coronary units, has been suggested. Blood pressure, pulse, and respiration may be readily registered. Methods of recording intracranial pressure have also been devised but their clinical application has been limited owing to a number of shortcomings. Unfortunately, as indicated by Jennett (1969), "the most important sign in the head injured patient is a changing conscious level and this is not yet susceptible to instrumentation." A report by Johnston et al (1970) deals with the simultaneous continuous monitoring of ventricular fluid pressure (indwelling catheter) and systemic arterial pressure in 32 patients with severe head injuries. The response of the blood pressure to raised ventricular pressure was variable. Aspiration of ventricular fluid was very effective in reducing intracranial pressure. The authors suggest continuous monitoring of the intraventricular and arterial pressure as a guide to treatment comprising the use of mannitol, hyperventilation, and ventricular drainage, in cases of trauma with progressive elevation of intracranial pressure not due to a surgically amenable lesion.

Observations on 90 cases of acute subdural hematoma evacuated within three days of injury were reported by McLaurin and Tutor (1961). The occurrence of a lucid interval was associated with a much more favorable prognosis. Only one of 16 patients who exhibited this feature (6 percent mortality) died; of the remaining 74 whose comatose state continued uninterrupted, 57 failed to survive (77 percent mortality). The mortality rose with the degree of pupillary abnormality. Changes in the level of consciousness, pupillary alterations, and motor signs were the factors that led to surgical intervention; observation of vital signs provided no useful guide in this respect. Necropsy performed in 34 cases disclosed cerebral contusion, laceration, or severe edema in most cases. Acute subdural hematoma was attributed to laceration of cortical blood vessels.

McKissock et al (1960 a) reviewed a series of 389 cases of subdural hematoma, subdividing their material into acute (occurring within three days of trauma), subacute (between four and 20 days), and chronic forms. The incidence of acute and subacute lesions increased with age. A striking feature was the nonspecific nature of the symptoms. Impairment of consciousness was a prominent feature, particularly in the first two groups, while headache was a common complaint in the chronic variety. The neurologic signs noted on admission were likewise of limited diagnostic value. Pupillary inequality was present in 116 cases, dilatation occurring on the side of the lesion in 79 percent and on the opposite side in 8 percent. Paresis (159 cases) was an even less reliable sign, being contralateral to the lesion in 59 percent and ipsilateral in 29 percent. Angiography was performed in only 21 patients, in all of whom it established the diagnosis. The most important prognostic factors were the state of consciousness and the rate of evolution of the clinical picture. Age also influenced the outcome. The overall operative mortality was about 20 percent, the figures for the acute, subacute, and chronic groups being 51 percent, 24 percent, and 6 percent respectively. Postmortem study often revealed associated lesions, especially intracerebral hemorrhage in the acute cases, as well as cerebral edema and changes in the brain stem. Of the 270 known survivors, 221 made a good recovery.

The overall mortality of 553 cases of subdural hematoma reported by Jamieson (1970) was 35 percent. There were 249 patients without associated cerebral lacerations and the mortality rate in this group was 22 percent; the mortality was over 50 percent in those with cerebral lacerations. The rapidity of evolution of the lesion was also of considerable importance in determining the outcome. Thus, the mortality rate of patients operated upon within 12 hours of injury was 76 percent; 38 percent of those operated upon in the next 36 hours died; thereafter the mortality was 13 percent. Angiography was performed in 40 percent of cases, its use being limited to those of slower evolution. In patients in whom an acute subdural hematoma was suspected on clinical grounds, a burr hole was sometimes made at the site of trauma to rule out an extradural clot, after which exploratory openings were made in the temporal region on one or both sides and enlarged to the size of a subtemporal decompression in the event a clot was found. Jamieson emphasized the change in pattern of the type of head injury resulting from traffic accidents in recent years in Australia, the trend being toward a higher incidence of inoperable lesions, and he stressed the necessity of devising a safer transport system and of preventing accidents.

Merwarth (personal communication) observed a case of subdural hematoma in which the neurologic deficit was similar to that noted following interference with the cerebral veins (Merwarth, 1940). In this particular instance the clinical manifestations consisted of weakness, maximal in the lower extremity and sparing the hand, gnostic sensory loss most pronounced in the lower limb, and retention of speech function.

Interhemispheric subdural hematoma is uncommon and is not associated with any distinctive clinical features. The diagnosis may be established on the basis of the angiographic or pneumoencephalographic findings (Clein and Bolton, 1969; Sibayan et al, 1970).

Subdural hematoma of the posterior fossa is of rare occurrence. Acute, subacute, and chronic forms have been described (Ciembroniewicz, 1965). The occipital region is the usual site of trauma. Following a lucid interval of varying duration, headache and vomiting develop followed by impairment of consciousness. Nuchal rigidity, cranial nerve palsies, and evidence of cerebellar dysfunction and of brain stem compression appear. Surgical intervention, preceded by ventriculography if time permits, is imperative. This type of lesion may occur in the newborn (Matson, 1969; Gilles and Shillito, 1970). Recognition of this fact is important since the resultant hydrocephalus may be cured following removal of the hematoma.

Seventeen cases of traumatic infratentorial hematomas observed over a 12-year period at the Massachusetts General Hospital were reviewed by Wright (1966). During this same period, 344 cases of traumatic supratentorial hematomas were encountered. The clot was extradural in location in six, subdural in five, and intracerebellar in six. Posterior fossa fractures were present in all cases of extradural hematoma, in four of the subdural hematomas, and in only one of the intracerebellar lesions. In all but one case the occipital region was the site of trauma. In one-third of the patients the diagnosis was not made during life; two patients were operated upon in a moribund state, and another died following surgery; eight patients recovered after operation. The common finding in all cases was impairment of consciousness. Acute cases were difficult to diagnose. Subacute and chronic cases gave rise to posterior fossa manifestations.

Acute subdural hematoma, an unusual form of cerebrovascular accident, may occur as a result of spontaneous rupture of a cortical artery. Eight such cases were reported by Talalla and McKissock (1971). In each instance the hemiparesis was on the side of the lesion. Drake (1961) also described 11 cases of subdural hemorrhage due to arterial rupture following trauma.

Intracranial hemorrhage is a well recognized complication of anticoagulant therapy. Seven cases of subdural hematoma occurring as a consequence of this form of treatment were reported by Wiener and Nathanson (1962).

Epidural and subdural bleeding complicating various intracranial surgical procedures has been described in a number of publications, including a recent article by Feiring (1968).

Subdural hematoma during infancy and childhood is discussed in detail elsewhere in this volume (Chapter 15), but will be dealt with briefly in this section. The frequency and importance of subdural hemorrhage during infancy is indicated by Mealey's statement (1968) that it "ranks second only to hydrocephalus as a major intracranial problem in the first year of life."

Utilizing the plan of treatment proposed by Ingraham and Heyl (1939) and further elaborated by Ingraham and Matson (1944), (subdural taps, followed by burr holes to determine the presence of a membrane, and craniotomy to remove the membranes and solid clot), a series of 537 patients with subdural hematoma under two years of age was reviewed by Matson (1969). The incidence was highest during the first six months of life, probably as a result of trauma sustained at birth or soon thereafter. The importance of excising the subdural membranes in order to avoid restricting the growth of the brain at this time of life was again emphasized. Unilateral or bilateral craniotomy was required in 75 percent of cases. Normal development subsequently occurred in about three-quarters of the patients. Children in the retarded group mostly had large chronic hematomas with advanced cerebral atrophy and thick membranes. The most common clinical manifestations were convulsions, vomiting, irritability, failure to gain weight, fever, hyperactive reflexes, bulging of the fontanel, anemia, enlargement of the head, and abnormal fundi.

The outcome in 92 cases of infantile subdural hematoma followed for periods of two to 15 years was reported by Yashon et al (1968). Seventy-one patients (73 percent) survived, of whom 55 (60 percent) were judged to have done well. Most of the latter were left with no residua other than minimal hemiparesis or an occasional seizure. The final outcome in nine patients was poor; all were mentally retarded and some were also left with a severe physical handicap. There were 21 deaths, six of which occurred postoperatively. No correlation could be drawn between the outcome and the specific type of treatment or the presence of membranes.

The frequency of parental abuse and deliberate trauma in the home as factors in the etiology of infantile subdural hematoma was emphasized by Mealey (1968). He also critically reviewed the principles of management, questioned the validity of some current therapeutic concepts, and expressed doubt concerning the detrimental effects of "the mere presence of subdural fluid and membranes" on the underlying brain. Evidence that removal of the membrane was not necessary in all cases of subdural hematoma had been presented earlier by Shulman and Ransohoff (1961) and by others referred to in their paper. These authors suggested that the prognosis in cases of subdural hematoma in infancy was related to the severity of the original trauma sustained by the brain rather than to the compressed effects of the effusion or membranes. In addition to raising questions concerning the advisability of removing subdural membranes routinely, Mealey pointed out that this form of treatment is not invariably effective, since recurrence of the subdural effusion not uncommonly follows craniotomy. Shunting procedures, notwithstanding their shortcomings, may be required in such cases. Mealey favors a plan of extended conservative treatment, that is, repeated subdural taps over a period of two to three months for symptomatic relief, anticipating spontaneous resolution of the subdural effusion.

The reports of Rabe et al (1968) and of McLaurin et al (1971) lend further credence to the idea that most cases of infantile subdural hematoma can be successfully managed by tapping alone. McLaurin et al suggest that the only indication for tapping following establishment of the diagnosis is persistence of intracranial hypertension.

It is not an uncommon experience to demonstrate by means of angiography small collections of fluid in the subdural space which displace the brain away from the inner table of the skull a distance of several millimeters. Assuming the patient's condition has stabilized at a satisfactory level, continued observation rather than operative intervention is probably indicated. While some such cases may subsequently deteriorate and require surgical treatment, many will improve and repeated arteriography will reveal that the fluid collection has diminished or disappeared (Hooper, 1969).

With regard to the policy of nonsurgical treatment of subdural hematoma proposed by some on the basis of the fact that spontaneous recovery may occur at times, Mackay (1963) commented as follows: "That subdural hematoma may resolve spontaneously is well known; that conservative therapy is generally inadequate and often fatal is equally well known. Elementary clinical judgment usually dictates burr hole exploration bilaterally." We fully concur.

Three cases of delayed intracranial hemorrhage following head injury were reported by Morin and Pitts (1970). In one, a 3-year-old girl, fatal subarachnoid bleeding occurred on the tenth day after injury. Each of the other two, a girl of eight and a man of 66, both of whom were operated upon successfully, sustained an intracerebral hemor-

279

rhage, on the thirty-fourth and ninth days respectively following trauma. The authors reviewed the literature and found that most patients were under 40 years of age, an observation that would tend to minimize the importance of cerebrovascular disease as an etiologic factor. In most cases the interval between the injury and the onset of symptoms, most commonly headache and hemiplegia, was less than 30 days.

Decerebrate rigidity following head trauma is a grave prognostic sign. It is indicative of injury to the brain stem either directly or as a consequence of tentorial herniation. Gutterman and Shenkin (1970) reviewed their experience with 52 such cases. Intracranial hematomas were evacuated in 29 patients, of whom 14 (48 percent) survived. Included in this group were 10 cases of epidural hemorrhage (7 survivors), 14 of acute subdural hematoma (5 survivors) and 5 with intracerebral clots (2 survivors). Two of the survivors had no neurologic sequelae, 9 had mild deficits, one a severe deficit, and 2 were left with behavioral disorders. Of the 23 patients who had no demonstrable intracranial hematoma, 15 survived (65 percent); of these 15 survivors 2 recovered fully in regard to neurologic function, and 3 were left with only a mild deficit. Thus the mortality of decerebrate patients with supratentorial hematomas was greater than that of those with direct trauma to the brain stem. The quality of survival, however, was better in the former group. Patients with epidural hematoma fared better than those with intracerebral and subdural hematomas, both as to mortality and morbidity. The longer the duration of the decerebrate state preoperatively, the higher the mortality in the surgical group. There was an increase in the mortality rate when decerebration lasted longer than a week, though there could be useful survival even after this state had existed for as long as 45 days. The mortality rate increased with age, the prognosis for recovery being best in patients under 20. (See also Robertson and Pollard, 1955; Scarcella and Fields, 1962; and Brendler and Selverstone, 1970). No benefit could be ascribed to the use of corticosteroids.

BIBLIOGRAPHY

(for the Addendum)

Alexander, G. L. Extradural Haematoma at the Vertex. *J. Neurol. Neurosurg. Psychiatry*, *24*, 381, 1961.

Brendler, S. J. and Selverstone, B. Recovery from Decerebration. *Brain*, *93*, 381, 1970.

Ciembroniewicz, J. E. Subdural Hematoma of the Posterior Fossa. *J. Neurosurg.*, *22*, 465, 1965.

Clein, L. J. and Bolton, C. F. Interhemispheric Subdural Haematoma: A Case Report. *J. Neurol. Neurosurg. Psychiatry*, *32*, 389, 1969.

Columella, F., Gaist, G., Piazza, G. and Caraffa, T. Extradural Haematoma at the Vertex. *J. Neurol. Neurosurg. Psychiatry*, *31*, 315, 1968.

Drake, C. G. Subdural Haematoma From Arterial Rupture. *J. Neurosurg.*, *18*, 597, 1961.

Feiring, E. H. Variations on the Theme of Postoperative Intracranial Hemorrhage. *Acta Neurochir.*, *19*, 129, 1968.

Gallagher, J. P. and Browder, E. J. Extradural Hematoma. Experience with 167 Patients. *J. Neurosurg.*, *29*, 1, 1968.

Gilles, F. H. and Shillito, J., Jr. Infantile Hydrocephalus: Retrocerebellar Subdural Hematoma. *J. Pediatr.*, *76*, 529, 1970.

Gutterman, P. and Shenkin, H. A. Prognostic Features in Recovery from Traumatic Decerebration. *J. Neurosurg.*, *32*, 330, 1970.

Hawkes, C. D. and Ogle, W. S. Atypical Features of Epidural Hematoma in Infants, Children and Adolescents. *J. Neurosurg.*, *19*, 971, 1962.

Hooper, R. Observations on Extradural Hemorrhage. *Brit. J. Surg.*, *47*, 71, 1959.

Hooper, R. *Patterns of Acute Head Injury.* Baltimore: Williams and Wilkins, 1969.

Ingraham, F. D. and Heyl, H. L. Subdural Hematoma in Infancy and Childhood. *J.A.M.A.*, *112*, 198, 1939.

Ingraham, F. D. and Matson, D. D. Subdural Hematoma in Infancy. *J. Pediat.*, *24*, 137, 1944.

Jamieson, K. G. Extradural and Subdural Hematomas. Changing Patterns and Requirements of Treatment in Australia. *J. Neurosurg.*, *33*, 632, 1970.

Jamieson, K. G. and Yelland, J. D. N. Extradural Hematoma. Report of 167 Cases. *J. Neurosurg.*, *29*, 13, 1968.

Jennett, W. B. Head Injuries. In S. Taylor (Ed.), *Recent Advances in Surgery*, 7th ed. Boston: Little, Brown & Co., 1969. Pp. 590-621.

Johnston, I. H., Johnston, J. A. and Jennett, B. Intracranial Pressure Changes Following Head Injury. *Lancet*, *2*, 433, 1970.

Mackay, R. P. Editorial Comment. In R. P. Mackay, S. B. Wortis, and O. Sugar (Eds.), *Yearbook of Neurology, Psychiatry and Neurosurgery, 1962-1963.* Chicago: Yearbook Medical Publishers, 1963.

Matson, D. D. *Neurosurgery of Infancy and Childhood. Springfield*, Ill.: Charles C Thomas, 1969.

McKissock, W., Richardson, A. and Bloom, W. H. Subdural Haematoma. A Review of 389 Cases. *Lancet, 1,* 1365, 1960 a.

McKissock, W., Taylor, J. C., Bloom, W. H. and Till, K. Extradural Haematoma. Observations on 125 Cases. *Lancet, 2,* 167, 1960 b.

McLaurin, R. L. and Ford, L. E. Extradural Hematoma. Statistical Survey of Forty-Seven Cases. *J. Neurosurg., 21,* 364, 1964.

McLaurin, R. L., Isaacs, E. and Lewis, H. P. Results of Nonoperative Treatment in 15 Cases of Infantile Subdural Hematoma. *J. Neurosurg., 34,* 753, 1971.

McLaurin, R. L. and Tutor, F. T. Acute Subdural Hematoma. *J. Neurosurg., 18,* 61, 1961.

Mealey, J., Jr. Acute Extradural Hematomas Without Demonstrable Skull Fractures. *J. Neurosurg., 17,* 27, 1960.

Mealey, J. Jr. *Pediatric Head Injuries.* Springfield, Ill.: Charles C Thomas, 1968.

Merwarth, H. R. Hemiplegia of Cortical or Venous Origin (Occlusion of Rolandic Veins). *Brooklyn Hosp. J., 2,* 193, 1940.

Merwarth, H. R. Personal Communication.

Morin, M. A. and Pitts, F. W. Delayed Apoplexy Following Head Injury ("Traumatische-Spät-Apoplexie"). *J. Neurosurg., 33,* 542, 1970.

Rabe, E. F., Flynn, R. E. and Dodge, P. R. Subdural Collections of Fluid in Infants and Children. *Neurology, 18,* 559, 1968.

Robertson, R. C. L. and Pollard, C., Jr. Decerebrate State in Children and Adolescents. *J. Neurosurg., 12,* 13, 1955.

Scarcella, G. and Fields, W. S. Recovery from Coma and Decerebrate Rigidity of Young Patients Following Head Injury. *Acta Neurochir., 10,* 134, 1962.

Schechter, M. M. Angiography in Head Trauma. Chapter XIV. In *Clinical Neurosurgery,* Vol. *12.* Baltimore: Williams and Wilkins, 1966. Pp. 193-220.

Schechter, M. M. and Zingesser, L. H. Neuroradiologic Aspects of the Posttraumatic Syndrome and of Posttraumatic Epilepsy. In A. E. Walker, W. F. Caveness and M. Critchley (Eds.), *The Late Effects of Head Injury.* Springfield, Ill.: Charles C Thomas, 1969. Pp. 228-260.

Shulman, K. and Ransohoff, J. Subdural Hematoma in Children. The Fate of Children with Retained Membranes. *J. Neurosurg., 18,* 175, 1961.

Sibayan, R. Q., Gurdjian, E. S. and Thomas, L. M. Interhemispheric Chronic Subdural Hematoma. *Neurology, 20,* 1215, 1970.

Stevenson, G. C., Brown, H. A. and Hoyt, W. F. Chronic Venous Epidural Hematoma at the Vertex. *J. Neurosurg., 21,* 887, 1964.

Talalla, A. and McKissock, W. Acute "Spontaneous" Subdural Hemorrhage. *Neurology, 21,* 19, 1971.

Wiener, L. M. and Nathanson, M. The Relationship of Subdural Hematoma to Anticoagulant Therapy. *Arch. Neurol., 6,* 282, 1962.

Wright, R. L. Traumatic Hematomas of the Posterior Cranial Fossa. *J. Neurosurg., 25,* 402, 1966.

Yashon, D., Jane, J. A., White, R. J. and Sugar, O. Traumatic Subdural Hematoma in Infancy. *Arch. Neurol., 18,* 370, 1968.

CHAPTER 9

GUNSHOT WOUNDS OF THE BRAIN AND THEIR COMPLICATIONS

EMANUEL H. FEIRING, M. D.

AND

LEO M. DAVIDOFF, M. D.

While gunshot wounds of the head are not uncommon in civil practice, our knowledge thereof is derived largely from war experience. During World War I, the management of craniocerebral injuries by specialists was initiated. Principles of treatment were formulated and accounts of their experiences published by Cushing (1918), Horrax (1919), and Jefferson (1919) among others. Sepsis was exceedingly frequent and, in a large measure, was responsible for the high mortality rate. In Cushing's series of 133 dural penetrating wounds, there were 55 postoperative fatalities (41.4 percent). Forty-three of these deaths were caused by infection (32.3 percent).

The treatment of intracranial wounds during the second World War was greatly facilitated as a result of the specialty status accorded neurosurgery and the availability of trained neurosurgeons. While the fundamental concepts established during the previous conflict continued to be adhered to, significant advances were achieved due to the introduction of antibiotics and its consequence, the abandonment of the open method for the delayed treatment of head wounds. The incidence of infection was lowered, the death rate appreciably diminished, and the period of morbidity considerably shortened. Thus, to illustrate, of 500 penetrating wounds treated by British surgeons during the European campaign of 1944 and 1945, the postoperative mortality was 16.4 percent (Small and Turner, 1947); the mortality from infection was only 5 percent. In a series of 2185 cases of penetrating head wounds operated upon by American surgeons, the postoperative mortality rate was approximately 14 percent (Matson, 1958). Comprehensive accounts of their experiences in the treatment of head wounds during

World War II have been published by the American and British military services.

The management of wounds of the nervous system during the Korean campaign differed in no essentials from that of the Second World War (Lewin and Gibson, 1955; Meirowsky, 1965), nor has it changed in Vietnam (Purvis, 1966; Jacobs, 1968; Hammon, 1971). Meirowsky reported an operative mortality of 9.6 percent in a series of 879 cases of penetrating brain wounds incurred in Korea. In an analysis of 1732 cases of wounds of the head treated surgically in Vietnam, Hammon (1971) reported a total operative mortality of 11.2 percent, the figure being even lower (9.7 percent) for U. S. military personnel; operation was not performed on 455 patients in a moribund state. A detailed description of the treatment of neurosurgical casualties in the Korean War may be found in a publication of the Office of the Surgeon General, *The Neurological Surgery of Trauma.*

The classification of gunshot wounds of the head proposed by Cushing in 1918 remains unsurpassed. It has been adopted by most authors and will continue to be utilized in this presentation. (See also Fig. 1):

    I. Wounds of the scalp.
    II. Cranial fractures without dural penetration.
    III. Cranial fractures with depression and dural penetration but without extrusion of brain.
    IV. Wounds (usually of gutter type) with brain extruding and indriven fragments of bone.
    V. Wounds usually of penetrating type with indriven bone fragments plus metal.
    VI. Wounds of type IV or V with penetration of bone or metal, opening cerebral ventricles.
    VII. Craniofacial wounds in which the ethmoidal or petrosal sinuses are opened.
    VIII. Perforating or traversing wounds.
    IX. Extensive bursting fractures.

SYMPTOMATOLOGY

The symptoms of gunshot wounds may be divided into those indicative of generalized cerebral dysfunction and those of focal origin caused by trauma to specific portions of the brain.

General Symptoms. In 1919 Frazier and Ingham stated that the commonest early general manifestation of cranial gunshot injury is loss of

I Wounds of the Scalp

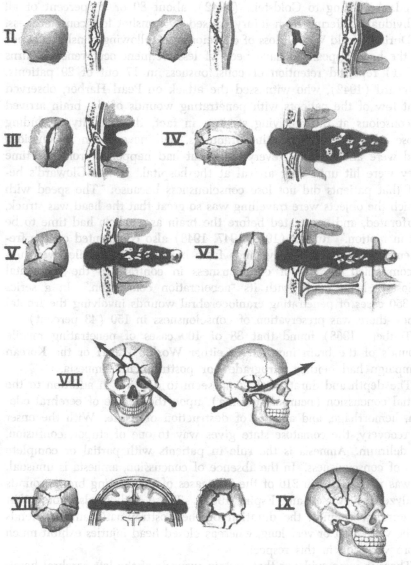

FIG. 1. GRAPHIC REPRESENTATION OF CLASSIFICATION OF GUNSHOT WOUNDS
OF THE SKULL AND BRAIN (CUSHING)

(From Courville, C. B.: Pathology of the Nervous System. Courtesy of Pacific
Press Publishing Association, Mountain View, California, 1937.)

285

consciousness, which may last from a few minutes to several weeks. Of 132 cases analyzed, these authors found only 22 in which there was no initial period of coma; the latter cases were not necessarily the least injured. According to Goldstein (1942), about 80 or 90 percent of all individuals suffering from injury caused by gunshot lost consciousness.

During World War II, loss of consciousness following gunshot wounds of the head appears to have been of less frequent occurrence. Cairns (1941) reported retention of consciousness in 17 out of 29 patients. Cloward (1942), who witnessed the attack on Pearl Harbor, observed that few of the patients with penetrating wounds of the brain arrived unconscious at the receiving station; in fact, the majority, excluding those with extensive bursting fractures, had never been unconscious and were able to recall everything that had happened from the time they were hit until their arrival at the hospital. It was Cloward's belief that patients did not lose consciousness because: "The speed with which the objects were travelling was so great that the head was struck, perforated, and penetrated before the brain as a whole had time to be set in motion." Russell (1945, 1947, 1948) also commented on the frequency with which head wounds from high velocity missiles were unaccompanied by loss of consciousness in contrast to the accidental (closed) head injury with its "acceleration concussion." In a series of 350 cases of penetrating craniocerebral wounds involving the frontal lobes, there was preservation of consciousness in 150 (43 percent).

Teuber (1968) found that 38 of 100 cases of penetrating missile wounds of the brain incurred in either World War II or the Korean campaign had neither retrograde nor posttraumatic amnesia.

The depth and duration of coma seem to depend, in addition to the initial concussion (neuronal trauma), upon the degree of cerebral edema, hemorrhage, and amount of destruction of tissue. With the onset of recovery, the comatose state gives way to one of stupor, confusion, or delirium. Amnesia is the rule in patients with partial or complete loss of consciousness. In the absence of concussion, amnesia is unusual. It was nonexistent in 216 of the 820 cases of penetrating brain wounds analyzed by Russell and Espir (1961). These authors also noted that in gunshot wounds, the duration of the posttraumatic amnesia tends to be very short or very long, whereas closed head injuries exhibit much more variation in this respect.

There is some evidence that certain wounds of the left cerebral hemisphere tend to cause a longer posttraumatic amnesia (P.T.A.) than corresponding wounds of the right cerebrum. Thus injuries affecting one optic radiation without sensorimotor involvement resulted in a more prolonged amnesia when the left side of the brain was the site of the lesion (Russell, 1948, 1971). Missile wounds reaching or crossing the midline in the region of the third ventricle may cause a severe temporary or permanent amnesia (Russell, 1963, 1971).

Jepson and Whitty (1947), who observed over 1000 cases of penetrating head injury, list as other early general manifestations, vomiting, urinary incontinence, and, not infrequently, a fine horizontal nystagmus and slight engorgement of the optic discs. In their experience, headache was rarely a spontaneous complaint, but did occur in patients with foreign bodies near the falx or tentorium. The pulse rate by itself proved to be no useful criterion of the nature of the intracranial pathology. Bradycardia, occurring in association with a small penetrating wound and a marked reduction in the degree of consciousness, however, suggested a clot under tension and constituted an indication for prompt surgical intervention. Transient cervical hyperalgesia, to which no special significance could be attached, was another fairly common finding. Roentgen examination of the cervical spine in such cases revealed no lesion.

The pulse, temperature, blood pressure, and respiratory rate, while frequently abnormal, do not, either singly or in combination, necessarily provide a reliable index of the intracranial pathology. Signs indicative of a poor prognosis include a deep and protracted state of coma; rapid, shallow or stertorous respiration, often with periodic variation; fixed, dilated pupils; profound hyperpyrexia; flaccidity with areflexia; decerebrate rigidity; and marked bradycardia or tachycardia.

General symptoms in cases that recover may persist for many months or even years. Among the sequelae of brain wounds, Russell (1947) commonly found intellectual impairment and an alteration of personality. These are important causes of persistent disability. Headache and dizziness are not infrequent residua, though occurring less often following penetrating wounds than after closed head injuries.

Reports as to the frequency of convulsive seizures following gunshot wounds are at variance. Sargent (1921) found an incidence of 4.5 percent, while Ascroft (1941) placed the figure at 34 percent. In Ascroft's series, seizures occurred twice as often (45 percent) in cases with dural penetration as in those with an intact dura (23 percent). Rolandic lesions accounted for the greatest incidence of fits, the percentage diminishing progressively in the temporal and parietal lobe injuries. In a series of 820 cases of penetrating brain wounds studied five years after injury by Russell and Whitty (1952), epilepsy occurred in 43 percent. They too observed a greater incidence of seizures following trauma in the vicinity of the central sulcus. Walker and Jablon (1961) reported the incidence of fits to be 35.8 percent in 472 cases of dural penetrating wounds followed for seven to eight years. Except for occipital wounds in which the incidence of posttraumatic epilepsy was significantly less, the location of the injury appeared to bear little relation to the development of seizures; in general, fits were more likely to occur in patients with wounds of greater severity and in those in whom healing was delayed due to such factors as infection, hemorrhage, and fungus formation. Convulsions developed within the first two years after injury in 36 percent of 279 cases reported by Watson (1947); most commonly the sensorimotor area was the site of trauma in those in which fits occurred. The incidence of epilepsy in 197 cases of missile wounds incurred in the Korean campaign, after periods varying between eight and eleven years, was found to be 42 percent by Caveness (1963); seizures developed in 28 percent of patients in whom the dura was intact, and in 50 percent of those with dural penetrating wounds. The incidence of fits was highest in parietal wounds. While focal manifestations commonly usher in an attack, generalized seizures develop in most cases (Watson, 1947; Walker and Jablon, 1961). Focal motor and somatic sensory fits comprise the largest group of focal epilepsies (Russell and Whitty, 1953). With regard to their temporal sequence, convulsions may occur soon after the infliction of trauma or may be delayed for many years. In 73 percent of cases observed by Russell and Whitty (1952), the onset of fits occurred within 12 months after injury; the region of the brain affected appeared to bear some relation to the time of onset of the seizures. Convulsions associated with frontal wounds developed relatively later than those resulting from injury to other areas. Caveness found that the onset of seizures occurred within two years of injury in 78 percent of his cases. Although not confirmed by the statistics of Caveness, the prognosis for the remission of the attacks is generally thought to be more favorable when they initially occur at an earlier stage. Other favorable prognostic factors, according to Walker (1957), are early cessation of attacks, infrequency of occurrence and the presence of gross neurological deficits.

Patients with large cranial defects often complain of persistent vertigo, a throbbing sensation and a feeling of insecurity, usually accentuated by bending forward.

Focal Symptoms. The specialized functions of different parts of the brain naturally lead one to expect a great variety of symptoms resulting from injury to these parts. After the concussion has subsided, edema receded and hemorrhagic deposits evacuated or absorbed, the focal

288

symptoms resulting from residual damage to specific portions of the brain can be studied without the complicating factor of increased intracranial pressure, which frequently accompanies the focal symptoms seen with brain tumor. The War of 1914-1918 furnished much material which permitted investigation of human neurophysiology under almost precise experimental conditions usually available only in the animal laboratory. The French particularly made good use of their material and the book by Chatelin (1918) based on a study of 5000 cases of injury to the brain is an outstanding contribution. The volume by Goldstein (1942) also contains a considerable amount of valuable information.

Exclusive of frontal wounds, Russell and Espir (1961) found the incidence of gross focal signs following gunshot injuries of the brain to be 75 percent in a series of 693 cases. These authors suggested that this high incidence of early focal signs might "depend partly on the spread of a shock effect from the site of wounding." Recovery occurred in many instances. Thus, less than half of the cases with early sensorimotor disorders were permanently affected and approximately one-third of those with visual or aphasic deficits recovered.

Accounts of the neurologic symptomatology caused by brain wounds incurred during World War II were published by Russell (1945, 1947), Jepson and Whitty (1947), Schiller (1947), Spalding (1952), Teuber, Battersby, and Bender (1960), and Russell and Espir (1961). Projectiles travelling at high velocity need not penetrate the skull to cause an injury to the underlying cortex (Russell, 1945). Thus an occipital "scalp" wound overlying the calcarine fissure may not only cause transient blindness, but may also produce permanent visual defects. Focal neurologic signs or symptoms were observed by Dodge and Meirowsky (1952) in 70 percent of 31 cases of tangential wounds of the scalp and skull; in only eight of 30 patients was there roentgenographic evidence of a fracture.

Eighteen cases of tangential head wounds were encountered by Jacobs and Berg (1970) in Vietnam. Loss of consciousness occurred in 16 and focal paralysis in 11; the usual x-ray finding was a comminuted depressed fracture.

Frontal Lobe. Focal signs are usually not in evidence following injuries to the anterior frontal lobe. In unilateral lesions, ataxia, apraxia, or ocular deviation is seldom observed. Abnormal postures and involuntary deviation toward the uninjured side have been described. Grasp reflexes may be demonstrable. According to Russell (1948), common symptoms resulting from frontal lobe injuries are "restlessness, inability

289

to maintain attention or to plan, lack of self-control, difficulty in learning, failure at technical or professional occupations, loss of interest in former hobbies or games, tactlessness, fatigability and, more rarely, nocturnal eneuresis." Bifrontal lobe involvement may produce a transient state of apathy very much like that following prefrontal lobotomy and characterized by profound inertia, somnolence, and incontinence. In such cases the ability to cope with problems of an abstract nature is commonly impaired. The prognosis for improvement in most frontal lobe lesions is good, though evidence of some personality alteration and intellectual deficit often persists.

Wounds in the frontal region may also be complicated by partial paralysis of the face due to injury of superficial branches of the seventh nerve. Cerebrospinal fluid rhinorrhea, with its attendant hazard of retrograde meningeal infection, occurs as a consequence of injuries involving the paranasal sinuses. Wounds of the orbit may injure the eye and optic nerve directly causing varying degrees of ocular damage and visual loss.

Motor Area (Precentral Convolutions). Injuries of the motor cortex result in a variety of paralytic phenomena, including facial palsy, brachial and crural monoplegias, hemiplegia, and disorders of speech. Paraplegia may occur as a consequence of a tangential wound of the vertex affecting both leg areas. A lesion in the mid-Rolandic area causes an immediate paralysis of the opposite arm accompanied by transient numbness. As a rule, such a *monoplegia of the upper extremity* is characterized at the onset by flaccidity and loss of the tendon reflexes (diaschisis of von Monakow). The state of areflexia may persist for several days. Eventually following their return, the deep reflexes become increasingly active. It is uncommon for the extremity to be uniformly paralyzed. Usually shoulder movements are retained, the weakness affecting the distal parts most severely. The extensors, lateral rotators, and abductors of the arm tend to be more involved than their antagonists. It may be possible to detect slight weakness of the face and lower extremity on the side of the monoplegia. Occasionally the paresis may be of a very circumscribed character, limited, for example, to movements of the fingers. Sensory disturbances occur commonly in association with brachial monoplegia. Superficial and deep sensation may be affected or the deficit may involve stereognostic perception. The sensory loss may assume a segmental pattern.

In *monoplegia of the lower extremity,* the paralysis may be complete affecting the flexors of the hip and knee and dorsal flexors of the foot predominantly, or it may be more limited in extent. Thus, the foot may be involved almost exclusively. Absence of reflexes, so frequently observed early in the course of a brachial monoplegia, is rarely noted in cases with paralysis of the lower extremity. Extensor hypertonus develops rapidly. This is a striking feature in missile wounds of the parasagittal Rolandic area (Russell and Young, 1969). As in paralysis of the upper limb, crural monoplegia is often accompanied by sensory disturbances. Paralysis involving the lower extremity occurs less often than brachial monoplegia.

According to Chatelin (1918), cerebral paraplegia resulting from tangential wounds implicating the paracentral lobules is seldom symmetrical. The distal parts are most severely affected. Sensory disturbances are also often evident. While voluntary dorsiflexion of the foot and toes may be abolished, these movements may nevertheless be executed on attempting to walk, owing to spinal automatism. Another type of cerebral paraplegia observed by Chatelin was one in which spasticity was associated with a disturbance of coordination, attributed by him to a contrecoup lesion of the cerebellum.

Hemiplegia due to gunshot injuries of the motor cortex or subcortical region is of frequent occurrence (Maltby, 1946; Walker and Jablon, 1961), and does not differ in essence from the neurologic deficit caused by cerebral vascular disease. The paralysis is at first flaccid, becoming spastic after a few weeks, at which time contractures develop. Varying degrees of sensory disturbances are usually evident.

Whereas wounds of the motor area generally give rise to sensory loss as well as paralysis, lesions situated anterior to the precentral gyrus may cause severe transient paralysis without any accompanying sensory impairment (shock effect). The closer the wound to the Rolandic area, the greater the probability of permanent disability.

In a study of war wounds of the brain, Russell and Espir (1961) found that of 145 cases of left cerebral lesions with some degree of persistent contralateral weakness or sensory loss, 119 exhibited evidence of aphasia. Patients with wounds in the parasagittal region were much less apt to be aphasic. Wounds involving the lower end of the central sulcus often caused motor aphasia, whereas those located farther back gave rise to a global aphasia.

Parietal Lobe. Lesions confined to the posterior parietal area may occasionally be unaccompanied by any neurological disturbances (Jepson and Whitty, 1947). Usually, however, some sensory loss can be detected, and this is often confined to one limb. Profound analgesia, usually of transient duration, may be observed, associated as a rule with a paralysis of the involved extremity. Persistent impairment of all modalities of sensation implies a severe lesion of the postcentral area. Not uncommonly, discriminative sensory function in one limb alone remains permanently defective. Astereognosis may be the sole manifestation or sequel of a parietal wound. As in cases with motor impairment, persistent sensory deficiencies tend to be most marked in the distal parts of the extremities. The affected area may, however, assume a pattern of segmental distribution. Transient hyperpathia and occasionally the occurrence of a phantom limb have been described following wounds of the sensory cortex. Double simultaneous stimulation may demonstrate the phenomenon of extinction (sensory inattention) (Bender, 1945).

Holmes (1918) observed that "lesions of the lateral surfaces of the hemispheres, particularly of the posterior parietal regions, may cause certain disturbances of the higher visual perceptual functions with intact visual sensibility, such as loss of visual orientation and localization in space, disturbance of the perception of depth and distance, visual inattention, and visual agnosia."

Aphasic and apraxic manifestations may result from lesions on the left side, and homonymous hemianopic defects from injury on either side. These disorders will be further discussed subsequently.

A detailed study of isolated focal fits and localized auras of major seizures of a motor and somatic sensory nature was made by Russell and Whitty (1953). Most focal motor attacks had both a tonic and clonic component. Motor phenomena initiating a seizure were of an adversive, tonic, clonic, myoclonic, or inhibitory variety. Comparable sensory phenomena included paresthesiae; numbness; pain; agnosia; thermal, electric shock; and phantom sensations. Noteworthy was the relative infrequency of attacks starting in the lower extremities. Whereas a sensory aura was often followed by a motor aura, the reverse sequence was uncommon. Clonic focal fits occurred most often in association with small wounds of the sensorimotor cortex; sensory auras were very uncommon in patients with hemiplegia.

An analysis by Russell (1951) of the disability caused by brain wounds disclosed that of 693 cases of penetrating injuries, 370 (53 percent) exhibited evidence of a sensorimotor deficit; in 169 cases (24 percent) the deficit persisted permanently. According to Walker and Jablon (1961) the likelihood of recovery from a hemiparesis following a penetrating head wound is about 25 percent.

Temporal Lobe. Homonymous visual field defects and disturbances of speech when the dominant hemisphere is the site of the lesion are commonly found in temporal lobe wounds. Slight facial weakness may also be observed. Injuries in the region of the superior temporal gyrus may also produce varying degrees of contralateral paresis and sensory deficit in addition to speech and visual disturbances. Involvement of auditory structures, including the external and internal ear, may occur in association with temporal lobe wounds.

Aphasia. It would be going too far afield to attempt to deal with the problem of aphasia in detail. Interpretation of disturbed speech mechanisms is no simple matter and, in fact, has been the subject of much controversy. In a study of the aphasic disturbances of 46 patients with penetrating wounds involving the dominant hemisphere, the generally accepted view that more than one aspect of speech is usually disturbed was confirmed by Schiller (1948). Impairment of word-finding ("nominal" or "amnesic" aphasia) was observed in all cases regardless of the location of the lesion within the "speech" area. It was further noted that wounds affecting the lower precentral area resulted in disturbances of articulation, inflection, and speed of enunciation (anarthria, motor or expressive aphasia). In patients with temporal lesions the understanding of spoken language was imperfect; paraphasia, jargon, and agrammatism resulted from a severely defective auditory control of speech. Posterior temporal and temporoparietal wounds were associated with disturbances of reading and writing (visual speech). Those aspects of speech related to orientation in space and appreciation of shape, including the ability to write, spell, read, calculate, and to construct (Kohs blocks test) were affected in parietal lesions. Perseveration and stammer were also commonly found in such cases.

Reference has already been made to the comprehensive study of aphasia resulting from war wounds, undertaken by Russell and Espir (1961). Their observations led them to conclude that, almost invariably, aphasia occurred as a consequence of involvement of the left side of the brain, even in left-handed individuals. They further noted that, as a rule, wounds affecting the left optic radiation anterior to the occipital lobe, caused aphasia. In addition to speech impairment, injury to the upper part of the left optic radiation in the parietal lobe produced an inferior quadrantic homonymous visual field defect with little or no motor or sensory loss. Lesions of the center of the left optic radiation in the region of the trigone of the lateral ventricle gave rise to homonymous sector defects and aphasia. Damage to the lower optic radiation in the left temporal lobe caused an upper quadrantic homonymous hemianopia and aphasia and, generally, spared motor and sensory functions. The duration of posttraumatic amnesia was prolonged in temporal lobe injuries associated with global aphasia, word deafness, and jargon. It was suggested that involvement of the fornix and hippocampal system might be responsible for the prolonged amnesia. Left temporoparietal wounds disrupted all aspects of speech, producing a central aphasia (global aphasia, jargon). Involvement of speech alone without concomitant motor, sensory, or visual deficits was observed when the lesions were located anterior to the motor cortex (motor aphasia), in the upper and posterior part of the left parietal lobe, in the left midparietal area, and in the left anterior temporal lobe. A relatively pure disorder of writing (agraphia) occurred in cases in which the wounds were posterior to the upper third of the left sensory cortex. Severe alexia, often with considerable intellectual dysfunction, was observed in patients with lesions of the left lower posterior parietal lobe (angular gyrus). Deep left posterior parietal parasagittal injury resulted in bilateral apraxia.

The treatise on Traumatic Aphasia by Luria (1970) is a scholarly analysis of speech and its disorders. Luria's position is that "damage to any area of the cerebral cortex which plays a role in the integration of one or another form of cerebral activity inevitably affects the overall system of psychophysiological processes," and "that almost any cortical lesion leads to some motor or perceptual deficit, some impairment of expressive speech or speech comprehension, or some reading, writing or computational disorder." Furthermore, "damage to a given cortical system may produce completely different symptoms depending upon the level of organization of various psychological processes at the time of injury." Luria points out that following trauma to the left (dominant) hemisphere, the relative frequency and persistence of speech disorders depends on the site of the lesion. Speech impairment resulting from injuries to the frontal and occipital poles is infrequent and hardly ever persistent. The most frequent, severe and persistent disturbances of speech are produced by damage to the principal speech areas (fronto-temporo-parietal, temporo-parietal and parieto-temporal). Injuries involving regions of the brain adjacent to the principal speech areas ("marginal zones") result in a large number of aphasic disturbances of lesser severity initially, many of which recover. Recovery from speech defects is considerably greater in cases of nonpenetrating than of penetrating wounds. In discussing recovery from traumatic aphasia, Luria indicates that only in cases of absolute dominance of the left hemisphere do gross lesions of the primary speech areas produce severe permanent impairment.

In their follow-up study of head wounds in World War II, Walker and Jablon (1961) found evidence of marked improvement or recovery in over half the patients rendered aphasic immediately after injury. Aphasic manifestations occurred in 217 (31 percent) out of a total of 693 cases of penetrating head wounds analyzed by Russell (1951); speech remained permanently affected in 135 (20 percent).

Occipital Lobe. The occipital lobe may be injured as a result of a direct wound or indirectly by a missile entering the skull elsewhere and coming to lodge in this region. As a rule, survivors of tangential wounds that cross the midline exhibit evidence of involvement of only the upper lip of the calcarine fissure; wounds that affect the lower lip are usually fatal due to concomitant injury to the transverse sinuses and structures of the posterior fossa. The disturbances associated with occipital lobe wounds are those referable to vision. Irritative phenomena in the form of sudden flashes of light may occur at the moment of impact. Unilateral lesions cause varying degrees of homonymous hemianopia.

Inferior altitudinal defects are produced by tangential wounds crossing the midline at a level above the tips of the occipital lobes. Destruction of the occipital poles results in loss of macular vision. Wedge-shaped sector scotomata that point toward the fovea, and paracentral quadrantic scotomata, occur more commonly in wounds of the occipital poles; paracentral scotomata are found very rarely in cases of injury involving the interior radiation. Lesions farther forward in the occipital region may cause bilateral hemianopia with macular sparing (peephole vision) or concentric contraction of the visual fields. Arc-shaped scotomata surrounding the macula combined with homonymous hemianopic field defects have been observed. Visuospatial disorders, abnormalities of color perception and visual extinction (visual inattention) may be demonstrable. Gunshot wounds involving the geniculo-striate system do not cause permanent total blindness as a rule, though transient bilateral amaurosis may occur immediately after injury.

Occipital wounds may be accompanied by lesions of one or both labyrinths resulting in various degrees of vertigo, disturbances of equilibrium, and loss of hearing.

A study of epilepsy with a visual aura, resulting from brain wounds, was made by Russell and Whitty (1955). Patients with wounds of the calcarine region, in whom fits were relatively infrequent experienced continuously moving unformed visual phenomena. Complex auras including formed visual hallucinations, distortion and extinction or blurring of vision as well as crude phenomena such as interrupted flashes, occurred in patients with lesions of the optic radiations. "A wide variety of visual phenomena ranging from crude hallucinations of flashes and colored lights, through more complex phenomena such as extinction of part or the whole of vision and distortion or disorientation of visual perception, to a highly integrated hallucination of a familiar remembered scene" was observed in cases of wounds of the "higher" visual cortex (i.e., parieto-occipital areas anterior to the calcarine cortex). Formed hallucinations, often associated with a feeling of familiarity, were also encountered in patients with injuries of the temporal lobes.

According to Rusell and Davies-Jones (1969) crude visual fits tend to occur in association with lesions that injure mainly the occipital or parioto-occipital region above the optic radiation and calcarine cortex but which are inadequate to produce a complete permanent hemianopia. Temporal-lobe wounds that disrupt the lower segment of the optic radiation, or those that result in complete division of one optic radiation or complete destruction of one calcarine cortex, rarely give rise to crude visual fits.

A good deal of our knowledge concerning the optic radiation and the occipital visual center has been obtained from a study of war injuries (Holmes and Lister, 1916; Holmes, 1918; Spalding, 1952; Teuber, Battersby, and Bender, 1960). Spalding found that "wounds involving the upper or lower margins of the anterior part of the visual radiation cause partial quadrantopia in which the horizontal meridian is spared and the field defect projects toward the fixation point in the vertical meridian; wounds involving the intermediate part of the anterior radiation cause narrow, sector-shaped defects in the horizontal meridian reaching to the fixation point." He concluded that "in the anterior radiation fibers subserving central vision lie on the lateral aspect tending to congregate at the intermediate part, and fibers subserving peripheral vision lie on the medial aspect, tending to congregate at the upper and lower margins." Evidence was presented to indicate that "central (macular) vision is represented unilaterally, that the horizontal meridian of the visual field is represented in the floor of the calcarine fissure, and that central vision within the 8° to 10° circumference (i.c., macular vision) is represented on that part of the striate cortex which faces posteriorly or posteromedially. The remainder which faces medially represents vision more peripheral than 10° from the fixation point." Teuber, Battersby, and Bender (1960) are essentially in agreement with the views of Spalding on the anatomy of the anterior visual radiation. Farther posteriorly in the geniculo-calcarine pathway, peripheral fibers congregate in its upper and lower portions, macular fibers being interposed. Teuber, Battersby, and Bender indicate that strictly quadrantic defects are rare following gunshot wounds, the defects more often being incomplete. They further stress the lack of congruence of homonymous field defects and the irregularity of the dividing line between the affected and spared field.

Visual defects still demonstrable a year after the occurrence of a penetrating wound may be expected to persist indefinitely. According to Walker and Jablon (1961), regression of a hemianopic deficit is likely to occur in about 30 percent of cases. In a series of 693 cases of penetrating wounds studied by Russell (1951) visual defects were present in 302 (44 percent); the defects proved to be permanent in 209 (30 percent).

Subcortical Areas. Penetrating wounds involving deep subcortical structures are associated with a high mortality. In addition to hemiplegia, survivors may exhibit sensory loss, ataxia, involuntary movements, and hemianopic defects. Although spontaneous pain of the sort occurring in the thalamic syndrome caused by vascular disease was described by Chatelin in 1918, it was not observed by Russell (1947).

Cerebellum. Owing to associated injury to the brain stem, gunshot wounds of the cerebellum are often fatal. The abnormalities resulting from unilateral injury to the cerebellum during the acute stage have been described by Holmes (1917); they consist of ipsilateral hypotonia, weakness, increased fatigability, slowness of movement and of relaxation, ataxia, asynergia, adiadochokinesis, deviation of the limbs, depression of the tendon reflexes and vertigo, nystagmus and an abnormal head attitude, together with disturbances of speech, ocular movement, equilibrium, and gait. The effects of involvement of the dentate nucleus were apparently similar though more pronounced in degree. Papilledema is a common manifestation of cerebellar wounds, according to Jepson and Whitty (1947).

DIAGNOSIS

The diagnosis of a gunshot injury of the head is usually self-evident, although there have been cases in which there was not only retention of consciousness, but the external evidence of trauma was so slight that the injury was completely overlooked.

Insofar as possible, a detailed history should be elicited. It is important to learn precisely when the injury occurred, the position of the wounded person when struck, whether a helmet was worn, whether

297

consciousness was lost and, if so, for what length of time. Inquiry should be made concerning any sensation experienced at the moment of impact and what deficit, if any, occurred immediately thereafter. A complete physical examination as well as an evaluation of neurologic function should be performed at the earliest opportunity. Injuries elsewhere must not be overlooked. While the external appearance of the head wound may give no indication of the extent of penetration and amount of brain damage, it must nevertheless be carefully inspected. Cerebrospinal fluid issuing from the wound is a grave sign, usually signifying penetration of the ventricle. Intracranial involvement should be suspected in wounds of the face, especially those of the orbit. It may be possible to detect a cerebrospinal fluid rhinorrhea in wounds of the fronto-orbital region.

Roentgenographic examination of the skull is of the utmost importance; whenever possible appropriate stereoscopic views should be obtained. X-rays show the location and extent of indriven bone and metal fragments and help enable one to estimate the probable degree of cerebral injury.

The existence of a number of special entities resulting from craniocerebral trauma is suggested by the presence of certain signs and symptoms (Jepson and Whitty, 1947). Drowsiness and marked papilledema occurring in a patient with a wound across the vertex and unaccompanied by abnormal neurologic signs or radiologic evidence of a bony lesion are, in all likelihood, caused by an obstruction to the superior longitudinal sinus. Contralateral hemiparesis and drowsiness often associated with papilledema in a patient with a temporal wound and roentgenologic evidence of a fracture involving the middle meningeal groove indicate a probable epidural hematoma. Intracranial hemorrhage on the side opposite the wound of entrance should be suspected whenever an ipsilateral hemiparesis is demonstrable and roentgen examination shows the missile to have crossed the midline and to be lying close to the opposite cortex. (See also Matson and Wolkin, 1946.) The possibility of a subdural or subcortical hematoma resulting from rupture of cortical vessels warrants placing an exploratory burr hole over the site of the retained projectile. Reference has already been made to the likelihood of an intracerebral clot under tension when bradycardia, a depressed state of consciousness, and possibly papilledema occur in a patient with a small penetrating wound. (See also Meirowsky, 1954.) A high incidence of hematomas in patients treated within eight hours was reported by Barnett and Meirowsky (1955).

The basic facts pertaining to treatment were clearly stated by Cushing in 1918:

"Every scalp wound, no matter how trifling, is a potential penetrating wound of the skull. Many penetrating wounds are met with even among the walking wounded. Only after an x-ray, after shaving the head, and possibly only after exploration, can one be assured that there is or is not a cranial fracture with or without dural penetration.

"If a case is operated upon and a penetration found, the operation must be completed, with a primary closure following the special debridement applicable to these injuries. In this respect wounds of the nervous system differ from other wounds which in times of rush should not be subjected to primary wound closure. 'All or nothing' is a good rule to apply to craniocerebral injuries — in short, evacuate hese cases untreated to the nearest base (except for shaving and the application of a wet antiseptic dressing) rather than do incomplete operations. Patients with craniocerebral injuries stand transportation well before operation; badly during the first few days after operation. This is true of all primary wound closures.

"The chief source of the high mortality in cranial wounds is infection — infection of the meninges; direct infection of the brain leading to encephalitis; infection of the ventricles. Wounds in which the dura has been penetrated are supposed to give a mortality of 50 to 60 percent, due to infection. It, however, has been shown that experienced neurological surgeons can lower this supposedly inevitable mortality to 25 percent if the operation can be done with reasonable promptitude in a forward area and the cases retained for a reasonable time after operation. These figure are capable of still further improvement."

Nothing that has been subsequently written on the subject of craniocerebral injuries has substantially added to or detracted from these basic principles. For example, Cairns (1940) and McKissock and Brownscombe (1941) again emphasized the importance of taking nothing for granted, even with the seemingly most trifling scalp wound, and Tönnis (1940), among others, called attention to the more favorable results in head injury cases when these were simply dressed and transported to a well-equipped base hospital for surgery than when a major operation was undertaken at a field hospital and the patient then transferred.

The one great innovation since the first World War has been the strongly reënforced weapon against infection in the form of antibiotics. It is still desirable to transfer the patient with a craniocerebral injury as quickly as possible to a hospital where neurosurgical facilities are available for operation, but in the event surgical treatment is delayed, infection is not inevitable thanks to the chemotherapeutic agents now available. Treatment may be divided into (1) initial or first aid, such as might be provided at a dressing station in a forward area, and (2) definitive, which is best performed by a neurosurgeon at a well-equipped hospital.

Initial treatment involves shaving and cleaning with soap and water a generous area of scalp surrounding the wound, controlling hemorrhage, and applying a firm dressing. In addition, shock, whenever present, must be treated, toxoid or human immune globulin administered for the prevention of tetanus, appropriate measures taken to deal with injuries involving other parts of the body, and prophylactic antibiotic therapy instituted. Head wounds are usually not accompanied by severe shock unless excessive loss of blood has occurred or there has been concomitant injury to other parts of the body. Comatose patients should be transported in a prone or semiprone position to avoid aspiration of blood or vomitus, care being also taken to prevent obstruction to respiration. A tracheotomy may be required to ensure maintenance of an adequate airway.

THE TREATMENT OF THE DIFFERENT CLASSES OF BRAIN INJURIES

Class I: Wounds of the Scalp. Scalp wounds produced by missiles are usually lacerations of the soft tissues, including the pericranium, although occasionally this structure remains intact. Frequently they are associated with cerebral concussion, occasionally with an underlying cerebral contusion. Scalp wounds must be meticulously debrided and sutured in order to avoid infection with the attendant hazard of secondary involvement of the skull, meninges, or brain. Hair, clotted blood and foreign matter are cut away and the head shaved for an appreciable distance from the wound. If a straight razor is not available, a safety razor blade held in a hemostat provides a very efficient substitute. The scalp is then thoroughly cleansed with soap and water, sponged with alcohol and ether, and finally painted with a dilute solution of an antiseptic such as 1:750 tincture of benzalkonium chloride. An area about 2 cm distant from the edges of the wound is infiltrated with a local anesthetic containing a small quantity of epinephrine, allowing a few minutes for the anesthetic to take effect. The ragged, dirty edges of the wound are then excised as cleanly and sparingly as possible. Hair and indriven particles are removed and damaged muscle debrided carefully. The wound is thoroughly cleansed with sterile saline and *tightly closed, without drainage, in separate layers with interrupted fine silk sutures applied to the galea and skin.* Defects up to 3 to 4 cm in diameter can be closed by undermining the scalp for some distance beyond the margins of the wound.

Class II: Cranial Fractures without Dural Penetration. Compound fractures of the skull without penetration of the dura may be linear or comminuted; in the latter variety there may or may not be depressed bone fragments. Extravasation of blood between bone and dura and local contusion of the underlying brain are commonly present. Sometimes the injury to the brain is considerable. A compound fracture, even of the linear variety, is a potential cause of osteomyelitis, meningitis, or abscess formation within the neighboring contused brain. An uncontaminated linear fracture may be left untouched, unless there is question regarding its cleanliness, in which case excision is the safer practice. Depending on the clinical course, in the presence of localizing neurologic signs, burr hole exploration of the extradural and subdural spaces may be indicated. Compound comminuted and depressed fractures are treated by removal of all loose fragments of bone and excision of the margins of the remaining defect. Radiating fissures which may coexist require no special treatment. Depressed fractures without loss of substance are usually associated with an intact dura. A defect in bone, on the other hand, regardless of size, usually signifies dural penetration. It is possible for a depressed fracture to affect the inner table alone, in which case a fragment of bone may be driven into the brain. Such a situation calls for exploration through a burr hole. The preliminary preparation of these cases, as well as the details of the cranial and intracranial operation, will be discussed in connection with the following groups.

Classes III and IV: Cranial Fractures with Depression and Dural Penetration but without Extrusion of Brain; Wounds (Usually of Gutter Type) with Brain Extruding and Indriven Fragments of Bone. The factor of dural penetration increases the seriousness of head wounds considerably and raises the mortality significantly. In non-penetrating wounds, those limited to the scalp and skull, there is a very low mortality. Thus, Meirowsky (1965) reported two deaths in 226 compound depressed skull fractures, mostly due to gunshot wounds treated during the Korean War. On the other hand, the mortality of 879 cases with penetrating wounds upon whom operation was performed was 9.6 percent.

High-speed missiles produce a relatively small opening when penetrating the skull. The scalp may be undermined and, characteristically, the inner table is more extensively disrupted than the outer table. Bone fragments are driven into the brain in the direction of the path of the missile. The resultant track contains blood clot, traumatized brain tissue, bone chips, hair, and other foreign particles, which collectively form a sort of plug at the site of entry of the missile. More distally the track narrows and is encroached upon by the surrounding brain.

The initial debridement of a penetrating brain wound largely determines the eventual outcome, and for this reason treatment should be carried out at a hospital adequately staffed and equipped to handle neurosurgical problems. Eden (1944) has wisely cautioned that "the surgeon who first operates on an open brain wound makes or mars it. There is no useful first-aid operation – ideally, the initial operation should be the final and complete one. Failure to obtain primary union or inadequate removal of indriven bone fragments, all too frequently spells the vicious circle of cerebral fungus, abscess, and meningitis."

The selection of cases for operation deserves comment. Operability is determined by the patient's general condition and is gauged by signs indicative of the degree of involvement of vital brain structures. Patients who are conscious present no problem. Likewise, whenever evidence exists of cerebral compression, the necessity for prompt surgical intervention as a lifesaving measure is clear. In some seriously wounded patients, however, evaluation of the surgical risk involved may be difficult. In obviously moribund cases, operation is contraindicated. Of grave prognostic significance are profound coma, a rapid respiratory rate, periods of Cheyne-Stokes respiration, tachycardia and a pulse of poor volume, decerebrate rigidity, fixed pupils, and hyperpyrexia – usually occurring in varying combinations. Patients in whom such signs are demonstrable have suffered severe brain injuries and most are probably inoperable. When there is doubt whether the severity of the intracranial damage is compatible with life, operation had best be deferred and treatment limited to supportive meassures. Usually after 12 to 24 hours, the issue will have been clarified and a decision as to the patient's operability reached. Even a longer delay may at times be justified by the condition of the patient.

As a preliminary to operation, the *choice of anesthesia* must receive consideration. Local anesthesia supplemented with a sedative agent such as one of the barbiturates has been employed extensively in the past. Intravenous morphine in conjunction with local anesthesia has been recommended for the treatment of patients with open head wounds, provided there is no respiratory problem (Matson, 1958). Because of impaired consciousness and restlessness, many patients require the use of a general anesthetic agent. Furthermore, wounds in some localities, such as the regions about the eyes and ears, do not lend themselves to satisfactory regional block. Currently the trend is toward the use of general anesthesia, employing intravenous thiopental sodium initially for induction and thereafter nitrous oxide and/or halothane and oxygen administered through an endotracheal tube.* The use of an endotracheal tube assures maintenance of a patent airway and permits the anesthetist to control respiration whenever necessary. In patients in whom increased intracranial pressure or cerebral edema may present a problem, the intravenous administration of urea or of mannitol or the use of dexamethasone may be salutary.

Preparation of the scalp is best performed under anesthesia or after sedation, and involves shaving the head completely. The administration of 5 percent dextrose in water or in one quarter strength saline intraveneously is begun prior to operation. Blood may be substituted thereafter as indicated.

The purpose of operative treatment is to thoroughly debride contaminated tissue, remove all indriven bone fragments, hair, debris, pulped brain, hematomas, and accessible foreign bodies, and to secure primary union. The procedure to be described will serve as a basic outline for operations applied even to the most complicated injuries.

The head should be draped so that the operative field exposed is adequate to allow for plastic closure if the amount of scalp lost is appreciable. It is well to keep in mind that poorly planned incisions may interfere with surgery at a later date for the purpose of repairing the skull defect. Figure 2 illlustrates satisfactory methods of closure, utilizing simple plastic procedures. (See also Converse, 1964.) If it is at once obvious that adequate closure of the wound will require rotating a scalp flap, this should be outlined on the skin before drapes are applied. The tripod and three-legged (isle of man) incisions advocated by Cushing frequently heal poorly and have been largely abandoned (Martin and Campbell, 1946; Woodhall, 1947). Procaine or lidocaine containing epinephrine may be infiltrated about the wound, even when general anesthesia is employed, and the dirty edges of the scalp excised throughly, though with an economy of tissue, down to skull. Not infrequently the fibro-fatty layer of scalp is damaged more ex-

*Alternatively anesthesia may be induced with droperidol and short acting narcotics (e.g., fentanyl) or meperidine and maintained with nitrous oxide and oxygen and fractional doses of narcotics.

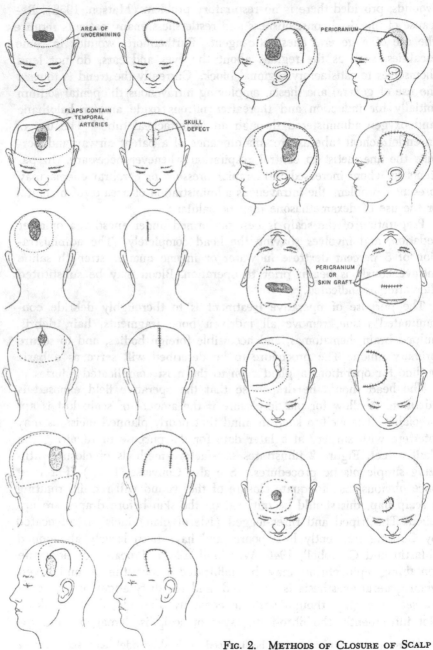

FIG. 2. METHODS OF CLOSURE OF SCALP DEFECTS (Medical Bulletin No. 31, May-June, 1945; Office of Chief Surgeon, European Theatre of Operations).

tensively than the more superficial tissues, in which case seemingly intact dermis must be sacrificed to secure a vertical wound edge. Contaminated periosteum is removed and damaged muscle thoroughly excised. The instruments employed in excising contaminated tissues are now discarded. Extruded brain substance and blood clot are evacuated with the aid of suction and detached bone fragments lifted out of the wound. Excision of bone edges is performed with rongeurs fully exposing the dural defect. Removal of bone en bloc is unnecessary judging from the experiences of most military neurosurgeons, though still advocated by some (Meirowsky, 1965). Large bone fragments attached to viable periosteum are permitted to remain.

Wounds belonging to Group II, in which the dura is intact, are treated at this point by irrigation with saline and closed with interrupted silk sutures in separate layers without drainage. In the presence of appropriate neurological signs, if the dura is tense and discolored, albeit intact, suggesting an underlying hematoma, this membrane must be opened for the purpose of evacuating the clot, especially if the operator feels that a thorough debridement has been accomplished. Should this be necessary, after the procedure is completed, the dura is closed carefully with fine silk sutures, threaded on small round needles that have no cutting edge. As an alternative, the clot may be evacuated through a separate incision and burr hole placed at a distance from the wound following its debridement and closure. Meirowsky (1965) recommends that the dura be opened in all cases of compound fracture of the skull because of the high incidence of intracranial hematoma. He reported finding a clot — extradural, subdural, or subcortical in location in 114 of 226 cases.

In the case of penetrating wounds, following excision of the fracture, the dural edges are trimmed sparingly, avoiding, whenever possible, further enlargement of the defect. Though indriven bone fragments are not invariably present, they nevertheless are a characteristic feature of penetrating brain wounds. They were demonstrable in 430 of the 500 patients treated by Small and Turner (1947). Retention of bone chips is distinctly hazardous since their presence constitutes a nidus of infection (Ascroft, 1943; Martin and Campbell, 1946; Meirowsky, 1965; Hagan, 1971; Hammon, 1971). The object of treatment, therefore, is to remove them completely, together with damaged brain tissue, blood clot, indriven hair, and foreign particles. This is most readily accomplished by excising the brain track with suction as indicated in Figure 3. Simultaneous use of the electrocautery by means of an

305

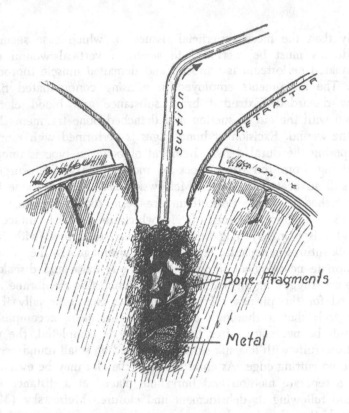

FIG. 3. DEBRIDEMENT OF BRAIN WOUND BY MEANS OF SUCTION.
The metal suction tip is attached to the electrosurgical unit and coagulates tissue simultaneously. (From Horrax, G.: The Treatment of War Wounds of the Brain; New Eng. J. Med 225, 855, 1941.)

attachment to the suction tip is of considerable help in achieving hemostasis. Visible bone fragments may be extracted with forceps. Occasionally the patient, if conscious, may assist in clearing the track by straining. The use of suction provides a much more efficient means of completely excising the brain wound than the catheter and syringe method employed by Cushing and has largely replaced it. Metallic foreign bodies are removed whenever they are encountered or are accessible. Attempts to pursue deeply situated metal fragments are ill advised. It is generally believed that they seldom give rise to infection and are best left alone. They are, nevertheless, a potential source of infection so that a more determined effort to remove them has been advocated by some (Meirowsky, 1965). At the conclusion of the operation, the brain cavity resulting from excision of the wound should remain open and exhibit pulsations, provided a thorough cleansing has been accomplished. The dura is tightly closed without drainage, a fascial or pericranial graft being utilized if necessary. The wound is then closed with interrupted silk sutures to galea and skin. It is important to avoid tension in approximating skin edges, since breakdown of the wound will otherwise result. In cases with excessive loss of scalp, closure may be accomplished by taking advantage of the ability of the scalp to stretch when undermined and freed from its attachment to pericranium. Should a gap still persist, it becomes necessary to resort to a rotation flap. The base of such a flap should be placed inferiorly to assure an adequate blood supply. Usually following rotation of the flap and undermining, it is possible to close the scalp entirely. Otherwise, the periosteum of the donor site may be covered with a split thickness skin graft, or left exposed to be grafted at a later date. Relaxing incisions are at times indicated though their usefulness is limited.

The treatment of posterior fossa wounds, according to Small and Turner (1947), must take into account the factor of edema with resultant medullary compression. They advise that a suboccipital craniectomy be performed following excision of an infratentorial wound, and that the lateral ventricle be tapped during and following operation for the relief of increased intracranial pressure.

Involvement of dural venous sinuses may give rise to severe hemorrhage during the course of an operative procedure, in anticipation of which certain precautionary measures should be adopted. Partial elevation of the head of the patient is desirable since it favors a reduction of cerebral venous pressure, although the danger of air embolus must be kept in mind. The use of a central venous catheter placed in the right atrium prior to operation so as to permit aspiration of air in the event such a catastrophe occurs, bears consideration. Continuous monitoring of heart sounds (oesophageal stethoscope), electrocardiogram, and blood pressure is essential for prompt diagnosis (Michenfelder et al, 1966, 1969). Muscle grafts and Gelfoam are useful hemostatic agents and should be available before operation is begun. In order to avoid bleeding before the dural

307

tear is adequately exposed, it is best to begin the removal of bone peripherally, approaching the sinus from all sides. Control of hemorrhage may be temporarily achieved by digital pressure over the defect. Ligation is a dangerous procedure and is indicated only when a complete severance exists, or when the site involved is the most rostral portion of the sagittal sinus well anterior to the motor area. The dural rent may be obliterated and bleeding effectively controlled by means of muscle stamps or bits of Gelfoam moistened with thrombin. These are held in place until they are securely fixed in position with sutures.

Lesions involving the paranasal sinuses and orbit, and the auropetrosal region are discussed later in this chapter.

The methods of treating head wounds in the past were necessarily influenced to a large extent by the amount of time which had elapsed before definitive therapy was instituted. It was recognized that the policy of early and thorough debridement with closure in layers minimized the danger of infection and of the development of a cerebral hernia. For wounds more than 24 hours old, however, the open method of treatment with resultant fungus formation and healing by granulation was deemed advisable (Horrax, 1942). The advent of antibiotics, especially penicillin, permitted a radical departure from this principle during World War II. It was no longer mandatory to adhere to the concept of an arbitrary time limit beyond which closure of wounds was not permissible. Favorable reports on delayed primary closure were published by a number of observers including Lebedenko (1943), Cairns (1944), and Schwartz and Roulhac (1945). The last named authors treated eight cases in which debridement and primary closure were performed between 36 hours and four days after injury. All healed by primary union. An additional six patients were successfully operated upon after much longer intervals (8 to 51 days). While early surgical treatment remains the procedure of choice, with the aid of antibiotics, debridement, removal of devitalized tissue and primary suture may be expected to yield good results in a large proportion of older wounds.

It is advisable following operation to reexamine the skull roentgenographically to determine whether there are any residual bone fragments. Even in the absence of symptoms, secondary wound debridement is indicated for the removal of large or clustered bone chips. If, however, the retained fragments are small, solitary, or inaccessible, and attempts at removal hazardous to neurologic function, operation may be withheld, provided there is no evidence of infection and the patient can be observed for some time thereafter. It has been demonstrated that in cases in which early debridement has been performed (2-4 hours after wounding) 55 percent of indriven bone fragments, and possibly even as many as 75 percent, are sterile (Carey et al, 1971). Wounds subjected to secondary operation should also be tightly closed.

Class V: Wounds Usually of Penetrating Type with Indriven Bone Fragments Plus Metal. The wounds in this group usually occur as a result of missiles striking the skull at approximately a right angle, and especially if of small size, entering the brain with relatively little damage to bone. Small penetrating missiles are frequently associated with intracerebral hematomas (Matson, 1958). Schorstein (1947) reported this occurrence in 32 cases of his series of 42 patients with deep penetrating wounds caused by small missiles weighing about 0.1 gm. The incidence of intracranial hematomas reported by Barnett and Meirowsky (1955) in a series of 316 cases of penetrating wounds treated within eight hours after injury during the Korean War was 46 percent. Intracranial hemorrhage, either subcortical or subdural, may be present on the side opposite the wound of entrance in cases in which the projectile has crossed the midline and lies near the opposite cortex (Matson and Wolkin, 1946). This possibility must be kept in mind and whenever its existence is suspected, exploration is indicated through a burr hole over the site of the retained foreign body. If a subdural hematoma is not disclosed, an intracerebral hemorrhage should be sought by means of a brain cannula.

The treatment of the wound is similar to that already described. With regard to the removal of the foreign body, several factors must be evaluated. If the missile is readily accessible, it should be removed. In the event it is deeply placed and its track crosses basal ganglia and internal capsule, attempts at removal are inadvisable. Even the most careful exploration and probing will increase the neurologic deficit and can result in hemorrhage and fatal edema, or a spread of infection into an area where it spells a lethal outcome. Should removal of a foreign body necessitate opening into a ventricle, it would be best not to make the attempt. On the other hand, if the track of the missile is superficial or involves a frontal lobe, more persistent efforts to remove the metal may be justified. It should be remembered that only infrequently do retained missiles become the seat of infection. In this connection it is of some interest that Ascroft (1941) reported a lower incidence of fits in patients with retained metallic fragments than in those from whose brains missiles have been removed. The study of Walker and Jablon (1961) indicated the very opposite however, while, according to Evans (1962), retention of metallic fragments appears unrelated to the development of epilepsy.

Class VI: Wounds of Type IV or V with Penetration of Bone or Metal Opening into Cerebral Ventricles. Ventricular penetration is suggested by leakage of cerebrospinal fluid from the depth of the wound, and by the disposition of bone fragments or missiles, as revealed by roentgenographic examination. Hyperthermia and a rapid decline of consciousness were frequently observed by Haynes (1945) in such cases. There is, however, no specific clinical syndrome characteristic of transventricular wounds (Wannamaker, 1965). In contrast to the high mortality rate noted by Cushing (1918), the incidence of recovery following operation on ventricular wounds during World War II was much greater. Haynes (1945) reported a postoperative mortality rate of 33.7 percent in his series of 77 cases; the mortality figures of Gillingham (1947), of Small and Turner (1947), and of Schwartz and Roulhac (1948) are about the same. Many fewer fatalities, 31, were reported by Wannamaker (1965) in a series of 214 transventricular wounds treated during the Korean War. Infection, and to a lesser extent, intraventricular hemorrhage and diffuse brain damage, accounted for the fatalities.

In the treatment of these cases, it is advisable that operation be performed as soon as possible in order to minimize the risk of infection or the effects of blood within the ventricles. The wound of entrance is debrided in the manner already described. Once the ventricle is exposed, blood clot and debris are thoroughly removed and the patency of a plugged foramen of Monro restored. It is important that all bleeding be controlled and that the ventricle be completely rid of blood clot. Foreign bodies are removed only when readily accessible. The wound is tightly closed, utilizing a dural graft whenever necessary. Removal of cerebrospinal fluid by repeated lumbar punctures may be required postoperatively.

According to Cairns (1947) patients recovering from ventricular wounds usually show profound mental changes and often suffer from recurrent attacks of meningitis.

Class VII: Cranio-facial Wounds in Which the Ethmoid or Petrosal Sinuses are Opened. Wounds with involvement of the paranasal sinuses and orbit may be divided into several groups (Calvert, 1947): those in which the missile enters the skull in the frontal region and emerges through the floor of the anterior fossa either by way of the orbital roof or the paranasal sinuses and nose; those in which the course of the projectile is a horizontal one resulting in a severe gutter wound of the

floor of the anterior fossae with destruction of the orbital roofs and paranasal sinuses; those in which the bullet or shell fragment traverses the
orbit, or nose and orbit, and enters the cranial cavity through the floor
of the anterior or middle fossa; penetrating wounds of the frontal sinus
in which the missile remains above the skull base; and those in which
entry takes place through the orbit or nose and, despite a downward
and backward course of the projectile beneath the base of the skull,
nevertheless result in associated fractures of the anterior fossae involving the paranasal sinuses.

In treating basal wounds, one is confronted with a more complex problem than is ordinarily the case in lesions involving the convexity of the
brain. Not only must the wound be debrided and closed, but dural
tears overlying fractures of the paranasal sinuses must also be repaired
and adequate drainage from the sinuses into the nose be established.
Stereoscopic roentgen examination provides an especially useful diagnostic adjunct in this group of cases, inasmuch as it may be possible
to determine with reasonable accuracy the relation of the missile track
to the paranasal sinuses. Such information is very useful as a guide to
treatment. The surgical approach to these compound fronto-orbital fractures varies with the individual case. In some instances one may advan-
tageously utilize the existing skin laceration, extending it as far laterally
as necessary. This plan may be adopted in cases with extensive scalp
wounds and considerable fragmentation of the frontal sinuses. More
often, perhaps, operation is best carried out through a separate frontal
bone flap, employing a coronal scalp incision. This approach is more
suitable for the treatment of dural lacerations overlying the ethmoid
cribriform area. Not uncommonly a bifrontal exploration is indicated.
Dural defects are repaired by fascial grafts preferably placed intradu-
rally rather than extradurally over the openings. When utilizing a bone
flap, one must, in addition, excise the wound of entrance and debride
the brain track. The approach by way of the direct route involves
exenteration of the comminuted walls of the frontal sinus and of its
mucous membrane. Detached fragments of bone from the orbital roof
and paranasal sinuses are removed, the brain track debrided, and the
extent of the dural tear ascertained. If the latter is situated in the region
of the cribriform plate, insertion of a fascial graft is performed, either
intra- or extradurally. Whenever possible, fascial grafts are sutured in
place. Dural defects in relation to the frontal sinus are closed separately
either by suture or by means of a fascial or pericranial graft placed
extradurally. Orbitofrontal wounds present formidable problems. Following enucleation of the eye, debridement of the brain track may be

311

performed through the dural laceration and the defect occluded by suturing the orbital tissues or by packing them against the undersurface of the opening. Communication of the subarachnoid space and paranasal sinuses may still be present and its obliteration necessitate an operative approach from above. Indeed it may be preferable to perform a bifrontal exploration and intradural repair initially and deal with the wounds of the orbit and sinuses thereafter. Orbitotemporal wounds are handled in a similar manner. Massive orbitocranial wounds may require a rotation flap for purposes of closure, together with a Thiersch graft applied to the bared area. Later on the unsightly hairy flap may be replaced by a tube pedicle graft. Webster, Schneider, and Lofstrom (1946) advise that a temporary fascia lata graft be used in the treatment of such massive wounds to be followed by a split-thickness skin graft at a later date.

Chemotherapy should be instituted in these cases at the earliest possible moment preoperatively and continued following operation. One must constantly be on the lookout for such complications as intracranial aerocele, cerebrospinal fluid rhinorrhea, meningitis, and brain abscess.

Dural defects associated with auro-petrosal wounds may be closed with temporal fascia grafts sutured in place.

The prognosis in cases of orbito-facio-cranial wounds treated by debridement and dural repair in conjunction with antibiotics is quite good, notwithstanding the severity of the trauma. There were only four deaths in Calvert's series of 57 cases.

Class VIII: Perforating or Traversing Wounds. It is characteristic of perforating lesions that the wound of exit is larger than the wound of entry (Matson, 1958). The amount of tissue destruction is greater in the region of the wound of exit, and indriven bone fragments may also be present at this site (Ascroft, 1943). These injuries are treated by separate excision of the wounds of entry and of emergence. The track of the missile is cleared from each end. While debridement of the entire length of the track is indicated whenever feasible, at times the danger of precipitating deep and uncontrollable hemorrhage may render it inadvisable to explore the innermost recesses of the wound. Matson and Wolkin (1946) stress the importance of operating on the exit wound first because of the frequency with which extensive hemorrhage is encountered in this region. Evacuation of a hematoma may improve the patient's condition considerably and convert a hazardous situation into one reasonably safe for further surgical treatment.

Experience with such wounds during the Korean War was reported by Harsh (1965).

Class IX: Extensive Bursting Fractures. Extensive bursting fractures of the skull are associated with such marked destruction of brain tissue and secondary hemorrhage that they are practically always fatal. Treatment is seldom undertaken because of the moribund state of the patient.

CHEMOTHERAPY

The value of antibiotics, especially of penicillin, in the treatment of penetrating brain wounds has been established beyond doubt. The lowered incidence of infection and, as a consequence, the decreased mortality rate of intracranial injuries during and following World War II were achieved, in a large measure, as a result of the use of intensive chemotherapy. It must be emphatically stated, however, that chemotherapy is no substitute for proper surgical treatment. Only when wounds have been thoroughly debrided are antibiotics effective in preventing infection.

During World War II it was the practice of most neurosurgeons to combine local and systemic chemotherapy, utilizing sulfadiazine and penicillin. Further experience with antimicrobial agents appeared to indicate that systemic administration alone was adequate. Transventricular wounds were considered an exception and local instillation of penicillin was advised in such cases (Woodhall, 1947).

In the Korean War reliance was placed upon a combination of penicillin and streptomycin. Systemic therapy alone was employed even in wounds involving the ventricles (Wannamaker, 1954).

In Vietnam (Hammon, 1971) antibiotics have been administered intravenously during the immediate postoperative period, usually aqueous penicillin, 40 million units and chloramphenicol, 2 grams, daily. Patients in whom the use of penicillin is contraindicated may be given instead a tetracycline, erythromycin or cephalothin.

THE COMPLICATIONS AND SEQUELAE OF GUNSHOT INJURIES TO THE HEAD AND BRAIN

Infection. The incidence of infection following initial operative repair of gunshot injuries to the head and brain incurred during the Second World War (European Theatre of Operations) was 37.7 percent, of which 16 percent were superficial infections (Spurling, quoted by Woodhall, 1947). Death resulting from infection, however, occurred in only 4.4 percent of cases.

313

The most virulent organisms isolated in cases of acute infection, especially meningitis, after brain wounds in World War II were non-B-hemolytic streptococci (Cairns et al, 1947). Other bacteria found in infected wounds included Staphylococcus aureus, coliform organisms, and less often pneumococci, H. influenza, and Neisseria. Clostridial infection, as a rule, was not severe, nor did it result in diffuse gas gangrene. Gram positive cocci, mostly hemolytic staphylococci and, to a lesser extent, beta hemolytic or non-hemolytic streptococci were the commonest organisms isolated from infected wounds during the Korean War (Wannamaker and Pulaski, 1958); combinations of gram positive cocci and gram negative bacilli (coliform, Proteus, and Pseudomonas) were also encountered.

Retention of intracranial foreign bodies necessitated re-operation in 68 of 506 cases of penetrating brain wounds incurred in Vietnam (Hagan, 1971). Positive bacteriologic cultures were obtained in 35 of 62 patients (56 percent) with retained bone fragments; the most common organism was Staphylococcus epidermis. All metallic fragments cultured were found to be contaminated by microbes. Superficial infection occurred in 32 cases. Eighteen patients had meningitis proven by culture; an additional 12 presumably had meningitis. The potential hazard of retained bone fragments is further revealed in the report of Hammon (1971). Of 40 patients with retained fragments who were reexplored, 16 had positive wound cultures while receiving antibiotics, and in 23 there was gross evidence of infection. Debris and/or necrotic tissue was present in all cases. Eight patients died following reexploration. The organisms cultured included Pseudomonas aeruginosa, Staphylococcus aureus and Staphylococcus epidermis.

A bacteriological study of craniocerebral missile wounds in Vietnam by Carey et al (1971) disclosed that organisms could be cultured from within the brain in only 11 percent of cases 2 to 4 hours after injury. Bacterial contamination, predominantly with Staphylococcus, was found in practically all cases. About one-half the skin wounds contained organisms capable of anaerobiosis. Debridement was performed within a few hours after injury and in 11 of 20 cases the indriven bone fragments were sterile.

Due to the influence of antibiotic therapy, the usual evidence of superficial wound infection is often lacking (Rowe and Turner, 1945). Thinning and darkening of the line of incision may provide the sole clues, and only probing with a pointed hemostat will indicate the presence of underlying pus. Minor wound infections usually respond favorably to adequate drainage, removal of sutures, and continued administration of antibiotics. The danger of wound necrosis resulting from closure under excessive tension has been referred to in a previous section.

The recognition of deeply situated infections may be difficult, especially in the early stages. Headache of constantly increasing severity, progressive neurologic signs, bulging of the wound, papilledema, mental torpor, and fever, either singly or in combination, should arouse suspicion. When, in addition to these manifestations, roentgenograms reveal the presence of retained bone fragments, the diagnosis of a deep infection is practically a certainty. Infections occur about ten times more frequently about bone chips than in their absence (Martin and Campbell, 1946). Metallic foreign bodies usually do not act as a nidus of infection, though occasionally they may do so. Treatment consists of redebridement with evacuation of all infected brain tissue, pus and bone fragments (Harsh, 1965). It is unnecessary, and hazardous, to await abscess formation and encapsulation. Closure is accomplished without drainage. Local instillation of penicillin is probably desirable. Infected wounds involving the cerebral ventricles, with abscess formation and ventriculitis, are handled in a similar manner (Schwartz and Roulhac, 1945). Appropriate systemic antibiotic therapy is administered.

Symptoms of brain abscess may be delayed for months or even years after gunshot injury to the brain. In some of these cases, the original wound may have healed completely, while in others a draining sinus may persist. Generally, incomplete debridement with retention of bone chips is the responsible factor. The clinical manifestations of brain abscess that develop late in the course of a penetrating wound are variable. Convulsions and recurrent attacks of meningitis, or headache, vomiting, and progressive focal neurologic signs and symptoms may dominate the picture. Occasionally, fulminating meningitis due to rupture of a "silent" abscess into a ventricle, is the first indication of the existence of the lesion. Electroencephalography, pneumoencephalography, arteriography, and radioisotope brain scans are valuable diagnostic adjuncts. Treatment consists of total extirpation of the abscess by means of an osteoplastic craniotomy (Fincher, 1946; Le Beau, 1946). After the brain is exposed, pus is evacuated from the abscess cavity by aspiration, care being taken not to contaminate the wound. This results in a diminution of the intracranial pressure and in collapse of the abscess, thereby facilitating its excision with the combined suction and cautery apparatus. Penicillin is placed in the wound and closure effected in layers without drainage. Antibiotics are continued postoperatively for a period of about four weeks, decreasing the dosage gradually. The sensitivity of the organism cultured from the wound to various antibiotics is determined as a guide to therapy.

The occurrence of meningitis following a penetrating head wound calls for eradication of the source of the infection, maintaining at the same time adequate chemotherapy. In the event meningitis complicates a fracture involving a paranasal sinus, repair of the dural defect should be delayed until resolution of the infection has occurred.

Cerebral Fungus. A postoperative fungus is a herniation of brain tissue through a defect in the scalp. The causes of fungus formation include failure to adequately close a wound after debridement, closure under tension with subsequent wound disruption, and increased intracranial pressure caused by an infection or hematoma. In the absence of deep infection, such herniae tend to recede and epithelialize of their own accord, provided superficial infection is controlled. Wet saline dressings for purposes of cleansing followed by the application of Vaseline gauze are all that may be required. Lumbar puncture may be resorted to in order to diminish the size of the protruding mass. Continued enlargement of the hernia should lead one to suspect the presence of an underlying abscess, and the presence of residual bone fragments affords confirmatory evidence. A draining sinus arising from a deep purulent collection may be present. Prompt evacuation of the abscess and bony fragments is imperative since otherwise the fungus will continue to enlarge, with the threat of meningitis and increasing intracranial pressure ever present (Schwartz and Roulhac, 1945; Campbell and Martin, 1946; Cairns, Calvert, Daniel, and Northcroft, 1947). Full doses of antibiotics should be administered until complete healing has occurred. Based on their experience during the Korean War with fungating cerebritis resulting from delayed or inadequate initial treatment, Meirowsky and Harsh (1953) advised resection of the mass and secondary closure of the wound after the infection had subsided.

Retained Foreign Bodies. Whenever feasible, foreign bodies should be removed at the time of the original operation. The technique of this procedure has already been discussed. Frequently, however, multiple small fragments are dispersed throughout the brain, or single deeply situated missiles are present, the removal of which is unduly hazardous. Cairns (1947), summarizing the experience of British neurosurgeons between 1939 and 1945, stated that intracranial missiles were removed in less than one-third of the cases in which they were present. While the incidence of abscess formation about metallic foreign bodies is small, assuming adequate debridement of the track, there is always the possibility that a latent infection may become active (Drew and Fager, 1954; Arseni and Ghitescu, 1967). As previously noted, Hagan (1971) found that cultures of metallic fragments invariably yielded bacterial growth. Should symptoms of brain abscess develop, operative intervention is, of course, mandatory. Reference has been made earlier in this chapter to the difference in opinion concerning the relative incidence of epilepsy in patients with and without retained missiles (Ascroft, 1941; Walker and Jablon, 1961; Evans, 1962). A number of patients are known to harbor intracranial projectiles varying in size from small fragments to steel bullets for as many as 20 years without symptoms. Not infrequently, however, after periods of quiescence of varying duration, epileptic seizures may occur. In the event the seizures remain refractory to adequate anticonvulsant medication, removal of the foreign body and its associated scar may be desirable. Craniotomy for this purpose is performed over the site of the missile, and the scarred track, the sclerotic tissue surrounding the foreign body, and the marginal cortical epileptogenic focus excised. Latent infection may be stirred up at the time of operation, for which reason antibiotics in full doses should be employed. Asymptomatic foreign bodies are best left untouched.

Localized Hydrocephalus Following Ventricular Wounds. Obliteration of the body of the lateral ventricle following parietal penetrating wounds involving the ventricle, with resultant obstructive hydrocephalus of the inferior horn, has been described by Cairns, Daniel, Johnson and Northcroft (1947). The symptoms produced by the progressive dilatation of the temporal horn resemble those of an expanding lesion so that abscess formation is at first suspected. The correct diagnosis is established by ventriculography together with the injection of air into the parietotemporal cyst after aspiration of its fluid contents. Ventriculographic examination reveals the ventricular system as a whole to be displaced away from the side of the wound; on the side of the lesion only the anterior horn and the anterior part of the body of the ventricle are filled with gas. Following the replacement of the fluid in the cyst with gas, a dilated non-communicating inferior horn is visualized, which obviously accounts for the ventricular shift. Excision of the choroid plexus contained within the inferior horn would appear to suffice as a means of effecting a cure of this condition.

Arteriovenous Aneurysm. An arteriovenous fistula involving the internal carotid artery and the cavernous sinus may result from trauma due to a gunshot wound, or more commonly, from a closed fracture of the middle fossa. Arterial blood entering directly into the cavernous sinus produces a pulsating exophthalmos, synchronous with the heart beat.

317

The earliest symptom is a bruit audible to the patient, and to the examiner on auscultation. At first the bruit may be intermittent, occurring only during systole, but subsequently it becomes a continuous roar, with a systolic accentuation. Thereafter pulsating exophthalmos makes its appearance, together with chemosis and engorgement of the vessels of the conjunctiva. Extraocular muscle palsies may occur with resultant diplopia. Due to the high venous pressure, papilledema also is to be observed. In a small number of cases, the proptosis and associated manifestations are present bilaterally. The diagnosis of an arteriovenous aneurysm is usually fairly obvious, pulsating exophthalmos being virtually a pathognomonic sign. In addition, compression of the ipsilateral carotid artery in the neck causes a cessation of the bruit. Confirmatory evidence may be obtained by means of angiography, which reveals a flow of the radiopaque substance from the internal carotid artery into the cavernous sinus and dilated orbital veins, and subsequently into the internal jugular vein through communicating channels (Wolff and Schmid, 1939). The cerebral arteries on the side of the injection either fail to fill with the contrast medium, or else visualize poorly, since their blood supply is derived mainly from the contralateral carotid and from the vertebral system, through the anterior and posterior communicating vessels respectively.

The treatment of this condition is operative and involves interrupting the arterial supply to the aneurysm. Ligation of the common carotid or the internal carotid artery may suffice to effect a cure. Symptoms may nevertheless persist, in which case it becomes necessary to occlude the internal carotid artery intracranially and in the neck, thereby "trapping" the aneurysm. It is advisable to clip the ophthalmic artery also at the time of the intracranial operation so as to completely deprive the fistula of an arterial blood supply.

Provided interhemispheric arterial communication is demonstrable, Hamby (1964, 1966) recommends a one-stage trapping operation, combined with embolization of the fistulous segment, as the procedure of choice.

Convulsive Seizures. Reference has already been made to the occurrence of convulsive seizures following head trauma and a more extensive account is presented in Chapter 17. Recent studies dealing with posttraumatic epilepsy have been published by Walker and Jablon (1961), Jennett (1962, 1969), Evans (1962), Caveness (1963), Caviness (1966), Russell (1969) and Walker and Erculei (1969). The report of Caviness concerns the course of posttraumatic epilepsy in 82 cases, mostly penetrating wounds, observed over a period of 20 years or longer. It was found that the more destructive the wound and the greater the neurologic deficit, the higher the incidence of seizures. Fits occurred most frequently following wounds in the parietal region. "Wounds of moderate severity in the frontal regions were associated with seizure disorders of decreasing frequency of attack. Wounds of greater severity in the central and posterior regions were associated with more intractable seizure disorders of increasing frequency of attack." Trauma involving the central region resulted in the highest proportion of neurologic deficits and seizures in such cases were of early onset and often focal.

A tendency towards a cessation of attacks in a substantial number of cases was reported by Walker and Jablon (1961), Caveness (1963), Russell (1969) and Walker and Erculei (1969). Among 560 survivors of penetrating brain wounds followed by Russell, the incidence of epilepsy (grand mal) was over 40 percent; 20 years later fits occurred in only about 25 percent and in only about 5 percent were they of frequent occurrence.

In a study of severely head injured men 15 years after wounding, 40 percent of 230 known to have had convulsions at some time had no seizures between the fifth and fifteenth year; eight others had no attacks from the tenth to fifteenth years; ten had only sporadic attacks (Walker and Erculei). Not only was there a tendency towards remission, but the pattern of the fits tended to change over the years. Generalized seizures occurred less often and the type of aura might vary.

Noteworthy is the observation of Walker and Jablon that the epileptic manifestations of a particular case may appear to be unrelated to the site of trauma. Thus an occipital wound may be associated with focal motor fits. It is suggested that the site of cranial trauma need not correspond to the location of the cerebral injury.

In a study of early traumatic epilepsy (331 nonmissile injuries) Jennett (1969) found that fits occurred most commonly during the first week following injury, were often of a focal motor pattern, and were much less likely to persist than seizures initially appearing at a later date. A smaller series of missile injuries showed similar trends. Of 41 cases of missile wounds with fits appearing during the first week, 19 (46 percent) developed late epilepsy. Convulsions first appeared between the second and eighth week following injury in 24 patients with missile wounds and of these, late epilepsy occurred in 19 (79 percent).

Since the likelihood of epilepsy increases with the severity of the injury, especially when dural penetration has occurred, the routine administration of anticonvulsant drugs to such cases would seem desirable as a prophylactic measure. The treatment of seizures once established is both a medical and surgical problem. Although patients with post-traumatic convulsions do not respond to medical therapy as well as those with idiopathic epilepsy, nevertheless anticonvulsant drugs, when administered in adequate doses, are usually effective in reducing, and occasionally even entirely arresting fits. Surgical treatment should be limited to selected patients who fail to obtain relief from a medical regimen (Penfield and Steelman, 1947; Walker and Johnson, 1948; Walker, 1949, 1958; Penfield and Jasper, 1954; Penfield and Paine, 1955).

Cranial Defects. The most visible sequel to a cranial injury following a gunshot wound is a defect in the skull. With the patient in the upright position, the site of the defect is characteristically drawn inward forming a pulsating hollow of varying depth, whereas when the head is held dependent, the overlying scalp exhibits a bulge. Patients with cranial defects frequently complain of local pain and tenderness, and of headache and dizziness precipitated by stooping or bending ("syndrome of the trephined"). The assumed danger to the unprotected brain in the region of the defect and an awareness of the unsightly appearance of the deformity contribute further to the patient's distress.

Treatment. For the above-mentioned reasons, cranioplasty is usually justified. Most surgeons prefer to wait at least six months after the wound has completely healed before undertaking repair of the defect. In cases in which the wound has become infected, it would appear advisable to defer operation for a minimum of one year after healing has taken place. Before cranioplasty is undertaken, the possibility of a latent brain abscess should be excluded, resorting, if necessary, to pneumoencephalography. Epilepsy per se does not constitute a contraindication. The advisability of cranioplasty in the face of a persistent severe neurologic disability will depend on a consideration of the individual case.

Various materials have been used for the repair of cranial defects, including bone grafts and alloplastic metallic and nonmetallic substances (Woolf and Walker, 1945; Reeves, 1950, 1958, 1965). Small defects may be readily repaired by autogenous bone grafts. These transplants are preferably taken from the skull itself, though other donor sites may be utilized, such as the tibia, ilium, and ribs. The advantages of a skull transplant are that it may be obtained simply by enlarging the original incision and that it conforms more readily to the contour of the remainder of the cranium. The operative procedure consists of incising the scalp at the site of the previous wound, excising the scar and exposing the defect. After separating dura from bone, the edges of the defect are bevelled with a fine chisel, and a pattern of the desired transplant prepared out of flat cotton. This pattern is then transferred to a neighboring area of skull, enlarging the exposure, if necessary, and outlined with a knife on the pericranium. If it is desired to hinge or rotate the graft on a pedicle of periosteum, the incision is not completed on the side closest to the defect. In the event a large transplant is needed, an area of skull may be exposed at a distance from the location of the defect through a separate incision. In either case, having incised the periosteum, a fine chisel is used to cut the outline into the bone itself and by directing the instrument through the diploe parallel with the surface, a layer of outer table attached to periosteum is lifted. The transplant consists of separate bone flakes arranged as a mosaic adherent to the intact pericranium. It is easily molded by pressure and can either be rotated on its pedicle or transferred as a free graft to the cranial defect. Fixation is accomplished by suturing the pericranium of the graft to that of the skull with interrupted silk sutures. The scalp edges are then undermined to secure coaptation and closure is effected in separate layers.

For linear defects, tibial transplants may be used with considerable advantage while larger rectangular defects are suitable for repair with split rib grafts. The inner table of the ilium provides another satisfactory donor site for large grafts properly curved to fit the contour of the skull (Money, 1946).

Of the various alloplastic materials suggested for the repair of cranial defects, tantalum has been used extensively in recent years. It is extremely well tolerated by tissues, in addition to which it possesses the desirable qualities of strength and malleability. Plates of tantalum may be fashioned at the operating table or preformed from an impression of the skull defect. Insertion of the plate is accomplished by fitting it into a ledge in the outer table of bone surrounding the defect. For purposes of fixation, tantalum wire sutures, screws, or triangular wedges may be utilized or it may be possible simply to spring the plate into the ledge. For a more detailed description of the techniques of preparation and insertion of such plates, the reader is referred to the publications of Gardner (1945); Hemberger. Whitcomb, and Woodhall (1945); Woodhall and Spurling (1945); Woolf and Walker (1945); Turner (1946); Woodhall (1946); Dahleen (1947); and Reeves (1950, 1958, 1965).

Stainless steel in the form of plates and wire mesh has also proved valuable for use in cranioplasty (Boldrey, 1945; Scott and Wycis, 1946). Our experience with this material has been most gratifying and we

321

prefer it to any of the other alloplastic substances available. The use of preformed steel plates is recommended since it facilitates the procedure considerably. Of the alloplastic nonmetallic substances used to repair skull defects, only the acrylic resins remain in vogue. Experience gained with methyl methacrylate indicates that it is a very satisfactory material for use in cranioplasty (Small and Graham, 1945; Elkins and Cameron, 1946; Mackay, 1947). A method of repairing cranial defects utilizing a methyl methacrylate resin molded into the skull defect was described by Spence (1954). Complications, most commonly infection or necrosis of the overlying scalp, may follow repair of a cranial defect, regardless of the type of graft employed (White, 1948). The long-term results of cranioplasty, as a rule, are very satisfactory (Scott, Wycis and Murtagh, 1962; Walker and Erculei, 1963).

CEREBROSPINAL FLUID RHINORRHEA AND SPONTANEOUS PNEUMOCEPHALUS

Cerebrospinal fluid rhinorrhea, i.e., a discharge of cerebrospinal fluid from the nose, occurs as a result of a communication between the intra- and extracranial structures. The most common cause is trauma, either blunt or penetrating. In closed head injuries rhinorrhea may appear soon after trauma, most commonly within 48 hours (Lewin, 1966) or after a delay of weeks, months, or even years. An incident of 2.3 percent was reported by Raaf (1967) in a series of 2194 cases of acute head injury. Other causes of cerebrospinal fluid rhinorrhea include neoplastic disease involving the base of the skull, especially pituitary tumors, infection, increased intracranial pressure, operative complications, and congenital defects of the cribriform plate or sella turcica (Ommaya, DiChiro, Baldwin, and Pennybacker, 1968; Rovit, Schechter, and Nelson 1969).

In most instances of rhinorrhea following closed head trauma, cerebrospinal fluid escapes as a result of a fracture of a paranasal sinus, usually the frontal or ethmoidal sinus, occurring in association with a tear of the overlying dura. Occasionally the fracture and dural rent involve the sphenoid sinus (Lewin and Cairns, 1951). Rarely the lesion involves the petrous bone in the middle or posterior fossa, fluid reaching the nose by way of the eustachian tube (Ecker, 1947). Facial trauma being a common cause of fractures of the paranasal sinuses, other injuries such as fractures of the maxilla and mandible and lacerations of the forehead may coexist.

Meningitis may be the first indication of a cerebrospinal fluid fistula. In all cases of posttraumatic meningitis, particularly recurrent meningitis, the possibility of a fistula should be suspected (Hand and Sanford, 1970).

The diagnosis of cerebrospinal fluid rhinorrhea is established by identification of the fluid issuing from the nose, most commonly by an analysis of its glucose content. Fluid may leak from one or both nostrils. Localization of the site of the fistula is largerly dependent on roentgenographic examination, including stereoscopic projections and laminagrams. Visualization of the fracture may be unsuccessful, however, and other procedures utilizing dyes, fluorescent substances, Pantopaque, radioactive tracers, and air insufflation during craniotomy have been proposed (DiChiro, Ommaya, Ashburn, and Briner, 1968; Ray and Bergland, 1969).

Treatment. In cases of closed head injury a trial of conservative treatment for a period of several days to a week is generally recommended in view of the high incidence of spontaneous cessation of the rhinorrhea. During this time it is advisable to confine the patient to bed with his head elevated, to caution him against blowing his nose, and to administer antibiotics prophylactically. There is some reason to believe, however, that even in the event the rhinorrhea ceases, spontaneous healing of the fistula is often imperfect so that the hazard of ascending infection and meningitis may nevertheless persist. It has, therefore, been suggested that all cases of rhinorrhea regardless of the time of onset, whether transient or protracted, be treated surgically (Lewin, 1954, 1966). After localizing the lesion as accurately as possible, the dural defect is exposed through a frontal craniotomy. An intradural exploration is preferred. A unilateral exposure will suffice provided the fracture and rhinorrhea are on the same side. Where doubt exists as to the site of the lesion or where there may be more than one lesion, a bilateral exploration is mandatory. Closure of the defect is accomplished by suture or the use of a graft, employing temporal fascia, fascia lata, or periosteum (Adson and Uihlein, 1949; Lewin, 1954, 1966; Schneider and Thompson, 1957).

In cases of rhinorrhea associated with fractures of the sphenoid sinus, the region of the tuberculum sellae is exposed, the defect plugged with muscle and covered over with dura or tissue (Lewin and Cairns, 1951). Ray and Bergland (1969) advise packing the sinus with muscle after detaching the mucosa from its posterior wall.

In cases of rhinorrhea or otorrhea due to petrous fractures, the defect is usually on the floor of the middle fossa, and treatment involves exposure of this region; exploration of the posterior fossa may be required.

The treatment of rhinorrhea caused by penetrating wounds is discussed elsewhere in this chapter.

Though multiple operations may be required to deal with the fistula and though not invariably successful, the results of surgical treatment are usually very satisfactory (Scheibert, 1965; Lewin, 1966).

Spontaneous pneumocephalus (aerocele) is frequently associated with cerebrospinal rhinorrhea, the mechanism responsible for both conditions being similar. Air enters through a dural defect and accumulates in the subarachnoid, subdural, or intraventricular spaces or within brain tissue. This condition is usually accompanied by severe headache and occasionally by mental disturbance and loss of consciousness. Air within cerebral tissue may collect under sufficient pressure to produce contralateral signs. Spontaneous pneumocephalus may be suspected on clinical grounds, but the diagnosis is unfailingly established by roentgen examination of the skull, which reveals the ventricular system outlined by gas, or else an area of decreased density within the cranium, obviously due to air. The treatment is similar to that of cerebrospinal rhinorrhea, namely, repair of the dural defect. Once the portal of entry of air into the cranial cavity is closed, nothing more need be done since the gas is rapidly absorbed. For a detailed review of this subject, the reader is referred to the article by Markham (*Acta Neurochirurgica, 16,* 1, 1967).

Residual Effects: Neurologic and Psychiatric. An analysis of the status of 364 men 15 years after they had suffered serious head wounds during World War II was undertaken by Walker and Erculei (1969). Not all injuries were sustained in combat. In well over two-thirds of the cases the wound extended beyond the scalp. Various elements of the posttraumatic syndrome, including nervousness, headache, irritability, easy fatigability, impaired memory, dizziness, defective mentation, and lack of concentration, were commonly present. Approximately two-thirds of all patients complained of nervousness or headache. It was found that "men with posttraumatic headache had a high hysterical, depressive and hypochondriacal score in the Minnesota Multiphasic Personality Inventory, although their formal intelligence was not lower than that of individuals without headache." Only 50 of the 249 patients examined were free of neurologic deficits. Hemiparesis was present in 118, hemihypesthesia in 121, hemianopia in 43, aphasia in 36, cranial nerve defects in 137, and mental impairment in 13. After the fifth posttraumatic year there was little change in the degree of motor or sensory deficit and, generally speaking, this was also true of visual and auditory disturbances. Speech, however, did appear to continue to improve beyond this time in some cases. Severe mental disturbances persisted only in a small percentage of the men. The more severely injured performed less well on all psychometric tests than did those less seriously wounded. Left cerebral lesions appeared to exert a more profound effect on intelligence than did injuries of the right side of the brain. Forty percent of those known to have had convulsions at some time (230) had no seizures between the fifth and fifteenth year following trauma. Eighty-seven percent of patients thought they had made a satisfactory adjustment from a social and marital standpoint. Thirty-nine percent were unemployed or not working steadily. Neurologic deficits and posttraumatic epilepsy were more frequent among the unemployed.

It should be clearly understood that the case material which provided the basis for the study of Walker and Erculei consisted of very serious brain wounds and is not representative of the ordinary civilian or even military head injury. By contrast, examination of 739 patients 5 to 9 years after they had suffered craniocerebral trauma during World War II (60 percent penetrating) revealed no neurologic deficit in 346, hemiparesis in 159, hemisensory deficits in 148, hemianopia in 68, aphasia in 59, mental impairment in 102, and cranial nerve palsies in 175 (Walker and Jablon, 1961). Headache was a symptom in 81 percent of cases. Over half of the patients rendered aphasic following injury improved or recovered, almost a third within the first six to eight months and nearly a quarter more in later years. The overall incidence of epilepsy was 28 percent; fits occurred in 36 percent of 472 patients in whom the dura had been penetrated and in 14 percent of 267 of those with an intact dura.

The results of a study of the posttraumatic sequelae of 467 men injured in Korea was presented by Caveness (1966). Missile wounds accounted for slightly more than half the cases. The dura was penetrated in about two-thirds of the missile wounds and remained intact in practically all the non-missile injuries. Over two-thirds of the cases (356) were followed for periods varying between eight and 11 years. Over an average period of ten years the incidence of central neurologic deficits decreased from 42 to 31 percent, and of peripheral deficits from 24 to 16 percent. A mild degree of emotional and intellectual impairment persisted in 13 percent. The overall incidence of epilepsy within the ten-year period was 31 percent; at the end of this time fits continued in 14 percent. Convulsions occurred in 50 percent of those in whom the dura was penetrated and in 20 percent of those in whom the dura remained intact. Five years after injury over half the pa-

325

tients complained of headache, nervousness, and irritability. Most were able to achieve a satisfactory social and economic adjustment, the incidence of failure being greatest in those with neurologic deficits or posttraumatic symptoms.

It is apparent that standard psychometric tests may fail to demonstrate the full spectrum of posttraumatic intellectual, memory, and other deficits. Special tests are required for a more objective and quantitative evaluation of various functional alterations. Noteworthy contributions in this area have been made especially by Teuber and his associates (1956, 1960, 1962, 1969) and a wealth of information has emerged from their studies. Only brief mention of some of their observations will be made here. These studies have demonstrated that brain wounds cause local as well as general effects, the latter unrelated to the site of injury. Thus, the ability to discover hidden figures is impaired following lesions in any lobe of the brain regardless of the presence or absence of sensory or visual symptoms. This is a nonspecific effect observed in penetrating brain wounds. The use of special tests has yielded information regarding the existence of deficits not demonstrated on routine examination. For example, the use of a test involving route finding by means of maps disclosed defective performance in patients with parietal lesions. Likewise, tachistoscopy has revealed visuoperceptual defects involving letters and numerals in patients with lesions affecting predominantly the left posterior hemisphere, and disproportionate difficulty with faces or complex line drawings when the lesions are on the right side. Differences have been noted between the effects of brain wounds involving the right and the left hemisphere. Subtle losses in complex perceptual achievements are more frequent or more pronounced following lesions of the nondominant hemisphere. Defects in tactile discrimination of three-dimensional size are greater when the right hemisphere is the one affected. Impairment of binaural sound localization is more marked following injury of the right parietotemporal region. Unilateral lesions may result in certain strictly contralateral effects or cause more diffuse bilateral changes (e.g., bilateral alterations in tactile discrimination following a unilateral parietal lesion). There is evidence to suggest that unilateral lesions may result in impaired interaction of both hemispheres.

Of considerable interest is the difference in functional representation in right and left hemispheres as revealed by studies of the sensory thresholds for pressure sensivity, two-point discrimination and point localization following brain injury. Threshold changes of the right hand were associated with lesions of the sensorimotor area of the opposite hemisphere In the case of the left hand, however, threshold changes were observed with lesions more widely dispersed over the contralateral and, in many cases, the ipsilateral hemisphere. Sensory changes in both hands were noted more often following lesions in the left cerebral hemisphere than the right one. Further evidence of asymmetry in functional representation of the hemispheres was revealed by the different kinds of sensory changes in the right and left hands. Whereas threshold changes involving the right hand tended to affect all sensory modalities tested, this was not so in the case of the left hand.

Employing the Army General Classification Test, Weinstein (1962) found relatively few patients with penetrating wounds who had incurred an intellectual loss. Some sustained a loss following injury to any area of the brain, but the greatest intellectual impairment occurred following trauma to the left parietotemporal area.

Important contributions in this field have also been made by Milner (1962, 1969). Her studies indicate that lesions of the dominant temporal lobe anterior to the critical speech area impair the acquisition and retention of verbal material, whereas right temporal lobe lesions affect nonverbal visual and auditory functions. Patients with post-traumatic epilepsy were found to exhibit specific deficits depending on the site of the lesion and the side of the brain involved. Thus, the performance of patients with frontal lobe injuries on a card-sorting test was significantly inferior to that of those with lesions elsewhere; the mean delayed verbal recall score was lowest when the left temporal lobe was the site of involvement.

The psychologic deficits resulting from unilateral cerebral lesions caused by penetrating wounds incurred during World War II were studied by Newcombe some 20 years later (1969). In a series of 97 men, the left side of the brain was found to be involved in 53, the right in 44. General intellectual function appeared unaffected though both groups responded more slowly in two visually presented tasks. The demonstrable deficits clearly indicated an asymmetry in the functional organization of the two sides of the brain. Defects of a verbal nature, regardless of the presence or absence of clinical dysphasia, were found only in patients with left cerebral lesions, whereas those in whom the right cerebral hemisphere was affected exhibited deficits in the field of visual spatial perception. The visual spatial impairment of the latter group was most striking in two tasks, visual closure and maze learning. The visual perceptual deficit was most pronounced in right temporo-parietal lesions, while the spatial maze learning deficit was greatest when the right parietal and parietooccipital areas were involved. This

327

dissociation of performance suggested the possibility of focal representation of function within the hemisphere. Impairment in some tasks of spatial orientation was also observed in some patients with left parietal lesions. It would seem that spatial orientation, though largely a function of the right hemisphere, is also dependent on the integrity of the left side of the brain. While the relationship between intellectual impairment and dysphasia was not clarified, the fact that some patients with marked expressive aphasia performed very well on many tasks, including standard intelligence tests, is noteworthy. The data appeared to indicate that visual field defects do not play a critical role in impaired visual spatial performance. The impression was also gained that appreciable improvement and restitution of function had occurred over the years.

A comprehensive account of the psychiatric disability of 670 patients with penetrating wounds observed over a five-year period was presented by Lishman (1968). Psychiatric disability was defined as a "disturbance in any area of mental life, as reflected by impaired intellectual function, disorder of affect, disorder of behavior, somatic complaints without demonstrable physical basis, and/or formal psychiatric illness." It was considered to be mild in 433 cases and severe in 144. There appeared to be significant correlations between the degree of psychiatric disability and the depth and amount of brain damage, the duration of posttraumatic amnesia and the occurrence of epilepsy, especially if it developed within one year of injury. An analysis of 345 patients with focal lesions indicated that the psychiatric disability was greater in those with involvement of the left side of the brain and in those with temporal lobe (principally left temporal lobe) wounds. Lesions, particularly of the left cerebrum (parietal and temporal lobes) resulting in sensory-motor and visual field deficits and those causing impairment of speech, were also significantly related to psychiatric disability. Analysis of the component features of the 144 patients with severe psychiatric manifestations disclosed that intellectual disorders as a group were more common following wounds of the left cerebrum, whereas affective and behavioral disorders and somatic complaints were more frequent after injuries involving the right side. Intellectual disorders especially were associated with lesions affecting the parietal and temporal lobes; affective and behavioral disorders and somatic complaints were relatively more frequent following frontal lobe injury. The "frontal lobe syndrome" was occasionally observed in other than frontal lobe lesions. With regard to the posttraumatic syndrome, the evidence favored a non-organic etiology.

BIBLIOGRAPHY

Adson, A. W. and Uihlein, A. Repair of Defects in Ethmoid and Frontal Sinuses Resulting in Cerebrospinal Rhinorrhea. *Arch. Surg.*, *58*, 623, 1949.

Arseni, C. and Ghitescu, M. Delayed Post-traumatic Cerebral Abscesses Due to Retained Intracerebral Foreign Bodies. *Acta Neurochir.*, *16*, 201, 1967.

Ascroft, P. B. Traumatic Epilepsy after Gunshot Wounds of the Head. *Br. Med.* (Eds.), *Head Injury*. Conference Proceedings. Philadelphia: J. B. Lippincott Co., 1966. Pp. 209-219.

Ascroft, P. B. Treatment of Head Wounds Due to Missiles. *Lancet, 2*, 211, 1943.

Barnett, J. C. and Meirowsky, A. M. Intracranial Hematomas Associated with Penetrating Wounds of the Brain. *J. Neurosurg.*, *12*, 34, 1955.

Bender, M. B. Extinction and Precipitation of Cutaneous Sensation. *Arch. Neur. & Psych.*, *54*, 1, 1945.

Boldrey, E. Stainless Steel Wire-Mesh in the Repair of Small Cranial Defects. *Ann. Surg.*, *121*, 821, 1945.

Cairns, H. Wounds of the Head in 1940. *J. Roy. Army Med. Corps, 76*, 12, 1941.

Cairns, H. Gunshot Wounds of the Head in the Acute Stage. *Br. Med. J.*, *1*, 33, 1944.

Cairns, H. Neurosurgery in the British Army, 1939-1945. *Br. J. Surg.*, *War Surg. Suppl. No. 1*, 9, 1947.

Cairns, H., Daniel, P., Johnson, R. T., and Northcroft, G. B. Localized Hydrocephalus Following Penetrating Wounds of the Ventricle. *Br. J. Surg.*, *War Surg. Suppl.*, No. *1*, 187, 1947.

Cairns, H., Calvert, C. A., Daniel, P. and Northcroft, G. B. Complications of Head Wounds with Especial Reference to Infection. *Br. J. Surg.*, *War Surg. Suppl.*, No. *1*, 198, 1947.

Calvert, C. A. Orbito-Facio-Cranial Gunshot Wounds. *Br. J. Surg.*, *War Surg. Suppl.*, No. *1*, 119, 1947.

Campbell, E. H. and Martin, J. Cerebral Fungus Following Penetrating Wounds. *Surgery, 19*, 748, 1946.

Carey, M. E., Young, H., Mathis, J. H., and Forsythe, J. A Bacteriological Study of Craniocerebral Missile Wounds from Vietnam. *J. Neurosurg.*, *34*, 145, 1971.

Caveness, W. F. Onset and Cessation of Fits Following Craniocerebral Trauma. *J. Neurosurg.*, *20*, 570, 1963.

Caveness, W. F. Posttraumatic Sequelae. In W. F. Caveness and A. E. Walker *J., 1*, 739, 1941.

Caviness, V. S., Jr. Epilepsy and Craniocerebral Injury of Warfare. In W. F. Caveness and A. E. Walker (Eds.), *Head Injury*. Conference Proceedings. Philadelphia; J. B. Lippincott Co., 1966. Pp. 220-234.

Chatelin, C. *Les Blessures du Cerveau*. Paris: Masson, 1918. (English translation: Chatelin, C. and De Martel, T. *Wounds of the Skull and Brain*. London: University of London Press, 1918).

Cloward, R. B. War Injuries to the Head. Treatment of Penetrating Wounds. *J. A. M. A., 118*, 267, 1942.

329

Converse, J. M. The Technique of Closure of Scalp Defects. *Clin. Neurosurg.,* *11,* 21, 1964.

Cope, Z. *Medical History of the Second World War. Surgery.* London: Her Majesty's Stationery Office, 1953.

Cushing, H. A Study of a Series of Wounds Involving the Brain and its Enveloping Structures. *Br. J. Surg., 5,* 558, 1918.

Cushing, H. Notes on Penetrating Wounds of the Brain. *Br. Med. I., 1,* 221, 1918.

Dahleen, H. C. Tantalum Cranioplasty, a Method for One-Piece Fixation. *Surgery, 21,* 546, 1947.

Di Chiro, G., Ommaya, A. K., Ashburn, W. L., and Briner, W. H. Isotope Cisternography in the Diagnosis and Follow-up of Cerebrospinal Fluid Rhinorrhea. *J. Neurosurg., 28,* 522, 1968.

Dodge, P. R. and Meirowsky, A. M. Tangential Wounds of Scalp and Skull. *J. Neurosurg., 9,* 472, 1952.

Drew, J. H. and Fager, C. A. Delayed Brain Abscess in Relation to Retained Intracranial Foreign Bodies. *J. Neurosurg., 11,* 386, 1954.

Ecker, A. Cerebrospinal Rhinorrhea by Way of the Eustachian Tube. *J. Neurosurg,. 4,* 177, 1947.

Eden. K. Mobile Neurosurgery in Warfare. Experiences in the Eighth Army's Campaign in Cyrenaica, Tripolitania, and Tunisia. *Br. J. Surg., 31,* 324, 1944.

Elkins, C. W. and Cameron, J. E. Cranioplasty with Acrylic Plates. *J. Neurosurg., 3,* 199, 1946.

Evans, J. H. Post-traumatic Epilepsy. *Neurology, 12,* 665, 1962.

Fincher, E. F. Craniotomy and Total Dissection as a Method in the Treatment of Abscess of the Brain. *Ann. Surg., 123,* 789, 1946.

Frazier, C. H. and Ingham, S. D. A Review of the Effects of Gunshot Wounds of the Head Based on the Observations of 200 Cases at U. S. Army General Hospital, No. 11, Cape May, N. J. *Trans. Am. Neur. Assn., 59,* 45th Annual Meeting, 1919.

Gardner, W. J. Closure of Defects of the Skull with Tantalum. *Surg. Gynec. Obstet., 80,* 303, 1945.

Gillingham, F. J. Neurosurgical Experiences in Northern Italy. *Br. J. Surg., War. Surg. Suppl., No. 1,* 80, 1947.

Goldstein, K. *After-effects of Brain Injuries in War.* New York: Grune and Stratton, 1942.

Hagan, R. E., Early Complications Following Penetrating Wounds of the Brain. *J. Neurosurg., 34,* 132, 1971.

Hamby, W. B. *Carotid-Cavernous Fistula.* Springfield, Ill.: Charles C Thomas, 1966.

Hamby, W. B. and Dohn, D. F. Carotid-Cavernous Fistulas: Report of Thirty-Six Cases and Discussion of Their Management. In *Clinical Neurosurgery,* Vol. 11. Baltimore: Williams and Wilkins, 1964. Pp. 150-170.

Hammon, W. M. An Analysis of 2187 Consecutive Penetrating Wounds of the Brain from Vietnam. *J. Neurosurg., 34,* 127, 1971.

Hammon, W. M. Retained Intracranial Bone Fragments: Analysis of 42 Patients. *J. Neurosurg., 34,* 142, 1971.

Hand, W. L. and Sanford, J. P. Posttraumatic Bacterial Meningitis. *Ann. Intern. Med., 72,* 869, 1970.

Harsh, G. R., III. Infection Complicating Penetrating Craniocerebral Trauma. In A. M. Meirowsky (Ed.), *Neurological Surgery of Trauma*. Washington, D. C.: Office of the Surgeon General, Dept. of the Army, 1965. Pp. 135-142.

Harsh, G. R., III. Through-and-Through Wounds. In A. M. Meirowsky (Ed.), *Neurological Surgery of Trauma*. Washington, D. C.: Office of the Surgeon General, Dept. of the Army, 1965. Pp. 161-164.

Haynes, G. W. Transventricular Wounds of the Brain. *J. Neurosurg.*, 2, 463, 1945.

Hemberger, A. J., Whitcomb, B. B., and Woodhall, B. The Technique of Tantalum Plating of Skull Defects. *J. Neurosurg.*, 2, 21, 1945.

Holmes, G. The Symptoms of Acute Cerebellar Injuries Due to Gunshot Wounds. *Brain*, 40, 461, 1917.

Holmes, G. Disturbances of Vision by Cerebral Lesions. *Br. J. Ophthal.*, 2, 353, 1918.

Holmes, G. and Lister, W. T. Disturbances of Vision from Cerebral Lesions with Special Reference to the Cortical Representation of the Macula. *Brain*, 39, 34, 1916.

Horrax, G. Observations on a Series of Gunshot Wounds of the Head. *Br. J. Surg.*, 7, 10, 1919.

Horrax, G. Treatment of War Injuries of the Skull and Brain. *Bull. Am. Coll. Surg.*, 27, 127, 1942.

Jacobs, G. B. Military Neurosurgery in Vietnam. In L. M. Davidoff Supplement to Vol. 26, *Proc. Rudolf Virchow Med. Soc.* New York, 1968.

Jacobs, G. B. and Berg, R. A. Tangential Wounds of the Head. *J. Neurosurg.*, 32, 642, 1970.

Jefferson, G. The Physiological Pathology of Gunshot Wounds of the Head. *Br. J. Surg.*, 7, 262, 1919.

Jennett, W. B. *Epilepsy After Blunt Head Injuries.* Springfield, Ill.: Charles C Thomas, 1962. P. 150.

Jennett W. B. Early Traumatic Epilepsy. *Lancet*, 1, 1023, 1969.

Jepson, R. P. and Whitty, C. W. M. The Neurological State and Postoperative Course in Penetrating Head Wounds. *Br. J. Surg.*, *War Surg. Suppl.* No. 1, 243, 1947.

Le Beau, J. Radical Surgery and Penicillin in Brain Abscess. *J. Neurosurg.*, 3, 359, 1946.

Lebedenko, V. Surgical Treatment of Brain Wounds in the Russian Army. *Trans. Am. Neur. Assn.*, 69th Annual Meeting, 17, 1943.

Lewin, W. Cerebrospinal Fluid Rhinorrhea in Closed Head Injuries. *Br. J. Surg.*, 42, 1, 1954.

Lewin, W. Cerebrospinal Fluid Rhinorrhea in Nonmissile Head Injuries. In *Clinical Neurosurgery*, Vol. 12. Baltimore: Williams and Wilkins, 1966. Pp. 237-252.

Lewin, W. and Cairns, H. Fractures of the Sphenoidal Sinus with Cerebrospinal Rhinorrhea. *Br. Med. J.*, 1, 1, 1951.

Lewin, W. and Gibson, R. M. Missile Head Wounds in the Korean Campaign. A Survey of British Casualties. *Br. J. Surg.*, 43, 628, 1955-1956.

Lishman, W. A. Brain Damage in Relation to Psychiatric Disability after Head Injury, *Br. J. Psychiat.*, 114, 373, 1968.

Luria, A. R. *Traumatic Aphasia. Its Syndromes, Psychology and Treatment.* The Hague: Mouton & Co., 1970.

331

MacKay, H. J. A Method of Cranioplasty Using Ready-Made Acrylic Craniopros-theses. *Surgery, 22,* 965, 1947.

Maltby, G. L. Penetrating Cerebral Injuries. Evaluation of the Late Results in a Group of 200 Consecutive Penetrating Cranial War Wounds. *J. Neurosurg., 3,* 239, 1946.

Markham, J. W. The Clinical Features of Pneumocephalus Based upon a Survey of 284 Cases with Report of 11 Additional Cases. *Acta Neurochir., 16,* 1, 1967.

Martin, J. and Campbell, E. H., Jr. Early Complications Following Penetrating Wounds of the Skull. *J. Neurosurg., 3,* 58, 1946.

Matson, D. D. *The Treatment of Acute Craniocerebral Injuries due to Missiles.* Springfield, Ill.: Charles C Thomas, 1948.

Matson, D. D. The Management of Acute Craniocerebral Injuries due to Missiles. In *Surgery in World War II, Neurosurgery,* Vol. *1.* Washington, D. C.: Office of the Surgeon General, Dept. of the Army, 1958. Pp. 123-182.

Matson, D. D., and Wolkin, J. Hematomas Associated with Penetrating Wounds of the Brain. *J. Neurosurg., 3,* 46, 1946.

McKissock, W. and Brownscombe, B. Apparently Trivial Head Injuries. *Lancet, 1,* 593, 1941.

Meirowsky, A. M. Wounds of Dural Sinuses. *J. Neurosurg., 10,* 496, 1953.

Meirowsky, A. M. Penetrating Craniocerebral Trauma. Observations in Korean War. *J.A.M.A., 154,* 666, 1954.

Meirowsky, A. M. Penetrating Wounds of the Brain. In A. M. Meirowsky (Ed.), *Neurological Surgery of Trauma.* Washington. D. C.: Office of the Surgeon General, Dept. of the Army, 1965. Pp. 103-130.

Meirowsky, A. M. and Harsh, G. R., III. The Surgical Management of Cerebritis Complicating Penetrating Wounds of the Brain. *J. Neurosurg., 10,* 373, 1953.

Michenfelder, J. D. and Terry, H. R., Jr. Current Practices and Trends in Neuro-anesthesia. In *Clinical Neurosurgery,* Vol. *13.* Baltimore: Williams and Wilkins, 1966. Pp. 252-263.

Michenfelder, J. D., Gronert, G. A., and Rheder, K. Neuroanesthesia. *Anesthesiology, 30,* 65, 1969.

Milner, B. Laterality Effects in Audition. In V. B. Mountcastle (Ed.), *Interhemispheric Relations and Cerebral Dominance.* Baltimore: Johns Hopkins Press, 1962. P. 294.

Milner, B. Residual Intellectual and Memory Deficits after Head Injury. In A. E. Walker, W. F. Caveness and M. Critchley (Eds.), *The Late Effects of Head Injury.* Springfield, Ill.: Charles C Thomas. 1969. Pp. 84-97.

Money, R. A. The Repair of Cranial Defects by Bone Grafting. *Surgery, 19,* 627, 1946.

Newcombe, F. *Missile Wounds of the Brain. A Study of Psychological Defects.* London: Oxford University Press, 1969.

Ommaya, A. K., Di Chiro, G., Baldwin, M., and Pennybacker, J. B. Nontraumatic Cerebrospinal Fluid Rhinorrhea. *J. Neurol. Neurosurg. Psychiatry, 31,* 214, 1968.

Penfield, W. and Steelman, H. The Treatment of Focal Epilepsy by Cortical Excision. *Ann. Surg., 126,* 740, 1947.

Penfield, W. and Jasper, H. *Epilepsy and the Functional Anatomy of the Human Brain.* Boston: Little, Brown & Co., 1954.

Penfield, W. and Paine, K. Results of Surgical Therapy for Focal Epileptic Seizures. *Can. Med. Ass. J., 73,* 515, 1955.

Purvis, J. T. Craniocerebral Injuries Due to Missiles and Fragments. In W. F. Caveness and A. E. Walker (Eds.), *Head Injury*. Conference Proceedings. Philadelphia: J. B. Lippincott Co., 1966. Pp. 133-141.

Raaf, J. Posttraumatic Cerebrospinal Fluid Leaks. *Arch. Surg.*, 95, 648, 1967.

Ray, B. and Bergland, R. M. Cerebrospinal Fluid Fistula: Clinical Aspects, Techniques of Localization, and Methods of Closure. *J. Neurosurg.*, 30, 399, 1969.

Reeves, D. L. Cranioplasty. In *Surgery in World War II. Neurosurgery*, Vol. 1. Washington, D. C.: Office of the Surgeon General, Dept. of the Army, 1958. Pp. 261-278.

Reeves, D. L. Repair of Cranial Defects. In A. M. Meirowsky (Ed.), *Neurological Surgery of Trauma*. *Washington*, D. C. Office of the Surgeon General, Dept. of the Army, 1965. Pp. 233-256.

Rovit, R. L., Schechter, M. M., and Nelson, K. Spontaneous "High Pressure Cerebrospinal Rhinorrhea" Due to Lesions Obstructing Flow of Cerebrospinal Fluid. *J. Neurosurg.*, 30, 406, 1969.

Rowe, S. N. and Turner, O. A. Observations on Infection in Penetrating Wounds of the Head. *J. Neurosurg.*, 2, 391, 1945.

Russell, W. R. Transient Disturbances Following Gunshot Wounds of the Head. *Brain*, 68, 79, 1945.

Russell, W. R. The Neurology of Brain Wounds. *Br. J. Surg., War Surg. Suppl.* No. 1. 250, 1947.

Russell, W. R. Functions of the Frontal Lobes. *Lancet*, 1, 356, 1948.

Russell, W. R. Studies in Amnesia. *Edinb. Med. J.*, 55, 92, 1948.

Russell, W. R. Disability Caused by Brain Wounds. *J. Neur. Neurosurg. Psychiatry*, 14, 35, 1951.

Russell, W. R. Amnésie de Mémoration Caused by Brain Wounds. *Trans. Am. Neur. Assn.*, 88, 43, 1963.

Russell, W. R. Epilepsy Following Brain Wounds of World War II — 20 Years After. *Proc. Soc. Br. Neurol. Surg.*, Sept. 19-21, 1968. Reported in *J. Neurol. Neurosurg. Psychiatry*, 32, 64, 1969.

Russell W. R. *The Traumatic Amnesias*. London: Oxford, 1971.

Russell, W. R. and Whitty, C. M. W. Studies in Traumatic Epilepsy. 1. Factors Influencing the Incidence of Epilepsy after Brain Wounds. *J. Neurol. Neurosurg. Psychiatry*, 15, 93, 1952.

Russell, W. R. and Whitty, C. M. W. Studies in Traumatic Epilepsy. 2. Focal Motor and Somatic Fits: A study of 85 Cases. *J. Neurol. Neurosurg. Psychiatry*, 16, 73, 1953.

Russell, W. R. and Whitty, C. M. W. Studies in Traumatic Epilepsy. 3. Visual Fits. *J. Neurol. Neurosurg. Psychiatry*, 18, 79, 1955.

Russell, W. R. and Espir, M. L. E. *Traumatic Aphasia*. Oxford: Oxford University Press, 1961.

Russell, W. R. and Davies-Jones, G. A. B. Epilepsy Following Brain Wounds of World War II. In A. E. Walker, W. F. Caveness, and M. Critchley (Eds.), *The Late Effects of Head Injury*. Springfield, Ill.: Charles C Thomas, 1969. Pp. 189-192.

Russell, W. R. and Young, R. R. Missile Wounds of the Parasagittal Rolandic Area. In S. Locke, *Modern Neurology*. Boston: Little, Brown & Co., 1969. Pp. 289-302.

Sargent, P. Some Observations on Epilepsy. *Brain. 44*, 312, 1921.

Scheibert, C. D. Cerebrospinal Fluid Fistula. In A. M. Meirowsky (Ed.), *Neurological Surgery of Trauma*. Washington, D. C.: Office of the Surgeon General, Dept. of the Army, 1965. Pp. 213-219.

Schiller, F. Aphasia Studied in Patients with Missile Wounds. *J. Neurol. Neurosurg. Psychiatry, 10*, 183, 1947.

Schneider, R. C. and Thompson, J. M. Chronic and Delayed Traumatic Cerebrospinal Rhinorrhea as a Source of Recurrent Attacks of Meningitis. *Ann. Surg., 145*, 517, 1957.

Schorstein, J. Intracranial Hematoma in Missile Wounds. *Br. J. Surg., War Surg. Suppl.*, No. *1*, 96, 1947.

Schwartz, H. G. and Roulhac, G. E. Craniocerebral War Wounds. Observations on Delayed Treatment, *Ann. Surg., 121*, 129, 1945.

Scott, M. and Wycis, H. T. Experimental Observations on the Use of Stainless Steel for Cranioplasty. *J. Neurosurg., 3*, 310, 1946.

Scott, M., Wycis, H., and Murtagh, F. Long Term Evaluation of Stainless Steel Cranioplasty. *Surg. Gynec. Obstet., 115*, 453, 1962.

Semmes, J., Weinstein, S., Ghent, L., and Teuber, H-L. *Somatosensory Changes after Penetrating Brain Wounds in Man*. Cambridge: Harvard University Press, 1960.

Small, J. M. and Graham, M. P. Acrylic Resin for the Closure of Skull Defects: Preliminary Report. *Br. J. Surg., 33*, 106, 1945.

Small, J. M. and Turner, E. A. A Surgical Experience of 1200 Cases of Penetrating Brain Wounds in Battle, N. W. Europe, 1944-45. *Br. J. Surg., War Surg. Suppl.*, No. *1*, 62, 1947.

Spalding, J. M. K. Wounds of the Visual Pathway. Part 1: The Visual Radiation. Part 2: The Striate Cortex. *J. Neurol. Neurosurg. Psychiatry, 15*, 99 and 169, 1952.

Spence, W. T. Form-Fitting Plastic Cranioplasty. *J. Neurosurg., 11*, 219, 1954.

Spurling, R. G. Quoted by Woodhall, B. Advances in Head Injuries. *J.A.M.A., 135*, 816, 1947.

Teuber, H-L. Effects of Brain Wounds Implicating Right or Left Hemisphere in Man: Hemisphere Differences and Hemisphere Interaction in Vision, Audition, and Somesthesis. In V. B. Mountcastle (Ed.), *Interhemispheric Relations and Cerebral Dominance*. Baltimore: Johns Hopkins Press, 1962. Pp. 131-157.

Teuber, H-L. Disorders of Memory Following Penetrating Missile Wounds of the Brain. *Neurology, 18*, 287, 1968.

Teuber, H-L. Neglected Aspects of the Posttraumatic Syndrome. In A. E. Walker, W. F. Caveness, and M. Critchley (Eds.), *The Late Effects of Head Injury*. Springfield, Ill.: Charles C Thomas, 1969. Pp. 13-34.

Teuber, H-L. and Weinstein, S. Ability to Discover Hidden Figures after Cerebral Lesiors. *Arch. Neurol. Psychiat., 76*, 369, 1956.

Teuber, H-L., Battersby, W. S., and Bender, M. B. *Visual Field Defects after Penetrating Missile Wounds of the Brain*. Cambridge: Harvard University Press, 1960.

Tönnis, W. Die Behandlung der Hirnverletzungen auf Grund der Erfahrungen im Feldzug gegen Polen. *Deutsche med. Wchnschr., 66*, 57, 1940.

334

Tönnis, W. Schussverletzungen des Gehirns. *Zent. f. Neurochirurgie,* 6, 113, 1941.

Turner, O. A. Repair of Defects of the Skull. With Special Reference to the Periorbital Structures and the Frontal Sinus. *Arch. Surg.,* 53, 312, 1946.

Walker, A. E. *Post-traumatic Epilepsy.* Springfield, Ill.: Charles C Thomas, 1949.

Walker, A. E. Prognosis in Post-Traumatic Epilepsy. *J.A.M.A.,* 164, 1636, 1957.

Walker, A. E. Posttraumatic Epilepsy. In *Surgery in World War II, Neurosurgery,* Vol. 1, Washington, D. C.: Office of the Surgeon General, Dept. of the Army, 1958. Pp. 279-317.

Walker, A. E. and Johnson, H. C. Surgical Treatment of Epilepsy. *Am. J. Surg.,* 75, 200, 1948.

Walker, A. E. and Jablon, S. *A Follow-up Study of Head Wounds in World War II.* Veterans Administration Medical Monograph. Washington, D. C.: Superintendent of Documents, Government Printing Office, 1961.

Walker, A. E. and Erculei, F. Late Results of Cranioplasty. *Arch. Neurol.,* 9, 105, 1963.

Walker, A. E. and Erculei, F. *Head Injured Men. Fifteen Years Later.* Springfield, Ill.: Charles C Thomas, 1969.

Wannamaker, G. T. Transventricular Wounds of the Brain. *J. Neurosurg.,* 11, 151, 1954.

Wannamaker, G. T. and Pulaski, E. J. Pyogenic Neurosurgical Infections in Korean Battle Casualities. *J. Neurosurg.,* 15, 512, 1958.

Watson, C. W. The Incidence of Epilepsy Following Cranio-cerebral Injury. *Proc. Assn. Res. Nerv. Ment. Dis.,* 26, 516, 1947.

Webster, J. E., Schneider, R. C., and Lofstrom, J. E. Observations upon the Management of Orbito-Cranial Wounds. *J. Neurosurg.,* 3, 329, 1946.

Weinstein, S. Differences in Effects of Brain Wounds Implicating Right or Left Hemisphere: Differential Effects on Certain Intellectual and Complex Perceptual Functions. In V. B. Mountcastle (Ed.), *Interhemispheric Relations and Cerebral Dominance.* Baltimore: Johns Hopkins Press, 1962. Pp. 159-176.

White, J. C. Late Complications Following Cranioplasty with Alloplastic Plates. *Ann. Surg.,* 128, 743, 1948.

Whitty, C. W. M. Early Traumatic Epilepsy. *Brain,* 70, 416, 1947.

Wolff, H. and Schmid, B. Das Arteriogramm des pulsierenden Exophthalmus. *Zent. f. Neurochirurgie,* 4, 241 and 310, 1939.

Woodhall, B. Cranioplasty. Chapter 4 in F. W. Bancroft and C. Pilcher, *Surgical Treatment of the Nervous System.* Philadelphia: J. B. Lippincott Co., 1946.

Woodhall, B. Advances in Head Injuries, *J.A.M.A.,* 135, 816, 1947.

Woodhall, B. and Spurling, R. G. Tantalum Cranioplasty for War Wounds of the Skull. *Ann. Surg.,* 121, 649, 1945.

Woolf, G. I. and Walker, A. E. Cranioplasty. Collective Review. *Inter. Abst. Surg.,* 81, 1, 1945.

The authors wish to thank the Pacific Press Publishing Association for permission to reproduce Figure 1, and the New England Journal of Medicine for permission to reproduce Figure 3.

CHAPTER 10

THE ROLE OF RADIOLOGY IN HEAD TRAUMA

M. M. SCHECHTER, M. D.

AND

MILTON ELKIN, M. D.

Along with heart disease and cancer, trauma is assuming an ever increasing role as a major maimer and killer of our time. In 1964 there were 10,200,000 disabling injuries in the United States of which almost a million resulted in death. Since high speed travel has become a routine in our daily lives most injuries in adults no longer result from military, industrial, or sporting accidents, but are sustained on the highway. In 1962 the death toll from motor injuries was 40,800. Three times this number ended up with permanent physical or mental impairment and 30 times this number were temporarily disabled. Seventy-five percent of the people involved in car accidents today receive head trauma and in 70 percent the cause of death is brain damage.

In 1900, only five years after the discovery of the roentgen ray, Borden published a monograph in which he described the use of radiography in diagnosing missile injuries of the head. Significant advances have been made since then. Contrast studies outlining the cerebrospinal fluid spaces in the head and the vascular tree have enhanced the management of patients who have suffered head trauma. In recent years radioactive isotopes have been added to the diagnostic armamentarium Roentgenographic methods now available for the evaluation of patients who have suffered head trauma include plain x-rays of the skull with particular projections, tomography, pneumography, angiography, gamma encephalography, and ultrasonography.

This chapter will deal with studies undertaken in acute injuries of the head and also with those relative to the late effects of head trauma.

RADIOGRAPHIC TECHNIQUE

Because films taken in most emergency rooms are often of poor quality and must usually be repeated, assuming there is no medical contraindication, patients with head injuries should be transported immediately to the radiology unit where studies of far better diagnostic quality can be obtained.

The particular projections requested will depend upon the preference of the physician, but will usually include both right and left lateral, AP, PA and Towne projections. Part of this routine should include a lateral film with the patient supine and the beam parallel to the table top. Fluid levels in the sinuses (CSF leaks) may thereby be recognized.

Particular views may be selected depending upon the clinical picture and suspicions of the radiologist. Displacements of the pineal gland are usually recognized in the AP film and the significance of this is usually obvious.

The types of intracranial expanding processes caused by acute head injury include subdural, epidural, and intracerebral hemorrhage, and brain contusion with edema.

Simultaneous biplane serial angiography is used in most institutions today. Since vital information may be elicited from any of the various phases of the angiogram, the span of radiographs should extend from the beginning of the arterial phase through the venous phase.

SOFT TISSUE INJURIES

Injuries to the soft tissues covering the calvarium are usually recognized by palpation and inspection. Air may enter the gaping margins of a scalp wound and resemble a fracture in the plain roentgenograms (Fig. 1). Foreign bodies such as gravel from the road, and metallic fragments may be recognized in the plain roentgenograms (Fig. 2). The changes associated with cephalhematoma, the result of difficult forceps delivery, may also be recognized. Aneurysms and arteriovenous fistulae of the soft tissues covering the skull may result from trauma; these lesions may be recognized in angiographic studies (Schechter and Gutstein, 1970). Traumatic aneurysms of the superficial temporal artery are infrequently encountered today although they were common in the days of dueling with foils and many case reports appear in the older German literature.

SKULL FRACTURE

Although it is generally recognized that much undue emphasis has been placed on the presence or absence of a skull fracture in the past, medicolegal practice continues to emphasize its importance. The occur-

337

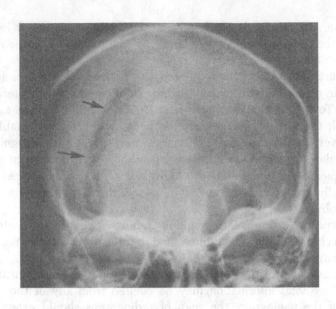

Fig. 1. Air trapped in a scalp wound outlined by arrows simulates a fracture of the skull.

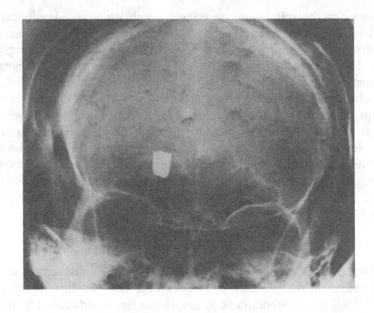

Fig. 2. A bullet lying within the head.

338

rence of a fracture is related to the force of the injury, yet skulls vary in their propensity toward fracture with any given trauma. In head trauma, what has happened to the brain is usually of greater import to the welfare of the patient than what has happened to the skull. The serious accompaniments of skull fracture include destruction of brain tissue, intracranial infection, and intracranial hemorrhage. The skull can be fractured with apparently no significant injury to the brain; on the other hand the brain may be severely injured while the skull remains intact. In general, the more severe the injury, the greater the possibility of brain damage and, in over three-quarters of all fatal head injuries, a fracture is found at autopsy. Depressed and compound skull fractures are likely to be associated with significant brain damage.

Skull fractures may be related to the type of trauma received. Thus the trauma may result from forces of acceleration or deceleration, from a slowly moving missile, or one of high velocity. The skull may also suffer crush injuries.

Skull fractures are classified as either simple linear or comminuted. Other descriptive terms refer to complications. Either type may be compound or depressed, although depression of a fragment occurs chiefly with comminuted fractures. Additional complications relating to the site of the fracture may also occur with either the linear or the comminuted fracture. When the fracture line crosses the middle meningeal artery or a major venous sinus, serious intracranial hemorrhage may ensue. The fracture may cross a foramen and possibly injure a cranial nerve, or, it may involve an accessory nasal sinus or the mastoid area with the possibility of a resultant cerebrospinal rhinorrhea or intracranial aerocele and infection.

The temporal and parietal regions are the sites most frequently involved by fracture, with the frontal and occipital areas being involved less commonly. Fractures in the base of the skull occur relatively infrequently; those that do occur are apt to be diagnosed by clinical criteria other than radiographic. Not only are fracture lines relatively difficult to see on a film of the base, but a base view is often omitted in an x-ray study of head trauma because the patient may be unable to cooperate adequately in regard to the more difficult positioning required for this view.

Mechanism of Skull Fracture

Gurdjian et al (1947 and 1950) have studied the mechanism of skull fracture by the "stresscoat" technique. Dry skulls were coated inside and out with "stresscoat" brittle lacquer and then subjected to deceleration impacts by being dropped onto a steel slab from varying heights. The lacquer cracked in the areas of greatest tensile deformation, the cracks appearing on the outside of the skull in the regions where the bone bent outward on the inside of the skull where the bone bent inward, i.e., the cracks occurred on the convexity of a bend. The location and direction of the cracks in the lacquer indicated the location and direction of fracture in the bone, if the blow had been struck with sufficient energy. They also produced fractures in embalmed cadaver heads with the fracture force applied to predetermined areas. A correlation was made between these experimental fractures and clinical fractures in which the site of the fracturing blow could be determined. Although the position of the fracture lines could be prophesied on the basis of location of impact, the size, shape and velocity of the injuring object, as well as the contour, thickness and "chance characteristics" of the bone structure, proved important in the mechanism of skull fracture. At impact, with forces insufficient to cause depressed fracture or to penetrate the bone, the area around the point of application of the blow bent inward with a simultaneous outbending of the bone peripheral to the bent-in region; the linear fracture was initiated by the resultant tearing-apart forces of outbending. On removal of the striking object, the bent-in zone rebounded with its outer surface becoming an area of tensile stress so that the already initiated linear fracture extended toward the point of impact. (In some specimens, a contrecoup type of outbending was observed approximately diagonally opposite the point of impact, suggesting the mechanism of contrecoup fracture.) With blows of greater energy, other tensile stress areas were produced with further fracture lines in additional regions of outbending, leading to comminuted fractures. In severe injuries resulting in stellate fractures, the stress caused by inbending of the bone also resulted in tearing-apart forces on the internal surface of the skull at the point of impact with fracture lines of stellate distribution. In depressed fractures, the more rapid the blow, the more localized the area of depression. Radial fracture lines in a depression were due to tensile stresses from inbending and were initiated on the internal surface of the skull. Anteroposterior or posteroanterior base fractures occurred from blows on the anterior and posterior aspects of the head; side-to-side base fractures occurred from parietal and lateral frontal blows.

Lines Mistaken for Fractures

The normal is often more difficult to diagnose than the abnormal. There may be normal or at least clinically insignificant radiolucent lines in the skull film which may be confused with linear fracture lines.

1. *Metopic Suture.* The fetal suture line in the frontal bone may persist in a small percentage of people even into adult life and in case of head trauma may be misinterpreted as a linear fracture line; its perfectly mid-sagittal position in the frontal bone as well as its serrated appearance should allow its true identification (Fig. 3).

2. *Arterial Channels.* In lateral films of the skull, fine branches of the

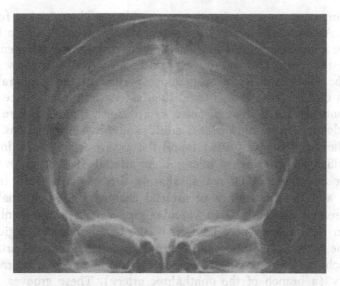

FIG. 3. Metopic suture. This fetal suture line in the frontal bone may persist in a small percentage of people and may be misinterpreted as a linear fracture. Its position and serrated appearance should lead to its identification.

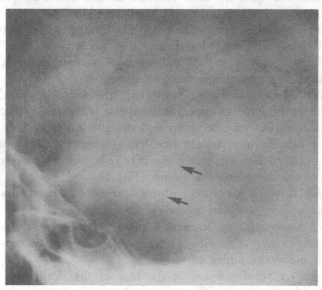

FIG. 4. The arterial vascular groove accommodating the middle temporal artery (a branch of the superficial temporal artery). These groves unlike other craniovascular channels, are on the outer table of the skull and are usually bilateral.

341

meningeal group, grooving the inner table, may be mistaken for fracture. An especially confusing vascular shadow is caused by a branch of the middle meningeal artery arising just distal to the foramen spinosum; this vessel courses upward and posteriorly in a shallow groove in the inner table of the squamous portion of the temporal bone for a distance of 4 to 5 cm and then enters the diploic space where it continues for a short distance in a definite channel before losing its identity. In a study of 996 adult skull x-ray examinations, Schumacher and Henesy (1957) found this groove in 38 skulls, in seven of which the groove was bilateral. An arterial channel, grooving the inner table, is usually not so sharply defined as a fresh fracture line, and the branchings of arterial channels will help make the differential diagnosis. Two vascular grooves not uncommonly mistaken for fractures may be seen in the temporoparietal region and in the frontal region accommodating the middle temporal artery (a branch of the superficial temporal artery) and the supraorbital artery (a branch of the ophthalmic artery). These grooves, unlike other craniovascular grooves are on the outer table of the skull (Fig. 4). When the markings are bilateral, they tend to be symmetrical and the question of a fracture should not arise (Schechter and Zingesser, 1969; Schunk and Maruyama, 1960).

3. *Venous Channels.* These channels are usually more tortuous, a good deal less well defined and more variable in width than fracture lines. Occasionally a stellate collection of venous channels in the parietal region may mimic fracture lines.

4. *The Normal Cranial Suture* (especially the sagittal suture) has a serrated, interdigitating appearance on the outer table, whereas its inner table aspect may be sharp and straight. An x-ray film of such a suture may show a straight fine line (its inner aspect) projected onto a serrated line (its outer aspect). This may be misinterpreted as a fracture line along the suture (Fig. 5).

5. *Wormian Bones.* Accessory sutures and bones (especially in the occipital region) may be mistaken for fractures.

6. *Unusual Projections of Normal Sutures,* or infrequently seen sutures, may cause difficulty (e.g., overlapping squamoso-parietal sutures; mendosal suture in children).

7. *Unrecognized Synchondroses* at the base of the skull may be mistaken for fracture, e.g., spheno-occipital synchondrosis.

It is not necessary to see a linear fracture line on all the views of the skull; as a matter of fact, it is not uncommon to see the fracture

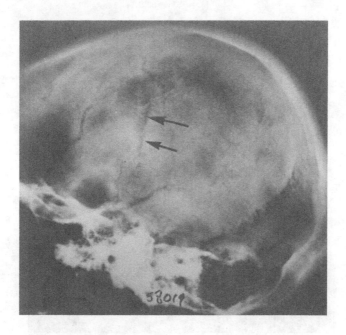

Fig. 5. The normal cranial suture has a serrated margin on the outer table of the skull whereas its inner table aspect is usually sharp and straight. The arrows point to a normal cranial suture having this appearance.

on only one or two of the projections. A temporoparietal fracture will usually be easily seen on the lateral films (stereoscopic best) and not visualized on the anteroposterior or posteroanterior projections. A fracture of the occipital bone (Fig. 6) (usually vertical) may be seen only on the Towne view. It is important to note whether a linear fracture line crosses a vascular channel (especially an arterial channel or dural sinus groove), since such a fracture may cause tearing of the vessel wall with production of an epidural hematoma (Fig. 7). It is also important to note whether the fracture line enters a paranasal sinus (Fig. 8), since such a fracture exposes the intracranial contents to bacterial invasion from the non-sterile sinus, with the possibility of development of meningitis. Another complication of such a fracture is intracranial aerocele. A linear fracture appears as a sharply defined line of diminished radio-opacity, sometimes of variable width, becoming narrower at its ends (Fig. 7). A fracture line may, of course, run in any direction, whereas suture lines and vascular grooves run in fairly constant directions.

343

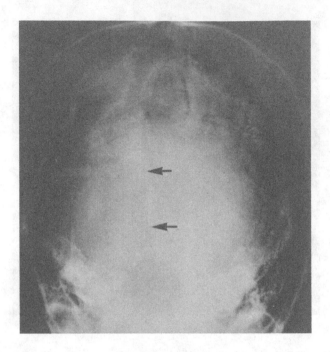

FIG. 6. A fracture of the occipital bone, usually vertical, may be seen only in the Towne view. Note that the line representing the fracture stops at the foramen magnum.

Comminuted Fracture

The presence of a comminuted fracture usually means that the injuring force was of greater magnitude than in the case of linear fracture (Fig. 9). With multiple fracture lines there is the increased possibility that one of them will cross a vascular channel. Also there is greater likelihood of wider separation of fragments with consequent slower healing or lack of healing of the fracture, as well as the greater likelihood of the presence of a depressed fragment. Comminuted fractures occur primarily in the vault, less commonly in the base.

Depressed Fracture

Gurdjian, Webster, and Lissner (1950, 1950) described six variations of depression based upon the velocity and, to a lesser extent, the shape of the injuring object:

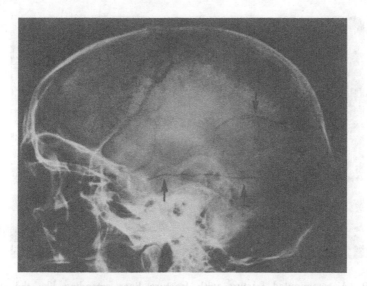

FIG. 7. A horsehoe fracture extending from one side of the skull to the other passing through the occipital or posterior parietal region. Note that the one limb of the fracture has a very sharp margin whereas the other limb is a little less distinct and a little wider. The sharp marginated fracture is on the side closest to the film. This fracture has crossed the groove of the middle meningeal artery.

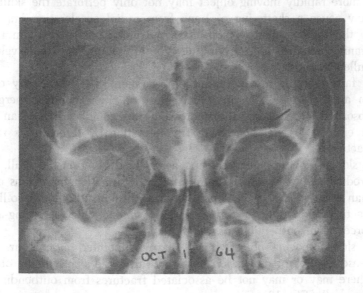

FIG. 8. Fracture through the paranasal sinuses with air in the subarachnoid spaces outlined by arrows.

345

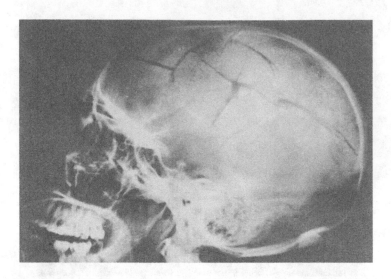

Fɪɢ. 9. A comminuted fracture with fracture lines extending like the spokes of a wheel from the center of the point of impact.

1. A rapidly moving missile may perforate the skull, resulting in fragments of bone being driven into the brain.
2. A more rapidly moving object may not only perforate the skull but may cause a shattering of bone from radial acceleration imparted to the skull contents, resulting in a tremendous increase in intracranial pressure, as in a bursting type of fracture with high-velocity bullet wounds.
3. A fairly rapidly moving blunt object, such as a brick, may cause an area of depression in which most of the expended energy is absorbed in producing the depression, i.e., an inbending of an oval or circular area of bone with fragmentation by three to six radial fractures.
4. A slowly moving object, causing a localized blow on the skull, may produce depression with simultaneous deformation in regions other than the area of impact. Thus, there may also result one or two linear fractures extending toward the area of impact due to tearing-apart forces from outbending of the skull.
5. A slowly moving object, fairly sharp or pointed in contour, may cause an area of depression patterned after the shape of the object. There may or may not be associated fractures from outbending of the skull (Fig. 10).

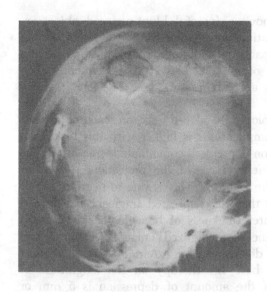

FIG. 10. Two depressed fractures with fairly circumscribed margins. The contour of the depressed fracture frequently suggests the type of force applied to the head.

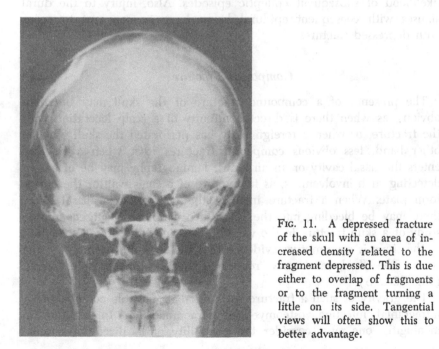

FIG. 11. A depressed fracture of the skull with an area of increased density related to the fragment depressed. This is due either to overlap of fragments or to the fragment turning a little on its side. Tangential views will often show this to better advantage.

347

6. Depression by a slowly moving, forceful blunt-surfaced object results in extensive comminution with radial fracture lines extending from the center of the impact and circular fracture lines at varying distances around the area of impact. This type is frequently seen and is often referred to as a crush fracture (see Fig. 9).

It is important for the radiologist to identify the presence of depression since the incidence of complications is higher with this type than with the simple linear or non-depressed comminuted fractures. The regular skull films show in one or more of the projections a zone of increased density related to the fracture. This is due to overlapping of the fragments, or to the fact that the depressed fragment has turned on its side, presenting a greater thickness of bone to the x-ray beam (Fig. 11). If such an appearance is recognized, tangential views should be obtained in an effort to determine the extent of the depression, since the neurosurgeon may base his therapy on the magnitude of the depression. In general, if the amount of depression is 5 mm or greater (Dyke, 1949), the depressed fragment should be elevated or removed, since such a depression may press upon the brain with the likelihood of subsequent epileptic episodes. Also, injury to the dural sinuses with consequent epidural hemorrhage is more apt to occur with depressed fractures.

Compound Fracture

The presence of a compound fracture of the skull may be quite obvious, as when there is direct continuity of a scalp laceration with the fracture, or when a foreign body has perforated the skull. On the other hand, less obvious compound fractures exist when a fracture enters the nasal cavity or an air sinus; laminography may be of aid in detecting such involvement, as in fracture of a sinus wall or the cribriform plate. When a fracture involves the wall of a paranasal sinus, there may be bleeding into the sinus; hence, in the roentgenographic study of a skull fracture in the vicinity of a sinus, the presence of fluid in the sinus is presumptive evidence that the fracture extends into the sinus. The fluid level may represent escaping cerebrospinal fluid (Fig. 12A, B).

The gravity of such a fracture rests upon its possible complications: intracranial infection, osteomyelitis, intracranial air. In addition to meningitis, one must consider the possibility of localized intracranial

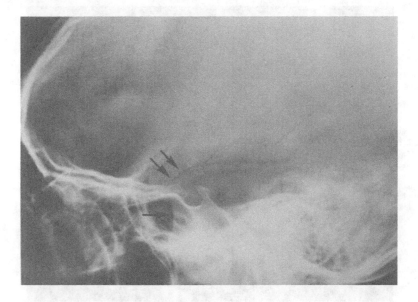

A

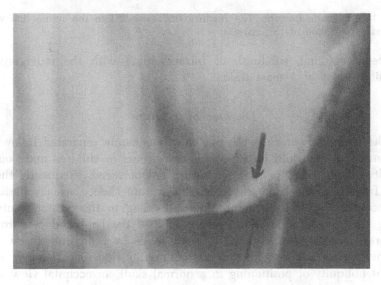

B

Fig. 12A, B. This is a lateral projection of the skull with the patient lying supine
and the beam horizontal to the table top (A). The presence of a fracture can be
seen, which in the tomogram (B), is seen to involve the base of the skull. A
fluid level in the sphenoid sinus suggests that the fracture has entered a nasal sinus.

349

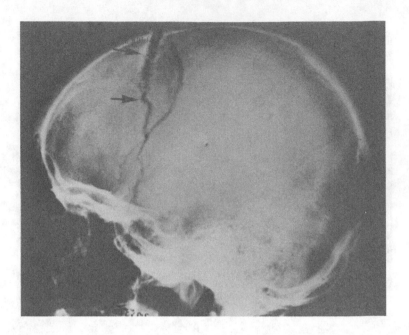

FIG. 13. Diastatic fracture. The fracture line extends into the suture line with resultant separation of the margins.

abscess (epidural, subdural, or intracerebral) with the radiographic manifestations of a mass lesion.

Diastasis of a Suture

The lambdoid suture is the one most commonly separated following trauma and, as would be expected, this occurs in children and young adults before bony union at the suture has occurred. Frequently there is a fracture of the bone adjacent to the suture (hence, usually parietal or occipital) with the fracture line extending to the diastatic suture (Fig. 13). If the separation involves one of the lambdoid or coronal sutures, radiographic diagnosis is easily made by comparing the width of the "sprung" suture with that of the opposite side. Occasionally, with slight obliquity of positioning in a normal skull, an occipital view will show the lambdoid sutures to appear to be of different widths. The apparently wider suture may be mistakenly interpreted as diastatic; a repeat film with proper positioning will settle the question.

As healing takes place, the margins of the fracture line become less sharply outlined and thus indistinct. There is no evidence of callus formation, the union probably being fibrous at first with the fibrous tissue later becoming ossified.

Glaser and Blaine (1940) studied the healing of skull fractures as followed by x-ray. Age of patient, width of fracture line, and location of the fracture seemed to be important variables. Fractures heal more rapidly in children than in adults. The narrower the fracture line, the more rapid the healing. In general, fractures located in the occipital area seem to heal more slowly than fractures in other regions of the vault. Linear fractures in children under six years of age disappear within six to twelve months after injury, except where separation of the fracture is extremely wide, as 5 mm or over, in which case the defect may persist permanently. Linear fractures in adults in the frontal, parietal and temporal regions begin to lose sharpness of outline in about four to five weeks, although complete disappearance rarely occurs under seven months, with the average time for complete disappearance being three to four years. Linear occipital fractures may take longer to disappear. In depressed fractures which have not been elevated, the fragments become rounded and unite with disappearance of the fracture lines, although the depression remains.

Vance (1936) studied follow-up films in 52 cases of linear skull fractures. He concluded that in adult skulls, fracture lines disappear in the roentgenogram in about two years and in children in about one year, although in very young children complete roentgenologic healing may occur as early as four months after injury. In adult skulls it takes on the average eight months for enough repair to occur to allow one to identify a linear fracture as old by its x-ray appearance.

HEMORRHAGE

Plain skull films may demonstrate a fracture, a shift of the calcified pineal gland or calcified glomus of choroid plexus, an intracranial opaque foreign body, intracranial calcification, or skull asymmetry. The presence of a fracture in the region of a vascular groove, especially the middle meningeal, will suggest the possibility of an epidural hematoma. Shift of the pineal body will help localize the side of the lesion but will not help greatly in the identification of its nature. The presence and location of an opaque foreign body intracranially may give some indication of the severity of the trauma, but will not differentiate the possible types of bleeding which may have occurred. Intracranial calcification or ossification will help identify a chronic subdural hematoma that has gone on to lay down calcium or bone in its walls, but this is an infrequent occurrence. Skull asymmetry may be a valuable clue to a long-standing subdural collection going back to infancy or early childhood.

Cerebral angiography has almost replaced pneumography in studying patients with intracranial hemorrhage. The angiogram may identify the exact site of the hematoma: intracerebral, subdural, or epidural. It may demonstrate concomitant lesions, such as the coexistence of an acute subdural hematoma with an intracerebral hematoma. It is worth noting

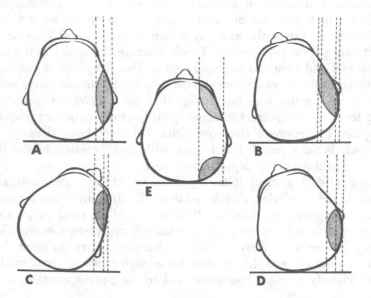

FIG. 14. The vertical dotted lines represent x-ray beams tangent to brain-hematoma-skull interfaces. These interfaces may or may not be recognizable angiographically in any given patient. In A there is an extracerebral hematoma at the widest part of the head. No vascularized brain is seen lateral to the "bare area." In B the patient's head has been turned away from the side that is being studied and the "bare area" that is seen angiographically is narrower and has a different configuration. In C an anteriorly situated extracerebral hematoma is demonstrated as a "bare area" by turning the patient's head to the side of the injection. In D a posteriorly situated extracerebral hematoma is demonstrated by turning the patient's head away from the side of the injection. In E an anteriorly and/or a posteriorly situated extracerebral hematoma may not be demonstrated, since no bare area is seen.

that posterior fossa hematomas of any type cannot be diagnosed by carotid angiography; however, hematomas in this location are relatively infrequent. Carotid angiography may however reveal ventricular dilatation without evidence of supratentorial pathology. This might be indirect evidence of a posterior fossa mass. Although vertebral angiography has been infrequently used in the evaluation of masses of a traumatic nature in the posterior fossa, a reevaluation of this modality is in order since reports have·appeared of changes in the vascular anatomy allowing the diagnosis of a posterior fossa epidural hemorrhage to be made. Perot, Ethier, and Wong (1967) reported displacement of the posterior meningeal artery from a posterior fossa epidural hematoma, and numerous reports have stressed the significance of displaced dural sinuses.

The avascular space, demonstrated by Lohr in 1936, is the keystone in the angiographic diagnosis of an extracerebral hematoma. There are certain pitfalls in the interpretation of this finding, and these may be divided into "false positives" and "false negatives." Care must be taken to obtain films with appropiate projections to obviate false positive and false negative conclusions (Fig. 14). Furthermore, bilateral collections of blood as well as collections in unusual sites, e.g., subfrontally and inter-hemispherically, must be given consideration. An evaluation of the total angiographic series, i.e., the arterial through the venous phase, is necessary since each phase may supply distinct information.

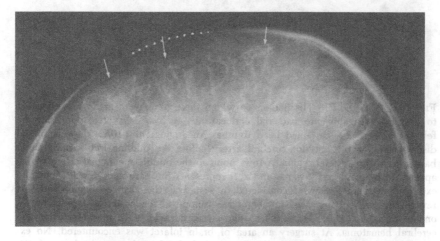

FIG. 15. Arrows outline a "bare area" over the top of the cerebral cortex in a very young child. No subdural collection was found at surgery. This appearance is not uncommon in infants and represents a large subarachnoid space.

353

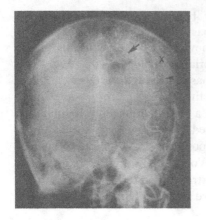

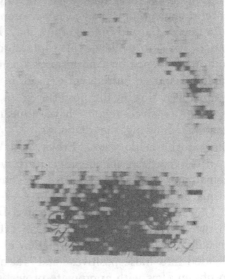

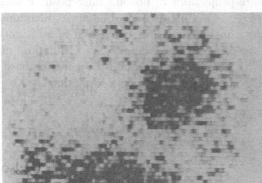

FIG. 16A, B, C, D, E. The patient on whom these films were made was admitted to hospital with subacute bacterial endocarditis. A few days after admission he fell out of bed and sustained head trauma. An angiogram (16A) shows minimal displacement of the anterior cerebral artery across the midline but a fairly large bare area in the parietal region. Arrows point to the middle meningeal artery which appears to be displaced inwards and a X represents the bare area. Since a possible extracerebral hematoma was considered, a scan was the next procedure and this revealed an area of increased uptake of the isotope in the posterior parietal region on the left side (16B, C). These changes were considered to represent an extracerebral hematoma. At surgery an area of brain infarct was encountered. No extracerebral hematoma was present. Scrutiny of the lateral arterial phase of the angiogram (16D) reveals occlusion of branches of the middle cerebral artery and the venous phase in Figure 16E shows vessels extending all the way to the periphery. This represents a false positive angiogram.

354

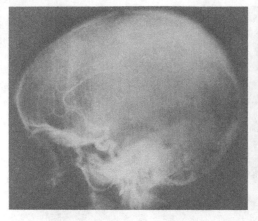 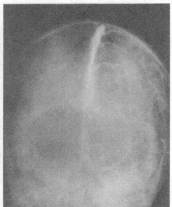

D   E

"False Positives"

The brain surface may be some distance away from the inner table of the skull for reasons other than traumatic extravasation of blood. This is more apt to be encountered in the early and in the late years of life. In children without an extracerebral hematoma, an avascular area may be present between the superior branches of the callosomarginal artery and the inner table of the skull. This is best seen in the lateral cerebral angiogram (Fig. 15). It represents a discrepancy between the size of the brain and the skull (e.g., due to brain atrophy or hypoplasia). Under these circumstances, however, the avascular space is usually (not always) narrow. Thus, even though there is a tendency for subdural hematomas in young children to collect high over the cerebral convexity (Fig. 15), the mere demonstration of an avascular space at the vertex in this age group may not be sufficient to warrant such a diagnosis if there are not additional features to support it. Furthermore, in this age group there is a tendency for the two hemispheres and the two anterior cerebral arteries to be slightly separated normally. This must be borne in mind when an avascular space between the hemispheres is to be evaluated for the presence of an interhemispheric subdural hematoma.

Late in life, atrophy of cerebral tissue may lead to recession of the brain from the inner table of the skull. This is important both in the etiology and in the diagnosis of subdural hematoma. The interhemis-

355

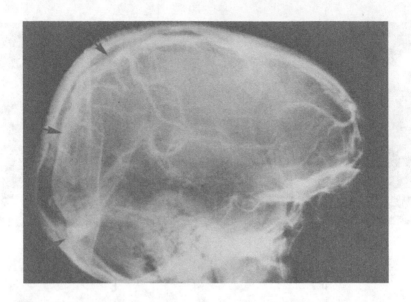

Fig. 17. An extensive epidural hemorrhage has stripped the superior sagittal sinus away from the inner table of the skull (arrows). Note that the transverse sinuses and the area of the confluence of sinuses have also been stripped from the inner table of the skull.

pheric space in this age group also may be widened due to atrophy. Such widening, however, can be differentiated from the widened interhemispheric space associated with an interhemispheric subdural hematoma. The callosomarginal artery is displaced ipsilaterally by the hematoma, while the pericallosal artery is displaced contralaterally. Still another pitfall in the diagnosis of extracerebral hematoma by means of the demonstration of an avascular space is illustrated (Figs. 16 A, B, C, D, E) in a case of occlusion of peripheral branches of the middle cerebral artery. The proximity of the veins to the inner table of the skull in the anteroposterior venous phase rules out a diagnosis of extracerebral hematoma.

In the posterior fossa, epidural hematomas may reveal themselves by stripping the torcular Herophili from the bone but this finding can be confused (Fig. 17) with the non-midline torcular Herophili in a normal patient due to rotation of the skull or merely to variation in anatomy. The fact that the torcular Herophili often lies on a prominent bony ridge also plays a role in simulating displacement. Separation of the superior sagittal sinus from the inner table of the skull, a sign of supratentorial epidural hematoma described by Wickbom in 1949, (Figs. 18 A, B) must also be differentiated from the non-midline superior sagittal sinus which only appears separated from the superior inner table of the skull (Friedmann, Schmidt-Witkamp, and Walter, 1959).

Displacement of the meningeal artery might be mentioned at this point as a sign which may be helpful in demonstrating an extracerebral hematoma even when there is no avascular space as such. However, the normal middle meningeal artery curving posteriorly along the inner table of the skull may appear displaced when it is not (see Fig. 16A).

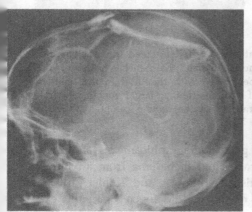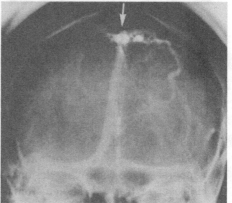

FIG. 18A, B. A large epidural hematoma which has separated the sagittal sinus and its branches from the inner table of the skull.

"False Negatives"

The absence of an avascular space on any one angiographic view does not rule out an extracerebral hematoma. Lateral angiograms may best reveal the anterior extracerebral hematoma, while oblique films (Lindgren, 1954) may be required to show the antero- or postero-laterally situated extracerebral hematoma (Figs. 19). There are also locations where the anatomical features of the area do not allow demonstration of an avascular space between the brain and the inner

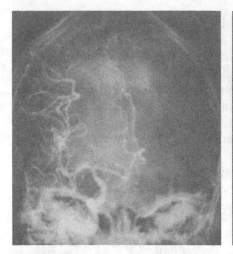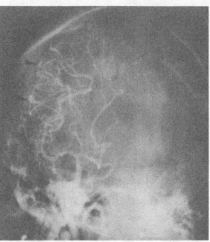

Fig. 19A, B.   Carotid angiogram of a patient who has sustained trauma. The anterior cerebral artery is displaced across the midline and the branches of the middle cerebral artery seem to extend to the periphery. With the head in the oblique position and turned towards the side of the injection, a large frontal subdural hematoma is outlined. The peripheral branches of the middle cerebral are indicated by arrows and the "bare area" by X.

table of the skull. For example, no good angiographic means of differentiating a purely subtemporal extracerebral hematoma from an intratemporal space-occupying lesion exists (Cronqvist and Kohler, 1963). However, extracerebral hematomas of the middle fossa commonly extend upwards along the lateral surface of the brain. Similarly, the angiographic diagnosis of an extracerebellar hematoma is difficult.

Norman (1956) laid down certain angiographic criteria for the differentiation of acute and chronic subdural hematomas based on the shape of the avascular space. He pointed out that a lentiform shape is associated with a chronic subdural hematoma and that a crescent shape is associated with an acute subdural hematoma. Our experience has led us to de-emphasize attempts to date maturity angiographically.

Epidural Hematoma

Epidural hematoma occurs most often in the temporoparietal region followed in frequency by frontotemporal and parieto-occipital sites.

Suboccipital epidural hematomas associated with fracture of the occipital bone have been infrequently reported. There is almost always a skull fracture, usually adjacent to the clot, with the fracture line crossing a vascular groove. However, there are case reports of middle meningeal hemorrhage without skull fracture, probably due to tearing of the vessel in its groove during the inbending of the skull by the injury, the trauma not being severe enough to produce a fracture. Associated intracranial lesions are quite frequent: brain laceration, subdural hemorrhage, and subarachnoid hemorrhage.

In patients with pineal calcification, the presence of a shift as seen on plain films may aid in the diagnosis and locate the side of the lesion accurately. Because of the acute nature of the lesion, the films do not reveal evidence of increased intracranial pressure as is seen in more slowly developing lesions such as tumors (e.g., demineralization of the sella turcica).

Cerebral angiography has almost replaced other radiologic modalities of investigation in such cases. If in the venous phase one can demonstrate displacement of the opacified superior sagittal sinus or a lateral sinus from the inner table of the skull following head trauma, the diagnosis is quite definite, since such a phenomenon localizes an extradural mass that is stripping the dura from the internal table (Wickbom, 1949). (See Figs. 17, 18 A, B). An important differential point from subdural hematoma is that in epidural hematoma from the very beginning there is considerable local expansion with the formation of a fairly well localized mass. This is due to the fact that unlike subdural bleeding, the extradural hematoma has no preexisting space in which to spread but must tear the dura away from the skull with consequent compression of the underlying brain. This localized epidural mass will lift surface vessels away from the inner table of the skull and the angiographic appearance will resemble that of a chronic subdural hematoma. Thus, if the patient has suffered head trauma only in the recent past (within a few days) and the angiogram shows a localized displacement of surface vessels from the inner table of the skull, the lesion is more likely an epidural hematoma than an acute subdural hematoma. Norman (1956) has illustrated this point nicely. The outline of the pure extradural hematoma is more or less irregular and faint without the smooth concavity characteristic of the chronic subdural hematoma; possibly clots adherent to the external surface of the dura are responsible for the irregularity. In addition, an epidural hematoma will displace the anterior cerebral vessels across the midline away from the

359

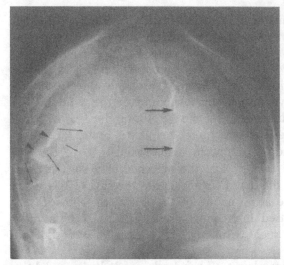

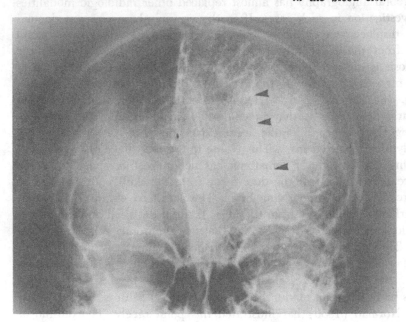

Fig. 20. Right carotid angiogram in a patient who sustained trauma a few hours before. The large black arrows show displacement of the anterior cerebral arteries across the midline. The arrows with thin shafts show the displacement of the middle meningeal artery inwards. The black arrow heads show the leaking of the mixture of blood and contrast medium from the torn meningeal artery. Films taken a few seconds later showed the leaking contrast dissipated, presumably within the blood clot.

Fig. 21. Angiogram of a patient with an epidural hemorrhage. Note that the surface of the "bare area" nearest the midline outlined by arrows is quite deep. The midline structures however are not displaced. In the venous phase of the cerebral angiogram, vessels in front of and behind the depth of the "bare area" are opacified.

360

side of the lesion; yet even with a large epidural hematoma, the degree of anterior cerebral shift is relatively small as compared to the anterior cerebral displacement seen with chronic subdural hematoma of comparable size (Figs. 20, 21).

Extravasation of contrast medium from a torn meningeal vessel during angiography is another sign of epidural hemorrhage (Fig. 20). Today it is generally accepted that the clinical spectrum seen with epidural hemorrhage is wide, and although the classic description of the symptomatology includes the "lucid interval," such a history is obtained less than 50 percent of the time, and although the classical description includes progression to a fatal outcome within hours, exceptions are fairly common in our experience and in that of others.

The explanation for this variability is complex. Certain anatomic

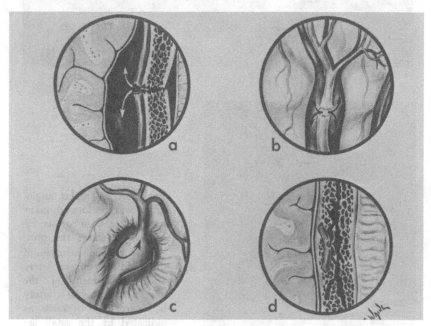

FIG. 22. In drawing a, the torn meningeal artery is leaking into the epidural space and through the fracture line into the subgaleal space. In drawing b, where the middle meningeal artery is accompanied by a venous channel, blood and contrast material pass out of the torn meningeal artery into the venous channel. This fistula is a type of "protective mechanism." In c, blood clot has sealed off a tear in the middle meningeal artery, forming a 'pseudoaneurysm." In d, a tear in the middle meningeal artery as it traverses the diploic space in the temporal area allows passage of blood and contrast material into venous diploic channels.

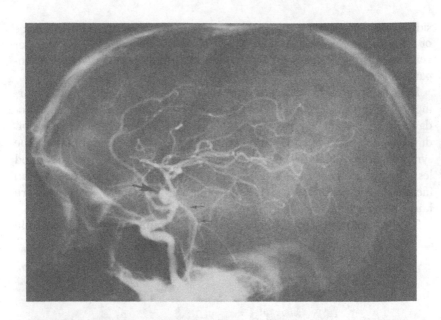

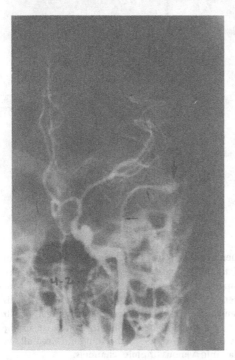

Fig. 23A, B. This angiogram was performed many hours after trauma was sustained. It shows the presence of a pseudoaneurysm of the middle meningeal artery and displacement of the middle meningeal artery backwards and inwards as indicated by the small arrows. The large arrow is directed towards the pseudoaneurysm. There is also elevation of the middle cerebral artery. At surgery a large epidural hematoma was encountered in the temporal fossa.

factors may be responsible in part. One such factor is the strength of attachment of the dura to the skull. The dura is more adherent in children, especially along suture lines, in females, and in elderly people. The dura of the posterior fossa is far less adherent. Bradley, commenting on this fact in 1952, observed that certain subjects seem to be "immune" to epidural hemorrhage. Another anatomic factor is the strength of the walls of the middle meningeal vessels. Hassler (1962) described congenital defects in the wall of the middle meningeal artery.

In addition to the anatomic factors mentioned above, certain pathologic features related to the injury influence the clinical picture. Two key ones are the site of the epidural hemorrhage (temporal location has the most rapidly progressive course) and the severity of injury to the underlying brain.

The use of angiography in epidural hemorrhage reveals certain other factors which influence the clinical course. Observations of contrast material which has extravasated from a torn meningeal artery (Fig. 22) has disclosed the following:

1. The extravasated contrast material may pass into the epidural space, the concomitant epidural hematoma progressively enlarging. No "protective" mechanism is operative here (Figs. 20, 22 A).
2. The extravasated medium may pass out of the epidural space through the adjacent fracture line into the subgaleal area (Fig. 22 A).
3. The extravasated contrast material may be walled off by the formation of a pseudoaneurysm (Figs. 22 C, 23 A, 23 B).
4. The extravasated contrast material may pass into adjacent venous channels, thereby indicating the presence of an arteriovenous fistula. These venous channels may be within the diploe of the skull or they may be the veins which accompany the meningeal artery (Figs. 22 B, 22 D, 24 A, 24 B, 24 C).

Reports on the extravasation of contrast material from the middle meningeal artery have been published by Jamieson (1952), Lindgren (1954), Lofstrom et al (1955), Vaughan (1959), Tiwisina and Stacker (1959), Huber (1962), and others. Arteriovenous fistulae involving the middle meningeal vessels as a result of trauma or "spontaneous" fistulae shown angiographically have been reported by Fincher (1951), Markham (1961), Leslie et al (1962), Berkay (1963), Ruggiero et al (1963), Wilson and Cronic (1964), Jackson and Du Boulay (1964), and Zingesser et al (1965) from 1951 to 1965. Pseudoaneurysm formation

363

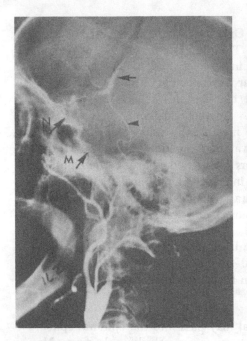

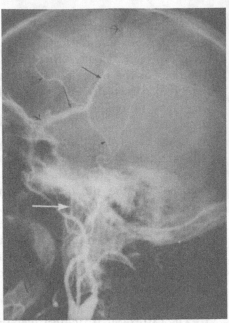

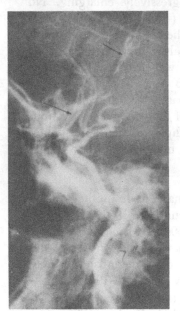

Fig. 24A, B, C.   A left common carotid angiogram in a patient who had sustained trauma.

The arrows indicated by the letters M and N are directed to the middle meningeal artery. The upper arrow points to the area of disruption where contrast fluid has passed into a venous channel.

In a film taken 2 or 3 seconds later (24B) the large white arrow is directed to the middle meningeal artery. There is further passage of contrast into the vein indicated by the black arrows; the arrowheads point to the superficial temporal artery.

Figure 24C is a film taken 7 seconds after the start of the injection. The contrast medium in this channel has cleared a little and there are now 2 parallel shadows representing the veins accompanying the middle meningeal artery.

involving the middle meningeal artery has been reported by Schulze (1957), Pouyanne et al (1959), Kia-Noury (1961), Markwalder and Huber (1961), Dilenge and Wuthrich (1962), Hirsch et al (1962), Ruggiero et al (1963), Paillas et al (1964), Kuhn and Kugler (1964), and Zingesser et al (1965).

Of particular importance is the time interval between the injury and the angiographic studies. It is of special importance also that in most of these cases large amounts of contrast material were seen to leave the torn meningeal artery. Certain anatomical factors are responsible for the pattern emerging in any given case in which torn meningeal vessels initiate an episode of hemorrhage. The determining factor, we feel, is the situation of the meningeal artery at the site of leakage. It may be encased by bone at this point, so that the extravasated material may find its way into diploic channels; the artery may be accompanied by venous channels at the site of the tear, resulting in fistula formation of the arteriovenous variety; finally, there may be no venous channel present adjacent to the torn meningeal artery, in which instance the extravasated material can accumulate only in the epidural space — unless the fracture site itself allows decompression. These anatomical relationships are illustrated in Figure 25.

The background for an understanding of what is involved in fistula formation lies in the work of Jones (1912). In seeking an anatomical basis for the grooves on the inner table of the skull he found that the major channels accounting for these grooves were the accompanying meningeal veins rather than the meningeal artery itself. According to Jones, this fact was discovered at an earlier date, but lost sight of for a time. Figure 24 illustrates passage of contrast material from a meningeal artery to an accompanying meningeal vein.

In pseudoaneurysm formation extravasated blood from a torn vessel becomes walled off by a covering made up of fibrinous clot. Thus the wall of the vessel does not form the wall of the aneurysm (Figs. 23 A, 23 B). The other "protective" mechanisms described above are self-explanatory. Angiography thus may reveal certain aspects of the mechanism of epidural hemorrhage and has been able to account for the fact that patients who sustained trauma many hours before angiography had at times insignificant hematomas in the epidural space, hematomas in no way commensurate with the expected amount of outpouring of blood as evidenced by the leaking of contrast material observed at angiography.

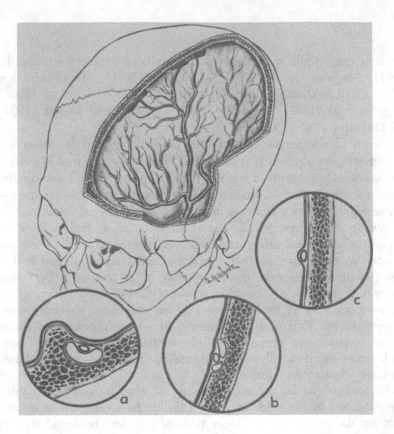

Fig. 25. The anatomical relationships between branches of the middle meningeal artery, the meningeal veins, the dura, and the inner table of the skull, are illustrated here. Note that the middle meningeal artery and its accompanying venous channels are often within the diploe (a) in the temporal area. More distally (b) the usual situation is that the middle meningeal arteries and veins groove the inner table of the skull. In certain areas more distally (c) the middle meningeal artery is not accompanied by venous channels. Note that some of the middle meningeal veins accompanying the middle meningeal artery are shown draining into lacunar channels in the region of the superior sagittal sinus.

Another pathway of drainage is through the spheno-parietal sinus and into the cavernous sinus, or along the floor of the middle fossa toward the foramen ovale, or into the superior petrosal sinus. Some venous channels still more posteriorly situated drain into the transverse sinus.

Certain lesions must be considered in the differential diagnosis of a torn meningeal vessel with its resultant fistula formation or pseudo-aneurysm formation:

1. Congenital aneurysms of the middle meningeal artery.
2. Traumatic pseudoaneurysm of a branch of external carotid artery in scalp.
3. Extravasation of contrast medium from a lacerated cerebral vessel such as the middle cerebral artery.

Cases of congenital "aneurysm" of the middle meningeal artery, a rare phenomenon, have been reported by Berk (1961), New (1965) and Zingesser et al (1965). Angiograms demonstrating a pseudoaneurysm of a branch of the external carotid artery in the scalp have been presented by Wortzman (1963). Such pseudoaneurysms result usually from open injury (Schechter and Gutstein, 1970), but may occur following closed injury. Clinically, there is generally no difficulty in determining whether such a pseudoaneurysm is present or not, but angiographically it may overlie a meningeal artery and simulate a pseudoaneurysm of the middle meningeal artery.

Case reports of extravasation of contrast medium from torn cerebral vessels are extremely rare (Lohr, 1936; Fincher, 1951; Schmidt and Rossi, 1961). To these we add a personal observation.

Subdural Hematoma

Subdural hematoma refers to a collection of blood in the subdural space. This may be large enough to cause signs and symptoms by compressing the underlying brain.

Although there may be adequate reason from the clinical viewpoint to divide subdural hematomas into acute, subacute, and chronic groups, the important feature, allowing the radiographic differentiation. In roentgenologic findings. The presence or absence of encapsulation is a division into acute and chronic will suffice for a discussion of the cases of more severe injury with an early onset of grave symptoms, a neomembrane has not yet formed; the blood lies free in the subdural space (acute subdural hematoma) presenting an angiographic picture different from that of the less severely injured group in which the blood has had an opportunity to become loculated (chronic subdural hematoma) and appear as a localized mass.

Acute Subdural Hematoma

Acute subdural hematoma is an accompaniment of severe head trauma with injury to cerebral vessels and consequent bleeding into the subdural space, the bleeding being both arterial and venous.

Skull fracture is commonly present, often compound or depressed; the fracture line does not always localize the site of the subdural hemorrhage. If the pineal gland is calcified, it will be shifted away from the side of the hematoma. In bilateral acute hematomas, roughly equal in extent, the pineal gland will not be displaced to either side. The hematoma is able to form freely in the preexisting subdural space in which it spreads quite uniformly with its pressure against the cerebral hemisphere being distributed over a fairly large area with hardly any localized deformity of the profile of the brain. The brain is pushed away from the inner table of the skull without any significant changes in the outline of the cerebral cortex, the hematoma forming a smooth layer of blood between the inner table and the brain. The cerebral angiogram in the anteroposterior view will thus show displacement of the peripheral vessels of the brain from the inner table in a rather uniform manner. In unilateral acute subdural hematoma this appearance of the peripheral vessels will be seen on the side of the bleeding, and there will be displacement of the anterior cerebral artery toward the opposite side (Figs. 26 A, B). In bilateral acute subdural hematoma

ACUTE SUBDURAL HEMATOMA

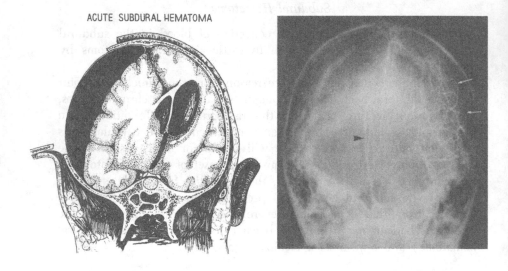

Fig. 26A, B. An acute subdural hematoma. The black arrowhead (26B) shows the displacement of the anterior cerebral artery across the midline with a step sign distally. The "bare area" shown by the two white arrows is crescentic in shape and represents an acute subdural hematoma.

the clear area between peripheral vessels and inner table will be seen on each side (if bilateral cerebral vessel filling is accomplished) and the anterior cerebral vessels are apt to be in the midline. Diffuse brain atrophy, in which the cerebral angiogram may show a symmetrical, clear area along the inner table of the skull with no shift of the anterior cerebral vessels, could produce a cerebral angiogram simulating bilateral acute subdural hematoma; however, in such cases of diffuse brain atrophy the same clear area can be seen in the lateral view whereas this appearance would not be present in the lateral angiogram of acute subdural hematoma. The lateral projection of the carotid angiogram usually distinguishes between displacement of vessels produced by a subdural collection and that resulting from a tumor since in the former the vessels appear crowded and in the latter stretched.

Chronic Subdural Hematoma

The presence of a membrane surrounding the extracerebral collection denotes chronicity. Membrane formation usually occurs about the tenth to the fourteenth day. The collection changes its shape so that the crescent shape now becomes lentiform (refer to previous pages) (Figs. 27 A, B).

Rowbotham (1964) states that there are three possible explanations for continued increase in size of the hematoma. The first involves a breakdown of the original contents of the hematoma increasing osmotic pressure therein with resultant absorption of cerebrospinal fluid. A second possibility is that fluid may escape into the center of the hematoma from the numerous thin-walled vessels in the organizing wall. Finally, there is the possibility of re-bleeding from these vessels into the interior of the clot. This last mechanism must frequently be of importance since fresh hemorrhage is often seen in histologic preparations. The passage of tagged red cells entering the clot from the peripheral blood was shown by Zingesser et al (1966). The growth in the size of the hematoma may be demonstrated angiographically or by a change in the position of metallic clips previously applied at operation to the dura and to the surface of the brain.

Regular skull films may or may not disclose a fracture. In a series of 65 cases reported by Gurdjian and Webster (1948), skull fracture was present in 21, and in a later group of 30 additional cases they found skull fracture on x-ray study in 10 (1953). In a series of 18 cases reviewed by Dyke and Davidoff (1938), there was no evidence of skull

CHRONIC SUBDURAL HEMATOMA

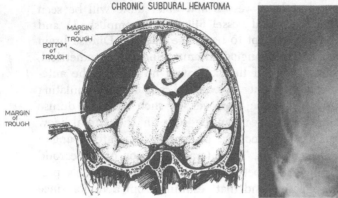

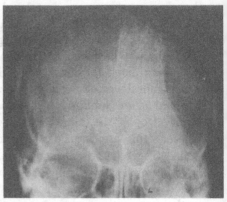

FIG. 27A, B. Chronic subdural hematoma. Note that the "bare area" is lentiform in shape. This denotes chronicity.

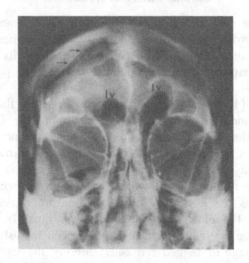

FIG. 28. Chronic subdural hematoma outlined by air along its medial margin, a classical picture. This 69-year-old male was admitted to hospital with a 3-month history of mental deterioration, headache, and drowsiness. His wife had noticed a change in his personal habits when he began to neglect washing and shaving in the morning, going as long as a week without doing so. In the differential diagnosis the following conditions were considered: metastatic deposits, a rapidly growing glioma, and an abscess. A pneumoencephalogram revealed shift of the ventricular system LV towards the left and a crescentic shadow of air (arrows) outlined in the chronic subdural hematoma. At surgery bilateral subdural hematomas were evacuated. Both had membranes. (Courtesy of the National Hospital, Queen Square, London, England).

fracture in any. Engeset (1950) found skull fractures in five patients of a series of 15. The site of the fracture does not necessarily indicate the side of the hematoma. Pineal shift, if visualized, will indicate the side, although in bilateral hematomas the pineal gland may not be shifted. In the lateral projection, the pineal body may be displaced downward or backward, or both downward and backward. Recognizable demineralization of the sella turcica is unusual in this condition.

Pneumoencephalography is used less and less today in the diagnosis of a chronic subdural hematoma. It is frequently performed when a mistaken diagnosis of another condition is made, and will help localize the lesion. If the ventricles are visualized, they are usually normal in size although dilatation (usually of the contralateral ventricle) may occur. There is a midline shift to the contralateral side. The homolateral ventricle is compressed diffusely, seldom showing any localized deformity, and is depressed. In 1936, Dyke reported a pathognomonic encephalographic sign of chronic subdural hematoma: air introduced via the lumbar route, collected subdurally, actually between the arachnoid and the inner membrane of the hematoma, with the dense soft tissue shadow lateral and dorsal to the finger-like collection of air representing the hematoma. This finding although pathognomonic, is infrequent (Olsson, 1948); the entry of gas into the subdural space during pneumography is a matter of chance (Fig. 28).

Cerebral angiography is most frequently used today and usually yields specific diagnostic information. As seen in the anteroposterior projection, there is a lens-shaped area devoid of blood vessels between the surface of the brain and the inner table of the skull; the clear area is more strikingly delineated in the late arterial, the capillary, or the early venous phases. The anterior cerebral artery is usually shifted across the midline away from the side of the hematoma. In case of bilateral chronic subdural hematomas about equal in size, bilateral angiography will show bilateral peripheral lens-shaped avascular areas with no shift of the anterior cerebral vessels; however (Figs. 29 A, B), if one of the collections is larger than the other, the anterior cerebral vessels will be displaced away from the side of the larger collection. Thus, the finding of a chronic subdural hematoma by angiography with displacement of the anterior cerebral vessels toward the opposite side does not exclude the possibility of another hematoma on the opposite side. It is advisable to obtain bilateral angiograms, in the anteroposterior view, either by compression of the opposite carotid artery during injection or by performing separate injections of opaque medium on each side.

Cerebral angiography is of greater specific diagnostic value than air studies in cases of chronic subdural hematoma. A posterior fossa collection of blood usually will not be identified by carotid angiography, although indirect signs may be present. Chronic subdural hematoma in the cerebellar region is, however, a rare lesion, usually diagnosed only by suboccipital trephine opening in a failing patient with or without an occipital fracture. With an appropriate history and displacement of the aqueduct and fourth ventricle, this condition may be suspected.

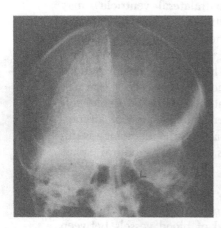

FIG. 29A. Right carotid angiogram showing a very large "bare area" with minimal shift of the anterior cerebral across the midline.

FIG. 29B. Left carotid angiogram in the same patient (29A) showing the very large "bare area" and the midline anterior cerebral artery. Here intracerebral collections about equal in size were balancing the midline structures between them.

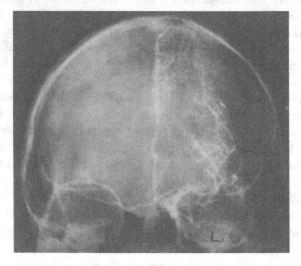

Criteria which allow angiographic distinction between epidural and subdural hematomas:

1. Displacement inwards of the meningeal arteries	— epidural — (Figs. 20, 21, 22, 23)
2. Displacement inwards of dural sinuses	— epidural — (Figs. 17, 18)
3. An irregular inner margin of the lentiform avascular space	— favors epidural — (Fig. 21)
4. Shape of a chronic subdural in presence of recent trauma	— favors epidural — (Figs. 20, 21)
5. Disproportionate (less) shift of the anterior cerebral artery	— favors epidural — (Figs. 20, 21)
6. Presence of fracture crossing meningeal groove	— favors epidural
7. Leaking of contrast medium from a torn meningeal vessel	— epidural — (Figs. 20, 22, 24)

Frequently a subdural and an epidural hematoma are present concurrently. Damaged brain tissue may further complicate the picture.

Calcified or Ossified Chronic Subdural Hematoma

Infrequently, calcification and even ossification will occur in the walls of a chronic subdural hematoma. Most, if not all, such cases probably represent hematomas that developed during infancy or childhood. With the skull being malleable at this early age, there may have been an increase in the size of the skull due to the hematoma. Dyke and Davidoff (1938) have suggested that with regression in the size of the hematoma, related to its becoming fibrotic and eventually calcified or ossified, the brain reacts to this "vacuum" by enlargement of the homolateral ventricle with pulling of the midline cerebral structures to the side of the lesion; the skull responds by thickening of the vault and hypertrophy of the air sinuses on the side of the lesion. In addition, of course, plain films of the skull show intracranial collections of calcium over a large part of a cerebral hemisphere (Fig. 30); sometimes a double layer of calcification may be visualized, one near the cortex (inner membrane) and the other near the inner table of the skull (outer membrane) (Fig. 30).

373

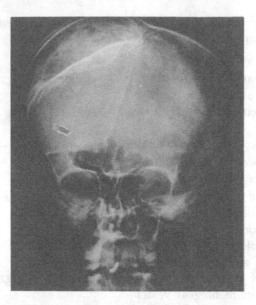

FIG. 30. Calcified subdural hematoma. Note that the calcification has occurred in the enveloping membrane (courtesy of the National Hospital, Queen Square, London, England).

Relapsing Juvenile Chronic Subdural Hematoma

In 1938 Davidoff and Dyke described this entity based on four cases. These patients were all young (ages 6, 14, 16, 18), with a history of early head trauma (5 to 11 years previously) and then more recent cranial trauma (2 to 12 months before admission) with evidence on admission of moderate increase in intracranial pressure and minimal localizing neurological signs. They exhibited changes in the skull which were explained on the basis of an old subdural hematoma with consequent resorption and then the occurrence of a recent injury with fresh bleeding into the sac of the hematoma.

The original chronic subdural hematoma, occurring in childhood, produced skull changes on the involved side due to the localized increased intracranial pressure: (1) elevation of sphenoid ridge, superior orbital plate, and superior orbital ridge; (2) deepening, widening, and lengthening of the middle fossa, and thinning of contiguous bone; (3) disappearance or indistinctness of the oblique line delineating the posterolateral wall of the orbit; and (4) atrophy of the inferior and lateral wall of the superior orbital fissure.

374

Due to subsequent resorption of the fluid content of the hematoma sac with localized "negative" intracranial pressure, adaptive (compensatory) skull changes occurred on the involved side: (1) hypertrophy of the frontal and ethmoidal sinuses; and (2) thickening of the skull.

Each case did not present all these changes on plain skull films. With the second head injury years later and fresh bleeding into the old sac, these patients showed current evidence of an expanding intracranial lesion with clinical findings of papilledema, headache, and vomiting. Air studies showed shift of the ventricle away from the site of the hematoma.

Chronic subdural fluid collections in children without episodes of recent injury may lead to localized thinning and localized bulging of the cranium (Childe, 1963). Untreated, the asymmetry may be discovered at a later age. In a series of eight cases reported by Childe one was a chronic subdural hematoma, the other seven were chronic subdural hygromas.

Subdural Fluid Collections in Infants

Subdural hematoma is of common occurrence during the first two years of life. It is a chronic slowly progressive serosanguinous liquid collection (hematoma, hygroma) pressing on the underlying brain. It reaches its highest incidence during the first 6 months of life (Matson, 1969).

Enlargement of the head occurs in about one third of the cases. X-rays may disclose separation of the sutures. The diagnosis is usually established by subdural puncture; in older children angiography or burr holes are necessary.

Intracerebral Hemorrhage

Our discussion here has to do with the massive type of intraparenchymatous hemorrhage rather than widespread small petechial bleeding.

Most cases do not show skull fracture. The pineal gland, if visualized, is usually displaced away from the side of the lesion.

Cerebral angiography will show distortion and displacement of vessels to a degree and of a sort dependent on the size and site of the intracerebral hematoma as well as on the presence or absence of associated lesions (e.g., subdural hematoma). Inasmuch as acute subdural hematoma usually produces a generally smooth displacement

375

of peripheral vessels from the inner table of the skull, the additional angiographic finding of considerable upward and medialward displacement of the middle cerebral artery suggests the presence of an additional lesion, either a basilar epidural hematoma or a temporal intracerebral hematoma. The differential diagnosis between these frequently cannot be made by angiography, although the intracerebral lesion (the intracerebral hematoma) is apt to cause local distortion and "draping" of vessels of the middle cerebral group as may be seen with a neoplasm of the temporal lobe, whereas the epidural hematoma produces the extrinsic pressure defect of an extracerebral lesion. Hemorrhage located deep in the frontal lobe will, of course, cause no differential problem from epidural or subdural hematoma; there will be displacement of the anterior cerebral artery across the midline toward the opposite side with lateral displacement and increased convexity of the vertical portion of the Sylvian group on the ipsilateral side.

Thus, intracerebral hematomas usually show the same angiographic changes as neoplasms and other expanding processes with the same localization. Associated radiological signs of increased intracranial pressure (e.g., demineralized sella turcica) are not present, however, with acute intracerebral bleeding. The breakdown products of damaged brain tissue may cause vasodilatation of vessels in the vicinity of the lesion.

CEREBRAL EDEMA

Considerable cerebral edema may occur as the result of cranial trauma without hemorrhage. Yet the x-ray findings may closely simulate those of intracerebral hemorrhage. There may be a shift of the pineal gland across the midline as well as of the ventricular system, as demonstrated by air study and of the anterior cerebral vessels as revealed by angiography. In case of edema, these changes will revert spontaneously to normal with subsidence of the swelling.

In pure cerebral edema, there is no extracerebral avascular zone as is seen with subdural hematoma (acute or chronic) or epidural hematoma. Also there is apt to be a generalized shift of vessels without a specific "local displacement" as one might see with an intracerebral hematoma. However, there are occasions when cerebral edema produces a more localized dislocation of vessels, simulating the changes produced by intracerebral hemorrhage; in such cases it is impossible to establish a differential diagnosis on the basis of the angiographic findings.

376

Head injuries may bring about a situation in which the cerebral blood flow proceeds quite slowly through the internal carotid artery because of thrombosis of that vessel or, more often, because of other factors. The pathogenesis of this phenomenon has been the subject of much controversy.

The fact that there is a more rapid passage of contrast medium through the external carotid system in the patient with no occlusion of the internal carotid artery has been suggested as a means of differentiating thrombosis from pseudothrombosis. Actually, the distinction may be difficult in many cases, for intracranial pressure may be so high that the internal carotid artery is effectively occluded. At the same time, systemic blood pressure may be extremely low so that contrast material passes through the external carotid system slowly. We have seen many bizarre examples of slow intracranial flow.

In our experience such slow circulation has invariably been a sign of impending death. However, when the intracranial vessels are not sufficiently well demonstrated in such cases, to exclude an extracerebral hematoma — a remediable condition — bilateral exploration is indicated. Agonal flow invariably involves both carotid arteries. The posterior circulation may not be involved (Figs. 31 A, B, C).

Local intracranial changes in flow occur in cases of trauma. The middle cerebral artery may be occluded (Wolpert and Schechter, 1966). When blood vessels become trapped between the herniated brain and dural reflections they may be temporarily occluded. Most commonly the anterior cerebral arteries are involved as they cross beneath the falx and the posterior cerebral arteries in the tentorial opening. We have encountered a case of thrombosis of the superior sagittal sinus from trauma.

CAROTID CAVERNOUS FISTULAE

The most common intracranial fistula involves the carotid artery and the cavernous sinus. The cavernous sinus is the only site in the body where an artery is bathed in venous blood and fistulae between the artery and the vein may result from disruption of the artery. Most often these fistulae result from a fracture involving the base of the skull. The wall of the carotid artery is torn as it passes through the cavernous sinus, or perhaps the tear involves branches of the internal

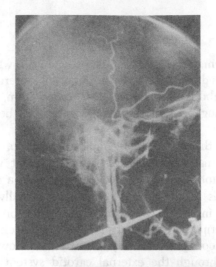

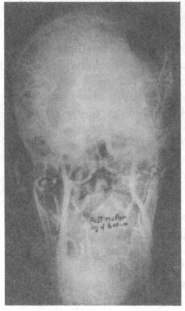

Fig. 31A, B, C. Patient sustained head trauma and the common carotid angiogram (31A) reveals very slow flow in the internal carotid artery due to raised intracranial pressure. The flow through the external carotid artery was normal. A film taken 8 seconds later (31B) showed only a few vessels of the middle cerebral artery filled, and a film taken 14 seconds later showed very little progression of the passage of contrast along these vessels. A similar situation was present on the opposite side. A postmortem angiogram (31C) revealed no disease in the vessels in the head and neck.

378

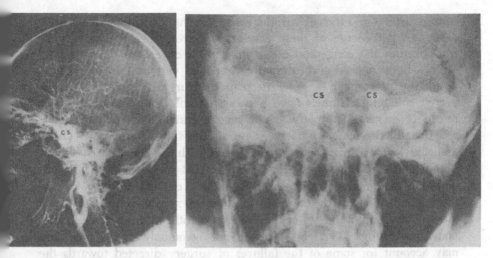

FIG. 32A, B. Patient sustained trauma at the side of the head and a few weeks later developed a whishing sound in her head with proptosis. The carotid angiogram shows filling of the cavernous sinus (C.S.) and of the orbital veins (O.V.) almost simultaneously with filling of the other arterial structures (32A). Figure 32B shows both sinuses filled via the circular sinus.

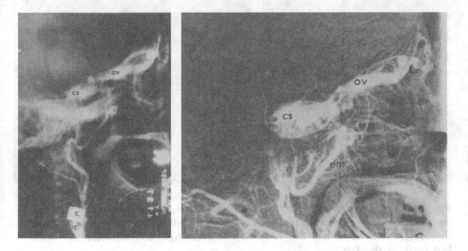

FIG. 33A, B. This patient had a ligation of the internal carotid artery both in the neck and in the head. Figure 33A shows filling of the cavernous sinus and orbital veins from branches of the external carotid artery. C.S = cavernous sinus; O.V. = orbital veins; C = clamp and IC = internal carotid artery. A subtraction study (33B) shows these structures to better advantage. Note the multiple vessels supplied by the external maxillary (E.M.) artery and other branches of the external carotid artery entering the cavernous sinus (C.S.).

379

carotid artery or external carotid artery in the cavernous sinus area. A certain percentage of these fistulae, however, are thought to arise from rupture of a congenital aneurysm into the cavernous sinus. Angiography — both internal and external carotid and vertebral angiography — should be performed in order to plan the surgical approach. Unsuspected collateral channels have been responsible for some of the poor results of surgery. The pathways of venous drainage are of some interest. Usually the major drainage is retrograde into orbital veins (Figs. 32A, 32B). There may be communications with the opposite cavernous sinus via the circular sinus (Fig. 32B), so that proptosis may be bilateral. Other venous drainage routes of less clinical interest include those connections with the petrosal and pterygoid sinuses. Fistulae may involve only branches of the external carotid artery and the cavernous sinus (Figs. 33 A, B). This is not commonly appreciated and may account for some of the failures of surgery directed towards the internal carotid artery. The unsuccessful treatment of carotid cavernous

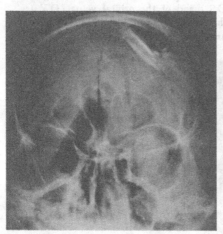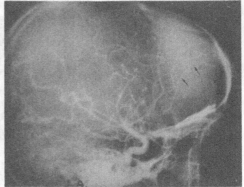

Fig. 34. Patient with multiple head injuries. Note the depressed fracture in the parietal region; other fractures have involved the air sinuses and air has passed through the torn dura into the ventricular system. Note the subdural air which had outlined the falx.

Fig. 35. This patient was involved in a motorcycle accident; films taken a few days later showed an air fluid level involving his frontal sinus. The small arrows are directed towards branches of the anteriorcerebral artery which are elevated by a mass. This mass turned out to be an epidural and subdural empyema, the result of organisms which entered through the fractured frontal sinus.

fistulae has been ascribed to the presence of small anastomotic channels (Hamby, 1952; Hayes, 1963). Another case illustrating these communications and the value of preoperative selective angiography was reported by Rosenbaum and Schechter (1969).

Traumatic intracranial pneumocephalus (or aerocele) may result from a compound fracture of the skull which permits access of air to the intracranial contents. Skull fractures involving mastoid air cells, the ethmoid bone and the cribriform plate, or the frontal bone through the posterior wall of a frontal sinus may produce intracranial pneumocephalus (Fig. 34). The first report of such an event in a living patient was made by Luckett in 1913; skull films made 12 days after fracture of the frontal bone disclosed air in the lateral ventricles. Since then, other reports of this condition have been contributed by Stewart (1913), Holmes (1918), Potter (1919), Horrax (1921), Dandy (1926), Lewis (1928), and many others. The entrance of air intracranially with its resultant symptoms may not occur for several days or even weeks after injury. Garland and Mottram (1945) reported a patient in whom intracranial air did not appear until nine weeks following a bullet wound in the frontotemporal region. The presence of intracranial gas may be due to infection by gas-producing organisms complicating a compound skull fracture (Fig. 35). In fractures involving a paranasal sinus connecting with the intracranial contents, a sudden increase in pressure in the upper respiratory tract, as may be produced by coughing, occurring days or weeks after the injury, may force air through the fracture into the cranial cavity. The resulting symptoms — severe headache, drowsiness, vomiting, and dizziness — are due to the sudden increase in intracranial pressure caused by the ingress of air. Depending upon the site and the severity of the fracture, air may be found in any of the following locations: (1) the extradural region; (2) the subdural space; (3) the subarachnoid space; (4) the brain parenchyma; and (5) the ventricular system. Osteomyelitis or meningitis may coexist.

The intracerebral, epidural, and subdural aeroceles are apt to be unilateral; when air is present in the subarachnoid space or ventricles, its distribution is bilateral.

Pendergrass, Schaeffer, and Hodes (1956) emphasize that in all cases of fracture of the skull involving the region of the mastoid and paranasal sinuses, repeated x-ray examination of the skull should be carried out in view of the possibility of the development of pneumocephalus, frequently days or weeks after the injury.

The diagnosis is quite apparent on plain skull films with no need for more complicated x-ray studies. Laminography may help locate the the entire extent of the fracture (e.g., cribriform plate).

LEPTOMENINGEAL CYST

Occasonally, in children, as a consequence of severe head trauma, especially in association with comminuted or depressed fractures of the skull, there may be laceration of the brain coverings (pia mater, arachnoid, and dura) with subsequent loculation of pockets of fluid within closed compartments of the subarachnoid space. Transmission of brain pulsations to these cysts may in the course of many months or years lead to circumscribed areas of rarefaction in the overlying skull. At the time of the initial injury arachnoid is believed to herniate through the dural tear, resulting in a progressively enlarging cyst which produces localized atrophy of the skull due to the water-hammer effect of cerebral pulsations; thus, instead of healing there is gradual widening of the fracture line.

The proper diagnosis can often be made from plain skull films (Figs. 36, 37). The original fracture may often still be visible with elongation and widening of the fracture line. The margins of the area may be rounded and smooth, although typically the inner table of the skull is scalloped due to pressure of the cyst. There may be several such leptomeningeal cysts. They occur most commonly, as might be expected, at the most frequent sites for skull fracture, i.e., the parietal, frontal and temporal regions.

DYKE-DAVIDOFF-MASSON SYNDROME

In 1933, Dyke, Davidoff and Masson reported a series of nine cases of cerebral hemiatrophy with changes in the skull believed due to the underlying brain damage. Since then many such cases, commonly called the D.D.M. syndrome, have been recognized. Inasmuch as the size and shape of the growing skull is dependent in large measure on the degree of development of its contained brain, injury to the brain at birth or early childhood with resultant cerebral atrophy may lead to secondary changes of the skull (Fig. 38).

The authors described the following changes associated with cerebral hemiatrophy dating back to childhood: (1) thickening of the cranial vault on the same side as the cerebral lesion (2) overdevelopment of the frontal and ethmoid sinuses on the side of the cerebral atrophy; (3) overdevelopment of the mastoids (air cells of the petrous pyramid of the temporal bone), the petrous pyramid on the affected

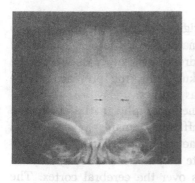
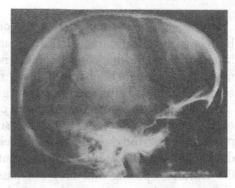

FIG. 36. A leptomeningeal cyst in a young infant. Note the indistinct and widely separated margins.

FIG. 37. A leptomeningeal cyst in an adult Leptomeningeal cysts are uncommon in adults.

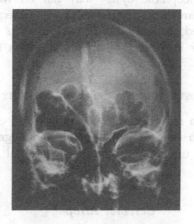

FIG. 38. This represents the Dyke-Davidoff-Masson syndrome. Note the elevation of the petrous bone, the well-developed frontal sinus, the thickening of the vault and the smaller cerebral compartment, all on the right side.

side being elevated; (4) enlargement of the lateral ventricle on the side of the cerebral lesion; (5) sometimes enlargement of the third ventricle; (6) displacement of the ventricular system and of the calcified pineal gland toward the affected side; and (7) coarse sulci or abnormal collections of air in the subarachnoid space, which may be present on the pathological side; owing to adhesions, however, no sulci markings may be seen on the abnormal side.

383

Of the nine cases reported in the original paper, four appeared to be related to infection and five to trauma as the cause of the cerebral hemiatrophy. The diagnosis of this syndrome can, of course, often be made from examination of the plain skull films, the presence of the cerebral atrophy being confirmed by gas studies.

Angiography has virtually replaced pneumography in the evaluation of the acute head injury, but gas insufflation remains a very useful procedure for studying the late sequelae of brain injuries. Air introduced via the lumbar subarachnoid route may not find its way beyond the tentorial opening and may not pass over the cerebral cortex. The absence of air over the surface of the cortex may suggest subdural collections of fluid. On the other hand areas of local atrophy may allow air to enter the adjoining dilated subarachnoid space. The lateral ventricles may be enlarged as a sequel of diffuse cerebral atrophy or a circumscribed area of atrophy may be revealed by local ventricular dilatation. These "porencephalic cysts" may not fill with air during the encephalographic examination but may do so subsequently. When this condition is suspected, patients should have a series of roentgenograms taken 24 hours after the injection of air, at which time the cyst may be visualized.

POSTTRAUMATIC CEREBRAL ATROPHY

Injury to the brain may be followed by atrophic changes, the extent and nature of which depend on the type and degree of the trauma. There may be (1) unilateral or bilateral cerebral atrophy, and (2) porencephaly.

Cerebral Atrophy

A localized, unilateral subcortical injury to the brain is apt to be followed by contracting scar tissue which causes unilateral dilatation of the ipsilateral ventricle as well as increased prominence of the cerebral sulci on the involved side. In closed head injuries, there is usually no shift of midline structures. In open head injuries with cranial defects and more severe trauma to the brain, there may be, in addition, a shift of the ventricles toward the side of the injury.

Troland et al (1946) described the following pneumoencephalographic findings in 143 cases of head injury: (1) shift of the ventricular system toward the side of the cranial defect, probably not due to fibrosis but to ipsilateral loss of cerebral substance, in 12 percent; (2) symmetrical enlargement of the lateral ventricles and of the third ventricle, probably caused by diffuse loss of cerebral tissue, in 8.5 percent; (3) symmetrical enlargement of both lateral ventricles without enlargement of the third ventricle, also resulting from diffuse cerebral atrophy, in 8 percent; (4) bilateral asymmetrical enlargement of the lateral ventricles, the more dilated one always being on the side of the injury, in 29 percent; and (5) enlargement of only one lateral ventricle, attributed to localized atrophy, in 29 percent.

Ventricular enlargement can be demonstrated usually within a short time after the injury, i.e., with subsidence of the cerebral edema. Thus in 33 cases examined within three months of the time of trauma, 20 (60 percent) showed ventricular enlargement of some type. Diminution of cerebral volume may occur as a consequence of impaired circulation, posttraumatic fibrosis and contracture, or loss of tissue due to the nature of the trauma and subsequent therapy, e.g., a penetrating wound requiring debridement. Pendergrass, Schaeffer, and Hodes (1956) also suggest that bilateral ventricular enlargement following cranial trauma may be the result of hemorrhage into the subarachnoid space with secondary basilar fibrosis causing obliteration of cerebrospinal fluid pathways and interference with the flow and absorption of the cerebrospinal fluid. This obstruction may involve the foramen of Magendie and/or the basilar cisterns and subarachnoid spaces over the hemispheres up to the arachnoid villi.

In some cases studied soon after injury (a week or so) there is apt to be absence or decreased prominence of the cerebral sulci on the side of the injury, probably due to cerebral edema, subarachnoid hemorrhage or arachnoiditis. Subsequently, as a result of atrophy, the cerebral sulci may become wider than normal and more prominent, either diffusely or in a localized distribution.

Dyke and Davidoff (1938) have pointed out that although cerebral atrophy may result from cranial trauma with consequent enlargement of one or both lateral ventricles, and encephalographic changes as described above, such atrophy is more commonly due to causes other than trauma — vascular insufficiency, for example.

According to Davies and Falconer (1944), ventricular dilatation appears more likely to be the result of intracerebral atrophic processes than of obstruction of cerebrospinal fluid pathways.

Ventricular enlargement may first appear within two to three weeks of injury and reach its maximum within a month. The presence of fracture of the skull is a factor, since focal dilatation tends to develop beneath the site of the fracture.

Porencephaly

Porencephaly refers to an abnormal cavity within the brain, which may communicate with the ventricular system (internal porencephaly) or with the subarachnoid space (external porencephaly). Occasionally there may be a "closed" porencephaly in which the cyst is separated from the ventricle by a thin membrane and does not communicate with the subarachnoid space.

A porencephalic cyst may be developmental or acquired, the acquired type representing loss of brain substance due to traumatic, vascular, or inflammatory factors. Trauma appears to be the most important causative factor, injury in some cases being incurred at time of birth; the patient may not develop symptoms for many years after the injury.

Pendergrass and Perryman (1946) reported 29 cases of porencephaly, most seeking medical attention because of epileptic attacks; the average age was 16 years, with a range of nine months to 34 years. The parietal region was involved exclusively or to some extent in 69 percent, the frontal lobes in 52 percent, and the occipital lobes in 26 percent of cases.

Porencephaly is a manifestation of cerebral atrophy, and it may be the underlying lesion in hemiatrophy or underdevelopment of the skull. When such a case occurs early in life, plain films of the skull will show the changes of the Dyke-Davidoff-Masson syndrome: the cranial vault on the affected side may be smaller and the bones thickened, together with elevation of the petrous ridge and increased pneumatization of the mastoid area as well as the frontal and ethmoid sinuses. If the pineal gland is calcified, it may be displaced slightly toward the affected side. Seven of the 29 cases in the series of Pendergrass and Perryman showed thickening of the skull on the side of the porencephaly; on the other hand, 15 cases of this series showed thinning of the bone on the side of the lesion, possibly due to the pressure effect of the pulsating intraventricular fluid transmitted to the vault through the contents of the cyst which lies against the bone.

Porencephaly can be definitely diagnosed only by pneumoencephalography or ventriculography, the defect in the brain being filled with gas and appearing as a sharply outlined gas shadow (Figs. 39 A, B, 40). Sometimes there are several communicating cavities. The "closed"

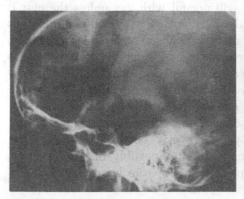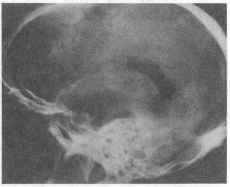

FIG. 39A, B. There is dilatation of the frontal horn of the lateral ventricle as a result of previous trauma (39A). The back of the ventricle (39B) is normal in size, shape and position.

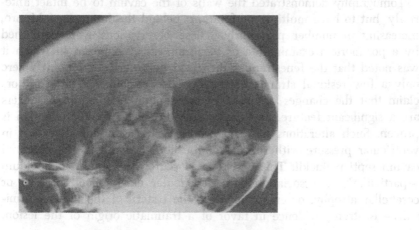

FIG. 40. Dilatation of the occipital horn in a patient who sustained trauma to the occipital region.

387

porencephalic cavity, of course, will not fill with gas unless the cyst is entered directly by the ventricular needle; this type of porencephaly is uncommon. Angiography may suggest localized ventricular dilatation.

In most cases there are other evidences of cerebral atrophy such as enlargement of the ipsilateral ventricle or increase in size of the sub-arachnoid sulci. Both lateral ventricles may be enlarged, the homo-lateral one usually to a greater extent. Most cases also show a shift of the ventricular system, usually toward the porencephalic side because of the accompanying atrophy; yet there may be displacement of the ventricular system toward the opposite side, possibly due to the pressure of the cyst or greater atrophy of the opposite hemisphere.

Effects of Repeated Injury (Boxing)

Encephalographic changes in prize fighters were first observed by Spillane (1962) in a study of five professional boxers. Isherwood et al (1966), conducted encephalographic studies in 16 ex-boxers, all of whom had evidence of neurological disease. Of the 16 patients, 3 had normal encephalograms, while the remaining 13 had a variety of abnormalities: (1) cavum septi pellucidi in 9 cases; (2) evidence of brain atrophy including generalized ventricular enlargement in 11 cases, cerebral atrophy in 2, and cerebellar atrophy in 4; (3) enlargement of the cistern of the lamina terminalis in 4 cases.

Tomography demonstrated the walls of the cavum to be intact anteriorly, but to have multiple perforations behind the foramen of Munro, increasing in number posteriorly. These observations were confirmed by a postmortem examination of the brain of an ex-boxer, in which it was noted that the fenestrations increased posteriorly to a point where only a few residual strands of the lamellae remained. These authors claim that the changes observed in the septum pellucidum in boxers are a significant feature, and the role of trauma in their production is proven. Such alterations may be produced by a sudden elevation in ventricular pressure with rupture of the floor or walls of the potential cavum septi pellucidi. This finding of a perforated septum pellucidum – particularly in association with ventricular enlargement, cortical or cerebellar atrophy, or enlargement of the cistern of the lamina termi-nalis – is strong evidence in favor of a traumatic origin of the lesion.

CEPHALHEMATOMA IN THE NEWBORN

Cephalhematoma in the newborn refers to a condition in which bleeding occurs subpericranially from injury at birth with elevation of the pericranium by the hematoma. Pressure of the blood clot causes depression in the underlying skull. New bone may be laid down by the elevated pericranium, so that a rim of calcium may be seen around the base of a cephalhematoma after two or three weeks. Cephalhematoma persists for several weeks or months and then usually disappears completely, although the bone in the region may remain thickened for months or years after the resorption of the hematoma.

Some cases of cranial deformity in the adult, consisting of a unilateral bulging of the anterior part of the skull, have been considered to represent late developmental complications of infantile cephalhematoma. This condition has been called "cephalhematoma deformans" (Schuller and Morgan, 1946). X-ray studies show extensive, irregular diploic hyperostosis. Reported cases of this condition are few in number and its direct relationship to infantile cephalhematoma is open to question.

In a series of 2774 newborn infants, Kendall and Woloshian (1952) found cephalhematomas in 69, an incidence of 2.49 percent. The incidence in other reported series is lower, varying from 0.41 percent to 1.66 percent (Ingram and Hamilton, 1950). Sixty-four of the 69 cases of Kendall and Woloshian had skull x-rays, fracture (parietal bone in all) being found in sixteen (25 percent). Except for one occurring in the occipital region, all the cephalhematomas were parietal in location, 11 being bilateral. They occurred more often in infants born of primiparous women, the incidence being higher in infants delivered with

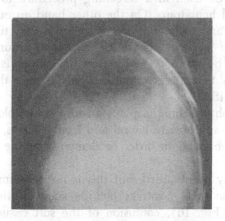

FIG. 41. Cephalhematoma in the parietal region.
Note that it does not cross the sagittal suture.
There is some calcification in the hematoma.

389

forceps than in those born spontaneously. In their 126 cases, Ingram and Hamilton found no cephalhematomas in the premature group; there was a greater incidence among the higher weight group of newborns. The fetal presentation had no etiologic significance.

Characteristically the boundaries of a cephalhematoma are limited by the periosteum adherent at suture lines of the individual bone involved; this is readily seen on x-ray. Thus the soft tissue swelling over the parietal bone does not cross the sagittal suture (Fig. 41), and the bilateral parietal cephalhematomas taper to the sagittal suture. This feature of a parietal cephalhematoma of not crossing the midline (the sagittal suture) should be contrasted with that of a cephalhematoma in the occipital region which may cross the midline because of the absence of a midline suture in this area.

GAMMA ENCEPHALOGRAPHY

Over the last 15 years many isotopes have been used in brain scanning, but none has worked so well in the demonstration of extracerebral hematomas as the radioactive mercury compounds (Zingessser et al, 1966) and, more recently, technetium — 99m pertechnetate. A few cases of subdural hematoma demonstrated with radioactive iodine-labeled diiodofluorescein, radioiodinated serum albumin (RISA), radioactive copper, and radioactive arsenic have been reported, but it is evident that these isotopes are not reliable for this purpose. In other words, they cannot be used in a screening procedure to rule out the presence of subdural hematoma. On the other hand, in our experience, radioactive mercury and technetium have served a very useful purpose in the evaluation of patients who have sustained trauma. The fact that the patient may be scanned shortly after the isotope is administered allows the work-up to proceed rapidly. This is not the case with radioisotopes like RISA.

As with angiography, technique plays an important role in the scanning procedure. The appropriate lateral and frontal views, either supine or prone, must be obtained in order to demonstrate the lesion (Figs. 42 A, B, C, D).

False positives may be obtained, but this is no criticism of a screening procedure. These false positives include such entities as peripheral infarction (See Fig. 16), contusion of the soft tissues (Fig. 43), peripheral metastatic disease, and intracerebral hematoma.

On the radioactive brain scan the extracerebral hematoma manifests itself as a hot "vascular rim." This is easily recognizable if it is

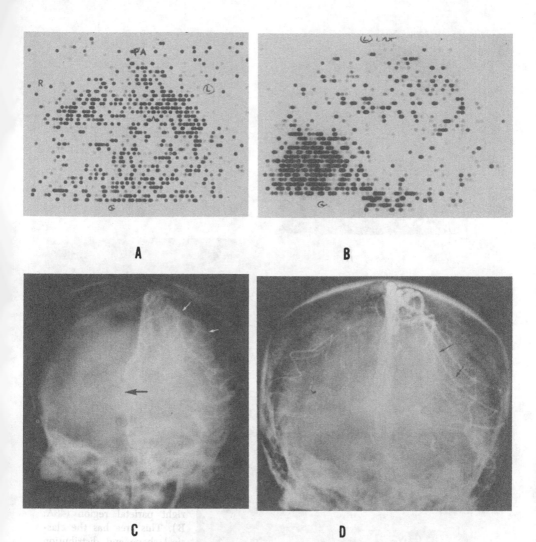

A **B**

C **D**

FIG. 42A, B, C, D. Radioactive scan of patient with cerebral trauma. Scan was made with the patient in the prone position, 3 hours after the administration of radioactive mercury. Abnormally high activity is seen over the brain bilaterally. The diagnosis of chronic subdural hematomas was made. The lateral projection (42B) shows the activity in the parietal region. A left carotid angiogram (42C) shows displacement of the anterior cerebral artery across the midline (large arrow) and the "bare area" (outlined with arrows). Although this "bare area" appears to be crescentic in shape, the next figure (42D), reveals the true situation. Here the veins have filled and line the depth of the crater representing a chronic subdural hematoma. This film was made with contralateral compression and some contrast is present in the middle cerebral artery on the right side. A subdural hematoma is present on this side also.

391

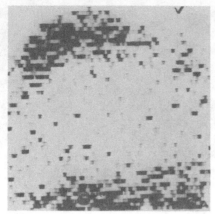

A

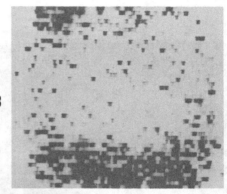

B

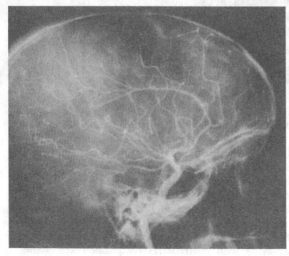

C

Fig. 43A, B, C. Radioactive mercury scan of a patient who had sustained head trauma reveals an area of increased uptake in the right parietal region (43A, B). This area has the classical shape and distribution of a subdural hematoma. An angiogram was then performed (43C) which excluded the presence of an extracerebral hematoma. It was then noted that the patient had a large subgaleal hematoma. When this was analyzed it was found to contain a high concentration of the isotope.

392

unilateral. When the vascular rim appears hot bilaterally, a situation in which the differential diagnosis involves bilateral subdural or epidural hematomas, renal disease, and Paget's disease the problem is resolved with a 24-hour scan; the extracerebral hematomas at the end of 24 hours will remain hot, while in cases of Paget's and renal disease the increased uptake will no longer be evident. This is so because the radioactive compound passes into the extracerebral collection and is not cleared as rapidly as from the blood, so that at the end of 24 hours, the blood-mercury level has dropped to a much greater extent than the contents of the subdural space.

ULTRASONOGRAPHY

Ultrasonography refers to A-scanning and B-scanning. In the A-scan the midline ideally is indicated as spike-shaped waves. The significance of a shift of this midline echo is the same as that of a displacement of a calcified pineal. In the absence of a characteristic midline echo one cannot be absolutely sure that the spike or spikes thought to represent the midline actually do so. However, when the examination is repeated from the opposite side, a shift of the suspected midline — in a commensurate direction, lends support to the interpretation of the spike or spikes as originating from the midline. Most authorities agree that echoencephalography is about 95 percent accurate in determining the midline. Thus when an extracerebral hematoma is present, and this hematoma has shifted the midline, echoencephalography proves its worth as a screening procedure. This procedure is apt to have more false negatives than radioactive scanning, however, although it has the edge over scanning in that it can be more rapidly performed. (This may not be true when technology involved in scanning has progressed a little further.) The false negatives are observed in cases in which a unilateral subdural or epidural hematoma has not caused a shift of the midline or in which where there are bilateral extracerebral hematomas which balance the midline. In our experience these situations are not at all uncommon.

Workers such as Schiefer and Kazner (1964) have claimed that they usually are able to demonstrate a hematoma echo with epidural hematomas and with chronic subdural hematomas. For this technique it is necessary that the transducer be situated opposite the extracerebral hematoma. When the transducer is placed so that the sound pulse is perpendicular to the hematoma, investigators claim that they are able to demonstrate a characteristic echo which they call the hematoma echo. Others have not been able to corroborate this observation very often.

Perhaps another disadvantage of echoencephalography relates to the fact that soft tissue trauma and the development of a subgaleal hematoma sometimes makes the technical aspects of achieving a satisfactory echoencephalogram difficult or impossible.

In regard to B-scanning (cross sectional "sound picture") the work of Adapon et al (1965), who have fairly extensive experience in this field indicates to us that it will probably be of little use as a screening procedure in the evaluation of a patient who has sustained trauma. First of all, the examination is more difficult technically than A-scanning; secondly, at this time it is evident that most extracerebral hematomas will be missed on B-scans for several reasons: (1) these extracerebral hematomas may not be found in the cross section impedances obtained at the interfaces of these extracerebral hematomas; and (2) they may not be sufficiently great to delimit their boundary from the adjacent membranes and brain.

BIBLIOGRAPHY

Adapon, B. D., Chase, N. E., Kricheff, I. I., and Battista, A. F. Cerebral Ultrasonic Tomography. *Radiology, 84*, 115-121, 1965.

Berk, M. E. Aneurysms of the Middle Meningeal Artery. *Br. J. Radiol., 34*, 667-668, 1961.

Berkay, F. A Rare and Interesting Case of Arteriovenous Fistula Between the Middle Meningeal Artery and the Greater Petrosal Sinus and Surgical Treatment. *Tip. Fak. Mec., (Istanbul), 26*, 61-71, 1963 (in Turkish).

Borden, W. C. *The Use of the Roentgen Ray by the Medical Department of the United States Army in the War with Spain (1898).* Washington Printing Office, 1900.

Bradley, K. C. Extra-dural Haemorrhage. *Aust. N. Z. J. Surg., 21*, 241-260, 1952.

Childe, J. W. Localized Thinning and Enlargement of the Cranium. *Am. J. Roentgenol., 70*, 1-22, 1963.

Cronqvist, S. and Kohler, R. Angiography in Epidural Haematomas. *Acta Radiol., 1*, 42-52, 1963.

Dandy, W. E. Pneumocephalus. *Arch. Surg., 12*, 949-982, 1926.

Davidoff, L. M. and Dyke, C. G. Relapsing Juvenile Chronic Subdural Hematoma. *Bull. Neur. Inst. N. Y., 7*, 95-111, 1938.

Davies, H. and Falconer, M. A. Ventricular Changes after Closed Head Injury. *J. Neurol. Psychiat., 6*, 52-68, 1944.

Dilenge, D. and Wuthrich, R. Traumatic Aneurysm of the Middle Meningeal Artery. *Neurochirurgia, 4*, 202-206, 1962 (in French).

Dyke, C. G. A Pathognomonic Encephalographic Sign of Subdural Hematoma. *Bull. Neur. Inst. N. Y.*, 5, 135-140, 1936.

Dyke, C. G. and Davidoff, L. M. Chronic Subdural Hematoma. *Bull. Neur. Inst. N. Y.*, 7, 112-147, 1938.

Dyke, C. G. (revised by L. M. Davidoff). The Roentgenological Aspects of Fractures of the Skull and Injuries of the Brain. In S. Brock (Ed.), *Injuries of the Brain and Spinal Cord and Their Coverings*, 3rd ed. Baltimore: Williams and Wilkins, 1949. P. 434-470.

Dyke, C. G., Davidoff, L. M., and Masson, C. B. Cerebral Hemiatrophy with Homolateral Hypertrophy of the Skull and Sinuses. *Surg. Gynec. & Obstet.*, 57, 588-600, 1933.

Engeset, A. On Roentgen Examination in Head Trauma. *Acta Radiol.*, 34, 288-298, 1950.

Fincher, E. F. Arteriovenous Fistula Between the Middle Meningeal Artery and the Greater Petrosal Sinus. *Ann. Surg.*, 133, 886-888, 1951.

Friedmann, G., Schmidt-Witkamp, E., and Walter, W. Zur diagnose des epiduralen hematoms in carotisangiogramm, *Dtsch. Z. Nervenheilk.*, 179, 603-613, 1959.

Garland, L. H. and Mottram, M. E. Traumatic Pnemocephalus. *Radiology*, 44, 237-240, 1945.

Glaser, M. A. and Blaine, E. S. Fate of Cranial Defects Secondary to Fracture and Surgery. *Radiology*, 34, 671-684, 1940.

Gurdjian, E. S., Webster, J. E., and Lissner, H. R.: The Mechanism of Skull Fracture. *J. Neurosurg.*, 7, 106-114, 1950.

Gurdjian, E. S., Lissner, H. R., and Webster, J. E. The Mechanism of Linear Skull Fracture: Further Studies on Deformation of Skull by "Stresscoat" Technique. *Surg. Gynec. & Obstet.*, 85, 195-210, 1947.

Gurdjian, E. S., and Webster, J. E. Traumatic Intracranial Hemorrhage. *Amer. J. Surg.*, 75, 82-98, 1948.

Gurdjian, E. S., Webster, J. E., and Lissner, H. R. Mechanism of Skull Fracture. *Radiology*, 54, 313-339, 1950.

Gurdjian, E. S. and Webster, J. E.: Chronic Subdural Hematomas. Diagnostic Considerations. *Med. Clin. North Am.*, 37, 430-449, 1953.

Hamby, W. B. *Intracranial Aneurysms*. Springfield, Ill.: Chas. C Thomas, 1952.

Hassler, O. Medial Defects in the Meningeal Arteries. *J. Neurosurg.*, 19, 337-340, 1962.

Hayes, G. J. External Carotid-Cavernous Sinus Fistulas. *J. Neurosurg.*, 20, 692-700, 1963.

Hirsch, J. F., David, M., and Sachs, M. Les Anevrysmes Arteriels traumatiques intracraniens. *Neurochirurgie*, 8, 189-201, 1962.

Holmes, G. W. Intracranial Aerocele Following Fracture of the Frontal Bone. *Am. J. Roentgenol.*, 5, 384-386, 1918.

Horrax, G. Intracranial Aerocele Following Fractured Skull. *Ann. Surg.*, 73, 18-22, 1921.

Huber, P. Die verletzungen der meningeal fasse beim epiduralhamatom im angiogramm. *Fortschr. a. d. Geb. d. Rontgenstrahlen*, 96, 207-220, 1962.

Ingram, M. D., Jr., and Hamilton, W. M. Cephalhematoma in the Newborn. *Radiology, 55,* 503-507, 1950.

Isherwood, I., Mawdsley, C., and Ferguson, F. R.: Pneumoencephalographic Changes in Boxers. *Acta Radiol., 5,* 654-661, 1966.

Jackson, D. C., and du Boulay, G. H. Traumatic Arterio-venous Aneurysm of the Middle Meningeal Artery. *Br. J. Radiol., 37,* 788-789, 1964.

Jamieson, K. G., Unusual Case of Extra-dural Haematoma. *Aust. N. Z. J. Surg., 21,* 304-307, 1952.

Jones, F. W. Vascular Lesion in Some Cases of Middle Meningeal Haemorrhage. *Lancet, 2,* 7-12, 1912.

Kendall, A., and Woloshian, H. Cephalhematoma Associated with Fracture of the Skull. *J. Pediatr., 41,* 125-132, 1952.

Kia-Noury, M. Traumatisches intracranielles aneurysma der arteria meningica media nach Schadelbasis-fraktur. *Zentralbl. f. Neurochir., 21,* 351-357, 1961.

Kuhn, R. A. and Kugler, H. False Aneurysms of the Middle Meningeal Artery. *J. Neurosurg., 21,* 92-96, 1964.

Leslie, E. V., Smith, B. H., and Zoll, J. G. Value of Angiography in Head Trauma. *Radiology, 78,* 930-939, 1962.

Lewis, A. J. Traumatic Pneumocephalus. *Brain, 51,* 221-243, 1928.

Lindgren, E. Rontgenologie. Band II. In H. Olivecrona and W. Tonnis (Eds.), *Handbuch der Neurochirurgie.* Berlin: Springer-Verlag, 1954.

Lofstrom, J. E., Webster, J. E., and Gurdjian, E. S. Angiography in the Evaluation of Intracranial Trauma. *Radiology, 65,* 847-855, 1955.

Lohr, W. Hirngefassverletzungen in arteriographischer darstellung. *Zentralbl. f. Chir., 63,* 2466-2482, 1936.

Luckett, W. H. Air in the Ventricles of the Brain Following Fracture of the Skull. *J. Nerv. Ment. Dis., 40,* 326-328, 1913.

Markham, J. W. Arteriovenous Fistula of the Middle Meningeal Artery and the Greater Petrosal Sinus. *J. Neurosurg., 18,* 847-848, 1961.

Markwalder, H. and Huber, P. Aneurysmen der Meningealarterien. *Schweiz. med. Wchnschr., 91,* 1344-1347, 1961.

Matson, D. D. *Neurosurgery of Infancy and Childhood.* 2nd ed., Springfield, Ill.: Charles C Thomas, 1969.

New, P. F. J. True Aneurysm of the Middle Meningeal Artery, *Clin. Radiol., 16,* 236-240, 1965.

Norman, O. Angiographic Differentiation Between Acute and Chronic Subdural and Extradural Haematomas. *Acta Radiol., 46,* 371-378, 1956.

Olsson, O. Subdural Hematoma Outlined with Air in Encephalogram. *Acta Radiol., 29,* 95-98, 1948.

Paillas, J. E., Bonnal, J., and Lavielle, J. Angiographic Images of False Aneurysmal Sac Caused by Rupture of Median Meningeal Artery in the Course of Traumatic Extradural Hematomata. Report of Three Cases. *J. Neurosurg., 21,* 667-671, 1964.

Pendergrass, E. P., and Perryman, C. R. Porencephaly. *Am. J. Roentgenol., 56,* 441-463, 1946.

Pendergrass, E. P., Schaeffer, J. P., and Hodes, P. J. *The Head and Neck in Roentgen Diagnosis,* 2nd ed., Springfield, Ill.: Charles C Thomas, 1956. P. 192, 1281.

Perot, P., Ethier, R., and Wong, A. An Arterial Posterior Fossa Extradural Hematoma Demonstrated by Vertebral Angiography. Case Report. *J. Neurosurg.*, *26*, 255-260, 1967.

Potter, H. E. A Case of Hydro-Pneumo-Cranium with Air in the Ventricles. *Am. J. Roentgenol.*, *6*, 12-16, 1919.

Pouyanne, H., Leman, P., Got, M., and Gouaza, A. Traumatic Arterial Aneurysm of the Left Middle Meningeal Artery. Rupture One Month after the Accident. Temporal Intracerebral Hematoma. Intervention. *Neurochirurgie*, *5*, 311-315, 1959 (in French).

Rosenbaum, A. E. and Schechter, M. M. External Carotid Cavernous Fistulae. *Acta Radiol.*, *9*, 440-444, 1969.

Rowbotham, G. F. *Acute Injuries of the Head.* Edinburgh: Livingstone Ltd., 1964.

Ruggiero, G., Calabro, A., Metzger, J., and Simon, J. Arteriography of the External Carotid Artery. *Acta Radiol.* (Diag.), *1*, 395-402, 1963.

Schechter, M. M. and Gutstein, R. A. Aneurysm and Arteriovenous Fistulas of the Superficial Temporal Vessels. *Radiology*, *97*, 549-558, 1970.

Schechter, M. M. and Zingesser, L. H. In A. E. Walker, W. F. Caveness, and M. Critchley (Eds.), *The Late Effects of Head Injury.* Springfield, Ill.: Charles C Thomas, 1969. P. 228.

Schiefer, W. and Kazner, E. Die echo-enzephalographie. *Dtsch. med. Wschr.*, *29*, 1394-1400, 1964.

Schmidt, H., and Rossi, U. Intrazerebrale extravasate nach hirnkontusion im karotis-angiogramm. *Fortschr. a. d. Geb. d. Rontgenstrahlen*, *94*, 505-508, 1961 (in German).

Schuller, A. and Morgan, F. Cephalhematoma Deformans; Late Developments of Infantile Cephalhematoma. *Surgery*, *19*, 651-660, 1946.

Schulze, A. Seltene verlaufsformen epiduraler hämatome. *Zentralbl. Neurochir.*, *17*, 40-47, 1957.

Schumacher, F. V. and Henesy, G. T. *Vascular Groove Simulating Skull Fracture.* Exhibit at 58th Annual meeting, The American Roentgen Ray Society, Washington, D. C., 1957.

Schunk, H. and Maruyama, Y. Two Vascular Grooves of the External Table of the Skull which Simulate Fractures. *Acta Radiol.*, *54*, 186-194, 1960.

Spillane, J. D. Five Boxers. *Br. Med. J.*, *2*, 1205-1210, 1962.

Stewart, W. H. Fracture of the Skull with Air in the Ventricles. *Am. J. Roentgenol.*, *1*, 83-87, 1913.

Troland, C. E., Baxter, D. H., and Schatzki, R. Observations on Encephalographic Findings in Cerebral Trauma. *J. Neurosurg.*, *3*, 390-398, 1946.

Tiwisina, T. and Stacker, A. D. The Fresh Cranio-cerebral Injuries in Vascular Picture. *Chirurg.*, *30*, 344-349, 1959 (in German).

Vance, R. G. The Healing of Linear Fractures of the Skull. *Am. J. Roentgenol.*, *36*, 744-746, 1936.

Vaughan, B. F. Middle Meningeal Haemorrhage Demonstrated Angiographically. *Br. J. Radiol.*, *32*, 493-494, 1959.

Wickbom, I. Angiography by Post-traumatic Intracranial Hemorrhages. *Acta Radiol.*, *32*, 249-258, 1949.

Wilson, C. B. and Cronic, F. Traumatic Arteriovenous Fistulas Involving the

Middle Meningeal Vessels. *J.A.M.A.*, *188*, 953-957, 1964.

Wolpert, S. M. and Schechter, M. M. Traumatic Middle Cerebral Artery Occlusion. *Radiology*, *87*, 671-677, 1966.

Wortzman, G. Traumatic Pseudo-aneurysm of the Superficial Temporal Artery. A Case Report. *Radiology*, *80*, 444-446, 1963.

Zingesser, L. H., Mandell, S., and Schechter, M. M. Gamma Encephalograms in Extracerebral Hematomas. *Acta Radiol.*, (Diag.), *5*, 972-980, 1966.

Zingesser, L. H., Schechter, M. M., and Rayport, M. Truths and Untruths Concerning the Angiographic Findings in Extracerebral Haematomas. *Br. J. Radiol.*, *38*, 835-847, 1965.

CHAPTER 11

THE ELECTROENCEPHALOGRAM IN CASES OF
HEAD INJURY

PAUL F. A. HOEFER, M. D.

Head injuries and their immediate and late sequelae constitute a large and important group of disorders in the practice of neurology and neurosurgery. Closed head injuries in most instances have a good prognosis but many require some form of medical care and, a few, surgical treatment in addition. Penetrating head wounds are rare in peace time but a large number of such war injured still require medical attention.

The final outcome in many cases depends on properly planned early measures, including the occasional anticipation of posttraumatic convulsive disorder. Furthermore, disability, compensation claims, and lawsuits often arise as a result of head injury. It is not always easy to evaluate the primary damage to the brain from consideration of original signs and symptoms, or to predict safely the final outcome in a given case.

For all these reasons, an objective measure of brain damage and of disturbance of brain function is desirable, and an attempt will be made, therefore, to correlate clinical and electroencephalographic (EEG) findings at various times after head injury.

Proper evaluation of data, as EEG findings after head injury, depends on statistical analysis of significantly large numbers of cases. Such data can only be gathered in large specialized civilian and military hospitals, where the case material is obviously weighted towards the more serious cases of trauma. Thus, our own findings and those presented by most authors must differ materially from those seen in general hospitals and even more so from the observations made in office practice. In order to offset this bias, a number of investigations will be reviewed, in which EEG findings after minor head injury are analyzed.

399

The electroencephalogram is a recording of electrical activity originating in the bodies, dendrites, and axons of cortical cells and of cells in subcortical gray matter. Conducted impulses in the long ascending tracts, especially from afferent receptor systems and from thalamic relays, contribute to the basic activity. This in turn is modified by excitatory and inhibitory synaptic processes in the cortex, by "recruitment" of participating elements, and by processes of summation and integration which are not yet fully understood. The degree of cortical and thalamic activity is furthermore controlled by the reticular formation in the brain stem.

The EEG, recorded after suitable amplification, consists of oscillations varying in frequency from 1 to 40 cycles per second (cps) and in amplitude from about 10 to 300 microvolts (one microvolt equals one millionth of a volt). This activity can be picked up through the intact skull and scalp; it may also be recorded from the exposed cortex during surgical operations or in laboratory experiments. It is then called an "electrocorticogram." Ink-writing oscillographs are used for recording. They are usually arranged for simultaneous tracings from several areas, with eight or even more channels combined in a single recording instrument. In spite of the structural complexity of the central nervous system and the continuous variations in its activity, a reproducible basic normal pattern exists in the EEG. This basic activity is obtained under certain conditions, which at first appear somewhat arbitrary. A normal adult pattern may be expected in healthy subjects who are physically and mentally relaxed and at ease, but fully awake, in a normal state of nutrition and adjusted to their physical environment. Sensory stimulation and the action of certain drugs may alter the basic pattern as do sleep and intensive mental activity. Conversely, if other than normal activity is recorded under normal conditions as defined, the subject is likely to have an abnormally functioning brain.

No clearly defined activity is found in the newborn. In infancy and childhood normal activity is slower than that seen in the adult. As the child grows older, organized adult type activity is first seen in the parietal and occipital areas. At this time the basic activity becomes faster and approaches the adult frequency range at the age of eight or ten and the incidence of adult activity increases during adolescence. It then spreads forward and is also seen in the more anterior areas of the head in the adult.

400

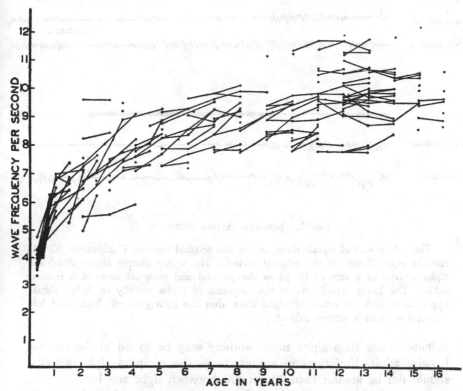

FIG. 1. Changes in average frequency of occipital rhythms observed in 132 children followed through several years of development. (After Lindsley.)

The mean frequency ranges of the normal EEG in the resting waking state are shown in Fig. 1 for the ages from 1 to 16 years. Some variations both in the faster and slower side of the frequency range are permissible, especially for the ages below 10. At 13, the normal adult pattern is reached in many instances, but in other normal subjects full maturation is not seen until the late teens. In old age, mild slowing is considered normal.

With drowsiness and different stages of sleep, characteristic changes are seen in normal subjects at all ages. The patterns of drowsiness in infancy are different from those of the adult. Sleep patterns show relatively less variation in different age groups. The normal waking resting record in the adult (Fig. 2) is well organized especially in the posterior leads, where the "alpha" activity (8 to 12 cps) is most prominent. In the more anterior leads low voltage rapid activity and some low

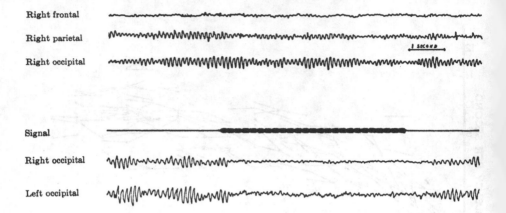

Right frontal

Right parietal

Right occipital

Signal

Right occipital

Left occipital

FIG. 2. NORMAL ALPHA ACTIVITY

Time: One second equals three cm. in the original records. Calibration: 50 microvolts equal 5 mm. in the original records. The upper sample shows dominant alpha activity at a rate of 10 cps in the parietal and occipital areas of a normal subject The lower sample shows the response of alpha activity to light (signal upper line), and the return of alpha soon after the light goes off. Right and left occipital areas of a normal subject.

voltage slower than alpha range activity may be found in the normal healthy adult. Variations in amplitude in the occipital alpha activity should not be greater than 30 percent between right and left.

Consistent depression of normal activity or its complete absence in one area may be considered an abnormal EEG finding, indicative of profound temporary or permanent depression of cortical activity and in some instances of destruction of cortical areas. Other EEG changes consist of deviations from the normal range towards the slower or faster side, and from the nomal amplitude towards larger deflections. Predominantly slow, often high voltage activity ($\frac{1}{2}$ to 4 cps) — which is often referred to as "delta" activity — is seen in a number of conditions in which a physiological or pathological decrease of brain cell metabolism is the common factor. This includes hypoglycemia (Fig. 3), anoxia, local or general impairment of blood supply to the brain, deep sleep, deep coma, and (in some patients as well as in normal young children) the vasoconstrictor response to over-breathing. Certain drugs, e.g., tranquilizers and alcohol, lead to slowing of the record. Mental retardation in children and adolescents is at times associated with activity slower than normal for the patient's age.

Predominantly rapid ("beta") activity, often to the exclusion of

402

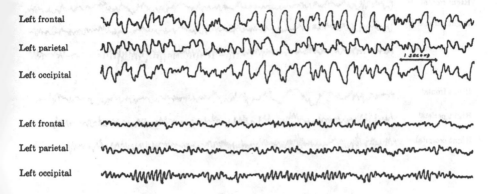

Left frontal

Left parietal

Left occipital

Left frontal

Left parietal

Left occipital

FIG. 3. HYPERINSULINISM

The upper sample is taken during a state of hypoglycemia. Note the very high irregular slow activity. The second sample is taken an hour after 100 gm. of glucose was given and is normal. Both samples were taken from the left frontal, parietal and occipital areas in monopolar leads.

recognizable normal activity, is recorded in conditions in which, for physiological or pathological reasons, cerebral activity is increased beyond the waking resting state. This may be the result of sensory stimulation in the appropriate cortical areas, as when light stimulates the retina (Fig. 2 lower record). It is seen in subjects who are tense or worried, and during intense mental activity. Some drugs, such as barbiturates and also Dexedrine, lead to the appearance of rapid activity in the EEG.

Changes from the normal pattern to slower and faster activity are seen as the result of many physiological alterations. As such they are not highly specific. On the other hand, if slow wave activity is repeatedly seen as a localized discharge against a background of otherwise normal or less abnormal activity, it may indicate the presence of a structural lesion of the brain, such as tumor, abscess, or a scar. Focal or diffuse slow wave activity is seen in inflammatory and degenerative processes, and also in many cases of vascular lesions.

A focal discharge of spike (i.e., high-voltage fast) activity may be the result of an irritative lesion leading to focal or generalized seizures. Spike discharges in some cases are seen only in sleep records and not during the waking state. Focal spike discharges may be considered as fairly specific paroxysmal abnormalities (Fig. 4). Other paroxysmal discharges consist of synchronous bursts of high-voltage slow wave activity in the resting, non-activated record. These discharges, abrupt both in onset and ending, may cover a large area of the brain or even

403

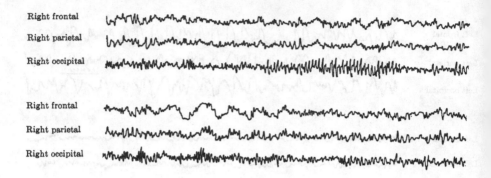

Right frontal

Right parietal

Right occipital

Right frontal

Right parietal

Right occipital

FIG. 4. Spike discharge from the right occipital area. Grand mal, inter-seizure record.

occur in all areas bilaterally. The most reliable seizure pattern is the spike-and-wave discharge consisting of an alternation of a fast and a slow wave usually of higher than medium amplitude and ranging in frequency from about 1 to 5 cps. Synchronous spike and wave discharges at a rate of approximately 3 cps are highly specific for petit mal epilepsy (Fig. 5). They occur in well over 80 percent of inter-seizure records of patients with this form of epilepsy. Spike-and-wave discharges may, however, occur in all other forms of epilepsy and may be occasionally seen in healthy, close relatives of epileptic patients.

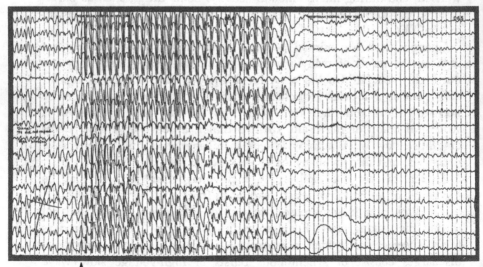

FIG. 5. Synchronous spike-and-wave discharge (3 cps). Onset of petit mal attack (↟).

404

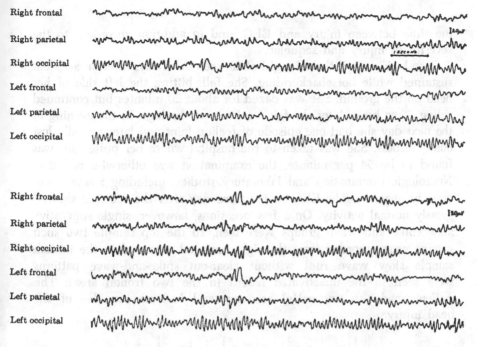

Right frontal	
Right parietal	
Right occipital	
Left frontal	
Left parietal	
Left occipital	

Fig. 6. Case I.

Very mild head injury, third day. Two samples in monopolar leads showing slow spike-and-wave group in the right occipital area (first sample) and a short bifrontal burst (second sample).

Approximately 15 percent of unselected normal subjects may show mildly abnormal EEG patterns, not explained by the physiological alterations which were discussed. Paroxysmal bursts on the other hand are extremely rare in normal subjects except in the close blood relatives of epileptics. The presence of normal activity in a single recording does not rule out seizures or structural lesions. Approximately 20 percent of unselected epileptics and a similar percentage of patients suffering from various cerebral hemispheric tumors show no focal or generalized abnormality.

In the interpretation of EEG findings after head injury the same criteria are applied for the evaluation of diffuse and focal abnormalities in general and for the evaluation of seizure discharges in particular.

Electroencephalographic Changes after Head Injury

Characteristic EEG changes seen in ten cases from the author's own material are presented. They are approximately arranged according to

405

the time between injury and EEG, and in addition according to the severity of injury and sequelae.

Case I (Fig. 6) is that of a girl of 20, seen three days after an accident sustained while horseback riding. She fell, hitting the left side of her head on the ground. She was dazed for about 20 minutes but continued riding. Two hours later she felt weakness of the legs. In the evening of the next day she had one episode of feeling faint and later actually lost consciousness. She was taken to the hospital where her pulse rate was found to be 54 per minute; the examination was otherwise negative. Neurologic examination and laboratory studies, including x-rays, were entirely negative. The EEG on the third day after the accident showed grossly normal activity. On a few occasions, however, single suggestive slow spike and wave groups were seen. In the top sample two such groups were recorded from the right occipital area and in the bottom sample slow wave runs without clear-cut spike-and-wave patterns were seen in the unactivated record in the two frontal areas. The patient made an uneventful recovery and had no sequelae of the head injury.

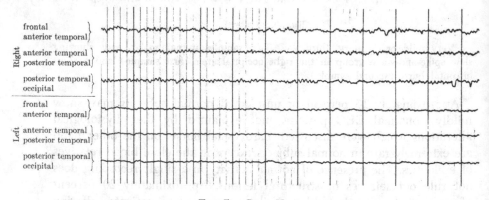

FIG. 7. CASE II.

Six-year-old boy with linear fracture of left parietooccipital area, five days after accident. Note general depression of activity on left side in three bottom leads.

Case II (Fig. 7) is that of a boy of six who was seen five days after head injury resulting in a linear fracture over the left parietooccipital area. The child was unconscious for an undetermined period of time, with amnesia for the accident. Neurologic examination revealed mild weakness of the right leg and bilateral Babinski signs. The EEG five days after the accident showed a depression of activity over the left side with occasional bursts of 2 to 4 cps slow wave activity and a single

406

suggestive slow spike-and-wave group during overventilation (not shown in Fig. 7). Four days later (record not shown) the depression of waking and sleep activity persisted on the left. Three weeks later the record was normal. Two months after the accident, however, a spike focus over the right occipital area was found which remained persistent; but the child had no clinical sequelae.

Case III (Fig. 8) is that of a man of 35 who sustained a head injury two months prior to the test. There were no neurologic complications other than unconsciousness lasting five minutes. At the time of the test

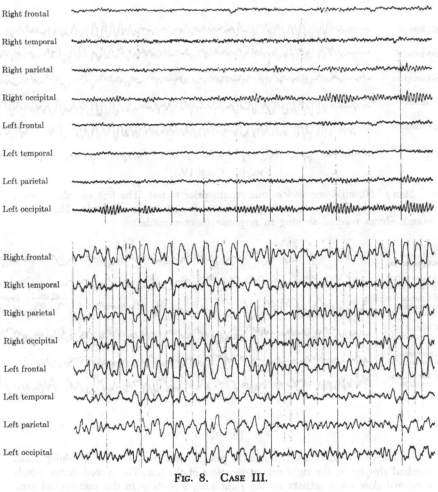

FIG. 8. CASE III.

Man of 35, mild concussion, two months prior to test.

407

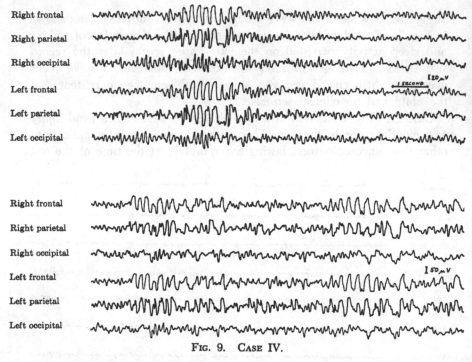

| Right frontal |
| Right parietal |
| Right occipital |
| Left frontal |
| Left parietal |
| Left occipital |

1 SECOND 120 μV

150 μV

FIG. 9. CASE IV.

Man of 50, mild concussion, one month prior to test. The first sample shows a synchronous burst of slow and spike-and-wave activity in all leads. The second sample shows marked slowing in response to overventilation.

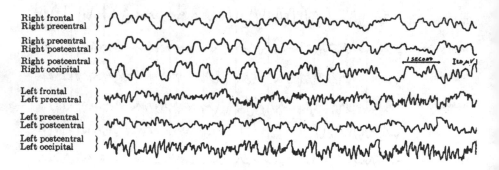

| Right frontal / Right precentral |
| Right precentral / Right postcentral |
| Right postcentral / Right occipital |
| Left frontal / Left precentral |
| Left precentral / Left postcentral |
| Left postcentral / Left occipital |

1 SECOND 100 μV

FIG. 10. CASE V.

Very severe head injury two months prior to test. Residual left hemiplegia and cerebral atrophy on the right side at the time of the test. The record shows grossly abnormal slow wave activity on the right side, especially in the post-central area. On the left side moderately abnormal activity is noted.

408

he complained of headache and episodes of dizziness. The resting record (top) is normal. During hyperventilation, however, the record (at bottom) shows synchronous bursts of high-voltage slow wave activity with frequent fairly typical spike-and-wave groups in the frontal and parietal leads bilaterally. The bursts last for up to 3 or 4 seconds and are not accompanied by clinical manifestations of any nature. There were no clinical sequelae.

Case IV (Fig. 9) is that of a man 50 years of age. He suffered a head injury with transient loss of consciousness about a month prior to the test. The head injury was followed by brief but frequent episodes of dizziness. The neurological examination and skull x-ray studies were normal. The EEG at rest (top) shows numerous spontaneous bursts of high-voltage slow wave and slow spike activity with a tendency towards synchronization in all leads, especially in the frontal and parietal runs. Marked additional slowing was seen with hyperventilation. There were no clinical sequelae.

Case V (Fig. 10) is that of a boy of 8 who was seen two months after a head injury — striking his head against a wall while running. He had no immmediate complaints but within two days developed headache, vomiting, stupor and finally deep coma. On admission to the hospital he had a left hemiparesis, including the left side of the face. He developed papilledema which subsided. When the coma subsided a left homonymous hemianopia was found. The spinal fluid showed many red blood cells. Two months later spasticity was found on the left side;

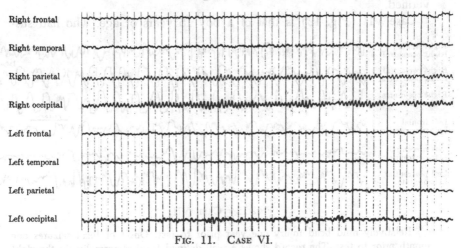

Right frontal

Right temporal

Right parietal

Right occipital

Left frontal

Left temporal

Left parietal

Left occipital

Fig. 11.   Case VI.

Subdural hematoma on left side. Compare right and left temporal, parietal and occipital leads, noting depression and slowing on the left side.

pneumoencephalograms, at that time, showed cerebral atrophy on the right side. The EEG shows high-voltage slow wave activity over the right side and somewhat less abnormal activity with some slow wave components on the left side as well. The presumptive clinical diagnosis was right intracerebral hemorrhage.

Case VI (Fig. 11) is that of a boy of 17 who sustained three head injuries while playing football during a period of about five weeks in October and November. Following the first injury, he developed a dull intermittent pain over the left side of the head. The second accident, four weeks after the first, was associated with amnesia for the remainder of the game, though he finished it. After the third injury he had an exacerbation of left-sided headache for three weeks. Five weeks later, in December, he had an episode of vomiting for three days. In January, one month prior to admission, he began having diplopia intermittently, which became persistent during the last two weeks. Eleven days before admission he had a sensory jacksonian attack on the right side, preceded by a twenty-minute episode of speech disturbance and followed by some weakness on the right side; after the attack he slept for almost a day. The only clinical finding on admission, in February, was marked bilateral papilledema with hemorrhages and exudates. There were no localizing motor or sensory signs.

The EEG showed completely normal activity on the right and depressed activity with disorganized 4 to 7 cps activity on the left. The diagnosis of left subdural hematoma was suggested and surgically verified.

Case VII (Fig. 12) is that of a boy 15 years of age, who had sus-

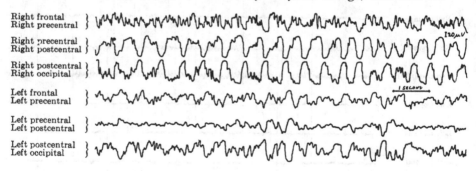

FIG. 12. CASE VII.

Relatively mild head injury one year prior to test. Onset of focal seizures one month prior to test. The record shows a well-defined focal abnormality in the right postcentral area consisting of continuous runs of high voltage slow waves at a rate of 1 to 2 cps.

410

tained a head injury one year prior to the examination, apparently without serious sequelae until 11 months after the head injury and one month prior to admission to the hospital. He then began to have generalized convulsive seizures which started with turning of the eyes to the left. He was admitted in status epilepticus which subsided after intravenous injection of sodium luminal. The neurological examination and pneumoencephalograms were negative. The EEG showed grossly abnormal activity bilaterally but the main finding was a very well-defined slow wave focus in the right parietal region, with suggestive spike-and-wave patterns superimposed. The boy continued having seizures for several years after onset.

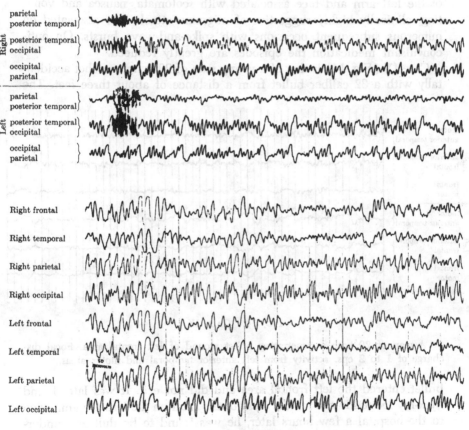

FIG. 13. CASE VIII.

A girl of 9 with injury of occipital region. Upper sample: Bi-occipital slow wave-and-spike and wave focus. Lower sample: Synchronous slow wave-and-spike and wave discharge with hyperventilation.

411

Case VIII (Fig. 13) is that of a girl nine years of age who fell at play, striking the occipital region. She did not lose consciousness but complained immediately of headache and a disturbance of vision. The EEG performed 18 months after the accident and on several occasions since showed a bi-occipital slow wave focus and spike-and-wave discharges in the same distribution. In response to a few minutes of hyperventilation, high-voltage slow wave-and-spike and wave bursts were seen, synchronous in all leads. About four years after the accident the record showed typical full-blown 3 cps spike-and-wave bursts in the resting record. The child has not developed generalized convulsions but for several years has had numerous episodes of transient numbness of the left arm and face associated with scotomata, nausea and vomiting, clinically highly suggestive of migraine attacks but associated on numerous subsequent occasions with spike-and-wave bursts. On anticonvulsant medication the episodes are greatly reduced.

Case IX (Fig. 14) is that of a young man of 20, who was shot accidentally with a 32 caliber bullet from a distance of about three feet. The

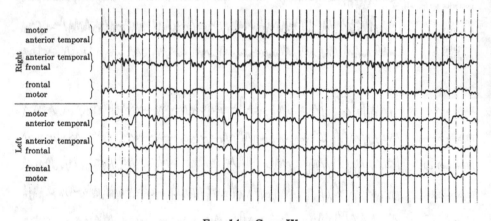

FIG. 14. CASE IX.

A man of 20 with a penetrating bullet wound of left frontal area. Focal discharge of 1 to 2 cps. activity from left anterior temporal and motor areas.

bullet entered the left frontal area and did not exit. It was later found by x-ray lodged in the middle fossa of the skull on the left. On admission to the hospital a few hours later, he was found to be dull and underproductive, but neurological examination at that time revealed no motor or sensory deficit, no aphasia or other form of cortical dysfunction, and no incoordination. The EEG on the ninth hospital day was basically disorganized with 8 to 10 cps activity, best seen in the pos-

412

terior leads and with 4 to 7 cps activity, best seen in the anterior leads. Against this background a focal discharge of partly high-voltage 1 to 2 cps activity was recorded from the left anterior temporal and motor areas.

The patient developed an abscess of the left frontal area which was treated by surgery and with antibiotics. At the time of discharge, seven weeks after the injury, he had a mild residual right hemiparesis. The EEG at that time was normal.

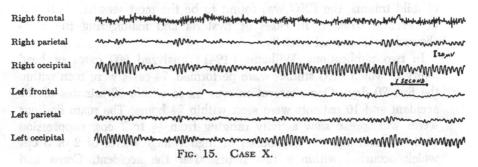

FIG. 15. CASE X.

Head injury four years prior to the test. Conversion hysteria. The record shows normal activity. In addition, muscle action potential artifact is seen in the tracing from the right frontal area.

Case X (Fig. 15) is that of a man 37 years of age. This patient had a head injury four years prior to the examination. He was reportedly unconscious for an unknown period. He presented numerous varying and unfounded complaints. Neurologic examination and complete x-ray work-up, including pneumoencephalograms, were negative. Clinical diagnosis of conversion hysteria was made. The electroencephalogram is completely normal. The record shows some muscle action potential artifact in the right frontal lead.

The earliest report on EEG changes in cases of head injury is by Williams and Gibbs (1939) who found signs of focal disorder in 12 out of 26 cases. In addition, they saw paroxysmal patterns in several of their patients.

Marmor and Savitsky (1940) attempted an analysis of 28 cases of head injury for the purpose of obtaining "objective criteria for the presence or absence of organic changes." They found no abnormal patterns in cases diagnosed as hysteria. Moderately slow activity was found in 5 out of 11 cases diagnosed as postconcussion syndrome; 3

413

other cases of this group showed normal findings. All 5 cases suffering from traumatic epilepsy showed abnormal records; two of these cases showed focal discharges of paroxysmal activity.

Jasper, Kershman, and Elvidge (1940) reviewed the EEG findings in 64 cases of head injury, 37 of which were acute. Paroxysmal activity was rare in this series. Subdural hygroma or hematoma led to a depression of activity over the lesion. In cases of severe trauma, all types of abnormal activity were found several years after the injury. In cases of mild trauma, the EEG was found to be the most sensitive indicator of cerebral damage. In cases of hysteria and malingering the EEG showed no abnormal activity.

In two publications, Williams (1941) analyzed 600 cases of head injury in which EEG studies were performed. 74 cases were seen within the first 20 days. One observation was made within 50 minutes of the accident and 10 patients were seen within 24 hours. The main findings were: widespread slow activity ranging from ½ to 7 cps, suppression of the normal activity, and bursts of high voltage waves of 2 or 3 cps which occurred within a few hours after the accident. Coma and states of confusion were accompanied by slow waves, with higher voltage in coma and increasing frequency in states of confusion. Severity of trauma and the amount of generalized abnormality in the EEG ran parallel. After an initial period, it was noted that the diffuse abnormality may subside and focal EEG signs may then appear. Six of the group of 74 patients had convulsive seizures shortly after injury. Two of these had severe, two moderately severe, and two mild injuries. Two had normal, two nonspecifically abnormal, and two had EEG records characteristic of epilepsy. None of these patients had persistent EEG abnormalities or clinical signs. In many instances, clinical and EEG improvement ran parallel; in other cases there was delay in the EEG improvement at a time when the patient had made complete clinical recovery. In 325 chronic cases, EEG findings were correlated with detailed clinical data; 50 percent of this group had abnormal records, some patients many years after the injury. Again, there was a positive correlation between severity of injury and persistence of symptoms, especially in cases where the dura was penetrated.

Hoefer (1943) analyzed the clinical and EEG findings of 244 cases in which complete clinical and laboratory work-up were available at the time of the accident and again at the time of the EEG. Of this group, 97 patients (40 percent) had normal and 147 (60 percent) abnormal records. In the abnormal group, 72 (30 percent) had gross

TABLE 1

The Incidence of Clinical Signs and Traumatic Pathology in 97 Cases of Head Injury with Normal EEG's in Relation to the Degree of Concussion

	Concussion		
	none	questionable	definite
No signs or seizures	13	3	14
Minor clinical signs	10	6	18
Major clinical signs	6	8	12
Severe clinical signs	2	0	0
Generalized seizures	2	1	2
Focal seizures	2	2	1
Psychomotor seizures	1	0	0
Fainting	2	0	2
Subdural hematoma	2	0	0
Subarachnoid hemorrhage	0	1	1
Fracture of skull	0	8	7
Cerebral atrophy, etc.	1	4	9

TABLE 2

Abnormal EEG Findings in 147 Cases in Relation to Fracture of Skull, Cerebral Atrophy, and Seizures

CONCUSSION	MARKEDLY ABNORMAL EEG			MODERATELY ABNORMAL EEG			FOCAL ABNORMALITY		
	NONE	QUES-TION-ABLE	DEFI-NITE	NONE	QUES-TION-ABLE	DEFI-NITE	NONE	QUES-TION-ABLE	DEFI-NITE
Fracture of skull	1	7	8	1	4	7	0	4	7
Atrophy of brain	2	3	10	2	2	7	2	4	7
Generalized seizures	2	5	15	1	1	3	2	2	9
Jacksonian seizures	0	3	5	1	0	1	1	1	4
Petit mal	0	0	1	0	1	0	0	0	1
Psychomotor equivalents	0	0	0	0	0	0	1	0	1
Fainting spells	0	0	4	0	1	4	0	0	1

diffuse abnormalities, 43 (18 percent) had moderate diffuse abnormalities, and 32 (13 percent) had gross focal abnormalities in the EEG. In both the normal and the abnormal groups the severity of clinical and x-ray findings and the incidence of seizures were in direct proportion to the degree of unconsciousness (concussion) sustained at the time of injury.

The clinical findings in patients with normal records are presented in Table 1, arranged in three columns in terms of absent, doubtful, and unquestionable concussion. The clinical data for patients with abnormal EEG findings are similarly arranged for three different types of abnormality in Table 2.

Of the 97 cases with normal EEG records, 59 percent had objective clinical signs at the time of the accident and only 17 percent had persistent clinical signs at the time of the test. 13 percent had skull fractures, and the same number developed cerebral atrophy. Twelve patients of this group developed seizures — 6 generalized, 5 focal seizures, and 1 psychomotor equivalent; two additional patients developed fainting spells.

Of the 147 cases with pathological EEG records 14 percent were clinically normal and had no seizures; 86 percent had clinical abnormalities or seizures or both. Persistent clinical signs were found in 90 percent of the patients who had clinical findings at the time of the injury. Of the 147 patients, 39 percent developed seizures; 27 percent generalized seizures, 11 percent focal seizures, 1 percent psychic equivalents.

The types of EEG abnormalities are presented in Table 3.

The EEG findings in 122 cases showing psychiatric signs are presented in Table 4.

Greenblatt (1943) reviewed a series of 263 patients, 48 percent of whom had abnormal EEG records. Skull fractures and concussion, as evidenced by a period of unconsciousness, did not appear as significant factors in the causation of abnormal activity. The incidence of abnormal activity was higher in cases with fits, lower in cases with posttraumatic headache. Posttraumatic psychoses showed a slightly higher incidence of EEG abnormalities than did other psychoses. Almost all cases showing focal EEG changes had evidence of severe trauma, such as depressed fractures and deformities of the skull, jacksonian seizures, etc.

In another study Williams (1944) reported observations on 1002 subjects, 234 with head injury but no seizures, 210 with posttraumatic epilepsy, 255 with idiopathic epilepsy, and 241 normal controls; 42 of the patients with head injury had EEG records before and after onset of posttraumatic seizures. All of his patients with head injuries were seen more than four weeks after the injury. The head injury group

TABLE 3

Types of EEG Abnormalities and Their Incidence
(Most records show more than one abnormal feature)

1. Records considered grossly abnormal (72 patients)

	Patients	Per cent
Purely slow activity	42	58
Purely rapid activity	7	10
Mixed rapid and slow activity	15	21
Very marked response to hyperventilation	11	15
Depressed activity	3	4
Spike-and-wave groups	13	18

2. Records considered moderately abnormal (43 patients)

Purely slow activity	14	32
Purely rapid activity	7	16
Mixed rapid and slow activity	9	21
Marked slowing in response to hyperventilation	4	9
Depressed activity	1	2
Spike-and-wave groups	3	7
Disorganized and borderline abnormal activity	11	25

3. Records presenting focal signs (32 patients)

In 24 patients of this group the EEG abnormality was confirmed by clinical signs, x-ray findings, and laterality of seizures. The remaining eight patients had focal slow wave discharges, not immediately correlated with other confirmatory signs.

Slow wave focus	21	66
Focal depression	2	6
Focal spike discharge	1	3
Focus on the opposite side	1	3
Background of slow activity	9	28
Background of rapid activity	5	16
Background of mixed activity	1	3
Marked slowing in response to hyperventilation	2	6
Spike-and-wave groups	5	16

417

TABLE 4

The Incidence of Psychiatric Abnormalities and Associated EEG Findings

122 patients had psychiatric abnormalities as follows:

Organic mental syndrome .... 46 patients
Emotional instability 36
Psychotic manifestations 29
Miscellaneous 11

EEG findings in 122 patients showing major psychiatric signs:

Normal .... 26 patients
Essentially normal 21
Low voltage rapid 4
Markedly abnormal 27
Moderately abnormal 21
Focal signs 8

included both open and closed injuries. The significant findings of this important paper are presented in Table 5.

The incidence of larval epileptic bursts (spike-and-wave groups without clinical manifestations) was three times higher in idiopathic than in traumatic epilepsy. The highest incidence of generalized abnormalities was found in the group of patients with head injuries and without fits. The group of 42 cases studied before onset of seizures did not differ from the group of posttraumatic epilepsy in the distribution of EEG findings.

TABLE 5

The Incidence of EEG Abnormalities in Cases of Head Injury, Idiopathic Epilepsy and Normal Controls, as Noted in Williams' Series (1944)

EEG FEATURES	NORMAL (241)	HEAD IN-JURY WITHOUT FITS (234)	HEAD IN-JURY WITH FITS (210)	RECORDED BEFORE ONSET OF FITS (42)	IDIO-PATHIC EPILEPSY (275)
Larval epileptic bursts	0%	0%	8.6%	5%	27%
Other paroxysmal bursts	0.8%	14%	17%	18%	29%
Other abnormalities	11%	46%	37%	38%	19%
Total abnormalities	12%	60%	63%	61%	75%
Normal	88%	40%	37%	39%	25%

As shown in Table 6, the incidence of traumatic epilepsy was three to four times higher in patients with paroxysmal EEG bursts, both for closed and penetrating injuries (Williams, 1944).

TABLE 6

The Prognostic Significance of Paroxysmal EEG Bursts in Closed and Open Head Injuries (Williams)

	Paroxysmal EEG bursts	Number of cases	Traumatic epilepsy	
			Number	Per cent
Closed head injuries	Absent	178	8	4.5
	Present	35	7	20
Open head injuries	Absent	75	6	8
	Present	28	7	25

Two important prognostic criteria suggested by Williams and based on his observations were: 1) in cases where the damaged part of the brain is surgically removed before seizures start and where EEG findings in the neighborhood of the affected area are normal, "dysrythmia is unlikely to appear;" and 2) when larval seizure patterns occur after injury, traumatic epilepsy is "virtually certain to supervene."

Jasper, Kershman, and Elvidge (1945) stressed the significance of unconsciousness and to an equal extent amnesia, confusion, irritability, and skull fractures in relation to the severity of EEG changes. In their series of 81 cases of closed injury, younger patients showed more profound EEG changes. In cases without loss of consciousness the EEG tended to become normal after 24 hours. After this period and within the first ten days after injury, a more reliable estimate of cerebral damage can be made from the EEG records. Cases with normal EEG immediately after injury have a good prognosis. Severe EEG changes rather than initial clinical changes point to a delayed recovery. Focal changes in their series persisted for many years.

Dow, Ulett and Raaf (1945) reported on a study of 213 patients, mostly with minimal injuries, seen within a very short time after the accidents at a first-aid station set up in a shipyard and equipped with recording apparatus. In this group only 11 percent had clearly abnormal records, 36 percent had borderline, and the remaining 53 percent had normal records. Lacerations of the scalp occurred in 201, skull fractures in only 2 cases.

Peuch, Fischgold and Verdeaux (1946) reported observations on 283 chronic and 55 acute cases with EEG studies. The highest incidence of EEG changes was seen within the first 2 weeks (70 percent). After this, a steady decline was noted with 19 percent abnormality seen three months after injury. After six months, another rise was seen up to 29 percent. This was due to the appearance of posttraumatic epilepsy. They concluded that in cases in which either no improvement or even deterioration of the EEG is noted after three months, posttraumatic seizures should be expected and the patients should be given prophylactic treatment.

A number of additional studies of EEG findings in open head injuries were reported on the basis of war experience. Roseman and Woodhall (1946) described their findings in 75 cases seen between one week to two years after injury: 20 percent had early convulsions, mostly focal; all of these had paroxysmal EEG changes, in some instances preceding the clinical fits. Another 20 percent had similar EEG changes without fits. The authors felt that anticonvulsant medication is indicated when the EEG shows abnormalities, especially of a focal nature. This opinion is held by others.

Maltby's report (1946) was based on 200 cases: 34 (17 percent) of these had seizures, some only for a short period but more than two-thirds continued to have fits. Only 14 of his patients had EEG studies. Seven of these had diffuse, the others mostly diffuse and in addition clearly focal abnormalities.

Laufer and Perkins (1946) found that convulsive seizures occurred in 11 percent of a group of 209 cases of closed and open head injuries. The highest incidence of abnormal activity was seen in 81 cases of open injuries with penetration of the dura. In this group 20 percent had a normal record, 21 percent diffusely abnormal and 13 percent focal EEG signs. The remainder were considered "borderline."

Busse (1947) was chiefly concerned with the correlation of EEG changes and posttraumatic headaches in patients with skull defects; 91 of his 116 cases (78 percent) showed evidence of abnormal cortical activity; 96 were unconscious at the time of the injury; and 92 had objective clinical findings at the same time. His patients were seen 3 weeks to 34 months after injury. The time interval in his experience did not bear any relation to the EEG findings.

Laufer and Perkins (1947) reported on the results of serial tests in 121 patients, 14 of whom had posttraumatic seizures. The authors stressed the improvement of the EEG records in time. Within six months 19 percent of their patients improved while 9 percent were found to be worse. In reexaminations 6 to 18 months after injury, they found improvement in 33 percent while 12 percent were worse. Marked voltage asymmetry was found in 58 percent of their cases. The voltage on the side of injury was higher in 93 percent, lower in 7 percent.

Kaufman and Walker (1949) studied a total of 324 cases of head injury, 241 with posttraumatic seizures, 83 without seizures. In the first group 91 percent had abnormal and 9 percent had normal EEG records. The figures for the group without seizures were 77 percent abnormal and 23 percent normal records. Focal abnormalities occurred in 84 percent of the seizure group and in 67 percent of the seizure-free group. The incidence of paroxysmal discharges was 22 percent (3 percent generalized) for the group with seizures, and 30 percent (2 percent generalized) for those without fits. Amplitude asymmetry was found in 18 cases with seizures, the higher amplitude being on the side of injury in 14.

The EEG may be activated by drugs, e.g., Metrazol, by physiological stresses, as overbreathing, and photic stimuli, i.e., strong flashes of light, and paradoxically, also by sleep. Metrazol activation was attempted in 106 of Kaufman and Walker's cases with focal abnormality; 72 had a focal, 4 a diffuse response. No response was obtained in 30.

Cramer, Paster, and Stephenson (1949) studied "cerebral blast concussion" in 441 cases. EEG abnormalities were found in about 60 percent; 107 patients had suppression of alpha activity, not leading to actual abnormal activity. This latter phenomenon occurred in 78 patients (73 percent) on the side of injury and in 29 (27 percent) on the opposite side.

Goetze (1950) found slowing of the EEG over the area of injury in patients as the result of breathing a mixture of 93 percent nitrogen and 7 percent oxygen for 2 or 3 minutes. This occurred in patients in whom complete depression of activity was found at the site of injury. The author reports that oxygen deprivation is a more sensitive activation test than overventilation.

421

Høncke (1951) reported on EEG findings in 100 patients with late concussion syndrome and with various complaints considered to be "functional," in the absence of objective signs. The EEG was abnormal in 38; the abnormality was "slight" in 29. Generalized slowing was found in 18, focal slowing in 11 and paroxysmal bursts in 7. There was no significant difference between patients seen within three months and those observed over two years after the injury.

Dawson, Webster, and Gurdjian (1951) described the serial electroencephalographic findings in 45 patients with mostly acute severe head injury. They found a delay in the appearance of EEG abnormalities as well as in their resolution after clinical recovery. Focal depression of activity was the most significant EEG abnormality in their opinion, even in cases without focal clinical lesions. Generalized depression of all activity occurred in three cases, all fatal. Delayed depression of activity was not considered to be of grave prognostic significance. Delta foci, in their experience, were unreliable. Epileptiform activity was found in all children and in only 13 percent of the adults.

Clark and Harper (1951), in a study of 186 cases of posttraumatic encephalopathy, were unable to find EEG evidence of the presence of convulsive disorders with any degree of accuracy.

Weil (1951), in a study of 50 patients with posttraumatic encephalopathy, found an 83 percent correlation of clinical and EEG abnormality.

Rodin, Bickford and Svien (1953) studied 45 cases of subdural hematoma, surgically verified. Focal slow wave discharges were the most significant EEG abnormality. Alpha asymmetry was noted in less than one-half of their cases. When present, it was found in anterior as well as in posterior hematomas.

Denker and Perry (1954) found 55 percent definite and 3 percent borderline abnormalities in the EEG records of 95 patients with postconcussion syndrome. All patients in this study were involved in litigation or compensation claims.

Müller (1955) reported on a correlation of clinical and EEG findings in 300 old cases of concussion and "contusion," excluding cases with seizures and subdural hematoma. Of his cases, 150 had focal EEG abnormalities, 150 had none. A little over one half of the patients with focal EEG changes had clinical neurological signs. The focus was found on the side of injury in 65 percent, on the opposite in 35 percent of the cases.

The report of Caveness (1955) dealt with serial EEGs in 366 cases of combat head injuries incurred in the Korean war. The necessity of early recording and of subsequent periodic follow-up was stressed.

Strauss (1956) evaluated the EEG records obtained on 600 patients with head injuries without gross neurological deficit. He found abnormal records in 20 percent of this group. When broken down by age groups, however, 50 percent of patients up to the age of 15 had abnormal records, with a considerable decrease of abnormalities in adults. Strauss also stressed the increase in abnormal records in cases with long-lasting initial unconsciousness (severe concussion). Only 10 percent of his cases without loss of consciousness at the time of the injury had abnormal records.

Kaplan, Huber and Browder (1956) presented a study of 30 cases of subdural hematoma and hygroma, verified at operation or autopsy. These authors recognized four groups of EEG abnormalities: (A) bilateral slow wave activity, but with slower frequencies, depression and poorer definition of activity on the side of the lesion (impeded activity); (B) bilateral abnormalities with depression and loss of definition; (C) unilateral slowing; (D) low-voltage fast activity with or without impeded activity. Patients with the most marked clinical findings and the greatest disturbance of consciousness fell into groups (A) and (B). Preoperatively alert patients were only found in groups (C) and (D).

Walker (1957), in a ten-year follow-up of craniocerebral injuries sustained in World War II, stated that while the EEG may denote cerebral damage, it does not reliably indicate or forecast the occurrence of convulsive complications. Even with serial records over a period of months such prognostication is usually difficult if not impossible. Walker also cautioned against using abnormal EEG findings in patients with dizzy spells or blackouts as an indication of epilepsy. Nevertheless the incidence of convulsive attacks was quite high in his group of 244 patients. Only one-third were free of attacks five years after injury, though seizures had become milder and less frequent in many instances. Medication appeared to play no significant part in the control of seizures in this group.

Beaussart et al (1960) studied the electroencephalograms of 52 boxers before and after engaging in a prizefight. Twenty-five exhibited changes after the fight consisting of depression of alpha, posterior slow wave activity, and fast activity. Nine were knocked out and of these, three showed changes; the others showed no abnormality.

Torres and Shapiro (1961) compared the electroencephalographic abnormalities following whiplash injuries with those occurring after closed head trauma. EEG abnormalities of moderate to marked degree were found in 46 percent of whiplash injuries and in 44 percent of cases of head trauma, suggesting to the authors a similar mechanism for the production of brain dysfunction.

Silverman (1962) studied 100 consecutive cases of head injury in patients below the age of 16 for up to four weeks after the accident. The main abnormality in his cases was posterior slowing in those between the ages of 4 and 11. This was not found in infants or older children. Another abnormality noted was the appearance of positive spikes during sleep in ten cases. He found a good correlation between the degree of injury and the EEG abnormality.

In a number of publications (Walker and Jablon, 1961; Marshall and Walker, 1961; Walker, 1962; and Walker and Erculei, 1969), Walker and his associates have recorded their observations, including electroencephalographic data in cases of head injury followed over a period of many years. Thus, in a series of 177 seriously wounded patients, the electroencephalograms 15 years later were normal or borderline in 43.5 percent; generalized abnormalities were found in 23.7 percent; and focal changes in 32.8 percent. The majority of non-epileptic patients had normal or borderline records; one-third of the normal records were from patients who had had more than one seizure; two-thirds of the electroencephalograms with generalized abnormalities were of patients who had had several attacks; focal abnormalities occurred almost entirely in patients who had had more than one fit. A high incidence of normal or borderline records was found in patients free of major seizures for 10 years. In general, the electroencephalographic findings within 5 years of injury were similar to those obtained 15 years following trauma. There appeared to be a significant correlation between the occurrence of focal EEG abnormalities and focal seizures which became generalized; otherwise the electroencephalogram did not correlate well with the type of attack. The degree of abnormality tended to correlate better with the frequency of major seizures (Walker and Erculei, 1969). A higher percentage of abnormal records was noted in patients with penetrating wounds and those with immediate neurologic deficits (Walker and Jablon, 1961). No specific electroencephalographic pattern was consistently associated with epilepsy, the highest correlation occurring in patients with focal abnormalities. Even spikes generally considered to be of convulsive significance were not found much more often in the records of patients with posttraumatic epilepsy than in those without fits (Walker, 1962).

424

Chatrian et al (1963) found EEG patterns resembling sleep with 14 cycle per second spindle activity, vertex sharp forms, and fairly typical K-complexes in eleven patients with severe head injuries resulting in loss of consciousness. The eventual outcome was favorable in all cases. This suggested to the authors a temporary reversible disturbance of function of the midbrain reticular formation.

Rodin et al (1965) analyzed the electroencephalographic records of 42 patients who died as a result of head injuries. No significant statistical differences in EEG variables were found between a group of 20 patients who died within the first 48 hours and the 22 who died later, but it was noted that the patients who died earlier had flatter records and fewer focal abnormalities.

Gutierrez-Luque et al (1966) analyzed the electroencephalograms of 179 cases of head injury, 97 uncomplicated and 82 with subdural hematoma. When the initial tracings were taken less than two weeks after injury, no distinctive EEG features were found. In later records bisynchronous projected rhythms and focal delta activity or alpha asymmetry were found in cases of subdural hematoma.

Lenard (1965) studied 636 EEG tracings obtained in 395 children with acute, mostly mild, trauma. The EEG changes in children were more marked and recovery slower than in adults. High voltage 2-4 per second symmetrical posterior slowing was typical for trauma in children. In infants under one year, on the other hand, the incidence of pathological changes was low and recovery faster. No seizure patterns were found in infants, while they were fairly frequent in older children.

Courjon (1966) cautioned against a too far-reaching interpretation of the electroencephalographic data as an indication of the likelihood of posttraumatic epilepsy, especially, as in his experience, the record may become normal in 40 percent of cases between the time of injury and the first attack. Moreover, the persistence of electrical abnormalities is not always associated with late seizures. He further stated that the risk of late epilepsy in closed head injury is small (2 percent), but rises in patients with localized spikes or waves of ictal discharges during the first weeks (15 percent).

Rodin (1967) recommended serial recordings, the first EEG to be taken as early as possible after injury. Both sleep and wake records were advocated, especially in children. This author pointed out that the initial record was of little value in differentiating between a simple closed injury and a complicating subdural hematoma. Initial improvement in the electroencephalogram with subsequent deterioration, especially in association with focal changes, is suggestive of a subdural clot, abscess or other expanding lesion. Rodin would discourage medicolegal testimony based on a single record.

Lie (1967) analyzed the EEG findings after head trauma in 156 children — 91 boys, 65 girls. Forty-seven percent were injured in traffic accidents and 30 percent at home. Thirty of the 66 patients with abnormalities were followed after six months; of these 8 were unimproved. Of 23 children with minimal trauma, 3 had seizure potentials and 2 "dysrhythmias." One hundred and twenty-three sustained concussion with or without fracture; of these 17 had amplitude asymmetries, 15 had depression of activity, 4 had seizure potentials, and 8 had dysrhythmia.

Naquet et al (1967) studied 100 patients in coma after head trauma. Forty-nine of these presented patterns of natural sleep, second stage. The others showed diffuse abnormalities.

In a series of 1925 cases of head injury in which 2560 electroencephalograms were done, Muller (1969) found that the incidence of abnormality varied depending on the severity of the trauma and the occurrence of localized lesions.

Discussion

EEG changes after head injury depend on a number of factors: severity of the original trauma, the resulting immediate and late structural changes in the brain, and the development of seizures in some cases. Another important factor is the time interval between trauma and test.

The severity of trauma is paralleled in many cases, though not always, by the duration of unconsciousness. Thus concussion may be an indicator, in a statistically significant fashion, of the degree of EEG abnormality to be expected. It correlates well with the degree of clinical abnormality and the incidence of seizures in most large series of cases. However, it was stated at the beginning of this chapter that large groups of hospital cases are of necessity weighted with a relatively high percentage of cases of severe trauma. The incidence of unequivocal EEG abnormality is uniformly high in all reports based on this type of case material.

The author's own series (1943) contained 60 percent abnormal records. The following incidence of abnormalities was reported by others: Greenblatt (1943), 48 percent; Williams (1954), between 60 and 63 percent in his various categories of patients; Peuch, Fischgold, and Verdeaux (1946), up to 70 percent; Kaufman and Walker (1949), 91 percent in cases with posttraumatic seizures and 77 percent in cases without seizures. The mean average of all these figures is 68 percent.

On the other hand, Dow, Ulett, and Raaf (1945) found only 11 percent unequivocally abnormal records in a series of ambulatory patients. Strauss (1956) in a large number of office patients without gross neurological deficit found 20 percent abnormal records on an average, but with 50 percent abnormality in patients below 15 years of age. Høncke (1951), in a series limited to patients with post-concussion syndrome, found only 9 percent grossly abnormal records, most of these having paroxysmal signs. Denker and Perry (1954), in a similar series, all litigation cases, had 55 percent clearly abnormal records.

EEG abnormalities in most large groups consist chiefly of slow wave activity with a high incidence of paroxysmal bursts. Hoefer (1943) found rapid activity in 10 percent and depressed activity in 4 percent, while 86 percent of the cases presented slow wave activity. The incidence of depression of activity was relatively low in this series, which consisted of mostly subacute and chronic cases. In the same series spike-and-wave or spike bursts were found in 14 percent; paroxysmal slow wave bursts occurred in an additional 12 percent. The corresponding figures in Williams' material (1944) are 26 percent total paroxysmal bursts in cases with posttraumatic seizures and 14 percent in cases without seizures. Kaufman and Walker (1949) found a higher incidence of paroxysmal bursts (30 percent) in patients without seizures and only 22 percent in the seizure group. This is contrary to the observations of most other authors.

The findings in subdural hematoma vary. In a small percentage, normal records are seen. Jasper, Kershman, and Elvidge (1940) first described depression of activity over the site of the hematoma. Hoefer (1943) saw focal slow wave discharges in most cases; depression of activity was rare. Rodin, Bickford, and Svien (1953) found slow wave foci in more than half of their cases, depression of activity and alpha asymmetry in the others. Kaplan, Huber, and Browder (1956) observed both abnormalities in their verified material, but depression of activity prevailed in the more severe cases.

Dawson, Webster, and Gurdjian (1951) considered depression of activity more significant than delta foci. Completely universal early depression was considered a sign of grave prognosis. Rodin et al (1965) came to the same conclusion.

Depression of activity as an early finding in cases of skull fracture and laceration of the brain on the side of the injury was reported in several papers.

Improvement of EEG abnormalities in time has been noted by all observers. In some reports normal EEGs have been found when clinical abnormalities persisted. Other authors found persistent EEG abnormality after clinical recovery. Williams (1944) stated that paroxysmal bursts occur three or four times as often in patients with posttraumatic seizures, as in those without convulsions. His material included a small series of posttraumatic cases in which EEGs were obtained before the onset of seizures — an important prognostic consideration. Puech and his co-workers found a high incidence of seizures in patients whose records failed to improve further or else deteriorated, after initial improve-

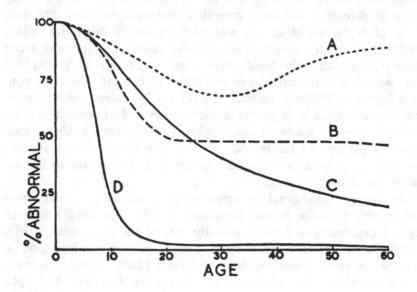

FIG. 16. Incidence of EEG abnormality. (A) Brain tumor; (B) chronic head injury; (C) idiopathic epilepsy; (D) normal. (From *Electroencephalography: A Symposium on its Various Aspects.* Dennis Hill and Geoffrey Parr, eds. Macdonald and Co. Ltd., 1950, p. 227).

The author wishes to thank Macdonald and Co. Ltd. for permission to reproduce Figure 16.

428

ment, three to six months following the injury. Walker (1957) pointed to the fact that posttraumatic seizures may be self-limited in time and advised caution in the use of the EEG alone for prognostication. In the author's own experience a high degree of correlation of EEG and clinical abnormality exists in adults. Most authors agree that EEG abnormalities in children may persist for a long time without major clinical abnormality, but clinical seizures may be expected in at least part of those showing paroxysmal activity in records obtained after the acute phase.

The relatively high incidence of abnormalities in children following head injuries has recently been stressed by several investigators. An abnormality apparently specific for children is the appearance of posterior slow waves, usually symmetrical in distribution. Several authors have found a similarity in pattern between sleep and subsiding posttraumatic coma.

The usefulness of the electroencephalogram is illustrated by Figure 16 which shows the variation with age of the percentage of cases showing abnormality in the EEG. This is based on: (A) 500 cases of verified brain tumor; (B) 1200 cases of chronic head injury; (C) 800 cases of idiopathic epilepsy; and (D) 500 normal subjects. It should be noted that while 25 percent of "normal subjects" show some abnormality, most of these are below the age of ten and that after 20 years of age, practically no abnormalities are found. The overall abnormalities in head injuries are 50 percent but, as several authors have stressed, the figures are much higher for children and teenagers. The probability for paroxysmal patterns in idiopathic epilepsy to appear after the age of 50 is only 25 percent.

BIBLIOGRAPHY

Beaussart, M., Niquet, G., Gaudier, B., and Guislain, F. L'electroencephalogramme enregistré immédiatament après traumatisme cranien dit benin. Etude comparative avec l'examen, effective avant combat, chez 52 boxeurs amateurs. *Press Medicale 68,* 913, 1960.

Busse, E. W. Electroencephalogram Associated with Post-traumatic Headaches (in Patients with Skull Defects). *Dis. Nerv. Syst.,* 8, 299, 1947.

Caveness, W. F. Electroencephalography in Head Injury. *Clinical Neurosurgery.* Baltimore, Williams and Wilkins, 1955.

Chatrian, G. E., White, L. E., Jr., and Daly, D. Electroencephalographic Patterns Resembling Those of Sleep in Certain Comatose States after Injuries to the Head. *EEG. Clin. Neurophysiol.,* 15, 272, 1963.

Clark, E. C. and Harper, E. O. Electroencephalographic Findings in 186 Cases of

Chronic Post-traumatic Encephalopathy. *EEG. Clin. Neurophysiol.,* 3, 9, 1951.

Courjon, J. A. Posttraumatic Epilepsy in Electroclinical Practice. In A. E. Walker, W. F. Caveness, and M. Critchley (Eds.), *The Late Effects of Head Injury.* Springfield, Ill.: Charles C Thomas, 1969. Pp. 215-227.

Cramer, F., Pastor, S., and Stephenson, C. Injuries due to Explosive Waves... "Cerebral Blast Concussion": Pathological, Clinical and Encephalographic Study. *Arch. Neurol. & Psychiat.,* 61, 1, 1949.

Dawson, R. E., Webster, J. W., and Gurdjian, E. S. Serial Electroencephalography in Acute Head Injuries. *J. Neurosurg.,* 8, 613, 1951.

Denker, P. G. and Perry, G. F. Post-concussion Syndrome in Compensation and Litigation: Analysis of 95 Cases with Electroencephalographic Correlation. *Neurology,* 4, 912, 1954.

Dow, R. S., Ulett, G., and Raaf, J. Electroencephalographic Studies in Head Injuries. *J. Neurosurg,* 2, 154, 1945.

Gotze, W. Der Sauerstoffmangelversuch als Provokationsmethode krankhafter hirnelectrischer Befunde bei Hirntraumatikern. *Nervenartz,* 21, 400, 1950.

Greenblatt, M. The Electroencephalogram in Late Post-traumatic Cases. *Am. J. Psychiat.,* 100, 378, 1943.

Gutierrez-Luque, A. G., MacCarty, C. S., and Klass, D. W. Head Injury with Suspected Subdural Hematoma, Effect on EEG. *Arch. Neurol.,* 15, 437, 1966.

Hoefer, P. F. A. The Electroencephalogram in Cases of Head Injury. In S. Brock (Ed.), *Injuries of the Skull, Brain and Spinal Cord.* Baltimore: Williams and Wilkins, 1943.

Høncke, P. Electroencephalography and Post-concussion Syndrome. 4th Internat. Neur. Congress. *Comptes rendus,* Vol. III. Paris: 1949. Pp. 48-52.

Jasper, H. H., Kershman, J., and Elvidge, A. Electroencephalographic Studies of Injuries to the Head. *Arch. Neurol. & Psychiat.,* 44, 328, 1940.

Kaplan, H. A., Huber, W., and Browder, J. Electroencephalogram in Subdural Hematoma. *J. Neuropathol. Exp. Neurol.,* 15, 65, 1956.

Kaufman, I. C. and Walker, A. E. The Electroencephalogram after Head Injury. *J. Nerv. Ment. Dis.,* 109, 383, 1949.

Laufer, M. W. and Perkins, R. F. Study of Electroencephalographic Findings in 209 Cases Admitted as Head Injuries to an Army Neurological-neurosurgical Center. *J. Nerv. Ment. Dis.,* 104, 583, 1946.

Laufer, M. W. and Perkins, R. F. Serial Electroencephalograms in Brain Injury. *J. Nerv. Ment. Dis.,* 106, 619, 1947.

Lenard, H. G. EEG — Veränderungen bei frischen schädeltraumen im kindesalter. *München. Med. Wschr.,* 107, 1820, 1965.

Lie, T. S. Schädelhirntrauma und EEG im Kindesalter. *Zbl. Chir.,* 92, 2458, 1967.

Maltby, G. L. Penetrating Cranio-cerebral Injuries. *J. Neurosurg.,* 3, 239, 1946.

Marmor, J. and Savitsky, N. Electroencephalography in Cases of Head Injury. *Trans. Am. Neurol. Assn.,* 1940. Pp. 30.

Marshall, C. and Walker, A. E. The Value of Electroencephalography in the Prognostication and Diagnosis of Posttraumatic Epilepsy. *Epilepsia,* 2, 138, 1961.

Muller, G. E. Early Clinical History, EEG Controls and Social Outcome in 1925

Head Injury Patients. In A. E. Walker, W. F. Caveness, and M. Critchley (Eds.), *The Late Effects of Head Injury*. Springfield, Ill.: Charles C Thomas, 1969. Pp. 414-422.

Müller, R. Corrélations électroencéphalographiques et cliniques dans les anciens traumatismes cranio-cérébraux fermés avec foyer de contusion corticale en EEG. *EEG. Clin. Neurophysiol.*, 7, 75, 1955.

Naquet, R., Vigouroux, R. P., Choux, M., Baurand, C., and Chamant, J. H. Etude électroencéphalographique des traumatismes craniens récents dans un service de réanimation. *Rev. Neurol.*, 117, 512, 1967.

Peuch, P., Fischgold, H., and Verdeaux, J. Utilization clinique et médicolégale de l'électroencéphalographie dans les traumatismes cranio-cérébraux anciens. *La Semaine des Hôpitaux de Paris*, 22, 1233, 1946.

Rodin, E. A. Contribution of the EEG to Prognosis after Head Injury. *Dis. Nerv. Syst.*, 28, 595, 1967.

Rodin, E. A., Bickford, R. G., and Svien, H. Electroencephalographic Findings Associated with Subdural Hematoma. *Arch. Neurol. & Psychiat.*, 69, 743, 1953.

Rodin, E., Wheland, J., Taylor, R., Tomita, T., Grisell, J., Thomas, L., and Gurdjian, E. The Electroencephalogram in Acute Fatal Head Injuries. *J. Neurosurg.*, 23, 329, 1965.

Roseman, E. and Woodhall, B. The Electroencephalogram in War Wounds of the Brain, with Particular Reference to Post-traumatic Epilepsy. *Res. Publ. A.R.N.M.D.*, 25, 200, 1946.

Silverman, D. Electroencephalographic Study of Acute Head Injury in Children. *Neurology*, 12, 273, 1962.

Strauss, H. The Electroencephalogram in the Evaluation of Head Injuries Without Gross Neurological Deficit. *J. Hillside Hosp.*, 5, 268, 1956.

Torres, F. and Shapiro, S. K. Electroencephalograms in Whiplash Injury. *Arch. Neurol.*, 5, 28, 1961.

Walker, A. E. Prognosis in Post-traumatic Epilepsy. *J.A.M.A.*, 164, 1636, 1957.

Walker, A. E. Post-traumatic Epilepsy. *World Neurol.*, 3, 185, 1962.

Walker, A. E. and Erculei, F. *Head Injured Men. Fifteen Years Later*. Springfield, Ill.: Charles C Thomas, 1969.

Walker, A. E. and Jablon, S. *A Follow-up Study of Head Wounds in World War II*. Veterans Administration Monograph. Washington, D. C.: Superintendant of Documents, U. S. Government Printing Office, 1961.

Weil, A. Electroencephalographic Findings in Post-traumatic Encephalopathy. *Neurology*, 1, 293, 1951.

Williams, D. The Electroencephalogram in Acute Head Injuries. *J. Neurol. & Psychiat.*, 4 (new series), 107, 1941.

Williams, D. The Electroencephalogram in Chronic Post-traumatic States. *J. Neurol. & Psychiat.*, 4 (new series), 131, 1941.

Williams, D. The Electroencephalogram in Traumatic Epilepsy. *J. Neurol. Neurosurg. & Psychiat.*, 7, 103, 1944.

Williams, D. and Gibbs, F. A. Electroencephalography in Clinical Neurology; Its Value in Routine Diagnosis. *Arch. Neurol. & Psychiat.*, 41, 519, 1939.

431

CHAPTER 12

POSTTRAUMATIC BRAIN ABSCESS

JOE PENNYBACKER, M. D., F. R. C. S.

Although improved methods of dealing with head injuries have resulted in a decrease in the number of posttraumatic brain abscesses, they still occur and are a hazard to life and function. In some respects the problems which they present are more difficult than those posed by abscesses due, say, to mastoid or frontal sinus disease, because the damage to the brain at the time of injury creates its own deficits, and it may be difficult to evaluate the changes due to subsequent infection. The common use of antibiotics in the treatment of open wounds, chest infections, etc., may also slow down the tempo of an intracranial infection and to some extent mask the evidence for an abscess. It is prudent to assume that any penetrating wound can cause an abscess, and any departure from the normal recovery process should be viewed in this light.

PREVENTION

Guidance in the proper management of open scalp, skull, and cerebral wounds in the acute stage is presented elsewhere in this volume. In essence this care amounts to thorough cleansing of the wound throughout its depth, with removal of devitalized tissue, bone fragments, foreign bodies, and blood clot, followed by accurate closure of the scalp. Bacteriological culture should be made at the time so that appropriate antiobiotics can be used subsequently, if there is any question of infection. If these measures are employed meticulously it is possible to prevent practically all brain abscesses as a complication of head injuries. Thus in the accident service of the Radcliffe Infirmary, Oxford, there has not been such an abscess among the last 10,000 head injuries, although, of course, not all of these had open wounds. On the other hand, we occasionally see patients such as the girl depicted in Figure 1, who was sent to the Radcliffe Infirmary ten days after a

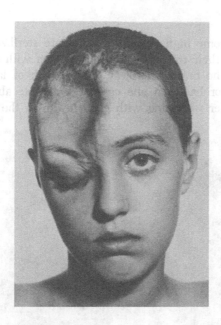

Fig. 1. Deformity consequent to excision of compound depressed fracture of frontal bone with acute cerebritis of frontal lobe.

severe compound depressed fracture of the right frontal bone had been treated in another hospital. She presented with a large boggy swelling of the scalp, and purulent brain was exuding through the suture line at several points. She was stuporous with the clinical features of meningitis, attested by some 2570 cells in the cerebrospinal fluid. A staphylococcus aureus was cultured from the cerebrospinal fluid. The infected skin edges were excised, and the necrotic frontal lobe containing pockets of staphylococcal pus, clot, and bone fragments sucked out until normal-looking white matter was reached. The resulting cavity was bathed in penicillin and the wound closed accurately. It healed by primary union and convalescence was uneventful but for the considerable physical deformity and disturbance of mentality consequent to the injury and the infection.

ETIOLOGY

Brain abscesses due to injury usually result from the direct implantation of organisms. Thus, non-lethal missile wounds may be followed by abscess formation, although it is remarkable that not all of them are. Presumably some high velocity missiles are sterilized by the heat generated during their trajectory, but any person with a retained missile fragment in the brain is subject to some risk of late abscess formation. The author has seen one case of a chronic abscess declaring itself 16 years after wounding with good health in the interval.

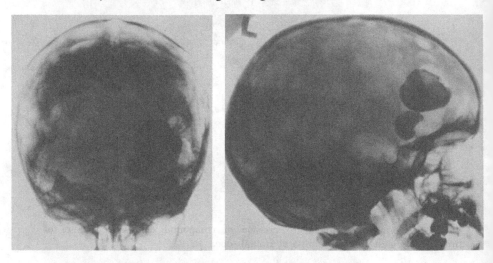

FIG. 2A, B. Multiloculated abscess of left frontal lobe (outlined by a contrast substance — thorotrast).

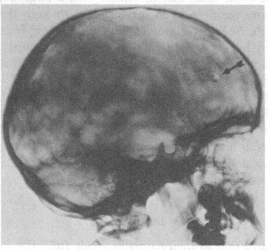

FIG. 3. Same case as Fig. 2 a and b. Plain x-ray showing cranial defect caused by penetrating wound (arrow).

In civilian life, any object sharp enough to pierce the skull can cause an abscess. The comparatively soft skulls of children are, of course, more vulnerable, and common objects such as knitting needles, scissors, pencils, or even flying splinters of wood can implant infection. Figure 2 shows a lobulated abscess in a child of seven who was watching his father chop wood and was struck by a splinter in the left frontal region just behind the hair line. There was a small puncture wound in the scalp, but the child did not appear to be hurt in any way and carried on with his normal activities for five days. Then, after he had a fit at school, he was admitted to the hospital where the puncture wound in the scalp was found to be infected, and x-rays (Fig. 3) showed an underlying penetrating wound of the skull.

A more obvious source of infection is an open wound of the scalp or skull as occurs in compound fractures, especially one in which the dura is torn and the underlying brain is exposed or lacerated. But it should be remembered that intracranial suppuration (extradural or subdural abscess, meningitis, or intracerebral abscess) can result from an infected scalp wound even though the skull is intact. In such cases the infection enters the cranial cavity by way of emissary veins (infectious thrombophlebitis). In other cases the scalp infection causes an underlying focal osteitis which in turn leads to intracranial infection. Thus, it is important that scalp wounds be treated properly initially, and that if they do become infected, they be treated energetically with these possibilities being borne in mind.

There is one rare type of abscess in which prevention is more difficult. Some cases of apparently closed head injury may be shown radiographically to have fractures involving the accessory air sinuses. It is well known that such fractures are often associated with cerebrospinal rhinorrhea, and the risk of meningitis is usually accepted as an indication for closure of the fistula. Occasionally such fractures are not accompanied by overt rhinorrhea, but even so they provide access for organisms to reach the brain and cause a brain abscess. The angiograms in Figure 4 relate to a boy of 14 who in September, 1962, sustained a linear fracture of the frontal bone in a motorcycle accident. The fracture extended into the left frontal sinus, but there was no rhinorrhea or aerocele and convalescence was uneventful. He remained well for six months, and then had a mild frontal sinus infection which led to meningitis and, although this responded clinically to antibiotics, the cerebrospinal fluid continued to show an increase of cells (30 per cu mm) and a slight excess of protein. He was admitted because of the

435

possibility of a chronic brain abscess, and although he looked very well, denied any symptoms, and had no significant neurological deficit — in particular no aphasia — the electroencephalogram revealed a delta wave focus in the left frontal region. An angiogram (Fig 4 a and b) showed a large avascular mass which proved to be a chronic abscess containing 100 cc of pus. It was treated by aspiration and was ultimately excised.

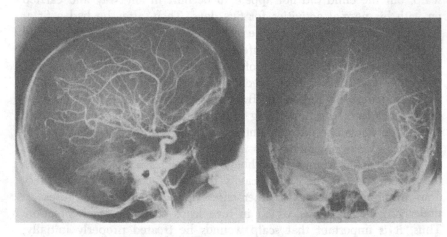

Fig. 4A, B. Left carotid arteriograms revealing displacement of anterior and middle cerebral arteries caused by a left frontal lobe abscess.

Some surgeons feel that this complication could be avoided by a uniform policy of operating on all skull fractures which involve the accessory air sinuses (frontal, ethmoid, and mastoid), whether or not there is any evidence of cerebrospinal rhinorrhea or aerocele, the two certain features of a fistula which indicate that organisms may have access to the cranial cavity. The author's view is that this policy would entail many "prophylactic" operations which in themeselves are not devoid of risk, and that in a civilized community it should be possible to diagnose and treat posttraumatic meningitis in the event this occurs. If meningitis develops, appropriate tests should be done to exclude the presence of an abscess.

Apart from skull fractures involving the frontal and ethmoidal sinuses or the mastoid, and leading to cerebrospinal rhinorrhea or otorrhea, a head injury without fracture may cause an infection in one of these cavities, or "light up" a preexisting chronic infection with the same

436

potentialities for intracranial extension as in non-traumatic cases. Thus, pain in relation to the sinuses or mastoid, or edema of the overlying scalp, requires investigation. It may be tempting to ascribe it to "the effects of injury" when in fact something more sinister is happening.

Finally, infection may reach the brain by the bloodstream from a distant focus such as the lungs or an infected wound in some other part of the body. Such a complication differs in no important way from blood-borne abscesses in non-traumatic cases.

PATHOLOGY

When pyogenic organisms reach the brain their first effect is to produce local necrosis and liquefaction. If they arrive in an already damaged and devitalized area, deprived of natural defenses, they proliferate rapidly and cause a diffuse "cerebritis" as in the first patient described. The affected part of the brain is swollen, soft, diffluent, and may contain little pockets of pus. There is little evidence of any natural effort to limit the infection and, in the pre-antibiotic era, most patients with this complication died within a few days of the injury; almost all of them had meningitis in addition to the cerebral infection. Nowadays with better primary treatment of head wounds and the common use of antibiotics, the tempo of the infection is slowed and defense mechanisms may have time to operate. Pari passu with the formation of pus there is a glial and vascular reaction around the infected area which tends to wall off the infection, and in time to allow the formation of a capsule around the abscess. The beginnings of en-capsulation may be seen as early as a week or ten days after injury and, although the abscess may continue to enlarge, the capsule becomes tougher, and by the end of five to six weeks may be 1 to 2 mm thick. There is some edema of the surrounding brain, and what with this and the increasing bulk of the abscess, the clinical effects of a rapidly growing tumor are reproduced. Thus there is evidence of increased intracranial pressure and of a progressive neurological deficit depending on the site of the abscess. In most cases, if the abscess is not treated it continues to increase in size until it causes death from in-creased pressure, or it ruptures into a cerebral ventricle or into the subarachnoid space to cause an overwhelming infection. It is possible that occasionally a small abscess may empty itself into the subarach-noid space and cause meningitis, which responds to treatment. It is also possible for an abscess to progress up to a point and then remain

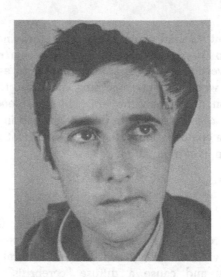

Fig. 5. Cerebral hernia due to posttraumatic brain abscess of left temporal lobe after debridement of compound fracture.

static, acquiring a thicker capsule as time goes on. Such abscesses may declare themselves months or years after the injury, and indeed some have been removed in the belief that they were solid neoplasms causing epilepsy, hemiparesis, and the like. Occasionally the capsule of a chronic abscess becomes calcified, and it would be easy to mistake this for calcification in a tumor if the possibility of an abscess is forgotten.

Two other pathological features should be mentioned. If there is a defect in the skull, e.g., if a number of comminuted fragments have been removed, the bulk of the abscess and the surrounding edema may force the brain out through the defect and produce a subcutaneous swelling, a cerebral hernia (Fig. 5). If the scalp is also deficient, the surface of the brain is exposed. If the patient survives long enough, this becomes covered with granulation tissue and is known as a cerebral fungus.

Almost any organism can cause an abscess, but the common ones are staphylococci, streptococci and pneumococci. Frequently there is a mixed infection with these and gram-negative organisms and, occasionally, gas-forming organisms which will produce a bubble visible in ordinary x-rays of the skull.

438

As with brain tumors, brain abscesses produce two groups of symptoms and signs: 1) the general effects of increased intracranial pressure, and 2) the local neurologic effects. Characteristic of the first group are headache, vomiting, incontinence, mental slowing, stupor, and coma. Most of these are common symptoms after a head injury, and to this extent it may be difficult to evaluate them in relation to the onset of infection. Speaking generally, however, if a person survives the immediate effects of an injury, the trend thereafter should be in the direction of improvement. If this is not the case, the possibility of a progressive lesion, whether vascular (e.g., a hematoma) or infectious, has to be considered. If there has been a penetrating or other kind of open wound of the scalp or skull, the likelihood of infection is enhanced. Fever and other systemic evidence of infection may be absent during the development of an abscess unless there is associated meningitis or sepsis elsewhere in the body. But help may be obtained from examination of the cerebrospinal fluid, since most brain abscesses are attended by an increase in the protein and cellular content of the fluid. As with the clinical features, it may also be difficult to evaluate these changes in the early days after an injury because of blood in the fluid. For this reason, the author thinks it advisable to do a lumbar puncture two or three days after an open injury so as to have a base line by means of which subsequent developments can be assessed.

Apart from the symptoms and signs of increased intracranial pressure mentioned above, there may be other objective evidence. If there is a defect in the skull and dura, the scalp may bulge due to the underlying cerebral herniation. If the dura is intact, papilledema may develop in time, but it should be stressed that this is not always the case; as with neoplasm, a brain abscess may cause death from increased intracranial pressure without any pathological changes in the optic fundi. The pressure of the cerebrospinal fluid as measured by lumbar puncture is usually elevated, and if the fluid is being withdrawn for analysis, as suggested above, the pressure should always be measured.

Another frequent feature of the genesis of a brain abscess is epilepsy. But again, epileptic attacks are not uncommon after head injuries in which there is contusion or laceration of the brain, or indeed simply subarachnoid hemorrhage. Nevertheless the onset of fits after a penetrating or other kind of open wound should cause some concern.

The focal neurological deficit depends on the location of the abscess;

439

characteristically, it is progressive. This is the important reason for determining the extent of the deficit as soon as possible after the injury so that a base line is established. There may be deficits of course, such as hemiparesis and aphasia, due to the injury. Some of these may persist if neurons and fiber tracts have been irreparably damaged. Others due to contusion may improve for a time and then regress as an abscess develops.

Abscesses in the frontal lobe may be remarkably silent, as in the third patient described (Fig. 4). In the speech-dominant hemisphere, slight manifestations of aphasia may be detected (and it should be remembered that disturbances of the language function are frequently mistaken for dementia, confusion, or delusions). Apathy, sullenness, and other alterations of personality are also common, but may be difficult to evaluate because of the injury. As the abscess expands it may involve the motor pathway and produce a progressive hemiparesis.

Abscesses in the parietal lobe produce defects in sensibility, often remarkably slight and affecting only the cortical modalities, e.g., discriminative sense, stereognosis, and the like, while crude sensation such as the ability to feel a pinprick may be preserved. The sensory examination of a patient who has had a severe head injury and is developing a brain abscess may be very difficult, but one feature which is very important and may be detected by a simple test is a lower quadrant homonymous hemianopia on the side opposite to the lesion. This is due to interruption of the upper fibers of the optic radiation as they traverse the parietal lobe. When the abscess is in the dominant hemisphere, aphasia is common.

Abscesses of the speech-dominant temporal lobe are usually accompanied by aphasia, and a homonymous upper quadrant hemianopia on the opposite side. The visual field defect is due to involvement of the lower fibers of the optic radiation as they sweep into the temporal lobe on their way to the lower lip of the calcarine fissure in the occipital lobe. In the non-dominant temporal lobe, this quadrantanopia may be the only sign, although as the abscess expands upwards it may involve the lower part of the motor cortex, producing first weakness of the opposite side of the face, then of the upper limb, and finally of the lower limb.

In the occipital lobes, an abscess may cause only a contralateral homonymous hemianopia, but in the dominant hemisphere, aphasia is common, and as the abscess expands there may be defects in sensation on the opposite side of the body.

Traumatic abscesses of the cerebellum are rare. When they do occur, the neurologic abnormalities are usually florid and unmistakable: nystagmus, which is slow and coarse on looking to the side of the lesion and more rapid and finer on looking to the opposite side, gross ataxia of the limbs on the side of the lesion, with hypotonia and dysdiadoko-kinesis, dysarthria, and dysphagia. Vertigo and vomiting are often early symptoms before these gross abnormalities are apparent.

DIAGNOSIS

For reasons set out above, it may be very difficult to evaluate the clinical features in a patient who has had a head injury and is developing an abscess. The essential feature is evidence of worsening at a stage when, in an uncomplicated injury, there should be improvement. The worsening may be in the general state, and it may be so subtle as to be hardly apparent from day to day. Or it may be that existing neurologic deficits become more marked, or that deficits appear for the first time. These are all manifestations of a progressive lesion, and the problem usually is that of deciding whether it is a vascular lesion (e.g., a subdural hematoma, cerebral thrombosis, etc.) or infective, e.g., an abscess. It should also be mentioned that in most neurosurgical clinics there are two or three cases a year in which a head injury calls attention to a brain tumor, and this possibility should be remembered.

As noted above, a developing abscess need not be accompanied by such systemic evidence of infection as fever, leucocytosis, and increase in the erythrocyte sedimentation rate. But almost always there is evidence of infection in the cerebrospinal fluid witnessed by an increase in the cellular and protein content. And there are other special diagnostic techniques which will usually provide the requisite information as to the nature and location of the lesion.

Plain x-rays of the skull are essential. They may reveal an unsuspected penetrating wound of the skull in what had been thought to be a simple scalp wound, as in the second case described (Fig. 3). Or, they may disclose a fracture involving one of the accessory air sinuses, with the attendant risks of meningitis, aerocele, and abscess as in the third case mentioned earlier. At a later stage, they may reveal retained bone fragments or foreign bodies in a wound thought to have been thoroughly debrided. Or, after three or four weeks there may be evidence of osteitis in relation to a fracture or in relation to an infected

441

scalp wound with an intact skull. Rarely, a bubble of gas may be seen in an abscess. If the pineal gland is calcified, displacement from the midline is good evidence of an expanding lesion in one hemisphere, but the fact that the pineal gland is in its normal position can not be taken as evidence that an expanding lesion is not present. This also applies to echoencephalography: If there is displacement of midline structures, there may be an expanding lesion in one hemisphere, but a midline echo does not exclude such a lesion.

Electroencephalography may provide useful information, although the record may be difficult to assess because of the effects of the injury. Repeated recordings in the hands of an expert may show evidence of a progressive lesion however. Similarly, isotope scans may reveal an abnormal uptake which may indicate either an abscess, a hematoma, or an area of infarction.

The most certain evidence of a space-occupying lesion is provided by contrast radiography — ventriculography or angiography. Angiography is probably the safer and more informative procedure — safer because it does not usually alter the pressure relationships within the cranium, and more informative because it usually reveals the precise site of the lesion. Ventriculography, whether the gas is introduced by lumbar puncture or direct puncture of the ventricles, may precipitate a crisis and should only be undertaken when surgical facilities are immediately available. It is sometimes the case that the ventricle in the affected hemisphere is so compressed by the abscess and associated edema that it is only possible to say that there is a space-occupying lesion in the hemisphere without evidence of its precise site.

For these reasons most surgeons prefer angiography for the primary investigation, but there are cases in which this may have to be followed by ventriculography for additional information.

In a suspected case of brain abscess the angiogram may reveal an avascular space-occupying lesion, which might be an abscess, a cystic tumor, or a hematoma and it may be that evidence for infection can only be obtained by examination of the cerebrospinal fluid. Rarely, as noted above, the angiogram may show the pathological circulation in an unsuspected tumor which has caused symptoms only after a head injury. Occasionally, it indicates some other pathological process such as dilatation of a part or the whole of the ventricular system from obstruction to the circulation of the cerebrospinal fluid, and it is in such cases that ventriculography may be required for further information.

Not all of the techniques mentioned above will be available in every

442

hospital. The two that will be of most help are examination of the cerebrospinal fluid and angiography.

TREATMENT

When the diagnosis has been made and the site of the abscess is known, the pus should be evacuated. Most surgeons nowadays prefer to do this by aspiration, repeated if necessary, rather than by continuous tube drainage as with abscesses in some other parts of the body. The reason is that tubes tend to become blocked, and thus act as plugs rather than drains. A burr hole is made at the site where the abscess is thought to most nearly approach the surface of the brain, a small incision is made in the dura, and a blunt brain cannula is passed carefully into the abscess. There is often a perceptible "give" when the cannula enters the abscess, and it should then be held absolutely steady. Gentle suction with a rubber bulb (Dakin) syringe is applied until all of the pus is evacuated. The cannula should not be moved to seek more pus, but rather while it is still in the collapsed cavity, a solution of penicillin (500,000 units in 2 cc) should be instilled. At the same time 2 cc of Steripaque (a suspension of barium sulphate) should be instilled for subsequent radiographic control. The cannula is then withdrawn and the scalp wound closed in the usual way. The bacteriology of the pus should be established as soon as possible, so that appropriate antibiotic treatment can be given systemically and topically if further aspirations of the abscess are required.

The initial aspiration of pus usually brings about a marked improvement. If there is headache, it is relieved to a large extent if not completely; if there is stupor, the patient becomes more alert; and if there are neurologic deficits, these become less marked — presuming that the deficits are due to the local pressure of the abscess and not to destruction of neurons and tracts. In some cases, a simple aspiration suffices, but more commonly it has to be repeated on several occasions. The indications for so doing are: 1) worsening of the general and neurological status, i.e., recrudescence of the symptoms and signs which led to the initial aspiration; and 2) radiographic evidence of expansion of the abscess. The Steripaque-filled cavity is usually crenated or crumpled-looking in x-rays taken immediately after an aspiration, and as pus reaccumulates, it assumes a more rounded contour and increases in size. This may not be accompanied by significant worsening of the general or neurologic status, but even so a further aspiration should be done. If a second aspiration is necessary within two or three days, it can be done with a blunt brain cannula introduced through the scalp wound, but thereafter it is preferable to use a sharp lumbar puncture needle with a fairly wide bore, such as the Greenfield needle. The needle should be introduced into the cavity and held perfectly still until as much pus as possible has been aspirated. The appropriate antibiotic should then be instilled, and if necessary, more Steripaque, before the needle is withdrawn.

There is one qualification that needs to be made about this method of treatment. Occasionally during an aspiration, the character of the pus alters and becomes watery. This usually means that a thin septum between the abscess and the lateral ventricle has ruptured and allowed the entrance of cerebrospinal fluid into the abscess cavity. It also means that pus may escape into the ventricular system, but this does not always happen because the fistula may seal off before the tension in the abscess has risen again. In these circumstances, however, it is important not to inject anything into the abscess, either a concentrated solution of antibiotic or Steripaque, which may get into the ventricular system with serious consequences. Lumbar punctures should be done at daily intervals to see whether there is any evidence of infection of the ventricular and subarachnoid systems, and if so, this should be treated by making burr holes to allow for intraventricular treatment with antibiotics, as well as by their instillation into the lumbar theca. Ventriculitis and meningitis are serious complications of a brain abscess, but they are not invariably fatal nowadays.

The treatment of abscesses by repeated aspiration is based on the assumption that the abscess contains only one loculus. Unfortunately this is not always the case. There may be two or more loculi. In some cases, as in that illustrated in Figure 2, the loculi may communicate with one another so that aspiration of one loculus will reach all. In others there is no such communication, and it is possible to treat one loculus effectively while others are continuing to expand. In such cases, despite encouraging progress of the known loculus as seen in x-rays, the patient continues to get worse. If that is so, another burr hole should be made close to the original one to allow exploratory aspiration in the vicinity of the known loculus. If another loculus is found, it should be treated along the same lines as the first one. If no pus is found, and the patient continues to get worse, angiography or ventriculography may provide the necessary information. If not, and the patient is suffering from increased intracranial pressure, a decom-

444

pressive craniotomy (osteoplastic flap) should be made over the site of the known abscess. Inspection of the exposed surface of the brain may indicate the site of the undetected loculus, but if not, the decompressive procedure in itself may save the patient's life until the abscess declares itself more eloquently.

In the majority of cases, however, the abscess will resolve with one or more aspirations. The patient improves in all respects and x-rays show the cavity to have become a small crenated mass of radiopaque material. Before pronouncing a cure, however, it is as well to have two further tests: 1) the cerebrospinal fluid should have reverted to normal; and 2) an air encephalogram should show that there is no residual or undetected loculus.

In some cases, the abscess keeps re-collecting and requires multiple aspirations. When this occurs, many surgeons feel that it is preferable to excise it by an open operation, much as with a solid neoplasm (Fig. 6). The capsule of the abscess is tough enough to make this feasible within five to six weeks of the onset of the infection, and if for any reason it is imperative to do it before then, the escape of pus during the removal is not disastrous. A solution of the appropriate antibiotic should be left in the cavity from which the abscess has been removed, and it is prudent to give intrathecal treatment by lumbar puncture for a few days afterwards.

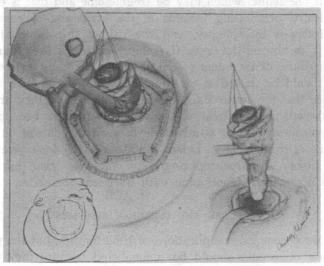

FIG. 6. Craniotomy and excision of left frontal abscess depicted in Fig. 2.

445

Even with the modern refinements of diagnosis and treatment described above, brain abscesses are sometimes fatal. Most commonly this is due to rupture of the abscess into the ventricular system or subarachnoid space resulting in a fulminating ventriculitis and meningitis. As mentioned above, all that can be done in these circumstances is to make burr holes to allow intensive intraventricular treatment with antibiotics and to support this with intrathecal treatment, by the lumbar route. Hope should not be abandoned until the patient's last gasp because the author has seen patients with thick pus in both ventricles who have made good recoveries.

If the patient does recover, the functional result will depend on the site of the abscess and how much of the cerebrum has been involved in the initial trauma and the complicating abscess. Thus, if an abscess in the Rolandic region has caused a hemiplegia, the patient is apt to be left with some weakness, possibly less than at the height of his illness because some of the deficit may be due to pressure of the abscess and edema around it rather than to destruction. Similarly, an abscess in the vicinity of the speech-dominant Sylvian fissure may leave the patient with some degree of dysphasia. But recovery from abscesses in less eloquent areas such as the frontal lobes or the non-dominant temporal lobe may be practically complete and allow the patient to return to a full and active life.

There is one sequel which may be troublesome and that is epilepsy. Uncomplicated penetrating wounds of the brain are, of course, frequently followed by epilepsy, and the risk of this is certainly not lessened if an abscess develops. If epilepsy manifests itself during the genesis or course of treatment of the abscess, a vigorous anticonvulsant regimen should be started in an effort to control the attacks, as there is evidence that the fewer the attacks the more likely they are to be controlled with medical treatment. Even if there have been no overt epileptic manifestations, it is advisable to keep the patient on a mild anticonvulsant regimen (e.g., Dilantin, 100 mg b.i.d.) for a year or two after the injury. Electroencephalography may give some information as to the necessity for continuing with treatment thereafter.

EXTRADURAL AND SUBDURAL ABSCESSES

These are uncommon complications of head injuries, but the possibility of their occurrence should be remembered because they may be difficult to diagnose and they have serious potentialities.

446

The commonest cause of an extradural abscess following a head injury is an infection of a scalp wound and of the underlying bone. Extradural collections of pus are usually more indolent and less eloquent than cerebral abscesses, and may not declare themselves until two or three weeks after the injury. There is usually local pain and tenderness at the site of the bony infection, but as more pus collects between the inner table of the skull and the dura, cerebral compression begins and the patient complains of generalized headache. As the volume of pus increases, focal neurologic deficits such as hemiplegia and aphasia may appear. The diagnosis can be made by angiography, which indicates an extracerebral collection which may be either extradural or subdural, but in either case a burr hole is called for. If it is an extradural adbscess pus will be encountered as soon as the inner table of the skull is breached. The pus is aspirated, and one or two small tubes are left in the cavity for the instillation of the appropriate antibiotic for four or five days. This is usually all that is required, although ıı the skull infection has led to sequestrum formation, a limited cranieo-tomy may be necessary.

Subdural abscesses are more serious: indeed in the pre-antibiotic era they were almost invariably fatal. They may result from a blood-borne infection from a distant source of sepsis, from suppuration in the accessory air sinuses or – in relation to trauma – from infected scalp and skull wounds. The author has seen one case, and has heard of others, in which a subdural abscess resulted from infection of the small scalp and skull wounds entailed in the application of calipers for skull traction in the treatment of spinal injuries. In terms of pathology the lesion is a collection of pus in the subdural space. It may be a thin and localized film at one extreme, to a layer of pus one or two centimeters thick disposed over the whole of one or both hemispheres including the medial surface and the base of the brain. Common symptoms are headache and general malaise, epilepsy, and various neurologic deficits such as hemiplegia and aphasia, depending on the area of the brain affected. The neurologic symptoms are usually due to cortical thrombophlebitis rather than to pressure, although with large volumes of pus, cerebral compression may be a factor. Examination of the cerebrospinal fluid may show evidence of infection manifested by an increase in the protein and cell content, but it is remarkable that with only the thin arachnoid membrane separating the pus from the cerebrospinal fluid, the changes in the fluid may be very slight and, in some cases, the fluid is perfectly normal.

447

The diagnosis may be made by angiography — as with extradural abscesses, there is evidence of an extracerebral collection. But with a thin film of pus, this may not be apparent, and the angiogram may appear to be quite normal. In such cases, and when there is a suspicion of a subdural abscess, multiple burr holes may have to be made before the pus is discovered. When this has been done two or three more burr holes are made over the abscess, as much pus as possible aspirated, and then two or three fine rubber tubes are inserted in various directions in the subdural space. These are not so much for drainage as for the instillation of the appropriate antibiotics, usually penicillin, when the bacteriology of the pus is known. As an example, a subdural abscess disposed over the anterior half of one cerebral hemisphere may require three burr holes, and eight or nine tubes in the subdural space. Into each of these a solution of penicillin (4000 units in 2 cc) is instilled every 4 hours for five days, every 6 hours for the next three days, and then every 8 hours for two days. Systemic treatment with antibiotics should be given from the outset, and it is advisable to give intrathecal treatment by the lumbar route as well. If the patient improves, all of the tubes can be removed by the tenth or eleventh day. The results of this regimen depend on the sensitivity of the organism to antibiotics and on the stage at which the diagnosis is made and treatment instituted. In late cases, when both hemispheres are bathed in pus, not only on the superolateral but also on the medial surfaces and at the base of the brain, treatment is unlikely to be effective.

CHAPTER 13

POSTTRAUMATIC MENINGITIS

EMANUEL APPELBAUM, M. D.

AND

CHARLES ABLER, M. D.

The increasing frequency of accidents makes it necessary to direct particular attention to the intracranial complications that may follow trauma. While posttraumatic meningitis occurs infrequently, it nonetheless assumes great importance, since it constitutes a serious complication of injuries to the head and face.

CLINICAL ASPECTS

Nature of the Trauma. It is well known that in many, if not most, instances of posttraumatic meningitis, the injury involves the frontal region of the head, resulting in fistulous communications which permit the entrance of organisms from the paranasal sinuses into the cranial cavity. In such cases fractures involving the frontal sinus or the floor of the anterior fossae of the skull (ethmoid sinuses), often in association with cerebrospinal fluid rhinorrhea, are commonly present. Less often the sphenoid sinus or petrous bone is implicated. The occurrence of cerebrospinal fluid rhinorrhea renders the meninges particularly vulnerable to infection. Fractures through the cribriform plate, where the dura is firmly adherent, may lead to meningeal involvement if there is a wide defect between fragments or displacement of pieces of bone through the dura. While complete healing of a dural tear may occur, in many cases the fracture line becomes covered only by a thin layer of fibrous and vascular tissue, the dural margins remaining adherent to the bony defect. The mucosal lining of the sinus may become attached to the dural margins or to brain tissue. Not uncommonly the defect will be found to contain a projection of dura or herniated brain tissue. Obviously this type of repair is imperfect and constitutes an

449

ineffective barrier against infection, even after a lapse of several years.

On occasion, an osseous defect produced as a result of chronic osteomyelitis in the region of the paranasal sinuses or petrous bone leads to cerebrospinal fluid rhinorrhea or otorrhea and, eventually, meningitis. At times, a skull fracture is followed by purulent otitis and mastoiditis or suppurative sinus thrombosis with subsequent meningeal infection. A fracture across a chronically infected mastoid, associated with an inflamed dura, may lead to meningitis even in the absence of a dural tear. Rarely meningitis may be brought about by spontaneous rupture of a posttraumatic abscess, or it may follow surgical intervention.

There are instances in which no fistulous tract can be demonstrated between the cranial cavity and the accessory nasal sinuses or ear, the adhesions at the site of trauma presumably serving as a pathway for infection.

The time interval between trauma and the onset of meningitis varies considerably. In a series of 91 cases of posttraumatic meningitis studied by the authors, the interval ranged from several hours to five years. In the majority of our cases, meningitis developed within two weeks following trauma. There are several case reports on the occurrence of meningitis 10 to 16 years after injury.

Symptomatology. While individual patients show considerable variation in the severity of the disease, most appear critically ill. Fever is uniformly present and headache, vomiting, and convulsions are quite common. Signs of meningeal irritation and a change in sensorium are almost always evident. Occasionally, however, the mental state is unaffected. There is fairly frequent involvement of the cranial nerves, particularly the second, third, sixth, and seventh. Monoplegia and hemiparesis are encountered occasionally. Bulging of the fontanel is an important sign in infants. Early in the course of the disease the tendon reflexes are apt to be brisk. Later they may become unequal, diminished and finally lost. The fundi often show congestion of the discs and, at times, papilledema. Cerebrospinal fluid rhinorrhea or otorrhea may be demonstrable. The presence of rhinorrhea is generally indicative of a fracture involving the frontal, ethmoidal, or sphenoidal sinuses. As previously noted, the risk of meningeal infection is considerably enhanced in the presence of rhinorrhea. However, there is no definite relationship between the time of the appearance of rhinorrhea and the time of the onset of meningitis.

Cerebrospinal Fluid. The analysis of the cerebrospinal fluid is the most important laboratory procedure in making a diagnosis of meningitis. The fluid is practically always under increased pressure and is usually cloudy. In some instances the fluid is bloody or xanthochromic. A clear or slightly hazy fluid may be found very rarely within the first 24 hours of onset and occasionally in cases of fulminating meningitis. The cells are usually greatly increased in number with a large preponderance of polymorphonuclear leucocytes. In our series, the cell count ranged between 210 and 11,000 cells per cubic millimeter. As patients improve the number of cells in the cerebrospinal fluid decreases, and the proportion of mononuclear cells increases. It is important that the differential cell count be done on a stained smear and not on the counting chamber.

The cerebrospinal fluid protein is increased to varying degrees. In our laboratory, 40 mg of protein per 100 cc of cerebrospinal fluid is regarded as the upper limit of normal. The sugar in the cerebrospinal fluid may be normal at the onset of meningitis. As the disease progresses, the amount of sugar usually decreases markedly or disappears entirely. With subsidence of the meningeal infection, the sugar returns to normal. The normal range of sugar in the cerebrospinal fluid is from 40 to 80 mg per 100 cc and may be higher in diabetic patients. It should be emphasized that a determination of the blood sugar level is essential to a correct interpretation of the cerebrospinal fluid sugar content, especially in borderline cases and in diabetic patients.

The bacteriologic study is by far the most important part of the cerebrospinal fluid examination. In many cases, varying numbers of organisms will be found in the smear. It has been our experience, however, that the stained smear alone is unreliable in the diagnosis of purulent meningitis, since the organisms often appear pleomorphic and irregular. It is necessary to base the diagnosis on the results of the culture of the fluid or on the identification of the organisms directly from the cerebrospinal fluid by the quellung reaction. The latter involves a swelling of the organism's capsule produced by a type-specific antiserum. It should be added that the test is useful only for the identification of pneumococcus, meningococcus, *H. Influenzae,* and Klebsiella.

Organisms Isolated from the Spinal Fluid in 91 Cases of Posttraumatic Meningitis

Organisms	No. of Cases
Pneumococcus	47
Streptococcus hemolyticus	11
Streptococcus viridans	2
Streptococcus gamma	1
Hemophilus influenzae	14
Meningococcus	9
Staphylococcus	5
Klebsiella pneumoniae	1
Listeria monocytogenes	1
Total	91

The accompanying table lists the causative organisms isolated in our cases of posttraumatic meningitis. It is obvious that the pneumococcus predominates as the etiologic agent in this form of meningitis. Reports from the literature show a distribution of organisms similar to that noted in our series. On rare occasions the meningitis may be caused by more than one organism, or by other, less common bacteria; at times the cause may remain undetermined because of a sterile cerebrospinal fluid.

Other Tests. Several other useful laboratory procedures are available. A blood culture should always be performed on every patient with pyogenic meningitis, since the etiologic agent can sometimes be recovered from the blood when the cerebrospinal fluid culture is sterile. In occasional cases of meningococcic meningitis, the organisms may be isolated from hemorrhagic skin lesions, the nasopharynx, the conjunctivae, or joint exudate.

In this connection it is pertinent to direct attention to the meningococcus agglutination test. In 1944, Falk and Appelbaum described a simple method for demonstrating agglutinins in the serum of individuals suffering from meningococcic infection. In subsequent studies, these authors found agglutinins in significant titers for one or more of the types of meningococci in a high percentage of bacteriologically proven cases of meningococcic infection as well as in clinically typical cases in which bacteriologic verification was otherwise lacking. Agglutinins were observed more regularly during the subacute than during the acute phase and reached their maximum titers early in the convalescent period. As recovery progressed, there was a decrease in the agglutinin titer. It thus became apparent that for optimum results

452

successive specimens must be tested during the various phases of the disease. When such serial tests were made on three or more specimens, the incidence of positive results exceeded 95 percent. These studies indicated the usefulness of the meningococcus agglutination test as a diagnostic procedure in cases of clinically typical meningococcic infection which lacked bacteriologic proof. The importance of performing serial tests to demonstrate the changes in the agglutinin titer cannot be overemphasized.

It is also advisable to make a roentgenogram of the skull in order to determine the presence, location, and type of fracture. Occasionally the roentgenogram will show the presence of air in the subdural or subarachnoid space, or in the ventricles. In cases in which there is a past history of trauma, it may be difficult to demonstrate a fracture, though this may be quite apparent at operation or at necropsy. In other instances the line of fracture may remain distinct for many months or even years.

The blood picture generally shows a leucocytosis, ranging from 13,000 to 30,000 white blood cells, with a predominance of polymorphonuclear leucocytes.

TREATMENT

The general treatment of meningitis is much the same as that of any other severe acute infectious disease. The patient should be kept absolutely quiet; restlessness and sleeplessness are controlled by appropriate sedation. Continued vomiting may cause dehydration, in which case the parenteral administration of physiologic solution of sodium chloride is indicated. There is evidence that acute hyponatremia may develop in some cases, accentuating the tendency toward vomiting and restlessness and even inducing convulsions. Such cases require a reduction in fluid intake. The nutrition of the patient must be supported by adequate nourishment, preferably in small amounts at frequent intervals.

Antibiotics and Chemotherapy

Prior to the advent of chemotherapy, many types of meningitis were almost invariably fatal. The introduction of sulfonamides and, subsequently, of the various antibiotics has resulted in a striking reduction in the mortality rate of such infections. Since specific drug therapy

453

varies with the etiologic agent, it is best discussed separately for each bacteriologic variety of meningitis.

Pneumococcic Meningitis. Penicillin is considered the drug of choice in the treatment of pneumococcic meningitis. However, there has been considerable difference of opinion regarding the need of administering the antibiotic intrathecally as well as systemically. Much light has been shed on this problem by Dowling and his associates who have shown that in treating pneumococcic meningitis with massive doses of penicillin administered systemically, adequate levels of the drug are demonstrable in the cerebrospinal fluid, thereby obviating the need for intrathecal therapy. These authors have recommended the administration of large doses of penicillin intramuscularly only. Most investigators generally are in agreement with this plan. In our earlier studies we favored the use of penicillin, both intramuscularly and intrathecally, but we too have since abandoned the intrathecal route.

There is no unanimity of opinion with respect to the adjunctive use of sulfonamides. We agree with Dowling and his collaborators who believe that sulfonamides are not necessary when large doses of penicillin are administered. However, some clinicians still prefer to employ sulfonamides as adjuvants.

There is also some uncertainty regarding the value of antibiotics other than penicillin in the treatment of pneumococcic meningitis. There have been several reports of the successful treatment of this form of meningitis with the tetracyclines, chloramphenicol, and erythromycin. We have not used any of these drugs alone, but we have used them in combination with penicillin in the treatment of a small number of patients with pneumococcic meningitis. The results of the combined therapy were not as satisfactory as those obtained with penicillin alone. This experience is in agreement with the work of Lepper and Dowling who concluded that penicillin and chlortetracyline (Aureomycin) are mutually antagonistic when employed together in the treatment of pneumococcic meningitis. There are also recent reports on the successful use of ampicillin, cephalothin sodium, and cephaloridine in pneumococcal meningitis.

At present it is our belief that pneumococcic meningitis is best treated with large doses of aqueous penicillin alone. We recommend the intramuscular administration of one million units every two hours. In infants and young children, one-half of this dose is generally sufficient. The total daily dose of the antibiotic may also be given intravenously, using a continuous infusion. Administration of the drug is, as a rule, continued for a period of five to seven days after clinical improvement is manifest, the cerebrospinal fluid no longer contains organisms, and its sugar content has risen to a normal level. This precaution is necessary because of the frequency of relapse in this form of meningitis. We have achieved a recovery rate of 78 percent with our regimen.

Generally, this program of intensive penicillin therapy succeeds in clearing up many of the primary foci of infection so that the latter rarely require further operative treatment. On occasion, however, it may be necessary to eradicate a primary focus in order to bring about complete recovery and to prevent a recurrence of the meningitis. This would apply particularly to cases of meningeal infection associated with brain abscess.

A report recommending the adjunctive use of steroids in this form of meningitis lacks confirmation.

Streptococcic Meningitis. The drug of choice in the treatment of this form of meningitis is also penicillin, employed in accordance with the schedule recommended for pneumococcic meningitis. In cases of infection caused by enterococci, which are more resistant to penicillin than are the other streptococci, it is advisable to combine the penicillin with 2 gm of streptomycin daily or to use ampicillin parenterally, in a dosage of 150 mg per kg per day. The treatment for streptococcic meningitis should be continued for five to seven days after the spinal fluid has become sterile and all clinical evidence indicates that the infection has subsided.

Meningitis Due to H. Influenzae. While encouraging results were obtained in the treatment of this disease with the use of sulfonamides and specific rabbit antiserum, it was not until the introduction of streptomycin and the broad-spectrum antibiotics that it became possible to cure almost all cases of *H. Influenzae* meningitis. Since the influenza bacillus is highly susceptible to the action of several antibiotics, the physician has at his disposal a number of effective agents for the treatment of meningitis due to this organism. Recently, ampicillin has also been found to be a highly effective therapeutic agent. However, in several instances of this form of meningitis, there was a failure of response to ampicillin. At present chloramphenicol and ampicillin are regarded as the agents of choice.

Chloramphenicol may be used intravenously or orally. It is often a good plan to administer the first three or four doses parenterally and then to continue the medication orally. The average daily dose of this drug is 100 mg per kg of body weight. At times it is necessary to raise the dosage to 150 mg per kg. Parenterally, chloramphenicol generally is given at 8- or 12- hour intervals, and orally at 6- or 8-hour intervals.

The dose of ampicillin is 150 to 350 mg per kg per day, administered intravenously or intramuscularly.

With all regimens, treatment is continued for a period of five to seven days after the temperature has become normal, the cerebrospinal fluid no longer contains organisms, and its sugar content has reverted to normal.

Meningococcic Meningitis. For more than 20 years the sulfonamides constituted the basis of therapy of meningococcic meningitis. The meningococci isolated during this period were usually group A strains, which were highly sensitive to the sulfonamides. In recent years, however, increasing numbers of sulfonamide-resistant group B and C strains of meningococci have been isolated in both the military and civilian population. Since there is ample evidence that the therapeutic results with penicillin in meningococcal infections are comparable to those with sulfonamides, it would seem reasonable to regard penicillin as the drug of choice currently in the treatment of meningococcal disease. It should be employed in accordance with the schedule recommended for pneumococcic meningitis.

It has also been shown recently that ampicillin may be as effective as penicillin G in the treatment of meningococcal infections. The dose of this drug is 150 mg per kg per day, administered intramuscularly or intravenously.

In patients allergic to penicillin, one may employ the sulfonamides if the strain of meningococcus isolated is sensitive to these drugs. Other antibiotics known to be effective include tetracycline, erythromycin, chloramphenicol, and cephalothin. However, the response to these agents may be suboptimal.

Staphylococcic Meningitis. Occasional recoveries in staphylococcic meningitis have followed the use of the sulfonamides. In most instances, however, the patients have not responded to this form of therapy. Penicillin has yielded more satisfactory results and for a number of years has appeared to be the drug of choice in the treatment of this type of meningitis. However, the sensitivity of staphylococci to penicillin has decreased steadily. Many investigators have called attention to the fact that the incidence of resistant strains is higher in hospital populations than in the community at large. For a while, penicillin-resistant staphylococci were susceptible to several new antibiotics as they became available. These included chloramphenicol, the various tetracyclines, erythromycin, bacitracin, novobiocin, kanamycin, lincomycin and vancomycin. However, with continued usage, most of the new antibiotics steadily became less effective in staphylococcic diseases. Recently, the semisynthetic penicillins, methicillin, nafcillin and oxacillin have largely replaced the drugs listed above. Of special interest are reports on the current decline in the incidence of antibiotic-resistant staphylococci.

The choice of antibiotic treatment in staphylococcic meningitis therefore depends on the results of sensitivity tests. If the staphylococcal strain is highly sensitive to penicillin, this antibiotic should be used in accordance with the schedule recomended for pneumococcic meningitis, namely, 12 million units or more of the drug daily, administered parenterally. When the causative staphylococcus is penicillin-resistant, it seems best to administer parenterally large doses of methicillin or oxacillin, preferably 2 gm intravenously every four hours. However, it is important to call attention to recent reports on the emergence of methicillin-resistant staphylococci. Of the newer antibiotics the more promising appear to be cephalothin, cephaloridine and gentamicin. The dose of cephalothin is 8 to 10 gm daily, given intravenously at 4-hour intervals or by continuous infusion. Cephaloridine is also administered intravenously in a daily dose of 3 to 4 gm. The dose of gentamicin is 3 to 5 mg per kg per day, given intramuscularly at 8-hours intervals. In patients allergic to penicillin, the drugs of choice at present appear to be cephalothin and vancomycin. The dose of the latter is 2 to 3 gm daily, administered intravenously. With all regimens treatment is continued for at least two weeks, even though clinical improvement may have become apparent earlier.

Unusual Forms of Meningitis. This category includes meningitis due to *E. coli, Klebsiella-Enterobacter-Serratia, Ps. aeruginosa, B. Proteus,* and *L. monocytogenes.* In these forms of meningitis it is of the utmost importance to plan the treatment in accordance with the organism's sensitivity studies. In *L. monocytogenes* infection, penicillin appears to be the drug of choice, but tetracycline and erythromycin also are effective. For a while meningitis due to the listed gram-negative bacilli responded satisfactorily to sulfonamides, chloramphenicol, streptomycin, tetracycline, and polymyxin. With the exception of polymyxin, these agents are at present ineffective against the majority of strains of these gram-negative organisms. The current drugs of choice in the treatment

457

of infections due to these bacteria are gentamicin, kanamycin, polymyxin, colistin, cephalothin, cephaloridine and ampicillin. The dose of kanamycin is 15 mg per kg per day, given intramuscularly in two divided doses. Polymyxin may be given intramuscularly or intravenously in a dosage of 2.5 to 3 mg per kg daily. Since polymyxin does not readily enter the subarachnoid space, it is often necessary to administer it intrathecally as well as parenterally. The daily intrathecal dose varies from 2 to 5 mg, dissolved in 10 cc of saline. The dose of colistin is 3 to 5 mg per kg daily, given intramuscularly. The dosages of the other drugs have already been indicated in connection with the therapy of other forms of meningitis. It is important to stress particularly the effectiveness of gentamicin, polymyxin, and colistin in Pseudomonas meningitis, and of ampicillin and gentamicin in Proteus meningitis. The intrathecal use of the enzymes streptokinase and streptodornase in these and other forms of purulent meningitis has been reported by several investigators. In our opinion the subject requires further study, and in the present state of knowledge the intrathecal use of enzymes is not recommended. It is important to emphasize that therapy in these forms of meningitis should be prolonged because of the danger of

Meningitis of Undetermined Etiology. In cases of purulent meningitis in which the etiologic agent cannot be isolated or accurately identified, it is essential to use a broad-spectrum antibiotic or a combination of drugs known to be effective against the more common pathogens. The combined regimen of penicillin and chloramphenicol or the use of ampicillin alone is recommended for this purpose. These drugs are administered in accordance with the schedule outlined for the forms of purulent meningitis of known etiology.

Toxic and Hypersensitivity Reactions

It is necessary to direct attention to the toxic and allergic potentialities of the sulfonamides and the various antibiotics. The most common toxic reactions following the use of sulfonamides are related to the urinary tract and consist of hematuria and oliguria or anuria. Other side-effects include drug fever, skin eruptions and encephalopathy. Allergic reactions to penicillin occur in about 2 per cent of patients and include fever, pruritus, urticaria, angioedema, arthralgia, and on rare occasion, a picture of anaphylactic shock with fatal terrelapse. Surgical drainage may be necessary in order to achieve complete recovery in cases that have a focal infection.

458

mination. Streptomycin, kanamycin, gentamicin and vancomycin are ototoxic. The potentially nephrotoxic drugs are bacitracin, polymyxin, colistin and vancomycin. Neurotoxic effects may follow the use of polymyxin and colistin. Of special interest is the occasional occurrence of neuromuscular blockade with apnea and respiratory insufficiency following the administration of large doses of colistin, particularly in the presence of impaired renal function. This reaction has been correlated with high serum concentrations of the drug. In this connection it is well to stress the importance of using a modified treatment schedule, with reduced drug doses given at prolonged intervals, in the presence of renal failure. The complication of aplastic anemia following the use of chloramphenicol has been well documented. The appearance of any of the untoward effects is an indication for the immediate withdrawal of the medication that is being employed and the substitution of another drug to which the causative organism is known to be susceptible. Hypersensitivity reactions may be further alleviated through the use of antihistamines or corticosteroids.

Complications and Sequelae

The more important complications of posttraumatic meningitis are arthritis, pneumonia, endocarditis, otitis, mastoiditis, cellulitis, osteomyelitis, infected extradural or subdural hematoma, subdural effusion, suppurative sinus thrombosis, and epidural, subdural, or brain abscess. As noted previously in connection with primary foci of infection, chemo- and antibiotic therapy generally succeed in clearing up complicating infections. Certain complications, however, notably infected hematoma, and epidural, subdural, or brain abscess, require surgical treatment.

Of special interest is the recognition in recent years of the not infrequent occurrence of subdural effusion as a complication of pyogenic meningitis. It has been stressed that this is most common with *H. Influenzae* meningitis. Most of the effusions have been observed in infants under one year of age. The fluid collections are usually sterile but may be purulent. Positive cultures yield the same organism responsible for the meningitis. An interesting and important feature is the development of fibrous membranes around the more chronic effusions.

The effusions usually appear towards the end of the first week of the patient's illness. The salient clinical manifestations of this complication are persistent irritability, lethargy, prolongation of fever after

459

72 hours of specific therapy, vomiting, focal convulsions, enlarging head, bulging fontanel, opisthotonos, and the development of focal neurologic abnormalities. An important laboratory finding is the presence of a positive cerebrospinal fluid culture after 48 hours of adequate treatment. These features have been regarded by most investigators as indications for performing subdural taps. However, it should be noted that subdural effusions frequently occur in the absence of the aforementioned manifestations.

With respect to therapy, these effusions are probably best treated by aspiration every day or two until no further fluid can be withdrawn. Surgical intervention involving excision of subdural membranes is advocated for the more chronic or persistent accumulations.

Serious neurologic residua, such as deafness, blindness, paralysis, and mental retardation, occur in a small percentage of cases. In some of these the brain damage resulting from the injury is an important contributory factor.

Recurrent Meningitis and Persistent Cerebrospinal Fluid Rhinorrhea

It is difficult to estimate the incidence of recurrent meningitis following head trauma. In our series of 91 cases there were three instances of recurrent meningeal infection. Each of these three cases was associated with a fractured skull and cerebrospinal fluid rhinorrhea. In most instances of recurrent meningitis, there is a dural defect, due usually to trauma, which leads to the establishment of a fistulous communication between the nasal cavity and the subarachnoid space. This in turn is responsible for the development of rhinorrhea and meningitis, which may come on spontaneously or may be precipitated by such factors as an upper respiratory infection, a forceful sneeze, an intranasal examination, manipulation of a facial fracture, and lumbar puncture. In the presence of rhinorrhea, meningitis may develop shortly after the occurrence of the trauma or many years later. There may be just two or three recurrent meningeal episodes in a relatively short period of time or there may be many recurrences scattered over a number of years, with long intervals between the attacks. Different organisms are, as a rule, isolated from the spinal fluid during various episodes. On occasion, however, the same organism may be recovered during different attacks. The most frequent etiologic agent is the pneumococcus. Not infrequently, no organisms are demonstrable. It is well known that recurrent meningitis may occur in the absence of rhinor-

Clark, E., Redish, J. and Jolliffe, N. Meningococcic Meningitis Complicating Fracture of the Skull. *Arch. Surg.*, *35*, 486, 1937.

Cooperstock, M. Pneumococcic Meningitis Following Head Injuries. *J. Michigan Med. Soc.*, *45*, 337, 1946.

Ditowski, S., Goldman, A. and Goldin, A. Pseudomonas Meningitis in an Infant Sucessfully Treated with Neomycin. *Pediatrics*, *9*, 101, 1952.

Dowling, H. F., Sweet, L. K., Robinson, J. A., Zellers, W. C. and Hirsh, H. L. The Treatment of Pneumococcic Meningitis with Massive Doses of Systemic Penicillin. *Am. J. M. Sc.*, *217*, 149, 1949.

Eagleton, W. P. Traumatisms of the Frontal and Temporal Regions and Their Relation to Meningitis from the Standpoint of the General Surgeon. *N. Y. State J. Med.*, *32*, 947, 1932.

Eickhoff, J. C. and Finland, M. Changing Susceptibility of Meningococci to Antimicrobial Agents. *New Engl. J. Med.*, *272*, 395, 1965.

Falk, C. R. and Appelbaum, E. Type Specific Meningococcic Agglutinins in Human Serums. I. Description of Method. *Proc. Soc. Exper. Biol. & Med.*, *57*, 341, 1944.

Falk, C. R. and Appelbaum, E. Type Specific Meningococcic Agglutinins. II. The Relationship of Titers to the Course of the Disease. *J. Clin. Invest.*, *24*, 742, 1945.

Falk, C. R. and Appelbaum, E. Type Specific Meningococcic Agglutinins. III. Application of the Test to Sporadic Cases and to Clinically Typical Cases Lacking Bacteriological Proof. *J. Clin. Invest.*, *32*, 39, 1953.

Feldman, H. A. Sulfonamide-Resistant Meningococci. *Ann. Rev. Med.*, *18*, 495, 1967.

Finegold, S. M. Toxicity of Kanamycin in Adults. *Ann. N. Y. Acad. Sci.*, *132*, 942, 1966.

Finland, M. and Haight, T. H. Antibiotic Resistance of Pathogenic Staphylococci. *Arch. Int. Med.*, *91*, 143, 1953.

Greenfield, S. and Feldman, H. A. Familial Carriers and Meningococcal Meningitis. *New Engl. J. Med.*, *277*, 497, 1967.

Griffith, R. S. and Black, H. R. Cephalothin - A New Antibiotic. *J.A.M.A.*, *189*, 823, 1964.

Hargraves, M. M., Mills, S. D., and Heck, F. J. Aplastic Anemia Associated with the Administration of Chloramphenicol. *J.A.M.A.*, *149*, 1297, 1952.

Harris, R. C., Buxbaum, L. and Appelbaum, E. Secondary Bacillus Pyocyaneus Infections in Meningitis Following Intrathecal Penicillin Therapy. *J. Lab. and Clin. Med.*, *31*, 1113, 1946.

Hoyne, A. L. and Schultz, A. Multiple Attacks of Meningitis. Report of a Case with Autopsy. *Am. J. Surg.*, *30*, 156, 1935.

Hurff, J. W. and Beling, C. A. Fracture of Temporal Bone through a Chronic Mastoiditis. *Am. J. Surg.*, *30*, 156, 1935.

Ivler, D., Thrupp, L. D., Leedom, J. M., Wehrle, P. F. and Portnoy, B. Ampicillin in the Treatment of Acute Bacterial Meningitis. *Antimicrob. Agents & Chemother.*, *3*, 335, 1963.

Jao, R. L. and Jackson, G. G. Gentamicin Sulfate, New Antibiotic Against Gram-Negative Bacilli. *J.A.M.A.*, *189*, 817, 1964.

462

Jensen, W. L. Treatment of Acute Meningococcal Infections with Penicillin G. *Arch. Inter. Med.*, *122*, 322, 1968.

Kaplan, K., Reisberg, B. and Weinstein, L. Cephaloridine. *Arch. Intern. Med.*, *121*, 17, 1968.

Kunin, C. M. and Finland, M. Restrictions Imposed on Antibiotic Therapy by Renal Failure. *Arch. Intern. Med.*, *104*, 1030, 1959.

Labby, D. H. Recurrent Pneumococcic Meningitis Following Sulfonamide Therapy. *J.A.M.A.*, *127*, 981, 1945.

Leedom, J. M., Ivler, D., Mathies, A. W., Thrupp, L. D., Portnoy, B. and Wehrle, P. F. Importance of Sulfadiazine Resistance in Meningococcal Disease in Civilians. *New Engl. J. Med.*, *273*, 1395, 1965.

Lepper, M. H. and Dowling, H. F. Treatment of Pneumococcic Meningitis with Penicillin Compared with Penicillin Plus Aureomycin. *Arch. Int. Med.*, *88*, 489, 1951.

Lepper, M. H., Dowling, H. F., Wehrle, P. F., Blatt, N. H., Spies, H. W., and Brown, M. Meningococcic Meningitis: Treatment with Large Doses of Penicillin Compared to Treatment with Gantrisin. *J. Lab. and Clin. Med.*, *40*, 891, 1952.

Levin, S. and Painter, M. B. The Treatment of Acute Meningococcal Infection in Adults. *Ann. Intern. Med.*, *64*, 1049, 1966.

Lewin, W. and Cairns, H. Fractures of the Sphenoidal Sinus with Cerebrospinal Fluid Rhinorrhea, *Brit. Med. J.*, *1*, 1, 1951.

Lewin, W. Cerebrospinal Fluid Rhinorrhea in Closed Head Injuries. *Brit. J. Surg.*, *42*, 1, 1954.

Linell, E. A. and Robinson, W. L. Head Injuries and Meningitis. *J. Neur. and Psychiatry*, *4*, 23, 1941.

Maegraith, B. C. Meningococcal Meningitis Following Fracture of the Skull. *Lancet*, *1*, 863, 1935.

Mathies, A. W. and Wehrle, P. F. Management of Bacterial Meningitis in Children. *Pediat. Clin. North Am.*, *15*, 185, 1968.

McKay, R. J., Jr., Ingraham, F. D. and Matson, D. D. Subdural Fluid Complicating Bacterial Meningitis. *J.A.M.A.*, *152*, 387, 1953.

McKay, R. J., Jr., Morrisette, R. A., Ingraham, F. D. and Matson, D. D. Collections of Subdural Fluid Complicating Meningitis Due to Haemophilus Influenzae (Type B). *New Engl. J. Med.*, *242*, 20, 1950.

Millar, J. W., Siess, E. E., Feldman, H. A., Silverman, C. and Frank, P. In Vivo and In Vitro Resistance to Sulfadiazine in Strains of Neisseria Meningitidis. *J.A.M.A.*, *165*, 222, 1957.

Morley, T. P. and Heatherington, R. F. Traumatic Cerebrospinal Fluid Rhinorrhea and Otorrhea, Pneumocephalus, and Meningitis. *Surg., Gynec. Obstet.*, *104*, 88, 1957.

Neal, J. B., Jackson, H. W. and Appelbaum, E. A Comprehensive Study of Meningitis Secondary to Otitic or Sinus Infection. *Ann. Otol., Rhinol., Laryngol.*, *43*, 658, 1934.

Norman, A. P. Recurring Pneumococcal Meningitis. *Lancet*, *257*, 281, 1949.

Nyhan, W. L. and Cooke, R. E. Symptomatic Hyponatremia in Acute Infections of the Central Nervous System. *Pediatrics*, *18*, 604, 1956.

Ory, E. M. Treatment of Pyogenic Meningitis in Adults. *Mod. Treatm.*, *4*, 918, 1967.

Parisi, A. F. and Kaplan, M. H. Apnea During Treatment with sodium Colistimethate. *J.A.M.A., 194,* 298, 1965.

Ribble, J. C. and Braude, A. I. ACTH and Steroids in the Treatment of Pneumococcal Meningitis in Adults. *Am. J. Med., 24,* 68, 1968.

Ross, S., Rice, E. C., Burke, F. G., McGovern, J. J., Parrott, R. H. and McGovern, J. P. Treatment of Meningitis due to H. Influenzae. Use of Chloromycetin and Sulfadiazine. *New Engl. J. Med., 247,* 54, 1952.

Tillett, W. S. *Studies on the Enzymatic Types of Fibrin and Inflammatory Exudates by Products of Hemolytic Streptococci.* The Harvey Lectures Series, 45. Springfield, Ill.: Charles C Thomas, 1952.

Traut, E. F. Recurrence of Pneumococcic Meningitis. *J.A.M.A., 129,* 273, 1945.

Trice, P. A. and Townsend, T. E. Meningitis Due to Klebsiella Pneumoniae. Report of Two Cases with the Use of Streptokinase and Streptodornase in One Case. *J.A.M.A., 149,* 1471, 1952.

Weinstein, L. and Perrin, T. S. Meningitis Due to Ps. Pyocyanea; A Report of 3 Cases Treated Successfully with Streptomycin and Sulfadiazine. *Ann. Int. Med., 29,* 103, 1948.

Weinstein, L., Kaplan, K. and Chang, T. W. Treatment of Infections in Man with Cephalothin. *J.A.M.A., 189,* 829, 1964.

Wolinsky, E. and Hines, J. D. Neurotoxic and Nephrotoxic Effects of Colistin in Patients with Renal Disease. *New Eng. J. Med., 266,* 759, 1962.

Wolf, R. E. and Birbara, C. A. Meningococcal Infections at an Army Training Center. *Amer. J. Med., 44,* 243, 1968.

Wysham, D. N. and Kirby, W. M. M. Micrococcic (Staphylococcic) Infections in a General Hospital. *J.A.M.A., 164,* 1733, 1957.

Young, L. M., Haddow, J. E. and Klein, J. O. Relapse Following Ampicillin Treatment of Acute Hemophilus Influenzae Meningitis. *Pediatrics, 41,* 516, 1968.

Young, R. C. and Murray, W. A. Post-Traumatic Streptococcus Viridans Meningitis. *Can. Med. Assn. J.,* 77, 223, 1957.

Chapter 14

CEREBRAL BIRTH INJURIES

BERNARD J. ALPERS, M.D.

AND

RICHARD G. BERRY, M.D.

Cerebral birth injuries are of great importance from two standpoints: (1) their recognition and treatment in the early stages of their occurrence, and (2) the determination of the sequelae or aftereffects in later life if survival takes place. Much is known concerning the acute manifestations of the various types of cerebral birth injuries, but very little can be said concerning their aftereffects. There has been much speculation among investigators concerning such effects, but no good data are available on which to base sound conclusions. Most of the subject matter in this chapter therefore will deal with the acute effects of cerebral birth injuries, but some consideration will be given to the sequelae insofar as it is possible to do so. Many types of injury may occur. The outcome of the case will depend largely of course on the nature and degree of the injury.

The available data are difficult to assess because of fallacies inherent in the methods of gathering information. These methods are: (1) Retrospective studies which may be clinical, or clinical and pathological. These studies rely, for the most part, on parental recollection of birth circumstances and, usually, an inadequate objective birth history. Nor are adequate statistical controls available in most studies. Unfortunately, even the small numbers of pathological studies usually depend on historical evidence. (2) Pathological studies. For the most part, pathological studies have been on those injuries severe enough to result in neonatal death. It is hardly justifiable to extrapolate such figures to those injuries which are compatible with life. (3) Statistical studies of patients with neurologic deficit have been correlated with

465

statistical data from hospital records at time of birth and show trends only. (4) Rarely, vertical studies of a series of birth-injured or asphyxiated patients are available. The need of a team of obstetrician, pediatrician, neurologist and neuropathologist cooperating in a carefully formulated study is evident.

DEFINITION OF CEREBRAL BIRTH INJURY

By this is meant any injury to the brain or its coverings sustained during the act of birth whether such injury is the result of direct trauma due to the application of forceps, or to indirect trauma resulting from forces exerted on the skull during normal or abnormal labor. It should be emphasized that the term *trauma* in the subsequent discussion will be applied not only to instances of direct but of indirect injury as well.

Defects of the brain and its coverings which result from malformations on a genetic basis (the remedy of which must be in the field of eugenics) must be differentiated from those lesions, the result of intrauterine or perinatal influences which are potentially preventable and which occasionally can be alleviated by surgical methods.

CLASSIFICATION

The various types of cerebral birth injuries may be classified as follows:

I. Injuries of the Skull
II. Injuries of the Meninges
    Extradural hemorrhage
    Subdural hemorrhage
    Subrachnoid hemorrhage
    Tentorial tears
III. Injuries of the Brain
    Lacerations
    Hemorrhage
    Softenings
    Sinus thrombosis
IV. Late Results of Cerebral Birth Injuries
    Cerebral diplegia
    Porencephalic cyst
    Epilepsy
    Choreoathetosis

This classification, like others, is not in itself complete, but it gives a general idea of the types of lesions which may result from injury of the brain or its coverings. It is for the most part a pathological rather than a clinical classification. It includes not only the immediate effects of cerebral birth injuries, but what is more important for patient, parents, and doctor, a grouping of some of the late effects of cerebral injury. How the latter extremely important group fits into the picture of the cerebral birth injuries will be discussed subsequently. Of the immediate effects of cerebral birth injury hemorrhage of one form or another is by far the most common.

INCIDENCE

The actual incidence of all types of cerebral birth injuries is difficult to ascertain accurately. Most of the studies which deal with this aspect of the problem have been made in cases of hemorrhage and on children which have been stillborn. The statement of Ford (1937) that at least one-third of all deaths within the first two weeks of life are the result of cerebral birth injury is no longer valid. The modern obstetrical stress on conservatism in operative techniques, and particularly the avoidance of trauma, is reflected in the decrease in percentage of deaths due to mechanical trauma in recent decades. At the Chicago Lying In Hospital the mortality rate for injuries incurred during delivery has been reduced from 5.6 deaths per 1000 total births in the years 1931-41 (14 percent of deaths and stillbirths) to 0.7 per 1000 total births (3 percent of deaths and stillbirths) (Potter, 1961). Mechanical trauma accounted for 13 percent of deaths in Morison's series (1963). The latter found trauma to cause 1.3 deaths per 1000 live births in term infants, but with prematurity the rate sharply increased giving 10 to 40 deaths per 1000 live births and was inversely proportional to the birth weights. Haller, Nesbitt and Anderson (1956) also noted an increase in anoxic brain hemorrhages in prematures at a time when overall mortality was decreasing.

Of far greater importance as far as the patient is concerned, is the incidence of remote sequelae as the result of birth injuries affecting the brain. Such an incidence is most difficult to estimate. As a matter of fact, it is extremely difficult to arrive at accurate statistics in such a study. Some of the late sequelae may be attributed safely to the effects of trauma at birth; however many conditions attributed to trauma have only a remote relationship to it; and finally many conditions

467

not attributed to birth trauma are probably due to this factor. These various possibilities will be discussed later.

An approach to such a vertical solution of incidence has been attempted by Denhoff and Holden (1955). The apparently significant factors in cerebral palsy were determined. These were divided into obstetrical (such as midforceps delivery, breech delivery, prolonged pregnancy and prolonged labor) and neonatal factors (prematurity, oxygen required, transfusions required, cyanosis, hypertonicity, and listlessness). On the basis of such presumptive causes of brain damage, they followed 15 patients for a period of 2½ years. Of this group, those whose mothers had not previously aborted developed normally. Previous abortion was found in the mothers' history in three of the four abnormal children in this group of suspected brain damage and in all three of those who showed neurological damage in a control group.

Keith, Norval, and Hunt (1953) investigated 4,464 infants and found no evidence that prolonged labor, asphyxia, or delayed respiration caused any neurological abnormality in those premature or term infants *who survived* and were followed over an average period of five years. Keith and Gage (1960) followed this group for up to 14 years and found no increased frequency of convulsions when compared to the control group.

ETIOLOGY

The various etiological factors which may produce cerebral birth injuries are best considered together since many of these factors are common to the several types of cerebral birth injury. Strictly speaking the term *cerebral birth injury* refers to injuries occurring at time of birth; since the factors which may occur before labor may definitely influence cerebral birth injury it seems advisable to consider under causative factors, influences which may occur before, during, and immediately after labor. This may seem to give too wide a connotation to the cause of cerebral birth injuries, but it is probably better to make the definition more inclusive than to confine it to too narrow limits.

Anderson (1952) reviewed the literature on causes of brain damage incident to the birth process and divided the factors into prenatal, paranatal, and postnatal or child factors. The following factors appeared to play a role in a decreasing order of incidence:

Prenatal factors. Primiparity, nausea and vomiting, premature sepa-

468

ration of placenta, hypertension, toxemia, vaginal hemorrhage, anemia, maternal trauma, maternal disease.

Paranatal factors. Forceps, version and extraction, pituitrin stimulation, holding head back, Cesarean section, precipitate delivery.

Postnatal and child factors. Cyanosis, birth injury and asphyxia, required O_2, convulsions, Rh incompatibility, neonatal jaundice, kernicterus, twins.

1. Influences Operating In Utero

Various influences which affect the fetus during pregnancy may be responsible for certain types of cerebral birth injuries by making the brain more susceptible to the traumatic factors associated with birth. It is well known that disease in the mother may be transmitted to the fetus via the placenta. This is true not only of infectious diseases, but also of intoxications of many sorts. Studies of Alpers and Patten show that there is good evidence that infectious diseases such as typhus fever, typhoid fever, anthrax, encephalitis, probably tuberculosis in some instances, and streptococcic infections in the mother may be transmitted to the fetus. Intrauterine infection with gas-forming orgamisms has been reported (Kemp and Stallworthy, 1942). In the great majority of instances the result of such infections is the production of a dead fetus, but sometimes survival takes place, and with it the development of a cerebral birth condition. The importance of fetal infection has been recognized by Wolf, Cowen, and Paige (1941) who believe that infantile cases of toxoplasmosis may begin in the fetus. They found neutralizing antibodies in the maternal circulation to support their concept and they point out that the calcified brain changes could hardly develop during the short extrauterine period during which these infants live. An intrauterine meningo-encephalitis resulting in the birth of a monster which died after 11 weeks has been recorded by Roback and Kahler (1941). Syphilis is of course known to be transmitted to the fetus through the mother. Its role in the production of cerebral birth injury is probably due to the fact that it is often associated with prematurity, which is often accompanied by cerebral hemorrhage. Intoxications such as eclampsia probably operate in a similar fashion, though it has been shown (Alpers and Patten) that eclampsia in the mother may be associated with toxic-degenerative changes in the infant's brain. The influence of such toxic substances as alcohol in the production of cerebral birth injuries is open to serious question. The role of trauma during pregnancy in the production of cerebral birth injuries is also open to question. It is difficult, if not impossible, to determine whether a serious physical trauma sustained by the mother will have a lasting effect on the fetus. Under ordinary circumstances, such a trauma is probably without effect on the fetus. If however, the trauma has been serious enough to cause uterine bleeding without miscarriage it is possible that damage to the fetus may have resulted from anoxemia even though it be temporary. The influence of injury to the fetus in utero has obtained greater recognition in recent years, so that at least as much consideration is now given to the factors operating before birth as to those at work during delivery. Aldridge and Meredith (1941) found in a study of fetal deaths occurring during a five-year period that approximately one-fifth of the deaths occurred during the antepartum period, a little more than one-fourth during the course of labor, and about one-half within one month after birth. The role of intrauterine fetal asphyxia must be recognized and it is possible that too much obstetrical analgesia and anesthesia may be contributory causes to fetal deaths.

Irradiation of the fetus from x-ray and from the effects of nuclear weapons, both in human subjects and experimentally in animals, causes defects in the central nervous system in the fetuses that survive. This is particularly true of irradiation during the first three months of pregnancy (Hicks, 1956; Plummer, 1952).

Drugs can penetrate into the fetus with resulting injury as shown by Heckel (1941) and by Ginzler and Chesner (1942) in the case of sulfanilamide, and by Taylor et al (1941) in the case of quinine – a presumed cause of nerve deafness produced in utero. In experimental animals, sulfhydryl reagents and ACTH damage neuroblasts (Hicks, 1952).

Rubella, especially in the first trimester, can produce intrauterine damage to the developing nervous system.

Premature infants are particularly prone to suffer damage to the central nervous system. There are numerous converging, occasionally conflicting, statistical and experimental analyses of the cause of prematurity. Pasamanick and Lilienfeld with various co-workers (1955, 1956) have postulated "a continuum of reproductive casualty" with a lethal component consisting of abortions, stillbirths, and neonatal deaths, and a sublethal component consisting of cerebral palsy and perhaps other related conditions. "Varying degrees of brain injury insufficient to cause death would result in corresponding degrees of

470

neurological impairment and serve as precursors to a number of neuropsychiatric disorders such as cerebral palsy, epilepsy, mental deficiency, and childhood behavior disorders."

From 38 percent (Anderson, 1952) to 50 percent (Drillien, 1957) of premature births have no known cause. Of those with a recognized etiology, 70 to 80 percent are associated with related (1) maternal toxemia, (2) congenital malformations and (3) placenta previa, and of course, in these the causes again are unknown. Drillien's study indicates that an inadequate customary diet before pregnancy is an apparent factor in prematurity. Statistically, the social class of upbringing and the efficiency of the grandmother are two important factors relating to the risk of prematurity.

Eastman and DeLeon (1955) analyzed the birth records of 96 infants who later developed cerebral palsy. A poor condition at birth was noted by the attending obstetrician or pediatrician in 41 percent of the cerebral palsy cases and in 2 percent of the controls. Neurologic conditions were infrequently observed during their stay in the hospital. There was no significant correlation with race, age, parity of the mother, syphilis, virus infection of the mother, type of pelvic outlet, or total duration of labor in these 96 cases. The high incidence of prematurity was the one and perhaps only etiologic factor which was established beyond doubt. The authors, however, raised the question whether the determining factor is the premature state itself or certain complications predisposing to prematurity, especially abruptio placentae and placenta previa. There can be no doubt, the authors concluded, that in many cases of premature birth, placental separation and the subsequent anoxia are responsible for the damage rather than the prematurity itself.

Denhoff and Holden (1955) suggested that acute birth anoxia may not be so important as long standing intrauterine anoxia in the cause of later brain damage. Mackay (1957), from studies on oxygen saturation of the cord blood, found that oxygen pressure is decreased in preeclampsia and that this is affected both by the duration as well as the severity of the toxemic process. A general anesthetic, especially nitrous oxide, nearly always is associated with a decreased oxygen pressure. Diabetic patients have low oxygen saturation.

It seems apparent that infections and toxic substances may penetrate the fetal circulation and that metabolic disturbances including hypoxia can result in intrauterine disease with consequent permanent damage to the brain and other organs.

471

2. Influences Operating During Birth

There is no question that trauma is an important factor in the production of cerebral birth injuries. The role of trauma appears to the obstetrician to be overemphasized, and undoubtedly far too much stress has been laid on this factor in all sorts of obscure neurological conditions dating from birth. Despite this, it is nevertheless true that in the various conditions to be discussed in this chapter trauma at birth is a very important cause. A study of 1000 consecutive fetal deaths made by D'Esopo and Marchetti (1942) showed that the most important causes of such deaths were asphyxia, birth injury, and pneumonia.

Benda (1945) suggested that 30 to 40 percent of cases of cerebral spastic infantile paralysis and 40 to 45 percent of cases of mental deficiency are the result of birth injury. On the basis of autopsies of 543 cases of mental deficiency, Malamud (1954) found 22 percent due to destructive processes. The specific causes of all full-term neonatal deaths show an almost equal division between birth trauma (23 percent), congenital malformations (22 percent) and anoxia (22 percent) as the cause of death. Anoxia, trauma, malformation, and pulmonary difficulties are the main causes of death in the premature group (Anderson, 1952). Thus certain contributory factors aid materially in the causation of cerebral injuries associated with birth trauma. The most important of these are (1) prematurity, and (2) asphyxia or anoxia. The importance of prematurity in the production of cerebral birth injuries has been well established by the studies of Yllpo (1922) who found cerebral lesions of some sort in 90 percent of premature infants. The importance of prematurity was emphasized also by Freud (1897) in his study of the cerebral diplegias. Browne (1921) found that intracranial bleeding occurred 16 times more frequently in premature infants than in full-term infants. Gröntoft (1954) found a mortality of 3.2 percent in 12,640 infants; 120 of the 319 autopsied cases had intracranial hemorrhage; 66 of these were premature; 54 were full-term infants. Intracerebral hemorrhage was rarely found in the full-term infants, all but five of those over 2,500 grams birth weight showing subdural hemorrhage. On the other hand, 38 of the 66 premature infants showed intracerebral hemorrhage. These and other postmortem studies show a high incidence of cerebral hemorrhage among premature infants. The exact role of the prematurity is not clear, but prematurity in itself is hardly responsible for the cerebral

472

birth injury. Many fetuses are premature because of some systemic disease of the mother or by virtue of other factors which would probably induce cerebral injuries. There is the additional possibility that the premature brain is poorly developed and hence more susceptible to the various forces and strains associated with birth. Its structure is softer, its water content higher, so that it is more easily damaged, either by direct or indirect force.

Difficult labor, breech presentation, and discrepancy between the size of the head and the pelvic outlet also contribute to the production of cerebral birth injury.

Trauma to the head sustained during labor is responsible for most of the cases of cerebral birth injury. The nature of the trauma, and the actual conditions which produce it are still matters of great controversy and there are many ideas concerning the factors associated with trauma sustained at birth. These will be discussed in detail in a consideration of cerebral hemorrhage in the newborn. It seems clear however that trauma need not necessarily be direct, i.e., due to the application of forceps or to manipulation by the obstetrician. It may be either direct or indirect. In direct trauma the brain injury results from the use of forceps or from the forcible compression of the skull by other methods. Many cases of cerebral birth injuries undoubtedly result from trauma of this nature. Their exact number has never been accurately determined. This much is true however: Not all the cases of cerebral birth injuries can or should be attributed to the technical difficulties encountered by the obstetrician. Without doubt many result from such trauma as compression of the skull during labor by a contracted pelvis or pressure against the pelvic floor during uterine contractions, breech delivery, or from injury to the skull and brain as the result of differences in atmospheric and other pressures resulting from the rupture of the placental membranes.

That trauma is by no means the only cause of intracranial injuries in the newborn however is shown clearly by occasional instances of cerebral hemorrhage found in children born by Cesarean section. Brander found in a review of the literature that there were 72 reported cases of intracranial lesions verified postmortem in children who had been delivered by abdominal (Cesarean) section. In some of these cases there was a tentorial tear. In others, mental deficiency, epilepsy, and paralyses of various sorts have occurred following Cesarean section. In these cases, the factor of heredity must be considered, although its role is not always clear. Furthermore, there may be a direct traumatic factor in cases delivered by Cesarean section. Thus the fetus may have been injured by attempted forceps extraction, or the head may have been injured by being tightly wedged in the inlet. In any event, Cesarean section may be associated with birth injuries in children, though the incidence is of course much lower than in normal deliveries.

SKULL INJURIES

Injuries of the skull during birth are frequently overlooked due to the presence of more important injuries to the brain substance itself. Their frequency is difficult to ascertain. It is safe to assert that incidence of skull injuries is probably quite low in comparison with the total number of births and the incidence of other forms of cerebral injuries. No statistics are available however on the actual incidence of skull injuries. That they are not too infrequent is shown by the studies of Hemsath (1934) who found 32 cases of injury of the occipital bone, and of Gfroerer (1914) who reported 26 cases of skull trauma during birth. Fleming and Morton (1930) reported 16 cases. Of these 9 involved the frontal bones, 5 the parietal bones, and 1 each the occipital and temporal bones. Potter found that skull fractures due to birth trauma are usually linear, that they extend most often from the superior margin of the bones of the calvarium to the base of the skull, that fractures of the base are extremely rare, and that many times fracture plays a role in the production of intracranial hemorrhage. More extensive studies of a similar nature are needed in order to determine the exact incidence of skull injuries during birth.

The nature of the skull injury is usually a fracture. Fissures along the lines of ossification in the skull bones are also encountered; they are often difficult to differentiate from fractures. Skull fractures sustained during birth are as a rule irregularly linear and depressed in type. Any part of the skull may be affected. Fractures have been found in the frontal, parietal, temporal, and occipital bones. Basilar fractures are not commonly encountered, and when found are usually fatal, due to the accompanying injury of the brain stem. Injuries to the occipital bone are also frequently fatal because of injury of the adjacent medulla oblongata. Hemsath reported 32 cases of separation of the occipital bone between the pars squama and the pars lateralis, all of them fatal. It is probable that, just as in adults, many of the cases of linear skull fracture are unassociated with injury to the brain. On

474

the other hand, severe cases of skull injury are probably always, or almost always, associated either with cerebral contusion or laceration.

In the majority of instances, the skull injury is the result of trauma sustained at birth. This trauma is usually caused by either severe traction with forceps or breech extraction. Forceps extraction is more apt to be associated with skull injury than other forms of delivery. In rare cases, however, skull injury has been found to be associated with spontaneous deliveries, without the use of forceps, and with relatively easy births. The mechanism of production of the fracture in such cases is obscure but it has been variously ascribed to sudden impact of the head against the pelvic floor at the moment of rupture of the membranes, pressure against the promontory, and rigid contraction of the cervix after ergot administration.

The symptoms of skull injuries are poorly defined and may remain unrecognized for some time. Linear fractures probably go unnoticed entirely. Even depressed fractures may not be recognized. It is only when the underlying brain tissue is injured that symptoms appear. Here too, there may be complete failure to recognize the presence of a skull injury except in severe cases. Only the formation of a cerebral cicatrix or an adhesive arachnoiditis secondary to the bone injury may call attention to the skull trauma some months after the injury has occurred. In such cases convulsions or weakness of one or more limbs may call attention to the presence of a cerebral injury.

The treatment of skull injuries is relatively simple. The linear fractures require no treatment except time and the opportunity to heal. The treatment of depressed skull fractures by elevation of the bone is recommended by most neurosurgeons (Matson, 1961). The procedure is simple and precludes further damage to the rapidly growing brain.

THE PATHOGENESIS OF INTRACRANIAL HEMORRHAGE

Undoubtedly, the most common lesion following cerebral birth injury is hemorrhage within the brain or its envelopes. This hemorrhage may occur in relation to the dural or arachnoid membranes or within the brain and the cerebral ventricles. The incidence of cerebral hemorrhage in different series varies from 9 to 70 percent (Gröntoft, 1954). In Gröntoft's own cases, the incidence was 37 percent but in only 17 percent of the total was it a "severe hemorrhage." In general, until recent years, the main cause of intracranial hemorrhage was thought to be mechanical trauma. Anoxia was considered a contributory cause but not a primary factor in severe hemorrhage.

475

Clinically speaking, it would seem wisest to discuss these various forms of hemorrhage separately in order to clarify their characteristics. They will be dealt with in this fashion subsequently, but first, it is necessary to discuss in general the pathogenesis of intracranial hemorrhage in the newborn since the mechanisms of production are the source of much confusion, and many theories have been evolved concerning its pathogenesis. The causative factors on which these theories are based may be summarized as follows:

1. Mechanical, due to
   (a) direct trauma
   (b) tentorial tears
   (c) suction effects
   (d) increased intracranial pressure
2. Nonmechanical, due to
   (a) anoxia and other metabolic changes
   (b) vasocirculatory factors

Mechanical Factors

(a) *Direct trauma.* Among the various theories as to the cause of intracranial hemorrhage in the newborn, the mechanical concepts have long held great sway. Trauma has been considered to have a very important role in the production of the hemorrhage. The trauma may be the result of the normal action of labor, it may follow the use of forceps, or it may result from abnormal deliveries. It has been assumed that when hemorrhage occurs in the normal process of labor it is the result of moulding of the head with undue stress on the cranial bones, overriding of the bones, and tearing of veins in the dura or within the brain. According to this theory, the action of forceps causes undue pressure on the cranial bones, and hemorrhage in the brain from direct tears of meningeal vessels. Presumably, abnormal deliveries such as breech presentations act in a similar fashion. Undoubtedly direct trauma from any one of these causes plays a role in the production of cerebral hemorrhage, but it hardly accounts for all the cases of intracranial hemorrhage in newborn infants.

Gröntoft (1954) was able to demonstrate a clear relation between birth weight (and larger than normal head size) and the extent of intracranial injuries in a series of neonatal deaths; fatal hemorrhage was higher in babies born at term than in the premature. Potter

476

(1941) found a direct connection between the type of delivery and the incidence of hemorrhage. Thus, she determined that one out of every 25 babies delivered by version or extraction was born dead or died in the neonatal period as a result of intracranial hemorrhage; one in every 33 cases died with mid- or high-forceps delivery; one in every 50 with breech delivery; one in every 110 by Cesarean section; one in every 330 delivered by low forceps; and one in every 500 after normal cephalic delivery. In a later analysis (1952), she stated that in the years from 1931 to 1941 the incidence of birth trauma was 5.6 per 1,000 total births which accounted for 14 percent of the deaths and stillbirths. However, in the same hospital, in the years 1947 to 1949, birth trauma accounted for 0.5 deaths per 1,000 total births and was responsible for only 3 percent of the deaths and stillbirths. Other studies have noted a similar reduction in the significance of mechanical trauma and subsequent intracranial hemorrhage, but at the same time, there has been an apparent and actual increase in incidence of premature births.

Studies from the brain registry of the American Academy for Cerebral Palsy by Josephy (1950) fail to indicate any evidence of hemorrhage in the residual lesions of the brain in cases of hemiplegic spastic cerebral palsy. He suggested that newborns with severe intracranial hemorrhage die and do not survive to become cases of cerebral palsy. Wolf and Cowen (1956) also noted a lack of evidence for hemorrhage as a cause of multiple cystic encephalomalacia.

(b) *Tentorial tears.* Tears of the tentorium have come to be regarded as an important cause of hemorrhage in the brain or meninges of the newborn. It is assumed that under some conditions of birth an undue stress is placed on the falx and tentorium due to severe lateral compression of the skull, thus causing a tear of the tentorium and hemorrhage (Beneke, 1910). The tear usually occurs at the point of bifurcation of the falx into the tentorium. This concept of the causation of intracranial hemorrhage in the newborn has been confirmed by experimental observations. Lateral compression of the head either during birth or even during first efforts to induce breathing has been found to be an adequate cause for the production of tentorial tears. In some instances longitudinal compression has also produced tentorial tears.

The most logical presentation of the role of tentorial tears in the production of intracranial hemorrhage was made by Holland (1922) who studied the problem in a large series of fetuses. His argument is as follows: during labor the head is in a state of stress consisting of 1) a general compression of the whole head and 2) a longitudinal compression acting at the ends of the long diameter of the head. This longitudinal compression is chiefly responsible for alterations in the shape of the head and the stretching of the falx. Excessive stress results in excessive moulding, and in stretching and tearing of the tentorium with rupture of blood vessels. The most common site of the tear is at the junction of the tentorium and the falx, and the vein usually torn is the great vein of Galen, resulting in subdural and cerebral hemorrhage.

Earle, Baldwin, and Penfield (1953) have suggested that one of the major causes of seizures resulting from birth trauma is "incisural sclerosis." Compression in travel through the birth canal results in a temporary herniation of the temporal lobe under the tentorial incisura. Compression of the branches of the posterior cerebral, the anterior choroidal, and the middle cerebral arteries against the free edge of the tentorium causes an acute local ischemia with resulting sclerosis, in any or all of the territories of supply. Lindenberg (1955) presented some confirming data in cases of acute head injury with edema.

(c) *"Suction" effects.* Schwartz (1927) propounded the theory that bleeding into the brain and its meninges is the result of suction or atmospheric effects. According to this theory the pressure on the head during the latter part of labor after the membranes have burst is atmospheric, the body itself being subject to intrauterine pressure. During the pains which are due to uterine contractions, blood is sent from the body to the presenting part of the head. The result, according to Schwartz is a suction effect which produces venous engorgement, stasis and, eventually, as the pressure increases, bleeding within the brain or its membranes.

(d) *Increased intracranial pressure.* Rydberg (1932) proposed the idea that hemorrhage in the newborn is the result of increased intracranial pressure. He assumes that due to the compression of the fetal head during the labor pains, the volume of the cranial cavity is reduced and blood flows from the head to the body. There is probably also a displacement of the brain and an expulsion of part of the cerebrospinal fluid. The increasing compression, furthermore, causes a rise in intracranial pressure which in turn is associated with a bradycardia which is especially noticeable during the pains. The increased pressure causes excitation of vasomotor centers producing a rise of blood pressure and hemorrhage if the pressure reaches a sufficient height.

Lindenberg (1955) found evidence that increased intracranial pressure from whatever cause can compress vessels, resulting in local ischemia and leading to a typical vascular sclerosis in the region of Ammon's horn as well as in other areas of arterial supply.

Nonmechanical (Anoxic and Vasocirculatory) Factors

Apnea itself may be the result of increased pressure from traumatic neonatal hemorrhage, but the role of anoxia in the pathogenesis of cerebral hemorrhage in the newborn has been a controversial subject. The role of neonatal hypoxia in the pathogenesis of such sequelae of birth trauma as cerebral palsy, mental retardation, and epilepsy has engendered even more discussion. There are no clearly defined and objective criteria upon which to base comparisons, often within a series and especially amongst several series of cases. Adequate controls are often lacking. Only recently have long term neurologic and neuropathologic studies been carried out in primates under controlled conditions of oxygen deprivation (Windle, 1960; Faro and Windle, 1969).

Although it is difficult to diagnose hypoxic lesions in the fetus and newborn on the basis of histopathology, Banker (1967) describes karyorrhexis of the cortex as typical of hypoxia, and Terplan (1967) refers to "bleaching" and necrosis of the cortex as characteristic of hypoxia. Such morphologic evidence of anoxic change in the cortex is infrequently found in the premature as compared with full-term infants. In his analysis of brains of handicapped children, Malamud (1963) found evidence of birth trauma primarily subcortical in location; cortical lesions were more frequently present in cases in which a convulsive disorder developed during infancy or early childhood.

On the basis of her pathological studies of neonates, Potter (1961) stated that mild subarachnoid hemorrhage is almost invariably anoxic in origin, that intraventricular hemorrhage occurs almost exclusively in premature infants, and that localized hemorrhage in the brain substance unaccompanied by external bleeding is predominantly anoxic and seldom traumatic.

Morison (1963) concurs with others in his finding that extrinsic anoxia, including the respiratory distress syndrome, is much more frequently represented in premature infant deaths than in term deaths. He emphasizes that prematurity is not a disease entity but rather a condition — with no single cause — which favors the operation of harmful influences.

479

Although Potter associated anoxic hemorrhagic lesions of the brain with pulmonary hyaline membrane disease, Windle (1969) suggests that the lung lesions found in his anoxic monkeys may have resulted from hypoxia rather than being the cause of it. Terplan (1967) found pure forms of hyaline membrane disease less frequently at fault in the lungs than a more inclusive pathological picture of "respiratory distress syndrome" with hemorrhages, atelectases, and exudates, but without hyaline membranes. In the premature he found this syndrome, with or without hyaline membrane disease, associated with either hemorrhagic or coagulative necrosis, but without the usual pattern of hypoxic cortical changes found in full-term infants. Cerebral capillary bleeding and, especially in the premature, periventricular (coagulation) necrosis of the white matter in the absence of hemorrhage or edema depend more on ischemia or vasocirculatory disturbances as Banker and Larroche (1962), Banker (1967), and Larroche (1964) have suggested. These findings were confirmed by Windle (1969) in his experimental monkeys. On the other hand, a variety of other pathologic conditions in early infancy are associated with lesions in white or grey matter in children who lack a history of abnormal birth or immediate perinatal distress (Terplan, 1967). These factors again underline the danger, ignored by some, of trying to bridge the gap between lethal lesions as observed in neonatal deaths and clinical or pathological cases which in retrospect seem similar.

Periventricular leukomalacia (Banker and Larroche, 1962; Larroche, 1964) is an ischemic necrosis of the white matter especially in the occipital, but also in other periventricular locations. These lesions may be "borderline" areas of necrosis due to arterial ischemia incident to hypotension (Walsh and Lindenberg, 1961) or may result from venous stasis and thrombosis (Larroche, 1964; Banker, 1967). A reconciliation of the theories of pathogenesis is less important than recognition of, and emphasis upon, the significance of the accompanying cardio-vascular and pulmonary pathology. Not only must the CNS findings be evaluated in the light of cardiopulmonary morphology but also in that of the metabolic milieu of the neonatal period. Larroche (1964) describes it as an "abuse" of the term anoxia to attempt to explain the CNS lesions on lack of oxygen alone, when other factors such as electrolyte imbalance, or respiratory and metabolic acidosis have not been monitered.

Although Windle (1950) found minimal hemorrhages in guinea pigs following nitrogen-induced pure anoxia, full-term monkey fetuses showed no such hemorrhages except when the animals had subsequent difficulty in breathing or when the birth was traumatic (Windle, 1961; Faro and Windle, 1969). Thus, he concluded that "brain damage by asphyxia neonatorum is not a function of anoxia alone." When CO_2 was allowed to accumulate, as animals were asphyxiated within their membranes, damage appeared which is not present in nitrogen asphyxiation. Metabolic acidosis appears as an important cause. Secondary, later respiratory distress and circulatory mechanical features are important factors in the pathogenesis of lesions in experimental primates, in neonatal death (Banker and Larroche, 1962), and in infants who survive to later develop diplegia (McDonald, 1963). R. E. Myers (1967) confirmed this when he demonstrated a monkey with ulegyria and status marmoratus several years after an acute episode of asphyxia subsequent to experimental neonatal hypoxia and acidosis. Experimentally produced neonatal anoxia consistently produced specific symmetrical lesions in the brain stem (Faro and Windle, 1969). Cortical lesions were found only once in monkeys with up to ten months survival. This lack of findings is in contrast to the experiences of Terplan (1967) and Walsh and Lindenberg (1961) in their studies of human lesions. Lindenberg suggests left heart failure as a cause of the cortical lesions. The discrepancy in findings presumably results from the fact that relatively pure hypoxia was responsible for the experimental lesion, whereas there were the added mechanical circulatory factors in the human. The lesions Windle found in his animals were most commonly in the inferior colliculus and thalamus, gracile and medial cuneate nuclei, and cerebellar roof nuclei, but not in the cortex, globus pallidus, or vestibular nuclei. According to Faro and Windle (1969), it was only after many months or years that cortical lesions were demonstrable, an expression of transneuronal degeneration consequent to primary thalamic lesions.

Courville (1953, 1959) made an extensive study of pathological material from anoxic cases. In comparing the lesions in such cases with certain so-called degenerative lesions of childhood, he theorized that many degenerative disorders of the brain with intrauterine or perinatal onset might be explained as a consequence of anoxemia. He suggested three stages in the development of lesions secondary to anoxemia. In the *first* or primary anoxemic phase there is a more or less generalized decrease in the oxygen supply to nervous tissue. This is followed by a *second* ischemic phase with local or regional damage, presumably due to vasospasm, which ultimately results in areas of localized atrophy. The *third* phase results from a disturbance in the balance of development because of the focal destructive processes and brings about a series of lesions which are ordinarily considered those of primary gliosis, such as ulegyria, or status marmoratus. In an extensive study of pathological specimens, Wolf and Cowen (1956) found much circumstantial evidence to indict hypoxic and ischemic processes as the cause of cortical and subcortical cystic and gliotic lesions, as did Towbin (1955, 1969) and Malamud (1963). Crome and Stern (1967) and Norman (1963) have critically reviewed much of the human pathological evidence.

The association of prematurity with hemorrhagic lesions, particularly those involving the drainage system of the great vein of Galen, has been accepted recently by many authors as evidence of anoxic damage to the brain. The available data, for the most part, are limited to the findings in pathological studies of infants who died in the neonatal period (Towbin, 1969; Banker, 1967). Although some clinical studies of survivors have failed to show significant evidence of residual neurological deficit (Keith and Gage, 1960), other studies (Lubchenko et al, 1963; Drillien, 1968) have revealed evidence of mental and neurologic deficits which could be expected from germinal matrix involvement in the premature (Towbin, 1969) or secondary cortical changes (Faro and Windle, 1969).

Meningeal Hemorrhage

Hemorrhage within the skull in newborn infants is invariably diagnosed as intracranial hemorrhage and no attempt is made to determine the exact form of bleeding present. This loose classification probably has its merits since the recognition of the various types of bleeding within the skull in infants is not as definite as in adults. Some effort is necessary however to work out the specific features of the various types of bleeding, for the prognosis is vastly different in some forms than in others. Thus, the outlook in subarachnoid hemorrhage is good; that in cerebral hemorrhage is poor. Failure to specify the type and location of the hemorrhage has resulted in hopeless statistical confusion concerning the prognosis of "intracranial hemorrhage." For this reason an effort will be made in the following pages to describe the various forms of intracranial hemorrhage under their separate categories.

Extradural Hemorrhage

Extradural hemorrhage in the newborn infant is extremely rare. It is surprising that its frequency is not greater in view of the numerous traumas to which the skull is subjected during birth. When it occurs it is the result of very severe trauma, usually with a depressed fracture, and severance of the middle meningeal artery somewhere along its course. Fracture of the skull is practically always present. The only important cause is direct trauma. Different coefficients of elasticity of dura and bone cause a shearing stress at the junction of the layers resulting in severance of arterial and venous channels of the dura (Campbell and Cohen, 1951). The blood clot is usually fresh since extradural hemorrhage is invariably fatal unless the bleeding is stopped by operation. The clot lies outside the dura, and causes a compression of the underlying brain substance. The clot is adherent in varying degree to the underlying dura. The middle meningeal artery may be torn high over the lateral surface of the cerebral hemispheres, or close to its emergence through the foramen spinosum.

The symptoms of extradural hemorrhage are quite dramatic. Stupor which becomes progressively deeper is characteristic. The fontanels bulge because of the increasing pressure within the skull. Convulsions are common and persistent. They may be unilateral and this may afford the only clue to the diagnosis. The pulse is slowed, and the temperature elevated. Death follows within 24 to 48 hours unless the bleeding vessel is tied. This is the only cure.

Subdural Hemorrhage

Acute subdural hemorrhage in the newborn occurs relatively often but it is quite different in its features from the subdural hematoma which is found in infants and children. The one is an acute subdural hemorrhage directly related to birth, the other a chronic subdural bleeding unrelated to the birth process.

The only important cause of subdural hemorrhage in the newborn is birth trauma. Other causes, such as an hemorrhagic diathesis, scurvy, and syphilis, may be responsible for such hemorrhage, but they are not as important as trauma. There is a clear statistical relationship between birth weight and extent of intracranial injury, the majority of tentorial tears and subdural hemorrhages being in the full-term infants (Gröntoft, 1954; Anderson, 1952). The condition occurs

483

most frequently in undernourished children. The trauma usually follows the use of forceps or abnormal delivery, such as a breech presentation, or it occurs in cases of contracted pelvis. Most frequently the hemorrhage is caused by a tear of the tentorium, although the studies of Capon (1922) have shown that the bleeding in subdural hemorrhage may result from the tear of small tentorial vessels, from the vena magna Galeni, or from cerebral veins at their point of termination in the superior longitudinal sinus. Although Holland (1922) found tentorial tears in 81 of 167 fresh fetuses (all but six cases associated with subdural hemorrhages), such tears are probably of less significance in recent years, occurring in only one of 2,060 births in a compilation by Nesbitt (1957). In his series, Gröntoft found subdural hemorrhages a significant cause of death in full-term neonatal deaths, but he emphasized that tentorial rupture and hemorrhage may occur after the death of the fetus and thus does not always signify vital injury, nor does the hemorrhage always arise during parturition. When subdural hemorrhages result from tentorial tears, they are found usually in the fossae at the base of the skull, particularly in the middle and posterior fossae.

As the name implies, subdural hemorrhage is found beneath the dura. It may be bilateral. In fresh cases the clot is usually soft and not organized. It is moderately adherent to the dura. If the clot has persisted long enough it may be enclosed by a new membrane which is probably derived from the fibroblasts on the undersurface of the dura. In such a case the contents may be fluid or solid. If solid they are usually old and organized.

The symptoms of subdural hemorrhage in the newborn infant are not easy to define. Since the hemorrhage is associated with quite severe and extensive cranial trauma there is usually a severe degree of shock. The fontanel bulges, the infant is restless and cries incessantly. Respirations are irregular. Convulsions occur quite frequently. They are usually generalized but they may be unilateral jacksonian convulsions if the hemorrhage is over one cerebral hemisphere. The convulsions may be quite persistent. Paralysis of one side of the body may result if the hemorrhage reaches a sufficient size to cause severe compression of the motor cortex. Since the bleeding in subdural hemorrhage is venous in origin, it may stop before it has attained a size great enough to cause death. On the other hand, if the hemorrhage reaches a size large enough to cause signs of increased pressure it is almost invariably fatal if not treated. Arteriography may be a useful diagnostic measure in some cases. The subdural hematoma pushes the surface of the brain away from the inner table of the skull.

The only effective treatment for subdural hemorrhage is removal of the clot. If the infant survives the hemorrhage it may not be necessary to remove the clot because it may be absorbed. A not uncommon procedure both for diagnostic and therapeutic purposes is aspiration at the lateral angle of the anterior fontanel. A needle is inserted through the dura and blood aspirated if there has been bleeding into the subdural space. The method is simple and in doubtful cases may be the only effective means of diagnosis of subdural bleeding. If blood is found successive taps may be necessary. Craniotomy is necessary if there is clot retention long enough for membranes to develop (2 to 3 weeks) (Schipke et al, 1954). The clot may eventually become organized, liquefied, or in rare instances calcified. It may be followed by atrophy of the underlying brain substance if it is not recognized and removed.

Subarachnoid Hemorrhage

Subarachnoid hemorrhage consists of bleeding into the subarachnoid space. Its incidence has been a matter of great dispute. Some authors such as Sharpe (1927) regard it as extremely common; others consider it relatively infrequent. Most of the cases described by Sharpe and others as intracranial hemorrhage are in reality cases of subarachnoid hemorrhage. The incidence of such cases is 9 percent (Sharpe) as proven by the occurrence of blood in the spinal fluid. It is probable that a small amount of blood in the spinal fluid is a relatively common finding among newborn infants and that the incidence would therefore be higher in a series of cases of newborn infants in whom routine lumbar punctures were performed. Other estimates of the incidence of subarachnoid hemorrhage vary widely; Waitz judged it to be 11 percent whereas Tasovaty estimated it at 0.05 percent (quoted by Riviere).

Although Levinson and Saphir (1933) found no evidence of organization in subarachnoid hemorrhage in newborn infants and thus assumed that blood in the subarachnoid space is absorbed and will give rise to no pathological sequelae, experimental (Bagley, 1928) and clinical data (Laurence, 1958; Foltz and Ward, 1956; Larroche, 1964) indicate that subarachnoid hemorrhage can be a significant cause of hydrocephalus.

Subarachnoid hemorrhage in the newborn is found with or with-

485

out evidence of hemorrhage elsewhere in the meninges or brain. It is probable that most of the cases with hemorrhage in the subarachnoid space alone survive without sequelae; those with subdural or cerebral hemorrhage are frequently fatal. According to Riviere there are several mechanisms concerned in the production of subarachnoid hemorrhage. These include (1) intracranial venous hypertension of circulatory origin, (2) sudden thrusts of the cerebrospinal fluid in the arachnoid spaces due to sudden increases of spinal fluid pressure, and (3) direct vascular lesions by spicules of broken bone. Potter (1952) considered mild subarachnoid hemorrhage almost invariably a result of anoxia, and not caused by mechanical injury.

The symptoms of subarachnoid hemorrhage are very similar to those of cerebral hemorrhage. They consist of prolonged cyanosis, drowsiness, poor attempts at nursing, irregular and labored breathing, rigidity of the neck or spine, and muscle twitchings involving the extremities. The anterior fontanel is often bulging. The spinal fluid contains blood in varying amounts; the fluid may be pinkish or may contain almost pure blood.

Subarachnoid hemorrhage is the one form of intracranial hemorrhage in which good recovery may be expected. In the infant, just as in the adult, it often results in complete recovery in contradistinction to the results in cerebral or ventricular hemorrhage both of which are invariably fatal. The outlook is far better, too, than in subdural hemorrhage.

INJURIES OF THE BRAIN

Injuries of the brain in the newborn may be grouped under the headings of contusion, laceration, and hemorrhage. Of these hemorrhage is by far the most important and, since contusion and laceration are found practically always in association with hemorrhage, all the cerebral injuries may be grouped under this one heading.

Cerebral Hemorrhage

The most recent statistics on the cause of death in the newborn period indicate that prematurity and its complications have surpassed hemorrhage and trauma as the most common cause of death in neonatal groups (Potter, 1952; Gröntoft, 1954; and Gruenwald, 1955). These figures are consistent for both pathological studies of neonatal mortality and for retrograde studies of clinical patients with evidence of brain damage related to the neonatal period (Eastman and DeLeon, 1955), or for pathological studies of central nervous system material in the so-called cerebral palsied children (Josephy; Benda, 1945; and Wolf and Cowen, 1956).

Arey (1952) in 100 postmortem examinations in neonatal deaths found that cerebral damage was the cause of death in 30 cases. In 11 of these, intraventricular hemorrhage occurred whereas in 5 kernicterus was the important pathological entity. In 17 other cases cerebral damage was a contributory cause of death. Arey noted that severe damage to the brain may occur in an apparently non-traumatic delivery.

Intracranial hemorrhage in premature infants is usually limited to bleeding in the intraventricular and subarachnoid spaces. Laceration of the tentorium, the commonest cause of fatal hemorrhage in the more fully developed infants is practically unknown in infants weighing less than 2,000 grams (Potter, 1952). According to Potter, the length of labor in itself does not contribute to an increased incidence of mechanical trauma; rather an increase in length of labor is associated indirectly with an increase in trauma, because the same factors responsible for abnormal labor are responsible for abnormal delivery and the incidence of operative delivery is always increased. She noted that hemorrhage from meningeal vessels is a rare cause of death in young infants; intraventricular hemorrhage occurs almost exclusively in premature infants when it is found alone. She concluded from her studies that localized hemorrhages in the brain substance unaccompanied by external bleeding are seldom traumatic, ordinarily being caused by anoxia.

Inertia and the subsequent management thereof (oxytocin, difficult forceps delivery, etc.) were the chief maternal complications found in association with traumatic brain hemorrhage, while uterine bleeding, intrapartum fever, and inertia were the important associated maternal factors in infants with anoxic brain hemorrhage. Breech delivery, indicated low forceps and mid-forceps deliveries were frequent methods of delivery in the group of infants with intracranial hemorrhage (Haller, Nesbitt and Anderson, 1956).

In 2,633 births Levinson (1939) found 12 with cerebral hemorrhage, an incidence of 0.45 percent, but in 1,527 premature infants, the incidence of cerebral hemorrhage was 292 or 19.1 percent.

The pathology of cerebral hemorrhage is relatively simple. Large cerebral hemorrhages are not common; when they occur they result from extremely severe trauma. The hemorrhage in such cases is usually found in one cerebral hemisphere. It may occupy only a small portion of the hemisphere, or involve a large part of it, destroying not only the subcortical white matter, but the structures at the base of the brain such as the basal ganglia. By far more common are the petechial hemorrhages which may be found anywhere in the cerebral white matter and at the base of the brain. Many of them are found beneath the ependyma (Patten and Alpers, 1933). These are small, minute hemorrhages often found around blood vessels everywhere in the brain. Hemorrhages in the medulla are quite common (Hemsath and Canavan, 1932).

The symptoms of cerebral hemorrhage are not specific. Some are suggestive; others indicate injury of the brain tissue. Marked drowsiness is often emphasized as an early symptom, but is not pathognomonic. The same may be said of the so-called cephalic cry. The occurrence of a sharp fretful cry, especially when the child is handled, is emphasized by Tyson (1931). Much more important is the occurrence of generalized convulsions which Tyson found in 58 percent of his cases, and which have been found by others to be very common. The convulsions are usually generalized, but may in some instances be unilateral. They are clonic or tonic, and persistent. They may be frequent and numerous or relatively infrequent. Intermittent cyanosis (Tyson) has been found frequently. Fever occurs very commonly. Regardless of its mechanism, whether due to irritation of the thermo-regulatory centers in the brain or to dehydration dependent on the cerebral hemorrhage, the fact remains that fever is a common and an important sign of cerebral bleeding. The pulse is at first rapid and later slowed. Pallor, dry skin, irregular respiration, and attacks of respiratory failure are common. Bulging of the fontanel is present in some cases, but is not common. A unilateral dilated pupil is found in some cases. The spinal fluid is clear, xanthochromic, or may contain blood.

Haller, Nesbitt and Anderson (1956) noted that the infant with anoxic brain hemorrhage initiates respiration more quickly than those with traumatic injuries. The following symptoms should be looked for clinically: apathy or restlessness, cyanosis or pallor, bulging fontanels, convulsions or twitching tremors, difficult resuscitation, feeble high-pitched cry, irregular breathing, unequal pupils or nystagmus, poor nursing or refusal to nurse, vomiting, rapid or slow pulse rate, exaggerated or absent Moro reflex, presence of altered blood in the spinal fluid and paralysis.

Very little can be done in the way of treatment once hemorrhage in the brain is diagnosed. The result is inevitable death.

Intraventricular Hemorrhage

The incidence of intraventricular hemorrhage varies from 2.2 to 8.5 percent of cases. It is rarely, if ever, found in term infants unassociated with other evidence of bleeding (Potter, 1952). The majority of the recent pathological studies of neonatal death (Haller, Nesbitt and Anderson, 1956; Potter, 1952; and Gröntoft, 1954) indicates its overwhelming occurrence with prematurity, presumably on the basis of hypoxic changes. It occurs principally as the result of subependymal hemorrhage from rupture of the terminal vein or from leakage from the choroid plexus into the ventricular system. Mechanical trauma is of secondary significance, in all probability.

The symptoms of intraventricular hemorrhage are those of cerebral hemorrhage and differ, as they do in the adult, only in the greater severity of the symptoms, and in the more profound evidences of shock. All cases of intraventricular hemorrhage are fatal. The spinal fluid is grossly bloody.

The Late Sequelae of Cerebral Birth Injuries

Many infants with cerebral birth injury will die, but it is difficult to estimate future neurologic and mental deficits in those infants who survive. In Eastman's (1962) series three-quarters of the babies subsequently showing cerebral palsy had no evidence of damage during the neonatal period and in one-third of the children the antenatal course, the process of labor, and the neonatal period *as recorded* were normal. When those with postnatal causes are eliminated from a series there is still a remaining group of handicapped children in whom recorded birth trauma in the broad sense is lacking. A certain number of these varying from 5 percent to one-third will show clinical or pathologic evidence of malformations. On the other hand malformations may actually cause the disability in some patients thought to have deficits that are purely "birth injury" in origin. It is apparent that a significant factor in the pathogenesis of some cases of prematurity and birth injury is the presence of malformation; in like manner additional cerebral damage may be caused by the malformation at the time of traumatic birth (Eastman et al, 1962; Bacola et al, 1966; Drillien, 1968; Gross et al, 1968; McDonald et al, 1963).

There is presumptive statistical evidence that socioeconomic or environmental factors may not only be in part causative in the constellation of "prematurity" but also additive to the deficit in postnatal life rhea and also when there is no history of trauma. However, in several such instances a fistulous communication was nevertheless demonstrated at operation or post mortem.

As previously noted, the natural repair of a posttraumatic fistulous communication is often imperfect. In order to effect a cessation of the rhinorrhea and prevent recurrence of meningeal infection, it is necessary to close the dural defect surgically, usually by means of a graft.

BIBLIOGRAPHY

Alexander, A. B. Fracture of the Skull Followed by Late Otogenic Meningitis. *J. Laryngol. Otol.*, 58, 372, 1943.

Appelbaum, E. and Nelson, J. Sulfadiazine and Its Sodium Compound In Treatment of Meningococcic Meningitis and Meningococcemia. *Am. J. M. Sc.*, 207, 492, 1944.

Appelbaum, E. and Nelson, J. Penicillin in the Treatment of Pneumococcic Meningitis. *J.A.M.A.*, 128, 778, 1945.

Appelbaum, E., Nelson, J., and Albin, M. B. The Treatment of Pneumococcic Meningitis with Penicillin. *Am. J. M. Sc.*, 218, 260, 1949.

Appelbaum, E. and Abler, C. Advances in the Diagnosis and Treatment of Acute Pyogenic Meningitis. *N.Y. State J. Med.*, 58, 204 and 363, 1958.

Appelbaum, E. Meningitis Following Trauma to the Head and Face. *J.A.M.A.*, 173, 1818, 1960.

Atuk, N. O., Mosca, A. and Kunin, C. M. The Use of Potentially Nephrotoxic Antibiotics in the Treatment of Gram-Negative Infections in Uremic Patients. *Ann. Intern. Med.*, 60, 28, 1964.

Barrett, F. F., McGehee, R. F., Jr., and Finland, M. Methicillin-Resistant Staphylococcus Aureus at Boston City Hospital. *New Engl. J. Med.*, 279, 441, 1968.

Benner, E. J. and Morthland, V. Methicillin-Resistant Staphylococcus Aureus: Antimicrobial Susceptibility. *New Engl. J. Med.*, 277, 678, 1967.

Berk, M. Traumatic Streptococcic Meningitis. *Am. J. M. Sc.*, 212, 18, 1946.

Brockway, C. E. and Jacobs, M. H. Streptococcal Viridans Meningitis Followed by Pneumococcal Meningitis in the Same Patient with Recovery. *J. Pediatr.*, 27, 273, 1945.

Browder, J. and Myerson, M. C. A Surgical Method for the Prevention of Thrombophlebitis of the Cavernous Sinus. *Arch. Otolaryng.*, 21, 574, 1935.

Bulger, R. J. and Sherris, J. C. Decreased Incidence of Antibiotic Resistance Among Staphylococcus Aureus. *Ann. Inter. Med.*, 69, 1099, 1968.

Bunn, P. A. and Peabody, G. Treatment of Pneumococcal Meningitis with Large Doses of Penicillin. *Arch. Int. Med.*, 89, 736, 1952.

Clandon, D. B. and Holbrook, A. A. Fatal Aplastic Anemia Associated with Chloramphenicol (Chloromycetin) Therapy. *J.A.M.A.*, 149, 912, 1952.

461

and thus be a factor in the prognosis of the organically damaged child (Drillien, 1968). A further factor to be considered is evidence from Windle's group of experimentally asphyxiated monkey fetuses. "If the infant's brain can be compared to the monkey's, asphyxia of such duration that resuscitation was required will certainly damage it." Although clinically well to usual appearance in the first 10 months of the postnatal period, severe loss of neurons in the infant's cortex can be demonstrated years later and definitive testing shows a significant memory deficit in association (Sechzer, 1969). Clinically, on the other hand, Lubchenco et al (1963) found improvement with time so that many "spastics" are nearly asymptomatic by school age.

McDonald (1963) followed 1128 children of low birth weight (1800 grams or less) for a period of 6 to 8 years. "Cerebral palsy" was diagnosed in 6.5 percent of which number 81 percent were designated "spastic diplegia" syndrome. The frequency of diplegia was inversely proportional to the length of pregnancy (cf Bacola et al, and Lubchenco). Postnatal cyanotic attacks, even in the absence of asphyxia during delivery, were found associated with diplegia. The history of these infants resembled that of Banker and Larroche's cases with periventricular leukomalacia.

The following conditions may be said to result sometimes from trauma to the brain at birth. The relative frequency of cerebral birth injury as a cause of these conditions will be discussed in a consideration of the individual diseases: 1) infantile hemiplegia; 2) cerebral diplegia; 3) porencephaly; 4) epilepsy; 5) mental deficiency.

Few serious studies on the late effects of cerebral birth injury have been made. Fleming (1931) found 5 out of 33 children who had signs of cerebral injury at birth, with sequelae at the end of one year. Ford (1937) has made a more extensive study. He collected a group of 33 cases of cerebral birth injury with a history of difficult labor and symptoms at birth. These patients varied in age from 4 to 15 years and showed a variety of clinical conditions. He found that the most common late sequela of cerebral birth injury was hemiplegia. Other sequelae included monoplegia, paraplegia, epilepsy, mental deficiency, and athetosis.

Other retrograde studies have, for the most part, emphasized either small groups of pathological entities or attempted from actual birth records to determine significant factors during the neonatal or perinatal period. One of these by Eastman and DeLeon (1955) is an analysis of 96 infants who later developed evidence of brain damage. Neurological conditions were infrequently noted during the prolonged stay in the hospital after birth. At the other end of the scale are the two studies previously quoted (Keith et al, 1953; Denhoff and Holden, 1955) in which a very low incidence of later neurological symptoms was found in those infants who survived but who were presumably damaged at the time of birth.

Infantile hemiplegia. Hemiplegia occurring in infancy may be the result of conditions existing before, during, or after birth. The prenatal hemiplegias may be the result of porencephalic cysts, defective development of the pyramidal tracts, or cerebral agenesis (Sachs, 1926). These have no relation to cerebral birth injury. The cases of hemiplegia occurring at birth are in the great majority of instances the result of trauma to the brain occurring during birth. Indeed, Ford maintains that hemiplegia is the most common late result of cerebral trauma in infants. Osler (1898) believed that all infantile hemiplegias were the result of birth injuries. The exact etiology of many of the so-called congenital hemiplegias is obscure. Out of 80 cases Gowers (1888) was unable to find an assignable cause in 50. In 140 cases of cerebral palsies of early life Sachs and Peterson (1890) found 105 with hemiplegia; 49 of these were analyzed carefully for the cause. This was found to be difficult labor (16), premature birth (4), asphyxia at birth (3), and acute trauma to the mother during pregnancy (5). The hemiplegias occurring in later infancy are the result of acquired diseases, usually some form of encephalitis following pertussis, measles, chickenpox and vaccinia, or tumors, or syphilis.

The pathology of cases of infantile hemiplegia is by no means uniform. The condition has been attributed to a variety of causes. Among them may be included porencephaly, subarachnoid hemorrhage, atrophic lobar sclerosis, cerebral hemiatrophy, and thrombosis of the dural sinuses due to cranial trauma. Of these only porencephaly, atrophic lobar sclerosis, and cerebral hemiatrophy are of any importance. Subarachnoid hemorrhage has been regarded by some as an important cause of infantile hemiplegia, but histological studies have failed to reveal that this sort of hemorrhage is capable of producing a permanent hemiplegia. As Levinson and Saphir have shown, subarachnoid hemorrhage in the newborn does not result in cerebral changes; the hemorrhage is absorbed without cerebral damage. Hence the assertions of MacNutt (1885) that subarachnoid hemorrhage may cause hemiplegias or diplegias in infants cannot be maintained. The role of porencephaly in the production of infantile hemiplegia will be discussed subsequently. Atrophic lobar sclerosis consists merely of focal atrophic changes in the cerebrum resulting from lacerations or focal damage due to circulatory or other causes, and may, if properly located cause hemiplegia in infants. Some cases of infantile hemiplegia are the result of cerebral hemiatrophy. This condition consists of atrophy of one cerebral hemisphere and is characterized by a syndrome consisting of hemiplegia, mental deficiency, and convulsions. The hemiatrophy of the brain may be almost complete or only partial. The condition is due to a variety of causes (Alpers and Dear, 1939). In rare cases infantile hemiplegia present from birth may be the result of a depressed fracture with the

491

subsequent formation of a cicatrix induced by the penetration of bone spicules into the brain substance; in other rare instances it may be the result of degenerative or vascular changes in the brain probably associated with birth or factors operating both before and during birth (Alpers, 1931 and Levin, 1936.) These cases are associated with areas of complete and incomplete necrosis of the brain related apparently to vascular changes.

Therefore, hemiplegia in the infant just as in the adult, is the result of a variety of causes. The cases occurring at birth or shortly thereafter are the rseult of porencephaly or atrophic lobar sclerosis from various causes, and rarely to thrombosis of the dural sinuses. Hemiplegias occurring later in childhood are the result of infections and are not considered here. The problem that then arises is: How many of the cases in infants are the result of trauma associated with birth? No percentages are available, but it is certain that some, if not many, are the result of cerebral birth injury. Some of the cases of porencephaly and atrophic lobar sclerosis undoubtedly are the result of trauma to the brain.

The clinical picture of infantile hemiplegia is quite readily recognized and is very characteristic. It usually consists of a spastic paralysis, partial or complete, of the upper and lower limb. In some instances monoplegias may be present, and if so, the lower limb is more usually involved than the upper. An ipsilateral facial weakness (central type), often dysarthria, a flexor spasticity of the upper limb, and extensor spasticity of the lower limb are also present. There is usually some degree of movement of the upper limb, and quite good use of the lower. Walking is possible, in the usual hemiplegic fashion, with the lower limb swinging out at the hip and the upper held in flexion. Sometimes choreoathetotic movements of the hands are present. Convulsions may occur and mental deficiency is sometimes found in varying degree.

In the last analysis infantile hemiplegias occurring at birth are usually caused by trauma to the brain during labor; the trauma results in a wide variety of conditions which are capable of producing hemiplegia. This does not include of course a large number of acquired infantile hemiplegias which are caused by cerebral infections of various sorts, as well as a smaller group resulting from a congenital change in the brain.

Cerebral diplegia. Cerebral diplegia is a condition occurring in infancy characterized by spasticity and paralysis of varying degree of all the extremities, and by mental deficiency and sometimes convulsions. Some doubt exists about the role played by trauma at birth in the production of this disease. There seems to be no doubt that the disease is caused by a variety of conditions, and that the pathological background of the disorder is extremely varied (Alpers and Marcovitz, 1938).

It is obvious from a review of the cases of cerebral diplegia in which autopsy has been performed that many kinds of lesions are seen in this disease. This apparently óbvious fact has been frequently overlooked. The following classification covers quite completely the various types of lesion associated with cerebral diplegia: 1) cerebral agenesis; 2) porencephaly; 3) atrophic lobar sclerosis with diffuse cerebral sclerosis; 4) status marmoratus; 5) meningeal hemorrhage; 6) relatively normal brain.

It may be desirable to consider these various types of lesions seriatim, in order to appraise their importance in the production of cerebral diplegia.

1. *Cerebral agenesis*. This accounts for not a few cases of cerebral diplegia. Its manifestations vary greatly. There may be almost complete failure of development of all parts of the brain and brain stem. Or there may be sufficient maldevelopment of only parts of the brain to produce cerebral diplegia. This is seen when there is absence of the pyramidal tracts or a focal lesion involving the precentral cortical areas. In these instances of cerebral agenesis the causative process is probably of intrauterine origin.
2. *Porencephaly*. In many cases cerebral diplegia is associated with porencephalic cysts. These are almost always bilateral. Many cases of cerebral diplegia are probably lost in the literature on porencephaly. The cause is intrauterine in some cases and extrauterine in others. In the latter case porencephaly results from softening, trauma, or an inflammatory lesion.
3. *Atrophic lobar sclerosis*. Many cases of cerebral diplegia have been reported under this heading. This type of sclerosis consists simply of focal atrophy of the brain, with loss of ganglion cells and replacement by astrocytes. The loss may be moderate, affecting only some of the cell layers, or it may be so complete as to wipe out almost the entire ganglion cell population of the affected area. Demyelination of the cortex is always present. The process is not confined to the cortex alone; it affects the subjacent white matter as well, causing demyelination, atrophy, or disintegration of the axis cylinders and glial scar formation. The lobar sclerosis usually involves the two hemispheres unequally. It affects single gyri or lobes of one or both hemispheres. It must be regarded as a secondary process in the majority of cases. It may be the result of inflammation, trauma, meningeal homorrhage, or vascular occlusion. In the majority of instances it is produced by extrauterine causes or factors associated with the process of birth.
4. *Status marmoratus*. This condition accounts for relatively few cases of cerebral diplegia, usually those in which there is athetosis. In most cases it must be regarded as having an intrauterine cause, probably a result of prenatal infection. It has been regarded by some authors as the result of birth trauma. It is difficult to know when status marmoratus is the cause of cerebral diplegia. The diagnosis is usually made post mortem, but it is safe to say that cerebral diplegia associated with idiocy and athetosis may be the result of status marmoratus. It is not possible to be more definite than this.
5. *Meningeal hemorrhage*. The role of meningeal hemorrhage is difficult to evaluate. No doubt subarachnoid hemorrhage occurs frequently in infants but usually it is of no serious consequence and causes no symptoms. In some cases, however, it is severe and forms a clot on the cortex which may produce atrophic lobar sclerosis by interference with the circulation of the brain beneath the clot. Eventually the clot becomes organized, and the result is marked adhesive meningeal fibrosis with atrophy of the underlying cortex. The evidence from MacNutt's necropsy material is not convincing. So-called atrophic lobar sclerosis was present, but the role of subarachnoid hemorrhage was proved only by inference and the results were not definite. Subarachnoid hemorrhage is probably not responsible for many cases of cerebral diplegia. Indeed, we should regard it as a rare cause of the condition.
6. *Relatively normal brain*. Cases of diplegia in which the brain is relatively nor-

493

mal form an important group. In a number of well-studied cases, a few lesions have been noted which could be regarded as responsible for diplegia. In a few instances nothing abnormal was seen; in others only minor changes in the cortico-spinal pathways were observed. How does one explain the cerebral diplegia in these cases? Infantile hemiplegias have been observed in some instances in which the pyramidal tracts were intact. Cases of this sort were studied particularly by Spielmeyer (1906) and by Bielschowsky (1918). In Spielmeyer's case there was spastic left hemiplegia without a Babinski sign. This condition was present for two years before the death of the patient. Histologic study revealed a completely intact corticospinal system; the Betz cells were not damaged, but there was com-plete loss of the upper cell layers of the lamina pyramidalis (III) in the motor cortex. In Bielschowsky's two cases hemiplegia had existed for about 21 and 16 years, respectively. In both instances the corticospinal systems were completely intact.

In such cases it is assumed (Spielmeyer) that the hemiplegia is due to isola-tion of the Betz cell layer from the other cortical layers. The hemiplegia is re-garded therefore as the result of interruption of intracortical connections between the cells of origin of the corticospinal tract and the cells of the lamina pyrami-dalis (III). Where this interruption takes place is not clear, but it must be on the afferent side.

Although it is possible that this mechanism is also operative in the cases of cerebral diplegia in which there are few changes in the corticospinal system, this is unlikely because the cell loss in the lamina pyramidalis is usually not so extensive as to lead to this type of paralysis.

Cerebral diplegia is characterized briefly by the following features: Concep-tion and maternal health are usually normal. In the great majority of instances the health of the mother is good during pregnancy, but sometimes there is a history of trauma such as a severe fall, or a story of a severe maternal illness. The part which such incidents play in the production of the diplegia is always diffi-cult to evaluate. The birth is normal in a surprisingly high percentage of cases. Frequently however delivery is difficult, instrumental, or precipitate. A high per-centage of cases of cerebral diplegia are born prematurely. Asphyxia seems to play no significant role in these cases. Some of the infants are cyanotic at birth and are revived with difficulty; others breathe easily at birth. Frequently there is difficulty in feeding and delayed dentition. Motor, mental, and general de-velopment are greatly impaired. It is often apparent soon after birth that those affected with diplegia are slower in general development than are normal chil-dren. They frequently do not learn to sit, or they are greatly delayed in sitting up. Their mental responses are impaired as well; they do not respond promptly, they are slower to comprehend, and they are frequently described as dull. Mental impairment may be pronounced or relatively slight. In exceptional instances, mental-ity may be perfectly normal. The motor manifestations vary somewhat. In the typical case there is spasticity of the four limbs. In contradistinction to the posture in hemi-plegia, these cases have greater involvement of the lower limbs rather than the upper. The lower extremities are held in extension, the upper in flexion. Often there is fairly good movement of the upper limbs. Sometimes athetotic move-ments are seen in the fingers and hands. The disability produced by the diplegia

494

may be so complete that no movement is possible, or there may be only moderate loss of movement. Many cases are ambulatory. Facial movements may be greatly impaired or may be relatively normal. Dysarthria is common due to spasticity of the muscles of speech. Difficulty in swallowing may develop late in the disease.

The role of trauma in the production of cerebral diplegia is problematical. Older concepts attributed many, if not most cases of cerebral diplegia to trauma. This is undoubtedly not sound. It is probable that some cases of cerebral diplegia, probably relatively few, result from trauma to the brain which occurs either with prolonged or precipitate labor. In such instances there may be sufficient damage to cause the development of a porencephalic cyst or a patch of atrophic lobar sclerosis. Meningeal hemorrhage plays no role in the production of cerebral diplegia for reasons which were given earlier in the discussion of congenital hemiplegia.

By far the great majority of cases of cerebral diplegia are the result of maldevelopment in utero. This is true of the cases which are due to cerebral agenesis, to many cases of porencephaly, some cases of atrophic lobar sclerosis, and most of the cases of status marmoratus. The reason for this maldevelopment is not clear, but there is good evidence that in addition to faulty heritage, there may be an added factor of infection or intoxication of the fetus in utero (Alpers and Patten, 1936). In any event it may be stated definitely that cerebral birth trauma plays only a minor role in the production of cerebral diplegia, and that intrauterine conditions of varying sorts are much more important.

PORENCEPHALY

Porencephaly is a condition characterized by cavity formation in the brain. The cavity may be small or it may occupy an entire lobe, is usually but not always continuous with the ventricle, and may extend from the cortex to the ventricle. Sometimes it is connected with the subarachnoid space. The cavity usually has a thin roof of cerebral cortex which is composed chiefly of neuroglia and contains a decreased number of ganglion cells, many of which are degenerated. Porencephaly or porencephalic cysts are sometimes the result of birth trauma. The symptoms vary with the area of brain affected; there may be hemiplegia, jacksonian convulsions, or other signs of focal brain disease. The symptoms may appear early in infancy, or not until the child is 5 or 6 years of age. There is often delay in mental development and evidence of mental retardation. The porencephalic cyst is frequently found in the frontal portions of the brain, hence jacksonian convulsions are a prominent feature of the disease. They may be the first symptom and may exist without other signs of focal brain damage. Frequently they are found in association with a hemiplegia or a monoplegia, the upper limb being more often affected than the lower. Sometimes aphasia is present if the cyst involves the speech centers in the brain. Hemianopsia may be found in cysts involving the temporal or occipital lobes.

This condition is frequently suspected, but the diagnosis must be confirmed by the injection of air into the subarachnoid space (pneumoencephalography).

THE EPILEPSIES AND CEREBRAL BIRTH INJURY

It is frequently assumed that birth injuries are commonly the cause of seizures. Convulsions in the neonatal period are always indicative of cerebral damage and usually carry a poor prognosis. Penfield and Jasper (1953) considered the commonest causes of seizures in the first two years of life to be birth injury, a congenital abnormality, or a degenerative process. To the age of 10 years, birth injury is an important cause of habitual seizures. These authors speak of the process of "epileptogenic ripening," a slow process during infancy and childhood, which characterizes the often long-delayed onset of recurrent fits due to birth injury. This interval of freedom from fits may be 10 to 30 years. Skull x-rays may show an asymmetry of the calvarium consequent to localized sclerotic microgyria which results from focal ischemic processes incident to birth trauma. Instead of rapid destruction with consequent cyst formation, a contracting sclerotic scar develops to an extent that it reduces the volume of the injured hemisphere to less than half that of the entire cranium. A smaller "half" of the cranium thus indicates cerebral damage in the first year of life.

The relationship of such damaged cortex to focal seizures is well established. The comparable relationship of Ammon's horn sclerosis to temporal lobe seizures later in life, and the origin of such sclerosis, be it compression and focal ischemia at birth (Earle, Baldwin, and Penfield, 1953) or subsequent to anoxia or cerebral edema and focal ischemia from trauma (Lindenberg, 1955), or status epilepticus or other causes (Meyer, 1956), is still debatable.

It is probable that some cases of convulsions are the result of birth injuries. These conditions are often associated with other evidences of brain damage such as hemiplegia or diplegia, but they may be found without any other sign of cerebral involvement. Probably only a small percentage of cases of convulsions or mental deficiency are due to brain damage associated with the process of birth, but in obscure cases of convulsions birth injury is often blamed in the absence of adequate proof.

Mechanical birth trauma per se probably accounts for a rare case of mental deficiency or retardation. In the broad sense of perinatal damage, including hypoxia, it is estimated that 2 to 5 per cent of cases of low grade mental deficiency result from birth injury (Crome and Stern, 1967). One prospective study of low-birth-weight infants showed no association between mental subnormality and either apnea at birth or the respiratory distress syndrome which responded to 40 percent oxygen inhalation. Those children who were mentally retarded had respiratory difficulties of the most severe form, late occurring apnea, or a toxemic mother (Bacola et al, 1966). Drillien (1968) interprets her analysis of obstetrical factors in the mentally handicapped to suggest that "severe complications of labor and delivery were not primarily responsible for the mental handicap in many cases but might have caused additional cerebral damage resulting in epilepsy and/or cerebral palsy." It is evident that socioeconomic and developmental anomalies are also of significance even in those with birth injury (Gross et al, 1968).

In full-term infants a correlation between degree of asphyxia and impairment of cognitive function three years later seemed to occur in the series of cases analyzed by Graham et al (1962). A hint as to the pathogenesis of some cases of late occurring retardation is contained in Windle's experimental monkeys as noted earlier in the discussion of anoxia (Faro and Windle, 1969).

BIBLIOGRAPHY

Aldridge, A. H. and Meredith, R. S. Obstetric Responsibility for the Prevention of Fetal Deaths. *Am. J. Obstet. & Gynec.*, 42, 373, 1941.

Alpers, B. J. Diffuse Progressive Degeneration of the Grey Matter of the Cerebrum. *Arch. Neurol. & Psychiat.*, 25, 469, 1931.

Alpers, B. J. and Dear, R. Hemiatrophy of the Brain. *J. Nerv. Ment. Dis.*, 89, 653, 1939.

Alpers, B. J. and Marcovitz, E. Pathologic Background of Cerebral Diplegia. *Am. J. Dis. Child.*, 55, 356, 1938.

Alpers, B. J. and Patten, C. A. Cerebral Birth Conditions. The Role of Intrauterine Infection and Intoxication in Man. *Am. J. Dis. Child.*, 52, 144, 1936.

Anderson, G. W. Obstetrical Factors in Cerebral Palsy. *J. Pediatr.*, 40, 340, 1952.

Arey, J. B. Observations on Some Causes of Cerebral Palsy Based on Postmortem Findings in Newborn Infants. *J. Pediatr.*, 40, 621, 1952.

Bacola, E., Behrle, F. C., de Schweinitz, L., Miller, H. C., and Mira, M. Perinatal and Environmental Factors in Late Neurogenic Sequelae. *Am. J. Dis. Child.*, *112*, 359, 1966.

Bagley, C. Blood in the Cerebrospinal Fluid. Resultant Functional and Organic Alterations in the Central Nervous System. A. Experimental Data. *Arch. Surg.*, *17*, 18, 1928.

Banker, B. Q. Neuropathological Effects of Anoxia and Hypoglycemia in Newborn. *Develop. Med. Child. Neurol.*, *9*, 544, 1967.

Banker, B. Q. and Larroche, J. C. Periventricular Leukomalacia of Infancy. A Form of Neonatal Anoxic Encephalopathy. *Arch. Neurol.*, *7*, 386, 1962.

Benda, C. Late Effects of Cerebral Birth Injuries. *Medicine*, *24*, 71, 1945.

Beneke. Über Tentoriumzerreissungen bei der Geburt. *Verh. d. deut. Pathol. Gesellschaft*, *14*, 128, 1910.

Bielschowsky, M. Ueber Hemiplegie bei intakter Pyramidenbahn. *J. Psychol., u. Neurol.*, *22*, 1, 1918.

Bound, J. P., Butler, N. R., and Spector, W. G. Classification and Causes of Perinatal Mortality. *Br. Med. J.*, *2*, 1191 and 1260, 1956.

Browne, F. J. Stillbirth: Its Causes, Pathology and Prevention. *Edinburgh M. J.*, *27*, 153, 1921.

Campbell, J. B. and Cohen, J. Epidural Hemorrhage and the Skull of Children. *Surg. Gynec. Obstet.*, *92*, 257, 1951.

Capon, N. B. Intracranial Traumata in the Newborn. *J. Obstet. & Gynec., Br. Emp.*, *29*, 572, 1922.

Cavanagh, J. B. and Meyer, A. Aetiological Aspects of Ammon's Horn Sclerosis Associated with Temporal Lobe Epilepsy. *Br. Med. J.*, *2*, 1403, 1956.

Courville, C. B. Antenatal and Paranatal Circulatory Disorders as a Cause of Cerebral Damage in Early Life. *J. Neuropath. Exp. Neurol.*, *18*, 115, 1959.

Courville, C. B. *Contributions to the Study of Cerebral Anoxia*. Los Angeles: San Lucas Press, 1953.

Crome, L. and Stern, J. *The Pathology of Mental Retardation*. London: J. and A. Churchill, Ltd., 1967.

Dekaban, A. *Neurology of Infancy*. Baltimore: Williams and Wilkins, 1959.

Denhoff, E. and Holden, R. H. Etiology of Cerebral Palsy: An Experimental Approach. *Am. J. Obstet. & Gynec.*, *70*, 274, 1955.

D'Esopo, D. A. and Marchetti, A. A. The Causes of Fetal and Neonatal Mortality. *Am. J. Obstet. & Gynec.*, *44*, 1, 1942.

Drillien, C. M. Social and Economic Factors Affecting the Incidence of Premature Births. *J. Obstet. & Gynec. Br. Emp.*, *64*, 161, 1957.

Drillien, C. M. Studies in Mental Handicap. II. Some Obstetric Factors of Possible Aetiological Significance. *Arch. Dis. Child.*, *43*, 283, 1968.

Earle, K. M., Baldwin, M., and Penfield, W. Incisural Sclerosis and Temporal Lobe Seizures Produced by Hippocampal Herniation at Birth. *Arch. Neurol. & Psychiat.*, *69*, 27, 1953.

Eastman, N. J. and DeLeon, M. Etiology of Cerebral Palsy. *Am. J. Obstet. & Gynec.*, *69*, 960, 1955.

Eastman, N. J., Kohn, S. G., Maisel, J. E., and Kavaler, R. The Obstetrical Background of 753 Cases of Cerebral Palsy. *Obstet. & Gynec. Survey*, *17*, 459, 1962.

498

Faro, M. D. and Windle, W. F. Transneuronal Degeneration in Brains of Monkeys Asphyxiated at Birth. *Exptl. Neurol.*, *24*, 38, 1969.

Fleming, G. B. and Morton, E. D. Meningeal Hemorrhage in the Newborn. *Arch. Dis. Childhood*, *5*, 361, 1930.

Foltz, E. L. and Ward, A. A. Communicating Hydrocephalus from Subarachnoid Bleeding. *J. Neurosurg.*, *13*, 546, 1956.

Ford, F. R. Cerebral Birth Injuries and Their Results. *Medicine*, *5*, 120, 1926.

Ford, F. R. *Diseases of the Nervous System in Infancy, Childhood and Adolescence*, 5th ed. Springfield, Ill.: Charles C Thomas, 1966.

Freud, S. *Die Infantile Cerebrallähmung*. Vienna: Alfred Holder, 1897.

Gfroerer, W. Zum Einflusz der Schädelimpression auf den Neugeborenen und seine körperliche und geistige Entwicklung. *Ztschr. f. Geburtshülfe u. Gynäkologie*, *75*, 101, 1914.

Ginzler, A. M. and Chesner, C. Toxic Manifestations in the Newborn Infant Following Placental Transmission of Sulfanilamide. *Am. J. Obstet. & Gynec.*, *44*, 46, 1942.

Gowers, W. R. Clinical Lecture on Birth Palsies. *Lancet*, *1*, 709, 1888.

Graham, F. K., Ernhart, C. B., and Thurston, D. The Relationship of Neonatal Apnea To Development at Three Years. Chapter 13 in *Mental Retardation*, Vol. 39 of the ARNMD. Baltimore: Williams and Wilkins, 1962.

Gröntoft, O. Intracranial Haemorrhage and Blood-brain-barrier Problems in the Newborn. *Acta Path. et Microbiol. Scandinav. Suppl.*, *100*, 1954.

Gross, H., Jellinger, K., Kaltenback, E., and Rett, A. Infantile Cerebral Disorders. Clinical-neuropathological Correlations to Elucidate the Aetological Factors. *J. Neurol. Sci.*, *7*, 551, 1968.

Gruenwald, P. The Pathology of Perinatal Distress. *Arch. Pathol.*, *60*, 150, 1955.

Haller, E. S., Nesbitt, R. E. L., Jr., and Anderson, G. W. Clinical and Pathologic Concepts of Gross Intracranial Hemorrhage in Perinatal Mortality. *Obstet. Gynec. Surv.*, *11*, 179, 1956.

Harrison, V. C., Heese, H. de v., and Klein, M. Intracranial Hemorrhage Associated with Hyaline Membrane Disease. *Arch. Dis. Childhood*, *43*, 227, 1968.

Heckel, G. P. Chemotherapy During Pregnancy. *J.A.M.A.*, *117*, 1314, 1941.

Hemsath, F. A. Birth Injury of the Occipital Bone. *Am. J. Obstet. Gynec.*, *27*, 194, 1934.

Hemsath, F. A. Cerebral Hemorrhage in the Newborn. *Am. J. Obstet. Gynec.*, *28*, 343, 1934.

Hemsath, F. A. and Canavan, M. Microscopic Cerebral Hemorrhages in Stillbirths and Newborn Infants. *Am. J. Obstet. Gynec.*, *23*, 471, 1932.

Hicks, S. P. Some Effects of Ionizing Radiation and Metabolic Inhibition on the Developing Mammalian Nervous System. *J. Pediatr.*, *40*, 489, 1952.

Hicks, S. P. Injury of the Central Nervous System Incurred During Fetal Life. *Res. Publ. A. Nerv. Ment. Dis.*, *34*, 86, 1956.

Holland, E. The Causation of Fetal Death. *Rep. Publ. Health & Med. Subjects*, No. 7. London, 1922.

Josephy, H. Cerebral Hemiatrophy. *J. Neuropathol. Exp. Neurol.*, *4*, 250, 1945.

Josephy, H. Pathologic Anatomy of the Brain in Cerebral Palsy. *Proceedings of the Scientific Sessions of the American Academy for Cerebral Palsy,* Feb. 17-18, 1950.

Kalbag, R. M. and Woolf, A. L. *Cerebral Venous Thrombosis.* London: Oxford University Press, 1967.

Keith, H. M., Norval, M. A., and Hunt, A. B. Neurologic Lesions in Relation to the Sequelae of Birth Injuries. *Neurology, 3,* 139, 1953.

Keith, H. and Gage, R. P. Neurologic Lesions in Relation to Asphyxia of Newborn and Factors of Pregnancy: Long-term Follow-up. *Pediatrics, 26,* 616, 1960.

Kemp, F. H. and Stallworthy, J. A. A Case of Intrauterine Infection of the Fetus by Gas-gangrene Organisms. *Br. Med. J., 2,* 94, 1942.

Larroche, J. C. Hémorragies cérébrales intra-ventriculaires chez le prématuré le partie: Anatomie et physiopathologie. *Biol. Neonat., 7,* 26, 1964.

Laurence, K. M. The Natural History of Hydrocephalus. *Lancet, 2,* 1152, 1958.

Levin, P. Cortical Encephalomalacia in Infancy. *Arch. Neurol. & Psychiat., 36,* 264, 1936.

Levinson, A. Cerebral Manifestation in the Newborn. *Arch. Pediatr., 56,* 210, 1939.

Levinson, A. and Saphir, O. Meninges in Intracranial Hemorrhage in the Newborn. *Am. J. Dis. Childhood., 45,* 973, 1933.

Lilienfeld, A. M. and Pasamanick, B. The Association of Maternal and Fetal Factors with the Development of Cerebral Palsy and Epilepsy. *Am. J. Obstet. Gynec., 70,* 93, 1955.

Lindenberg, R. Compression of Brain Arteries as Pathogenic Factor for Tissue Necrosis and Their Areas of Predilection. *J. Neuropathol. Exp. Neurol., 14,* 223, 1955.

Lubchenco, L. O., et al. Sequelae of Premature Birth. *Am. J. Dis. Childhood, 106,* 101, 1963.

Lund, C. J. The Relation of Inhalation Analgesia and Anesthesia to Asphyxia Neonatorum. *Am. J. Obstet. Gynec., 43,* 365, 1942.

Mackay, R. B. Observations on Oxygenation of the Fetus in Normal and Abnormal Pregnancy. *J. Obstet. Gynec. Brit. Emp 64,* 185, 1957.

Malamud, N. Recent Trends in Classification Of Neuropathological Findings in Mental Deficiency. *Am. J. Ment. Defic., 58,* 438, 1954.

Malamud, N. Recent Trends in Classification of Neuropathological Findings in Schade and W. H. McMenemey (Eds.), *Selective Vulnerability of the Brain in Hypoxemia.* Philadelphia: F. A. Davis Co., 1963. P. 211.

Matson, D. C. Craniocerebral Trauma in Childhood. *Am. J. Surg., 101,* 677, 1961.

McDonald, A. D. Cerebral Palsy in Children with Very Low Birth Weight. *Arch. Dis. Childhood, 38,* 579, 1963.

McNutt, S. J. Double Infantile Spastic Hemiplegia with the Report of a Case. *Am. J. Med. Sci., 89,* 58, 1885.

McNutt, S. J. Seven Cases of Infantile Spastic Hemiplegia. *Arch. Pediatr., 2,* 20, 1885.

Meyers, R. E. Effects of Asphyxiation in the Fetal Monkey. *Diag. Treat. Fetal Disorders,* 1967.

Morison, J. E. *Fetal and Neonatal Pathology.* London: Butterworths, 1963.

Nesbitt, R. E. L. *Perinatal Loss in Modern Obstetrics.* Philadelphia: F. A. Davis Co., 1957.

Norman, R. M. Malformations of the Nervous System, Birth Injury and Diseases in Early Life. Chapter 6 in Greenfield, J. G. *Neuropathology.* Baltimore: Williams and Wilkins, 1963.

Osler, W. *The Cerebral Palsies of Childhood.* Philadelphia: P. Blakiston's Sons & Co., 1898.

Patten, C. A. and Alpers, B. J. Cerebral Birth Conditions with Special Reference to the Factor of Hemorrhage. *Am. J. Psychiat., 12,* 751, 1933.

Penfield, W. and Jasper, H. *Epilepsy and the Functional Anatomy of the Human Brain.* Boston: Little, Brown & Co., 1953.

Plummer, G. Anomalies Occurring in Children Exposed in Utero to the Atomic Bomb in Hiroshima. *Pediatrics, 10,* 687, 1952.

Potter, E. L. Birth Injuries. *Proc. Am. Cong. Obstet. Gynec., 1,* 331, 1941.

Potter, E. L. *Pathology of the Fetus and the Newborn.* Chicago: Year Book Publishing Co., 1952.

Potter, E. L. and Adair, F. L. *Fetal and Neonatal Death* (2nd. ed.) Chicago: Univ. of Chicago Press, 1961.

Riviere, M. Meningeal Hemorrhages of the Newborn. *J. de. Med. de. Bordeaux, 114,* 129, 1937.

Roback, H. N. and Kahler, H. F. Monstrosity Due to Intrauterine Purulent Meningoencephalitis. *J. Nerv. Ment Dis., 94,* 669, 1941.

Rydberg, E. *Cerebral Injury in Newborn Children Consequent on Birth Injury.* Copenhagen: Levin and Munksgaard, 1932.

Sachs, B. The Cerebral Palsies of Early Life. *Am. J. Med. Sci., 171,* 376, 1926.

Sachs, B. and Peterson F. A Study of Cerebral Palsies of Early Life Based Upon an Analysis of One Hundred and Fifty Cases. *J. Nerv. Ment. Dis., 17,* 295, 1890.

Schipke, R., Riege, D., and Scoville, W. B. Acute Subdural Hemorrhage at Birth. *Pediatrics, 14,* 469, 1954.

Schwartz, P. Traumatic Injury of the Brain at Birth. *Deutsche med. Wochnschr., 50,* 1375, 1924.

Schwartz, P. Die Traumatischen Schädigungen des Zentralnervensystems durch die Geburt. *Ergebn. inn. Med. u. Kinderh., 31,* 165, 1927.

Schwartz, P. *Birth Injuries of the Newborn.* New York: Karger, 1961.

Sechzer, J. A. Memory Deficit in Monkeys Brain Damaged by Asphyxia Neonatorum. *Exper. Neurol., 24,* 497, 1969.

Sharpe, W. Intracranial Hemorrhage in the Newborn. *N. Y. State J. Med., 27,* 296, 1927.

Spielmeyer, W. Hemiplegie bei intakter Pyramidenbahn. *Münch. Med. Wschr., 53,* 1404, 1906.

Srsen, S. Intraventricular Hemorrhage in the Newborn and "Low Birth Weight." *Dev. Med. Child. Neurol., 9,* 474, 1967.

Taylor, H. M., Dyrenforth, L. Y.., and Pollard, C. B. Absorption of Quinine into Cerebrospinal Fluid of Fetus in Utero. *J. Florida Med. Assn., 27,* 487, 1941.

Terplan, K. L. Histopathologic Brain Changes in 1152 Cases of the Perinatal and Early Infancy Period. *Biol. Neonat., 11,* 348, 1967.

Towbin, A. Pathology of Cerebral Palsy. II. Encephaloclastic Processes. *Arch. Pathol., 59,* 529, 1955.

Towbin, A. Mental Retardation due to Germinal Matrix Infarction. *Science, 164,* 156, 1969.

Tyson, R. M. Intracranial Hemorrhage of the Newborn. *Am. J. Obstet. Gynec., 21,* 694, 1931.

Walsh, F. B. and Lindenberg, R. Hypoxia in Infants and Children: A Clinical-pathological Study Concerning the Primary Visual Pathways. *Bull. J. Hopkins Hosp., 108,* 100, 1961.

Windle, W. F. *Asphyxia Neonatorum.* Springfield, Ill.: Charles C Thomas, 1950.

Windle, W. F. Effects of Asphyxiation of the Fetus and Newborn Infant. *Pediatrics, 26,* 565, 1960.

Windle, W. F. Anoxia and Asphyxia: Experiments in Fetal and Neonatal Monkeys. In W. S. Fields and M. M. Desmond (Eds.), *Disorders of the Developing Nervous System.* Springfield, Ill.: Charles C Thomas, 1961. Pp. 144-155.

Windle, W. F. Brain Damage by Asphyxia at Birth. *Sci. Am., 221,* 76, 1969.

Wolf, A. and Cowen, D. The Cerebral Atrophies and Encephalomalacias of Infancy and Childhood. *Res. Publ., A. Nerv. Ment. Dis., 34,* 199, 1956.

Wolf, A. and Cowen D. Perinatal Infections of the Central Nervous System. *J. Neuropathol. Exp. Neurol., 18,* 191, 1959.

Wolf, A., Cowen D., and Paige, B. H. Fetal Encephalomyelitis: Prenatal Inception of Infantile Toxoplasmosis. *Science, 93,* 548, 1941.

Yllpo, A. The Pathology of Premature Babies. *Klin. Wochnschr., 1,* 1241, 1922.

CHAPTER 15

HEAD INJURIES IN INFANTS AND CHILDREN

KENNETH SHULMAN, M.D.

INTRODUCTION

The mortality and serious morbidity of head injuries in infants and children warrant separate consideration within a text on cranial and spinal injuries. Accidents kill more children than the three most common diseases of childhood combined, and one-fourth of these violent accidental deaths are the result of head injuries. Despite the fact that child care has resulted in a decrease in other major childhood illnesses, head injuries are increasing in both frequency and seriousness, partly as a result of increased automotive accidents and partly — in major urban areas — as the result of falls from newly constructed high-rise apartment buildings. It is estimated that 200,000 children per year are hospitalized because of such injuries; 3,000 die, and up to 20,000 have prolonged or permanent impairment of neurological or mental function (U.S.P.H.S., 1963). Effective accident prevention measures are the ultimate solution and should be the concern of parents, educators, manufacturers, and governmental authorities. The medical aspects of pediatric head injuries are of interest not only because of their complexity but also because of the effects of injury upon the growing brain — with its vulnerability on the one hand and its plasticity on the other — as compared with similar injuries in adults. Finally, there are a number of conditions that are unique in children as, for example, chronic subdural hematoma, the growing skull fracture, and birth injury.

The general approach in this chapter will be through the citation of personal experiences of the author in two different settings: that of a large municipal hospital with a very active trauma service and which tends to be the primary care hospital, and that of a children's referral hospital that does not have an acute trauma service. Emphasis will

503

be placed on injuries in the infant and young child. Modern patho-physiologic concepts of brain trauma will be discussed as they apply specifically to the developing brain and the metabolic milieu of the child.

PERINATAL INJURIES

The head is subjected to considerable force during delivery. Recent measurements of intrauterine pressure have recorded pressures of 60 + mm Hg during labor (Schulman and Romney, 1970). The sudden release of this applied pressure in cases of rapid delivery would seem to be the major causative factor in intracranial hemorrhage. Such intracranial hemorrhage accounts for 10 to 20 percent of all neonatal deaths, including stillborns and those dying within the first two weeks (Dekaban, 1959). Although perinatal anoxia may be of importance in the premature, direct mechanical stress is the major cause of head injury in full-term infants.

Cephalhematoma

The collection of blood beneath the pericranium or galea – cephal-hematoma – is a frequent cause of request for neurosurgical consul-tation. The swelling is most often parietal, and unilateral and, when below the pericranium, is confined by the attachment of the periosteum at the cranial sutures. Parietal skull fractures have been found in 25 percent of infants with cephalhematomas (Kendall and Woloshin, 1952). Cephalhematoma may be accompanied by a decrease of hematocrit and an elevated leukocyte count, but the infant will be normal on neurological testing. There is no specific treatment; needle aspiration is inadvisable because of the hazard of infection. Calci-fication may develop within a cephalhematoma, but such calcification will generally resolve without surgery and without causing an abnor-mality of skull shape or size.

Skull Fracture

The newborn skull is elastic and can be distorted, thus tending to resist fracture. The bones are thin and membranous, with loose junc-tures at the suture lines, and are made more pliable by the periosteal to dural bridging at these sites. As already indicated, linear fractures may complicate cephalhematoma. The characteristic fracture of the

504

newborn membranous skull is a depression without a break in bone continuity, the so-called "Ping-Pong," "derby-hat," or indented fracture. Many fractures of this variety, generally thought to be due to placement and stress of obstetrical forceps, are due rather to blunt compression of the infant's head against the sacral promontory in a contracted pelvis. Rarely are such fractures compounded; however, inappropriate forceps application can lacerate the scalp.

It has been our policy to elevate depressed infantile fractures when they involve the parietal or frontal bones, in order to allow the child to attain a normal cosmetic appearance and to remove any possibility of focal cortical compression. Attempts to manipulate the fractures through the skin by compression of the skull are not successful and operative elevation is necessary. This can be done electively in the first few days of life under local or general anesthesia. The use of local anesthesia has been proposed by Mealey (1968) who stresses judicious use of small amounts of procaine. However, the newborn usually tolerates general anesthesia well and, since competent pediatric anesthesiologists are readily available, intubation can easily and safely be done. In this author's opinion, general anesthesia is preferable.

Injuries to Cranial Nerves at Time of Delivery

Forceps application to the face can compress the facial nerve at the stylomastoid foramen or in its course through the parotid. The paralysis produced is of the peripheral type, affecting all muscles of the face. The diagnosis of facial paralysis in a newborn is difficult but is suggested by facial asymmetry during crying and an unequal, inefficient suck. Often, other findings such as extreme moulding or a cephalhematoma, give evidence of a difficult delivery. Generally, conservative management is indicated, the tendency being towards recovery beginning within the first two weeks of life and steadily progressing to full return of function by three months. The mother should be instructed to protect the conjunctiva by irrigating it with a mild antiseptic solution if the eye cannot be completely closed during sleep.

Extradural Hematoma in the Newborn

This rare condition has not been encountered in our clinic. The case reports in the literature (Campbell and Cohen, 1951; Courville, 1945) stress the unusual clinical presentation with neurologic symptoms delayed for days in an infant who has had a difficult delivery, a skull fracture and, usually, an unstable hematocrit. The classic signs of temporal lobe herniation associated with extradural hematoma in the older child and adult are not found in the majority of infantile cases, because the extradural collection is outside the middle fossa. Most cases have been diagnosed at the time of exploration of a fracture site in the vault. Fontanel puncture is negative. Carotid angiography demonstrates the lesion when one remembers that oblique views are needed to demonstrate frontal clots.

Subdural Hematoma

Fatal bleeding into the subdural space associated with birth trauma from moulding of the head is most frequently due to tearing of the tentorium at its junction with the falx. Such an injury is a common finding in postmortem studies of birth injuries, and represented the major cause of deaths in Courville's series (1945). In such fatal injuries, bleeding into the subarachnoid space and around and into the midbrain also occurs along with primary and secondary intraventricular hemorrhage. In such cases, the infants are acutely ill and irritable with seizures, poor Moro and sucking reflexes, opisthotonus, and a tense bulging fontanel. Subhyaloid hemorrhages may be visible early on funduscopic examination. Fontanel taps may be non-revealing or yield very bloody fluid. Ventricular puncture discloses hemorrhagic cerebrospinal fluid. The hematocrit is unstable with a decreasing level, a feature characteristic of the newborn with significant intracranial bleeding.

The management of these infants whose long-term prognosis is poor due to mental retardation, seizure disorders, and hydrocephalus, taxes one's judgment. That craniotomy is feasible was demonstrated by Cushing (1905), but a more conservative approach involving subdural taps and general supportive measures has been adopted in most centers (Schipke et al, 1954). However, in instances in which a solid clot over the hemisphere cannot be evacuated through an 18-gauge needle, burr hole exploration is indicated. Failure to demonstrate blood in the cerebrospinal fluid by lumbar puncture is generally an indication that bleeding is confined to the subdural space and that it has occurred from bridging veins rather than from a tentorial tear. In such cases, craniotomy for persistent effusion may be indicated. One should keep in mind also that the infant with a neonatal bleeding disorder may present with a subdural hematoma.

Finally, Lourie and Berne (1965) and Reigh and Nelson (1962) have produced evidence that non-fatal bleeding into the subarachnoid and subdural spaces over the brain stem due to injury to the vein of Galen and the straight sinus at birth may contribute to the development of communicating hydrocephalus.

Subarachnoid and Intraventricular Hemorrhage of the Newborn

In addition to the mechanical factors cited, perinatal anoxia is an important cause of this type of intracranial bleeding which tends to predominate in the premature. Following the rupture of a subependymal vein, a solid clot forms within the ventricle. The accompanying damage to the germinal cell layer with subsequent mental deficiency has led to a well-accepted policy of conservatism. In our clinic, it is the practice to perform ventricular and lumbar taps to remove bloody fluid, place the child on anticonvulsants, and provide supportive care. When the ventricular fluid is very bloody, the invariable result is a fibrous arachnoidal obstruction of the CSF pathways and hydrocephalus. In such instances, at the age of seven days, provided the infant is improving, a local anesthetic is administered and a Rickham reservoir is placed in a parietal burr hole to facilitate daily ventricular taps and thus limit the number of cortical punctures for the purpose of removing bloody fluid in order to minimize the reactive arachnoiditis and ependymitis that such fluid produces. At 10 to 12 days, a ventriculogram is performed through this same system and a decision whether or not to perform a shunt is made. In our experience with the use of a low-pressure Holter valve, cerebrospinal fluid containing some blood and an increase of protein can be successfully shunted; many infants have benefited from such a program, and have achieved reasonable growth and development.

Birth Injury to the Spinal Cord and Brachial Plexus

Traumatic rupture of the spinal cord at the cervicothoracic junction, as a consequence of excessive traction applied in delivering the shoulders and head of a breech presentation, is well recognized (Leventhal, 1960). However, the clinical diagnosis of traumatic paraplegia in the infant is difficult and must be distinguished from diffuse anterior horn cell involvement (Werdnig-Hoffman disease), which is manifested by paralysis with preservation of sensation. In cases of spinal cord disruption, plain x-rays of the spine are usually unremarkable because of the elasticity of the ligaments and muscles supporting the spinal column. Myelography may show a complete spinal block of the mixed variety and extravasation of pantopaque is possible. Although we cannot cite an instance of benefit from early surgical exploration, laminectomy may still be indicated on occasion in order to decompress the cord and at the same time determine the nature and extent of the lesion — observations of prognostic value.

Brachial plexus injuries are by far more frequent and are mostly of the upper plexus variety (Erb's) with the major deficit occurring proximally in the extremity. Unless there is a significant hematoma in the supraclavicular area, conservative care and orthopedic splinting, rather than neurosurgical exploration of the plexus, is the treatment of choice.

HEAD INJURIES IN INFANCY AND CHILDHOOD — DIAGNOSTIC PROCEDURES

Skull X-rays

Every child admitted to the hospital after a head injury should have posterior-anterior, right and left lateral, and half axial (Towne's) plain x-rays of the skull. These should include anterior-posterior, projections to visualize the occipital bone and the foramen magnum. The hazard of radiation is considered of lesser importance than the information to be gained by roentgenologic study. Only radiographs can demonstrate the nature, location, and extent of skull fractures — whether linear, comminuted, or depressed — or whether suture diastasis has occurred. If a neck injury is suspected, cervical spine x-rays should also be taken. Pseudosubluxation of the second on the third cervical vertebra so frequently observed in children should be kept in mind.

Fontanel Puncture

During infancy fontanel puncture remains the primary exploratory neurosurgical procedure utilized to establish the diagnosis of subdural hematoma and to initiate treatment for this condition. This procedure may also be employed in an emergency to drain the rarely occurring traumatic intracerebral hematoma as a life-preserving measure preceding angiography and definitive surgery. It may also permit ventricular drainage in cases of severe contusion and edema, thereby affording some degree of immediate decompression. The possibility of a false negative subdural tap, because of the presence of a solid clot that will

508

not pass through the needle (18- or 19-gauge), should be borne in mind. A false positive subdural tap with a flow of fresh blood that clots is usually the result of direct puncture of a cortical vein.

Technique. The anterior one-third of the head is shaved, care being taken not to nick the skin. After preparation of the skin with an antiseptic solution, a towel is placed over the head behind the fontanel, leaving the forehead and face uncovered so that the needle can be properly directed. An 18- or 19-gauge two-inch needle with a short bevel is used to puncture the skin slightly behind the point at which the dura is to be penetrated so as to make a longer tract which can close and prevent persistent leakage of fluid. It is desirable to puncture the dura in an oblique fashion, parallel to the brain surface at the lateral edge of the fontanel or, in an 8- to 10-month old child with a small fontanel, to perforate the coronal suture 2 to 3 centimeters from the midline. The stylet is removed and the needle slowly advanced an additional millimeter so as to place the entire bevel within the subdural space. The needle is not aspirated. If clear fluid is obtained, a lumbar tap should be done subsequently for the purpose of comparing the protein content of the respective fluids and thereby determine whether the fluid from the subdural tap differs from CSF. If a hematoma is encountered, as much subdural fluid as flows freely should be collected while carefully observing the baby's pulse and color, because it is possible to produce vasomotor collapse with drainage of large amounts of fluid. Should this occur, drainage is of course terminated and the child's condition allowed to stabilize. To limit drainage to a small arbitrary amount does not make sense, particularly when one is dealing with a well-established hematoma. In such cases repeated taps aim to remove enough fluid to allow the subdural membranes to come together and obliterate the intervening space, which occurs only when as much fluid as flows freely is allowed egress. Hematocrit and protein determinations are done regularly on each fluid specimen so as to follow the progress of successive taps.

In the case of a critically ill infant whose fontanel is tight, and in whom subdural taps have been negative, tapping the frontal horn of the lateral ventricle on one side to obtain CSF and perhaps proceeding — as the clinical state dictates — to ventriculography, is fully warranted.

Exploratory Burr Holes Including the Twist Drill Exploration

Currently in this clinic burr hole exploration under general anesthesia before angiography is not frequently performed. However, the use of twist drills in children and adolescents has been helpful as an emergency life-preserving procedure on many occasions. The usual clinical circumstance leading to such a measure is an extremely ill child with such focal findings as anisocoria, a depressed sensorium, or full decerebrate posturing upon arrival in the emergency room. Bitemporal, bifrontal, and biparietal holes are placed without anesthesia using a ⅛" twist drill attached to a Cone-Barton hand drill. With practice, the operator becomes deft in advancing the tip of the drill no further than the epidural space. Then the instrument is removed so as to permit any accumulation of blood to escape, prior to perforating the dura. In our experience, this drainage is sometimes all that is required. In most cases, however, some uncertainty arises concerning the adequacy of twist drill drainage and, accordingly, burr holes are usually made thereafter. Or, more frequently, the patient is routed to the neuroradiology department for angiography and then, if a significant intra- or extradural space-occupying lesion is found, to surgery.

Cerebral Angiography

The paramount importance of this diagnostic procedure in the care of head-injured children has been established over the past decade. On a busy neurosurgical trauma service that cares for 50 children and adolescents with severe head injuries every year, it is estimated that 90 percent of such patients will be studied by angiography. General anesthesia is not used for cerebral angiography. If the patient is a child with a depressed sensorium, atropine premedication and a small (1 mg) intravenous dose of meperidine just prior to injection of the contrast medium will suffice. For the awake child, a "cocktail" of sodium phenobarbital (10 mg/kg), meperidine (0.8 to 1.0 mg/kg), and chlorpromazine (0.5 – 1.0 mg/kg) is given intramuscularly one hour prior to study. The child arrives in the neuroradiology suite with the intravenous administration of fluid having been started, and small supplementary doses of meperidine are given if needed. With this technique, the x-ray suite must have at hand the necessary equipment to deal with respiratory depression, though this is of rare occurrence. Of considerable importance also is the availability of a recovery room so that small children can be observed for two to three hours after the procedure for evidence of impaired respiratory function.

In the infant, it is our practice to puncture the femoral artery by the Seldinger technique and place the catheter in either the carotid or vertebral artery. In the newborn, the umbilical artery may be catheterized. The femoral route may also be employed in older children and adolescents, but direct carotid puncture with a #20 gauge thin-walled Cournand needle is frequently' feasible. A biplane film series is obtained, followed by an anterior-posterior series with cross compression. This allows for complete supratentorial study with 10 to 15 cc of contrast material. In addition to providing evidence of a space-occupying lesion, the size of the ventricles may be determined, especially in the venous phase; dilated ventricles suggest a posterior fossa mass.

The angiographic appearance of an extradural hematoma, including the extravasation of dye from the torn vessel, has been well described by Schechter (1966). Frontal epidural clots that have a much slower clinical evolution are best visualized in oblique projections, the head being turned towards the side of the lesion.

In the angiogram, subdural collections in children differ from the adult variety only by virtue of their large size and the presence of the "brain stain" described by Leeds et al (1968). Angiography does not provide useful information, however, concerning the presence or absence of membranes surrounding the subdural collection.

Of major importance in the management of serious closed head injuries in children is the fact that angiography clearly establishes the presence of such non-surgical lesions, as multiple contusions and areas of cerebral swelling.* These lesions frequently occur at the frontal or temporal tips, areas that are forced against the sphenoid wing upon impact. Angiography will also demonstrate herniation at the tentorium, in which case it may be necessary to remove contused, swollen temporal lobe in order to decompress the brain stem as a lifesaving measure.

Finally, cerebral angiography in conjunction with well designed studies of regional cerebral blood flow in head-injured children will undoubtedly provide greater understanding of the underlying pathophysiology (Kasoff et al, 1972).

Air Study

Pneumoencephalography has a minimal to nonexistent role in the management of acute head injuries in children. Ventriculography is

* Angiography does not readily distinguish between cerebral edema or contusion and hematoma. (Ed.)

511

occasionally useful in demonstrating supratentorial clots but is of greater value in the diagnosis of posterior fossa hematomas. The presence of an infratentorial clot is revealed by a deformity of the aqueduct and fourth ventricle, obliteration of the cisterna magna, and acute ventricular dilatation.

Electroencephalography

This procedure, like pneumoencephalography, is reserved essentially for the study of special secondary problems following head injury, such as seizures. The electroencephalogram will usually show voltage depression over a chronic subdural hematoma, but it does not replace angiography in establishing such a diagnosis.

Other Diagnostic Procedures

Lumbar Puncture. This procedure is generally not of help in distinguishing between surgical and non-surgical problems following head injuries, and may be dangerous. When there is increased intracranial pressure and lumbar puncture is necessary, e.g., to rule out meningitis, a careful tap can be done.

Ultrasonic Brain Scanning (Echoencephalography). This technique involves the transmission of a pulsed beam of ultrasonic waves with frequencies of greater than 20 kc/sec into the head and recording the echoes reflected from a tissue interface within the cranium. It has found widespread use in neurosurgery as a screening technique in trauma (Ford and Ambrose, 1963; Kazner et al, 1965), but has not been used in our clinic.

Radioactive Brain Scanning. When Tc99m is used, the radiation hazard to the child is not significant. However, the real value of this form of investigation after head injury remains unproven. False negative results have been obtained in cases of chronic infantile subdural hematoma, while contused scalp overlying a skull fracture often contributes to a false positive scan. It would seem that this mode of study should be used more widely in association with angiography in order to establish its usefulness and limitations.

CLOSED HEAD INJURY

A closed head injury is one in which there is blunt trauma to the head without disruption of the skin; basilar skull fractures are included in this category. The management of closed head injuries in children is primarily non-surgical, close observation being maintained for the possible occurrence of intracranial bleeding. Such an injury may or may not be associated with a linear or comminuted fracture and, in fact, many severe closed head injuries are not accompanied by fracture. Much of the experimental study of head injuries has been based upon a closed-head injury model and has led to various supportive measures (hypothermia, steroids, hyperventilation, dehydrating agents) to control what is thought to be the pathophysiology, i.e., progressive cerebral swelling.

Closed head injuries vary from mild concussion with transient loss of consciousness and rapid complete recovery to prolonged states of coma with severe neurological sequelae. For every obviously severe head injury that is a threat to life or results in serious neurologic sequelae, there are many of a minor nature. Immediately following trauma, there is no reliable way to separate a minor bump from a more serious intracranial lesion, and each injury in a child must for a while be looked upon with concern by the pediatrician and neurosurgical consultant. The experience of any pediatric neurosurgical unit with regard to the type of trauma will vary, depending largely upon its source of referrals and its geographic location. In a large metropolitan area where an indigenous, underprivileged population lives in crowded conditions, and where children play on rooftops and in streets, there will be 35 to 50 cases of severe closed head injury and perhaps 100 of mild injury admitted to the unit every year. Such injuries will be the result of falls from a considerable height, vehicular and pedestrian accidents, and flying missiles, rocks, etc. Purposeful assault, the so-called battered child syndrome, should be suspected in a child with unexplained injury or if several young members of the same family are admitted sequentially. It is of great importance to investigate such cases with the aid of a social worker in order to prevent children from being injured further. Severe injuries are characterized by profound depression of consciousness often lasting for more than 12 hours whereas in milder cases clouding of the sensorium is of shorter duration. Our experience is in sharp contrast with that of a large children's referral center where 86 percent of all patients were conscious when admitted and only 9 percent were comatose or failed to exhibit purposeful responses to stimulation (Hendrick et al, 1964).

Minor Closed Head Injury

The minor closed-head injury group comprises those children who exhibit transient loss of consciousness, lethargy, irritability, and vomiting. Such symptoms are usually grouped together as the concussive syndrome. Loss of consciousness is often difficult to document in a child, the history frequently being that of a youngster who falls while playing with a friend and is "dazed." By the time the parent reaches the child, he is crying but after a short while wants to sleep, may vomit, or complain of headache. A third to a half of the children who sustain head injuries do not lose consciousness (Hendrick et al, 1964; Hjern and Nylander, 1964; Hooper, 1962). These absence of an initial effect on consciousness is most notable in infants. In only seven of 50 infants hospitalized for skull fracture, was a clearly documented history of unconsciousness elicited (Selley and Frankel, 1961).

At the time of impact, or shortly thereafter, even in the case of a child with minor head injury, a seizure may ensue – the so-called "impact seizure." Such a seizure may be focal, but this does not always imply a localized cerebral lesion. It has been our practice, however, to place such a child on anticonvulsant medication (phenobarbital, 5 mg/kg/24hrs.) for 4 to 6 weeks. If the EEG remains abnormal after this period, the child is maintained on this medication for six months to a year.

Otherwise, the management of the mild variety of closed head injury in children involves the usual general, supportive measures. A lumbar puncture is less often of medicolegal importance in children than in adults, and generally is not done. An electroencephalogram and skull x-rays are, of course, obtained in all hospitalized patients. The child is encouraged to be up as soon as possible and enter into the play program. If possible, in 2 to 5 days, he is allowed full activity, and returns to school generally in the second week.

The frequently encountered post-concussional syndrome of dizziness, easy fatigability, and headache, observed in adults and teenagers, is rare in children. Serious sequelae such as epilepsy and mental impairment are also exceedingly uncommon and personality disorders infrequent in children who are well adjusted prior to injury. Dencker (1960) has shown that psychometric scores, EEG, and personality integration were no different among 117 minor head injured and control twins.

Severe Closed Head Injury

Severe closed head injuries manifested by prolonged unconsciousness result from a combination of concussion, contusion, and laceration which may be followed by cerebral swelling and increased intracranial pressure. The mechanical forces operating at the time of impact are acceleration and deformation. In the unfused, more pliable skull of young children and infants greater deformation is possible, and more of the force of the impact is absorbed. On impact, motion is imparted to the brain producing, for example, the characteristic frontal and temporal tip injuries after a blow to the back of the head. When the head is struck, there is a sudden increase in intracranial pressure lasting a few milliseconds (Gurdjian and Webster, 1958; Scott, 1940; Sellier and Unterharnscheidt, 1963; Walker et al, 1944), and reaching levels of 750 to 5000 mm Hg close to the site of the impact (Gurdjian et al, 1966; 1955) with the lowest levels, and indeed a negative pressure, opposite the site of the blow. As a result of deformation and acceleration, the brain is subjected to compression and shear stresses, the latter being maximal at the level of the craniospinal junction. Distortion and shear strains are the cause of widespread neuronal damage and hemorrhage; a cavitation effect has been attributed to a negative pressure factor (see Chapter 1).

Contusions and lacerations are superficial hemorrhagic lesions resulting from deformation at the site of impact or else occurring as a consequence of contrecoup trauma. Studies of pathologic material (Courville, 1965; Lindenberg et al, 1955) suggest that contusions are less common after head injury in young children, especially in those less than two years of age. The eventual tissue damage in contused brain at any age is a result of acute hemorrhagic infarction. Brain lacerations are usually associated with skull fractures, occurring either as a result of penetration of the dura by bone fragments or inbending of the more pliable young skull. A laceration over the Sylvian fissure may produce a tearing and thrombotic occlusion of major middle cerebral vessels with secondary infarction. Traumatic intracerebral hematomas result from such contusions and lacerations, their increase in size being associated with liquefaction necrosis of adjacent white matter.

Following an injury, the brain undergoes a series of secondary reactive changes, all of which tend to cause an increase in brain bulk and be associated with increased intracranial pressure. By comparison with adults, little is known of the specific reaction of the developing, not fully myelinated brain to injury. It is not certain whether cerebral edema is different in children or whether vasomotor paralysis occurs.

The treatment of the seriously head injured child includes measures of both an emergency and definitive nature. Emergency care involves those measures designed to assure an adequate airway, whether this be intubation or tracheotomy, respiratory assistance, treatment of associated pulmonary and chest lesions, and monitoring of blood gases with special emphasis upon pCO_2. It is the author's belief that more lives of children have been saved by such measures than by any other form of treatment. External bleeding must be controlled, and if the child is in shock, its cause must be determined. Hypovolemic shock is not a characteristic feature of craniocerebral trauma except in the very young child in whom arterial scalp bleeding and intracranial clot formation can deplete blood volume enough to cause a fall in blood pressure and a lowered hematocrit. A suitable vein is exposed surgically and fluid administered through this route. A nasogastric tube is inserted if the abdomen is distended, an indwelling catheter introduced into the bladder, and the child's body temperature stabilized. After an hour or two of observation of the child's state of consciousness, skull x-rays are obtained, and a decision made with regard to angiography. In this clinic, it has been the policy to perform angiography on most severely injured children whose state of consciousness is appreciably depressed in order to: (1) rule out a space-occupying blood clot; (2) document cerebral contusion and laceration; and (3) evaluate cerebral circula-. tory dynamics. If there are focal neurologic findings, particularly anisocoria with contralateral hemiparesis, angiography is done immediately. On the other hand, if the child appears to be awakening, angiography is delayed for 6 to 12 hours until his general condition has stabilized, assuming a persistent neurologic abnormality. This program has taught us that cerebral angiography is well tolerated, and has permitted a more conservative policy, when indicated, to be adopted with confidence.

If, by angiography, the child is shown not to be a surgical candidate, supportive measures are continued. These include intensive nursing care, maintaining the patient in the 3/4 prone position and turning him every two hours, keeping the head elevated 15°, periodic nasotracheal suction and proper care — including high humidification — of the endotracheal tube or tracheotomy. We have been able to maintain a child on a cuffed endotracheal tube with periodic deflation of the balloon for up to ten days without subglottic stenosis and, in general, prefer this method of intubation to tracheotomy, especially in the young child. The urinary output is measured and the child weighed daily to guard against overhydration. Anticonvulsants (phenobarbital 5 mg/

516

kg/24 hrs., or diphenylhydantoin 7 mg/kg/24 hrs.) are given by mouth, gastric tube, or intramuscularly as prophylaxis against seizures. Although seizures are rare, should they occur, they may obscure an important sign of a surgical lesion, i.e., a depressed state of consciousness. The anticonvulsants in the dosage suggested do not impair the level of consciousness. If there is clear clinical evidence of a basilar fracture or CSF otorrhea or rhinorrhea, it is our policy to place the child on Ampicillin for a period of 14 days; otherwise antibiotics are not used in the general supportive care of the seriously head injured child.

Hypertonic solutions (urea, mannitol) and oral glycerol have a major role in the management of the increased intracranial pressure that accompanies head injury. Because of its tendency to remain extracellular in the brain, causing less rebound, mannitol is the preferred agent in a dose of 2 to 3 gm/kg as a 20 percent solution administered intravenously in 30 to 40 minutes. Such a rapid infusion can cause increased venous pressure and circulatory overload in the young child. The administration of mannitol may be repeated every 12 to 16 hours, in which case electrolytes must be monitored every 24 hours; potassium is replaced as necessary.

It has also been the policy of this service to use steroids liberally in seriously injured children to control cerebral swelling. Unfortunately gastric and duodenal bleeding has occurred as a complication in some cases so that we now introduce a nasogastric tube and initiate an ulcer regimen in all comatose children receiving steroids. Young children are given 0.25 mg/kg/day of dexamethasone. Steroids need not be tapered if administered for only five days; if prescribed for a longer time, the dose should be gradually decreased over a period of four to five days to allow the adrenal to resume the synthesis of adequate amounts of endogenous steroid.

Despite the interest in hypothermia in this clinic (Rosomoff, 1961; Rosomoff et al, 1960 and 1965), we are well aware of the difficulty of translating data obtained from animals maintained at 25°C to the patient maintained at a temperature of 32°C. We limit the use of hypothermia to those cases in which other measures have failed.

It should be recognized that especially in children, prolonged states of coma are compatible with full recovery provided supportive care is employed assiduously and with discretion. Although each patient must be treated individually, our experience in dealing with a large number of seriously injured children has fully justified early angiography in order to delineate the surgical cases and to gauge the need for dehydrating agents, steroids, and other measures to deal with cerebral edema. The use of twist drills as an emergency measure has undoubtedly saved the lives of some children with hematomas who would otherwise have promptly succumbed or failed to survive the delay entailed in the performance of a more elaborate surgical procedure in the operating room. While the prognosis for survival is grave in patients with prolonged coma and decerebrate rigidity, this is certainly less so in children than in adults with head injuries. In a recent report of 46 patients aged 2 to 18 years, with an average duration of coma lasting 7 weeks, independence in ambulation and self care was achieved in 87 percent. However, severe deficits were observed in the intellectual level as measured by intelligence test scores, with children in the younger age group showing greater impairment than the adolescents. The eventual degree of recovery of both motor function and intellectual ability was related to the duration of coma (Brink et al, 1970).

SKULL FRACTURES

Breaks in skull continuity are frequent in the head injured child. Special problems arising from such injuries in the pediatric age group include the diagnosis and management of depressed fractures and of growing fractures, the treatment of epilepsy and cranial defects, and cranial nerve palsies.

Depressed Fractures

Depressed fractures in children are diagnosed on the basis of an x-ray examination of the skull. Frequently tangential views are required. Whenever a fragment is depressed the depth of the skull thickness, we generally prefer to elevate it. If the injury is a compound fracture, debridement and elevation are best done within 24 hours. Bone fragments can be replaced after thorough washing in saline and aqueous Zephiran. All foreign bodies are removed. The dura, if torn, is repaired in watertight fashion, the wound closed per primum and ·the child maintained on antibiotics (Ampicillin, methicillin) for ten days. All children with such fractures in the region of the frontoparietal junction are routinely placed on anticonvulsants. If, for one reason or another, treatment has been delayed for more than 24 hours, operation is performed as soon as possible thereafter under antibiotic coverage.

518

In the event bone fragments are not replaced for any reason, primary cranioplasty with stainless steel mesh is done.

Penetrating craniocerebral wounds are one variety of compound depressed fracture and occur in children as a consequence of accidental gunshot injuries or falling upon hard pointed objects. Immediate exploration and debridement, with closure of dura and scalp, is the preferred method of management.

Growing Fractures

In the case of a linear fracture in the parietal region, the dura may be torn due to inbending of the relatively elastic bone at the time of impact. If the arachnoid is also disrupted, a growing fracture or leptomeningeal cyst may develop. This is not a true cyst but a fluid-filled space between the brain and arachnoid; communication with the subrachnoid space allows the ingress of CSF into the cyst but since more fluid enters than leaves, the lesion expands. The initial break in the skull is usually a long, parietal, diastatic fracture occurring in a child less than five years of age. A soft tissue swelling coming on weeks or months after an injury should arouse suspicion of the diagnosis, although rarely the cyst remains within the skull and is manifested by seizures or an increasing neurological deficit (Matson, 1969). On subsequent x-rays, the edges of the fracture will appear to spread and on tangential view it can be seen that the fracture is being expanded from within. Surgical repair is designed to bring about dural closure, using pericranium or a synthetic dural substitute, followed by cranioplasty with wire mesh and acrylic. Meticulous dissection of the cyst wall and dural closure must be done.

Cranioplasty

As a general rule, cranioplasty for posttraumatic skull defects in children should be postponed for at least a year on the assumption that new bone formation may accomplish closure of the defect. Such regeneration has been observed up to the age of five, particularly in the temporal region. Should cranioplasty be required, we favor the use of acrylic because it can be molded and is radiolucent. For small defects, wire mesh may be used.

Basal Skull Fractures

Basal skull fractures in children are mentioned here primarily to underline the diagnosis and management of persistent CSF leakage.

519

At best, such leaks are difficult to localize, and in a less than cooperative child it may be impossible to do so. Experience with rhinorrhea and otorrhea in children is limited to ethmoidal cribriform plate and petrous injuries, because the frontal and sphenoidal paranasal sinuses do not develop for a number of years. Skull laminagrams are useful and should be done to locate defects in the bone. Isotope studies have not helped in our hands. The technique of surgical exploration and repair is not different from that employed in adults.

Posttraumatic Epilepsy

Posttraumatic epilepsy has been reported in 6 to 14 percent of pediatric patients with head injuries of all types (Dugger, 1964; Hendrick et al, 1964). Seizures occurring on impact or during the acute phase (up to one month after injury) are less likely to persist than those occurring later. Mealey (1968) states that children who develop posttraumatic epilepsy do so after a longer interval than adults, the first seizure not occurring for a year or more in about 50 percent of cases. The risk of epilepsy is under 2 percent in cases in which consciousness is retained or impaired for less than one hour, increasing to 5 to 10 percent if consciousness is lost for more than one hour. Posttraumatic epilepsy following a depressed fracture and brain laceration is much more apt to occur in the adult than in the child (Jennett, 1962). In our experience of dealing with a large number of depressed fractures each year, posttraumatic epilepsy is unusual.

Cranial Nerve Injury

Cranial nerve injuries may occur in association with basal skull fractures. Of importance are injuries of the facial, oculomotor, abducens, and acoustic nerves. Fractures of the petrous temporal bone are relatively common in children, occurring in 6 to 10 percent of cases (Hendrick et al, 1964); bloody drainage from the ear or hemotympanum is the usual clinical manifestation. Damage to the middle ear is due to a fracture of the tegmen tympani; fortunately, persistent hearing loss or vestibular disturbance is not a common consequence. The facial nerve may be injured within the facial canal of the temporal bone, or, rarely, at or distal to the stylomastoid foramen; facial paralysis occurs in 3 to 5 percent of head injuries (Gurdjian and Webster, 1958; Hughes, 1964; Turner, 1943) and, although usually present immediately following trauma, its appearance may be delayed for several days. Usually spontaneous recovery occurs, particularly when the paralysis is incomplete or delayed in onset. When the paralysis is complete and fails to improve, exploration of the facial canal should be considered. When to proceed with endotemporal exploration is a difficult decision to make, and electrodiagnostic tests of nerve conduction and neuromuscular response to aid in the selection of cases for early operation have been described (Taverner, 1965). Those cases with total loss of electrical activity indicating a complete lesion, are perhaps best explored within a month or less; the usual finding at exploration is nerve compression or edema with anatomic continuity (Jongkees, 1965).

Impairment of ocular motility after head injury is particularly common in children when there has been trauma to the orbit as well as to the cranium. Third nerve palsy present immediately after injury usually indicates such an injury rather than temporal lobe herniation, but the differential diagnosis is at times difficult and requires careful observation. Third or sixth nerve paralysis is reported in 1 to 7 percent of injuries (Gurdjian and Webster, 1958; Hughes, 1964; Turner, 1943) with a 75 percent recovery rate (Hughes, 1964). With a blow-out fracture of the orbit, the inferior oblique muscle is trapped and the eye cannot move upward or inward; such an injury can be corrected by exploration and repair of the orbital floor.

EXTRADURAL HEMATOMA IN CHILDREN

The rarity of this condition in the perinatal period has already been indicated. This is due to the firm adherence of dura to bone at the suture lines, the elasticity of the infantile skull protecting against fracture, and the fact that the middle meningeal artery has not yet grooved the bones of the vault but lies chiefly on the dura and hence is not liable to injury if there is a fracture. Extradural hemorrhage, though less frequently encountered in infancy and childhood than among adults, is of major importance as a complication of closed head injury in the pediatric patient. In children, 1 to 2 percent of closed head injuries will be complicated by extradural hematoma (Hendrick, et al, 1964; Ingraham et al, 1949) and 31 percent of all extradural hematomas occur in the pediatric age group (Pia, 1964). The relative rarity of the condition and the atypical presentation in the child only emphasize the necessity of being constantly aware of the possibility of extradural hematoma if the diagnosis is not to be missed. Unless the condition is recognized early and surgical therapy instituted quickly, the mortality rate is high.

Extradural hemorrhage is of two types; arterial, of middle meningeal origin, caused by a fracture of the squamous temporal bone, and venous, resulting from injuries involving emissary veins or the major sinuses. In extradural hemorrhage of venous origin, symptoms may be slowly progressive, several days elapsing before the condition is clinically evident. Moreover, the classical syndrome of initial loss of consciousness followed by recovery (the lucid interval) with subsequent progressive deterioration, pupillary enlargement, and crossed hemiparesis, is rather unusual in the reported pediatric cases (Hawkes and Ogle, 1962). Because of the rapid loss of blood into the extradural space, the blood volume of the infant or young child may be depleted with a resultant drop of hematocrit and clinical evidence of shock despite the rising intracranial pressure. Skull fracture need not be seen in the child with extradural hematoma (Jacobson, 1885-1886); and this lack of fracture is particularly characteristic of the adolescent (Mealey, 1960). Angiography may be required to make the diagnosis (Ingraham et al, 1949).

Surgical treatment is not different from that of the adult with extradural hematoma, except that in the child the clot is confined to the middle fossa. The results in children are generally excellent if the hematoma is removed before brain-stem hemorrhages occur. Blood loss can be a major problem and must be corrected by means of transfusion during surgery.

In summary, extradural hematoma in the infant, child, or adolescent is a curable lesion if the diagnosis can be made before irreversible brain-stem damage occurs. In a child who remains comatose from the time of injury with a focal neurologic deficit, the diagnosis must be reached by means other than clinical signs. In this type of case, cerebral angiography at an early stage is strongly recommended. By this means, we may be able to reduce the theoretical minimal or inevitable death rate of 10 percent that has been postulated (Hooper, 1959; McKissock et al, 1960).

Finally, posterior fossa extradural hematomas have been reported in children from 18 months to 16 years of age (Campbell et al, 1953; Fisher et al, 1958; Hooper, 1954; Lemmen and Schneider, 1952; Meredith, 1961; Wright, 1966). There is no typical clinical picture but in the conscious child, severe and persistent headache after head injury should make one suspicious of this diagnosis. Also, ventricular dilatation revealed by carotid angiography suggests a posterior fossa clot.

The bleeding is usually of venous origin, occurring as a result of a sinus tear associated with an occipital fracture. Again, results are quite satisfactory if the diagnosis can be made before brain-stem decompensation occurs.

INFANTILE SUBDURAL HEMATOMA

Traumatic subdural effusion in infants is a unique condition (Table). Its etiology, pathogenesis and management are all of considerable interest (Gardner, 1932; Zollinger and Gross, 1934).

CLINICAL CHARACTERISTICS OF 53 CHILDREN WITH SUBDURAL HEMATOMA *

Age	Less than 3 months	37%
	Less than 1 year	88%
Symptoms	History of trauma	41%
	Skull fracture	20%
	Retarded development	22%
	Seizures	65%
	Vomiting	52%
	Enlarging head	39%
	Hyperirritability	37%
Duration of symptoms	Less than 1 week	46%
	More than 6 months	5%
Signs	Enlarged head	42%
	Bulging fontanel	36%
	Retinal hemorrhages	38%
	Neurological loss	36%
	Anemia	70%
	Increased intracranial pressure (roentgen ray)	52%

* Reproduced, by permission, from the *Journal of Neurosurgery*, XVIII, No. 2, pp. 175-181, 1961.

The mistreated or battered infant has become clearly defined as a clinical entity during the past few years. In a home setting of inadequate parental personality development, acts of commission and omission place such infants in continual jeopardy. Infantile subdural hematoma is a significant component of the battered syndrome, occurring in up to 28 percent of such babies (McHenry et al, 1963); each infant

523

with a traumatic subdural effusion must be carefully examined for other injuries, e.g., rib and long bone fractures.

A definite history of trauma or one highly suspicious of it may be elicited in 75 percent of cases of infantile subdural hematoma. Often the trauma is insignificant, however, and does not require immediate medical attention or hospitalization.

The source of bleeding is generally thought to be a torn cortical bridging vein, the resultant hemorrhage spreading over the convexity and along the falx. Such blood is not absorbed but evokes a response by the dura in an attempt at encapsulation through the formation of a membrane. This membrane is most highly developed on the dural side (outer membrane) but eventually completely surrounds the effusion with the inner membrane in apposition to the arachnoid. Fresh red blood cells are continually added to such a chronic effusion from large vessels in the outer membrane. These blood vessels undoubtedly also contribute to the high protein (albumin) content of the effusion. The exact reason for the expansion of the effusion to produce symptoms of increased intracranial pressure and head enlargement is, however, not completely understood. Radioactive tracer studies employing tagged albumin suggest that blood, effusion contents, and CSF are separate compartments with gradients of diffusion that encourage transudation of albumin into the subdural compartment, both from the blood and the CSF (Rabe et al, 1962, 1964). It is these factors of membrane formation and persistence of effusion which have been thought to restrict brain expansion during the infantile period of rapid growth; the rationale of surgical treatment has been based on this concept (Ingraham and Matson, 1944).

Craniotomy and membrane stripping in persistent effusions have yielded good results in 80 percent of patients; the failures did not succumb to the effusion, but remained neurologically impaired, mentally subnormal, or incapacitated by seizures. We (Shulman and Ransohoff, 1961) have questioned the necessity of craniotomy in all cases of persistent effusion and whether membrane stripping always prevented reaccumulation of the effusion. A more conservative plan of therapy has been adopted during the past decade in a number of clinics. The effusion is tapped and continuous drainage via a shunt from the subdural space to the peritoneum, chest, or bloodstream instituted for a period of three to four months (Sayers, personal communication). McLaurin et al (1971) believe that in most instances subdural hematomas can be successfully treated by tapping alone;

their indication for tapping, once the diagnosis has been verified, is persistence of increased intracranial pressure. There still remain some 10 to 20 percent of patients who do poorly regardless of the form of therapy. These are thought to be either infants with preexisting brain atrophy in whom an effusion has developed to fill the enlarged subdural space or infants who sustained a severe cortical contusion or other intracerebral lesion at the time of the injury, which also produced the subdural hematoma. These considerations have led us to adopt a program as follows: fontanel taps are done for five to seven days and if fluid persists, a cerebral angiogram is done. If there is considerable brain-skull disproportion with a very large subdural collection and a small brain with a capillary stain [brain stain (Leeds et al, 1968)], a shunt from each subdural space into the peritoneum is performed, using silastic tubing without a valve. If, on the other hand, the subdural effusion is relatively small but symptomatic despite repeated tapping, craniotomy and membrane stripping are done with drainage (1/2" Penrose drain) of the subdural space for at least 48 hours. If the subdural taps are subsequently negative, the child is discharged on anticonvulsants and followed at monthly intervals. Finally, with regard to infants who respond favorably to fontanel taps alone, no further fluid being aspirated after five to seven days, we have been content to follow such children on an outpatient basis without further study, being guided by measurements of their head circumference and by their general development. The false negative Tc99m pertechnetate scans in infantile subdurals have already been mentioned.

REFERENCES

Brink, J. D., Garrett, A. L., Hale, W. R., Woo-Sam, J., and Nickel, V. Recovery of Motor and Intellectual Function in Children Sustaining Severe Head Injuries. *Dev. Med. Child Neurol. 12*, 565, 1970.

Campbell, E., Whitfield, R. D., and Greenwood, R. Extradural Hematomas of the Posterior Fossa. *Ann. Surg., 138*, 509-520, 1953.

Campbell, J. B. and Cohen, J. Epidural Hemorrhage and the Skull of Children. *Surg. Gynec. Obstet., 92*, 257-280, 1951.

Courville, C. B. Contrecoup Injuries of the Brain in Infancy. *Arch. Surg. 90*, 157-165, 1965.

Courville, C. B. *Pathology of the Central Nervous System*, 2nd. ed. Mountain View, California: Pacific Press, 1945.

Cushing, H. Concerning Surgical Intervention for the Intracranial Hemorrhages of Newborn. *Amer. J. Med. Sci., 130*, 563-581, 1905.

Dekaban, A. *Neurology of Infancy*. Baltimore: Williams and Wilkins, 1959.

Dencker, S. J. Closed Head Injury in Twins. *Arch. Gen. Psychiatry, 2,* 569-575, 1960.

Dugger, G. S. Head Injury. In T. W. Farmer (Ed.), *Pediatric Neurology*. New York: Hoeber Medical Div., Harper, 1964. Pp. 392-442.

Fisher, R. G., Kin, J. K., and Sachs, E., Jr. Complications in the Posterior Fossa Due to Occipital Trauma — Their Operability. *J.A.M.A., 167,* 176-182, 1958.

Ford, R. and Ambrose, J. Echoencephalography — Measurement of the Position of Midline Structures in the Skull with High Frequency Pulsed Ultrasound. *Brain, 86,* 189-196, 1963.

Gardner, W. J. Traumatic Subdural Hematoma. With Particular Reference to the Latent Interval. *Arch. Neurol. Psychiat. 27,* 847-855, 1932.

Gurdjian, E. S., Lissner, H. R., Hodgson, V. R. and Patrick, L. M. Mechanism of Head Injury. *Clin. Neurosurg., 12,* 112-128, 1966.

Gurdjian, E. S. and Webster, J. E. *Head Injuries. Mechanisms, Diagnosis and Management*. Boston: Little Brown & Co., 1958.

Gurdjian, E. S., Webster, J. E. and Lissner, H. R. Observations on the Mechanism of Brain Concussion, Contusion, and Laceration. *Surg. Gynec. Obstet., 101,* 680-690, 1955.

Hawkes, C. D. and Ogle, W. S. Atypical Features of Epidural Hematoma in Infants, Children and Adolescents. *J. Neurosurg., 19,* 971-980, 1962.

Hendrick, E. G.., Harwood-Hash, D. C. F., and Hudson, A. R. Head Injuries in Children; a Survey of 4465 Consecutive Cases at the Hospital for Sick Children, Toronto, Canada. *Clin. Neurosurg., 11,* 46-65, 1964.

Hjern, B., and Nylander, I. Acute Head Injuries in Children. Traumatology, Therapy and Prognosis. *Acta Pediatr.* Suppl. 152, 1964.

Hooper, R. Head Injuries in Childhood. *Aust. N. Z. J. Surg., 32,* 11-22, 1962.

Hooper, R. S. Extradural Haemorrhages of the Posterior Fossa. *Br. J. Surg., 42,* 19-26, 1954.

Hooper, R. S. Observations on Extradural Haemorrhage. *Br. J. Surg., 47,* 71-87, 1959.

Hughes, B. J. The Results of Injury to Special Parts of the Brain and Skull. In G. F. Rowbotham, *Acute Injuries of the Head. Their Diagnosis, Treatment, Complications and Sequels,* 4th ed. Baltimore: Williams and Wilkins, 1964. Pp. 408-433.

Ingraham, F. D., Campbell, J. B., and Cohen, J. Extradural Hematomas in Infancy and Childhood. *J.A.M.A., 140,* 1010-1013, 1949.

Ingraham, F. D. and Matson, D. D. Subdural Hematoma in Infancy. *J. Pediatr., 24,* 1-37, 1944.

Jacobson, W. H. A. On Middle Meningeal Haemorrhage. *Guy's Hosp. Rep., 43,* 147-308, 1885-86.

Jennett, W. B. *Epilepsy After Blunt Head Injuries*. Springfield, Ill.: Charles C Thomas, 1962.

Jongkees, L. B. W. Facial Paralysis Complicating Skull Trauma. *Arch. Otolaryngol., 81,* 518-522, 1965.

Kasoff, S. S., Zingesser, L. H. and Shulman, K. Compartmental Abnormalities of Regional Cerebral Blood Flow in Children with Head Trauma. *J. Neurosurg.*, *36*, 463-470, 1972.

Kazner, E., Kunze, St., and Schiefer, W. The Importance of Echoencephalography in Recognizing Epidural Hematomas (English reprint). *Arch. Klin. Chir.*, *310*, 267-291, 1965.

Kendall, N., and Woloshin, H. Cephalhematoma Associated with Fracture of the Skull. *J. Pediatr.*, *41*, 125-132, 1952.

Leeds, N. E., Shulman, K., Borns, P. F., and Hope, J. W. The Angiographic Demonstration of a "Brain Stain" in Infantile Subdural Hematoma. *Am. J. Roent.*, *104*, 66-70, 1968.

Lemmen, L. J. and Schneider, R. C. Extradural Hematomas of the Posterior Fossa. *J. Neurosurg.*, *9*, 245-253, 1952.

Leventhal, H. R. Birth Injuries of the Spinal Cord. *J. Pediatr.*, *56*, 447-453, 1960.

Lindenberg, R., Fisher, R. S., Durlacher, S. H., Lovitt, W. V., Jr., and Freytag, E. The Pathology of the Brain in Blunt Head Injuries of Infants and Children. *Internat. Congr. Neuropath. Proc.*, *1*, 477-479, 1955. Amsterdam, Excerpta Med.

Lourie, H. and Berne, A. S. A Contribution on the Etiology and Pathogenesis of Congenital Communicating Hydrocephalus. *Neurology*, *15*, 815-822, 1965.

Matson, D. D. *Neurosurgery in Infancy and Childhood* (2nd. ed.). Springfield, Ill.: Charles C Thomas, 1969.

McHenry, T., Girdany, B. R. and Elmer, E. Unsuspected Trauma with Multiple Skeletal Injuries During Infancy and Childhood. *Pediatrics*, *31*, 903-908, 1963.

McKissock, W., Taylor, J. D., Bloom, W. H., and Till, K. Extradural Haematomas. Observations on 125 Cases. *Lancet*, *ii*, 167-172, 1960.

McLaurin, R. L., Isaacs, E., and Lewis, H. P. Results of Non-operative Treatment in 15 Cases of Infantile Subdural Hematoma. *J. Neurosurg.*, *34*, 753-759, 1971.

Mealey, J., Jr. Acute Extradural Hematomas without Demonstrable Skull Fractures. *J. Neurosurg.*, *17*, 27-34, 1960.

Mealey, J. *Pediatric Head Injuries*. Springfield, Ill.: Charles C Thomas, 1968.

Meredith, J. M. Extradural Hemorrhage in the Posterior Fossa. Diagnosis and Treatment with a Report of Two Surgically Treated Patients. *Amer. J. Surg.*, *102*, 524-531, 1961.

Pia, H. W. Die traumatischen hirnblutungen des kindersalters. Acta Neurochir., *11*, 583-600, 1964.

Rabe, E. F., Flynn, R. D., and Dodge, P. R. A Study of Subdural Effusions in an Infant. With Particular Reference to the Mechanisms of Their Persistence. *Neurology*, *12*, 79-92, 1962.

Rabe, E. F., Young, G. F., and Dodge, P. R. The Distribution and Fate of Subdurally Instilled Human Serum Albumin in Infants with Subdural Collections of Fluid. *Neurology*, *14*, 1020-1028, 1964.

Reigh, E. E. and Nelson, M. Posterior-fossa Subdural Hematoma with Secondary Hydrocephalus. Report of Case and Review of the Literature. *J. Neurosurg.*, *19*, 346-348, 1962.

Robson, F. C. and Dawes, J. D. K. Delayed Facial Paralysis of Lower Motor

Neuron Type Following Head Injury. *J. Laryngol.*, *74*, 275-289, 1960.

Rosomoff, H. L. Effects of Hypothermia and Hypertonic Urea on Distribution of Intracranial Contents. *J. Neurosurg.*, *18*, 753-759, 1961.

Rosomoff, H. L., Clasen, R. A., Hartsock, R., and Bebin, J. Brain Reaction to Experimental Injury after Hypothermia. *Arch. Neurol.*, *13*, 337-345, 1965.

Rosomoff, H. L., Shulman, K., Raynor, R., and Grainger, B. S. Experimental Brain Injury and Delayed Hypothermia. *Surg. Gynec. Obstet.*, *110*, 27-32, 1960.

Sayers, M. P. Personal communication.

Schechter, M. M. Angiography in Head Trauma. *Clin. Neurosurg.*, *12*, 193-220, 1966.

Schipke, R., Riege, D., and Scoville, W. B. Acute Subdural Hemorrhage at Birth. *Pediatrics*, *14*, 469-474, 1954.

Schulman, H. and Romney, S. L. Variability of Uterine Contractions in Normal Human Parturition. *Obstet. Gynec.*, *36*, 215-221, 1970.

Scott, W. W. Physiology of Concussion. *Arch. Neurol. Psychiat.*, *43*, 270-283, 1940.

Selley, I. and Frankel, F. B. Skull Fracture in Infant. A Report of 50 Cases. *Acta Chir. Scand.*, *122*, 30-48, 1961.

Sellier, K., and Unterharnscheidt, F. *Mechanik und Pathomorphologie der Hirnschaden nach stumpfer Gewalteinwirkung auf den Schädel.* Berlin: Springer, 1963.

Shulman, K. and Ransohoff, J. Subdural Hematoma in Children. The Fate of Children with Retained Membranes. *J. Neurosurg.*, *18*, 175-181, 1961.

Taverner, D. Electrodiagnosis in Facial Palsy. *Arch. Otolaryng.*, *81*, 470-477, 1965.

Turner, J. W. A. Indirect Injuries of the Optic Nerve. *Brain*, *66*, 140-151, 1943.

U. S. Public Health Service. *Accidental Death and Injury Statistics.* Publication No. IIII. Washington, D. C.: U. S. Public Health Service, October, 1963.

Walker, A. E., Kollros, J. J., and Case, T. J. The Physiological Basis of Concussion. *J. Neurosurg.*, *1*, 103-116, 1944.

Wright, R. L. Traumatic Hematomas of the Posterior Cranial Fossa. *J. Neurosurg.*, *25*, 402-409, 1966.

Zollinger, R. and Gross, R. E. Traumatic Subdural Hematoma. An Explanation of the Late Onset of Pressure Symptoms. *J.A.M.A.*, *103*, 245-249, 1934.

CHAPTER 16

BRAIN INJURIES IN BOXERS

JOHN D. SPILLANE, M. D.

In the West Cloister at Westminster Abbey, London, England, is the tomb of Jack Broughton (1705-1789), the first boxing champion of England, father of professional boxing, founder of the famous "Code" and inventor of the boxing glove. He enjoyed exceptional health with unimpaired faculties until his death at the ripe old age of 84 years. In the past 200 years many other professional boxers have enjoyed health and long life. From time to time, however, boxers have died after contests; in Britain there have been six fatal accidents in professional boxers since 1945. Death is usually due to intracranial hemorrhage. I have personal experience of two such cases.

Case 1. Hemiparesis one hour after winning a four-round fight; died one day later; autopsy showed tearing of the intima of both internal carotid arteries, with subsequent thrombosis and softening of the frontal lobes and pontine hemorrhages.

Case 2. Knocked out in the third round of a fight; failed to regain consciousness and died several hours later; autopsy disclosed a large subdural hematoma.

Acute brain injury may be non-fatal, with or without residual deficit. I have seen two such cases with a hemiparesis. In both, there was an onset of acute hemiplegia in the dressing room immediately after the fight. In both angiography showed occlusion of one internal carotid artery. There was good recovery in the first case, but a permanent hemiplegia in the second.

Further examples of mild intracranial injury are as follows:

529

Case 3. Knocked out in first round; unconscious 15 minutes; recovery complete. but with persistent (three years) parietal occipital slow-wave focus in the EEG.

Case 4. Diplopia for one year after a fight in which the boxer was severely punished and the fight was stopped in the fourth round.

Case 5. Knocked out in the first round; collapsed one hour later; recovered. Headaches, giddiness, and mental slowness for six months. Persistent (four years) bilateral occipital slow-wave focus in the EEG. CSF protein 70 mg/ml.

THE PUNCH-DRUNK SYNDROME

The facts concerning *acute* brain injury in boxers may be undeniable, but it is not so with the so-called *punch-drunk* syndrome. Martland introduced this term to medical literature in 1928. No one knows who originally coined the term. Martland examined five out of 23 cases of the syndrome and found that the cardinal features were tremors, ataxia, dysarthria and a parkinsonian facial expression. In some there was increasing dementia and many patients ended their days in a mental hospital. He knew that some, including "eminent neurologists," denied the existence of the syndrome but he was convinced that what was generally recognized in the boxing world would in due course be confirmed scientifically. "The condition can no longer be ignored by the medical profession or the public. Is is the duty of our profession to establish the existence or nonexistence of *punch-drunk* by preparing accurate statistical data as to its incidence...."

Forty years were to pass before this was done. The existence of the syndrome has usually been denied by those with a financial interest in professional boxing and also by those concerned only with amateur boxing. Some medical investigators, often those who have some connection with the boxing world, have satisfied themselves that the syndrome is a myth. But in the 1930's, reports from the United States (Parker, 1934; Carroll, 1936), Germany (Jokl and Guttmann, 1933), France (Ravina, 1937), and England (Winterstein, 1937) all indicated that *chronic traumatic encephalopathy of boxers* was a recognizable clinical syndrome. Carroll's paper, a graduation thesis, was based on a two-year 'field' study of the boxing scene. He thought that 5 percent of boxers who fought for five years were affected and no less than 60 percent of those who continued longer in the professional ring.

Twenty years later these clinical opinions were assailed on the basis of more detailed "scientific" investigations at the ringside. Kaplan and Browder (1954) reported the findings of a four-year study of 1,043 professional boxers in New York. Ringside observations (one of the writers attended at the ringside once a week for three years), slow-motion cinematography, and electroencephalography were the three main procedures. Their conclusions were interesting. Clinical observations "failed to reveal any abnormal neurological features, even in those contenders who lost their bouts by a knock-out." Slow motion cinematography "confirmed one major impression gained at the ringside, namely that most blows to the head were short of their mark or deflected by their recipient." Electroencephalography "primarily serves its purpose in professional fighters in the detection of grossly disorganized electroencephalograms." All the effects of cerebral concussion are reversible, stated these doctors. McCown (1959 a), medical director of the New York State Athletic Commission, wrote that between 1952 and 1957 among 9,871 boxers there were 259 knockouts and nine serious head injuries requiring admission to hospital; 138 boxers retired or were denied license — we are not told why. He stated that in an average ten-round contest, 1,000 punches are exchanged. These New York "investigations" failed to disclose any examples of the *punch-drunk* syndrome. "It has never been proved to be a neurological syndrome peculiar to boxers and produced by boxing . . . a slick medical cliché" (McCown, 1959 b).

The naïvete of these opinions is amazing. Surely enquiries such as these do not tell us what happens to the brains of professional boxers in later years. One might just as well say that regular medical and radiological examination of young cigarette smokers for four or five years, on failing to reveal any examples of pulmonary carcinoma, means that cigarette smoking does not cause that disease. The problem centers on the delay in the appearance of symptoms.

In England, Critchley (1957) reported on 69 cases of chronic neurological disease in boxers, the majority being examples of the *punch-drunk* syndrome. On the other hand, Blonstein and Clarke (1954) said "it has never been observed in amateur boxers."

I became interested in this subject during World War II. During those years many service neurologists saw ex-professional boxers whom they considered were suffering from the *punch-drunk* syndrome. Perhaps we accepted the diagnosis somewhat uncritically. The roles

531

of epilepsy, alcoholism, syphilis, arteriopathy, or presenile dementia were not always critically examined. Air encephalography was not usually performed. Clinical diagnosis was based on the existence of such symptoms and signs as dysarthria, ataxia, tremors, and cerebral impairment. In some cases it progressed to dementia. Cerebral atrophy was generally acknowledged to be the basis of the disorder, but up to 1962 there were only three published autopsy reports – a meagre pathological basis for the syndrome (Brandenburg and Hallervorden, 1954; Grahmann and Ule, 1957; Neuberger, Sinton and Denst, 1959). These authors suggested that repeated injury may upset the normal colloid equilibrium of the brain and induce premature aging. Holbourn's (1943) studies of the mechanics of head injuries led him to conclude that shear-strains set up by rotational forces were the probable cause of cerebral damage. The "knockout" blow to the chin in boxing produces just such a rotational movement. Pudenz and Shelden (1946) were able to demonstrate swirling rotatory movements of the brain in experimental injuries in monkeys. It is difficult to believe that repeated blows to the head often of a degree to produce concussion would not eventually damage the brain. Common sense is a better guide in this judgment than electroencephalography and slow motion cinematography.

The prevalence of traumatic encephalopathy in ex-professional boxers has been the subject of investigation by a Committee on Boxing of the Royal College of Physicians of London (Roberts, 1969). The investigation was based on a random sample of 250 boxers who had been licensed for three years or more in the years 1929 to 1955. It was in 1929 that the British Board of Boxing Control was established in order to supervise the interests of the professional sport in the United Kingdom. Of the 224 ex-professional boxers examined, 37 showed evidence of brain damage which was disabling in 13. One in six of the boxers studied showed evidence of some damage to the brain attributable to boxing. There was no suggestion of any direct relationship between boxing and the cause of death in 16 ex-boxers of the series who had died. The prevalence of brain injury increased with increasing "occupational exposure" measured by the length of the professional career. Among ex-boxers aged 50 years and over, who had boxed professionally for more than ten years, 47 percent showed evidence of brain damage; 17 percent of those who had boxed from six to nine years, and 13 percent of those who had boxed five years or more were affected. In the younger age group between 30 and 50 years of age, the percentage with brain damage was lower, but there was a similar trend; 25 percent showed brain injury if they had boxed more than ten years, 14 percent if they had boxed between six and nine years, and 1 percent if they had boxed five years. *The investigation revealed that the prevalence of the clinical signs of brain injury increased with increasing exposure to boxing.*

The brain has been likened to a gel, with characteristic response to strains (Lindgren, 1964), although Dodgson (1962) thought that it lacked both the rigidity of a gel and the plasticity of a paste. Correlation of the physical effects of brain injury with the biological results has yet to be achieved. The effects of pressure waves and acceleration changes are widespread; they make it difficult to judge the nature of concussion itself, whether it is a widespread neuronal paralysis or a selective lesion of the brain stem and basal frontal and temporal structures.

In 1962, the year when a bill to prohibit the promotion of boxing for money was introduced in the House of Lords, I published an account of five ex-professional boxers with chronic neurological disability. In four, air encephalography demonstrated the presence not only of cerebral atrophy but also of *injury to the septum pellucidum*. I wrote that "before the existence of the syndrome is denied — as in some quarters it has been — follow-up studies of former professional boxers will be necessary." In 1965 I reported that in a series of ten ex-professional boxers, a clinical diagnosis of the *punch-drunk* syndrome could be made in six; in two there was alcoholic dementia, in two a psychopathic personality. Air encephalography in these ten patients showed no abnormality in the alcoholics or in the psychopaths. In the six *punch-drunk* cases the septum pellucidum was normal in only one; cerebral atrophy was present in four out of the six. In another 100 consecutive cases of idiopathic cerebral atrophy, I found no example of injury to the septum pellucidum. I suggested that *injury to the septum pellucidum may be a feature of the punch-drunk syndrome,* i.e., a sign indicating that cerebral atrophy in an ex-boxer may be due to repeated injury and not to some unrelated disorder. To date, air encephalography in ten personal cases of the *punch-drunk* syndrome has revealed injury to the.septum pellucidum in each one.

These observations were confirmed by Mawdsley and Ferguson in 1963 and 1965 and by Isherwood, Mawdsley and Ferguson in 1966. Mawdsley (1969) has now examined 32 ex-professional boxers, all of whom showed chronic neurological disorder; clinical evidence of

dementia was present in half the group; air encephalography performed on 28 showed evidence of brain atrophy in 21; and injury to the
septum pellucidum was found in 23. In four autopsies the cerebral
atrophy was found to be most marked over the frontal lobes and the
most striking histological finding in all four specimens was the presence
of Alzheimer's neurofibrillary changes in the cortex and midbrain.

Johnson (1969) has described the psychiatric disorders in 16 ex-
professional boxers some 22 years after the end of their career in the
ring. The neurological features in ten of these cases were previously
reported by Mawdsley and Ferguson (1963). All had had between 200
and 300 professional fights. There were five main psychiatric syndromes: (1) chronic amnesic state; (2) dementia; (3) morbid jealousy
syndrome; (4) rage reactions and personality disorder; and (5) psychosis. Air encephalography was carried out in 15. Ruptured septum
pellucidum was found in ten cases and was almost invariably associated with ventricular dilatation. The electroencephalogram was abnormal in 11 out of the 16 cases. There were two main types of abnormal
record: (1) a flat low voltage record with minimal or no alpha activity (3 cases); and (2) a diffuse abnormality of slow and intermediate
slow wave activity in an alpha-dominated record (8 cases). These
changes are similar to those described in presenile dementia. Psychometric evidence of brain injury was present in 11 out of 16 cases. In
eight cases there was no sign of progression of the disability.

This accumulating clinical, radiological, and pathological evidence is
sufficient to establish the authenticity of the *punch-drunk* syndrome as
a chronic, traumatic encephalopathy.

The Clinical Features

The insidious development of chronic, traumatic encephalopathy
recalls the words of James Parkinson in his famous essay "On the
Shaking Palsy" (1817). He wrote, "So slight and nearly imperceptible
are the first inroads of this malady and so extremely slow is its progress,
that it rarely happens that the patient can form any recollection of the
precise period of its commencement." The typical patient with chronic,
traumatic encephalopathy usually started boxing in his teens and fought
in the lighter weight divisions. He rarely achieved fame, although there
are a few exceptions. The patient whose pneumoencephalograms and
brain are shown in Figures 3, 9, 21, and 22 was a world-title holder,
one of the most famous boxers of all time. Too many fights too soon

is the common story. A fighter more often than a boxer, his fans soon recognize his courage and his ability to "take a punch," but after 350 or more contests and encouraging reports of his prowess, he begins to lose fights. He is often knocked out or badly beaten. He takes days or weeks to recover from a bout. He begins to slow up. At this stage his wife usually notices a change in his behavior. He may complain of nothing, but she finds that he is quieter, slower, sleeps more, and perhaps shows traces of mood swing which worry her. When challenged he protests that he feels well. He ridicules the idea that boxing is harming him; he will not see a doctor. As time passes others notice these subtle changes, but comment is rarely frank or helpful to him. Not until he experiences symptoms does he usually seek advice. Headaches and dizziness are the commonest of his complaints, but his lack of awareness may be complete in respect to any intellectual or personality change. He might admit to a little shakiness at times, or intolerance to alcohol, or transient obscuration of vision, but he usually has no insight into the mental symptoms that are appearing. He becomes irritable, moody, and liable to outbursts of rage. Or he may be merely forgetful and euphoric, childishly reassuring his family and friends that he feels like a "champion." Progressive failure of memory may make him an unreliable worker. Impotence, suspicion of infidelity on the part of his wife, and chronic paranoid deterioration may wreck his marriage. He may suffer an occasional epileptic attack, lose a number of jobs, require admission to a psychiatric unit for impulsive acts of violence, or he may take to alcohol.

Against this background of alteration of personality and cerebral enfeeblement, signs may appear. One of the earliest involves speech. It is usually the wife who first notices that at times this is indistinct and slurred, especially after alcohol. At first the dysarthria may be intermittent, so that others whom she questions cannot confirm it, but gradually it becomes generally recognized. Along with it tremors develop, giving the appearance of clumsiness, or early parkinsonism, or alcoholic intoxication. Formal examination may reveal no more than the evidence of the dysarthria and the tremors, but, if the wife is interviewed, these telltale signs become all-important. At this stage in a non-boxer, such affections as multiple sclerosis, parkinsonism, frontal lobe tumor, presenile dementia, cerebral arteriosclerosis, or subdural hematoma might be viewed as possible diagnoses. Critchley (1957) remarked that "the neurologist may encounter almost any combination of pyramidal, extrapyramidal and cerebellar signs." Disability may be mild, moderate or marked, and either stationary or progressive. There is general agreement that if boxing ceases when there are only mild cerebellar and striatal symptoms and signs, progression is unlikely, but if the change goes unrecognized and the fighter pursues his career, there is grave danger ahead. A few thrashings may have a lasting effect on his brain.

Electroencephalography

This is likely to be abnormal, as already stated, but there are no specific patterns. As in the presenile dementias, the abnormality depends on the stage of the disease; in the early stages there may be merely a reduction of alpha rhythm with a flattening of the record. Later, the tracings are more strikingly abnormal with rhythmical theta and delta discharges predominating. It may be recalled that in Alzheimer's disease the electroencephalogram is invariably abnormal whereas in most other types of presenile dementia, the record is frequently normal (Gordon and Sim, 1967). In chronic, traumatic encephalopathy there is a closer correlation between electroencephalographic abnormality and cerebral atrophy as demonstrated by air encephalography than with "clinical" dementia.

Air Encephalography

This is the most important investigation. It enables one to detect the presence of *injury to the septum pellucidum* thereby differentiating the encephalopathy from other forms of cerebral atrophy. Evidence of injury to the septum pellucidum is obtainable in 80 percent of cases of chronic, traumatic encephalopathy.

In the majority of cases there is evidence of brain atrophy as revealed by symmetrical enlargement of the lateral ventricles. This is sometimes associated with pools of air in dilated sulci over the frontal, parietal, or temporal lobes. Cerebellar atrophy may also be detected. Normally, on air encephalography the septum pellucidum is seen as a narrow white shadow, 1 to 1.5 cm in height, 2 to 3 mm in width, stretching from the corpus callosum above to the anterior commissure and fornix below. In chronic, traumatic encephalopathy the two leaves of the septum are usually separated and perforated; air encephalography discloses a *cavum septi pellucidi*. Normally, an anteroposterior view with the patient lying on his side shows some of the air trapped

536

in the lowermost ventricle below the septum pellucidum (Figs. 15, 16). In chronic, traumatic encephalopathy the air escapes through the ruptured septum into the uppermost ventricle (Figs. 17, 18, 19, 20). Tomography is of particular value in demonstrating the details of the communicating septi pellucidi. It often reveals the extent of the injury to the leaves of the septum; this tends to be more marked posteriorly (Figs. 7, 8, 9). Rarely, air encephalography reveals complete absence of the septum pellucidum (Fig. 12).

Congenital absence of the septum pellucidum is very rare (Dyke and Davidoff, 1935). Normally the two leaves of the septum are in close apposition, with a potential space between them. The incidence of cavum septi pellucidi at autopsy has been variously reported at 60 percent (Van Wagenen and Aird, 1934) 20 percent (Schwidde, 1952), 85 percent (Hughes et al, 1955), and 60 percent (Schunk, 1963). The majority of these are mere slits in the septum 2 to 3 mm in width. On the other hand, cavae which fill with air on routine encephalography are very rare. Schunk, reviewing one thousand normal air encephalograms, found that in only six cases (0.6 percent) was the width of the septum 5 mm or more. (He did not say whether any of these six septa contained an air-filled cave.) A communicating cavum septi pellucidi is not a feature of *idiopathic* cerebral atrophy and neither is it a known sequel to *acute* head injury.

Injury to the septum pellucidum must be a feature of chronic, traumatic encephalopathy of boxers.

Pathology

Cerebral atrophy (Figs. 21 and 22) is the basis for the cerebral impairment and dementia. Histological examination has revealed the presence of Alzheimer's neurofibrillary changes. Mawdsley (1969) has found these changes, together with a cavum septi pellucidi, in four other brains of demented boxers.

Air encephalography in chronic, traumatic encephalopathy of boxes, with particular reference to rupture of the septum pellucidum.

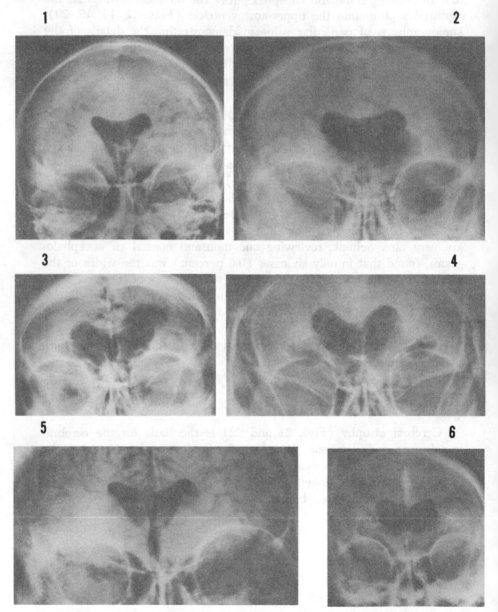

FIGS. 1, 2, 3, 4, 5, 6. Anteroposterior views. Absent septum pellucidum in Fig. 1 (Case 1). Cavum septi pellucidi in Figs. 2, 3, 4, 5, 6 (Cases 2, 3, 4, 5, 6.).

7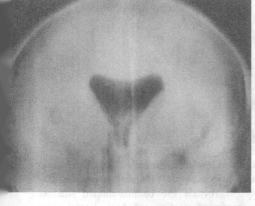

8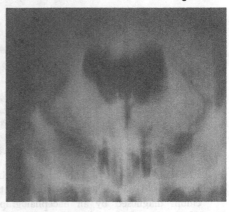

9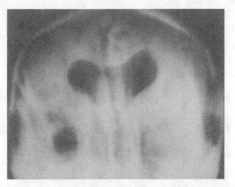

FIGS. 7, 8, 9. (Cases 1, 2, 3). Anteroposterior tomography to show cavum septi pellucidi Figs. 8 and 9.

10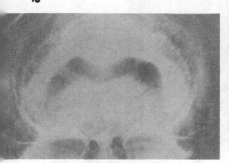

11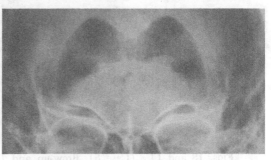

FIGS. 10 and 11. (Cases 1 and 4). Posteroanterior views. Absent septum pellucidum in Fig. 10 (Case 1). Cavum septi pellucidi in Fig. 11 (Case 4).

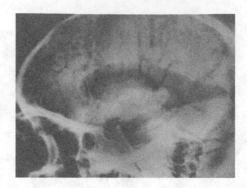

Fig. 12. (Case 1). The lateral horizontal view recommended by Dyke and Davidoff (1935) when they reported their first example of absent septum pellucidum diagnosed by air encephalography. It reveals the comma-shaped shadow which they described. It represents the confluent portions of both lateral ventricles at the midline.

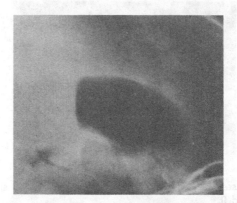

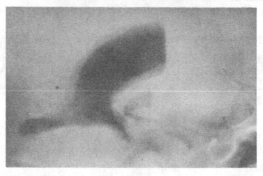

Figs. 13 and 14. (Case 5). Brow-up and brow-down views showing the dense shadow within that cast by the lateral ventricles, resulting from the presence of a communicating cavum septi pellucidi.

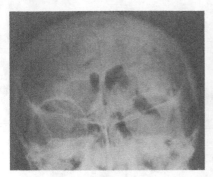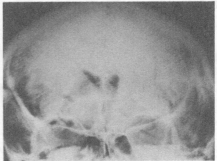

Figs. 15 and 16. Anteroposterior views taken with the patient lying on his side, the head horizontal. These are the *normal* appearances. With an intact septum some air remains in the lowermost ventricle.

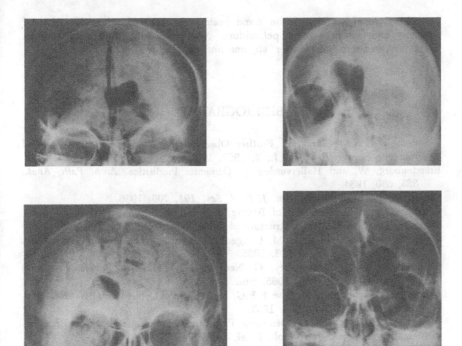

Figs. 17, 18, 19, 20. (Cases 1, 2, 5, 6). Anteroposterior views taken with the patient lying on his side. In each case all the air collects in the upper lateral ventricle. It has passed through the ruptured septum pellucidum.

541

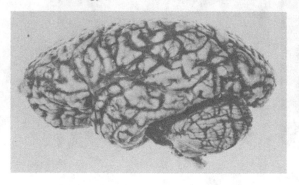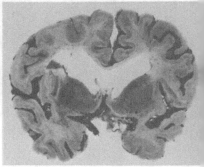

FIG. 21. Lateral view of the brain of a boxer who suffered from gross organic dementia for over 20 years. He was a former world-title holder. Air encephalograms, Figs. 3 and 9. Gross diffuse cerebral atrophy.

FIG. 22. Coronal section of the same brain (Fig. 21) showing dilatation of ventricles and absent septum pellucidum. Note remaining strands of septum. Death occurred ten years after air encephalography was performed.

BIBLIOGRAPHY

Blonstein, J. L. and Clarke, E. Further Observations on the Medical Aspects of Amateur Boxing. *Br. Med. J.*, *2*, 1523, 1954.

Brandenburg, W. and Hallervorden, J. Dementia Pugilistica. *Arch. Path. Anat.*, *325*, 680, 1954.

Carroll, E. J. Punch Drunk. *Am. J. Med. Sci.*, *191*, 706, 1936.

Critchley, M. Medical Aspects of Boxing, Br. Med. J., *1*, 357, 1957.

Dodgson, M. C. H. Colloidal Structure of Brain. *Biorheology*, *1*, 21, 1962.

Dyke, C. G. and Davidoff, L. M. Congenital Absence of the Septum Pellucidum. *Am. J. Roentgenol.*, *34*, 573, 1935.

Ferguson, E. R. and Mawdsley, C. Neurological Disease in Boxers. *Proc. 8th Internat. Cong. Neurol.*, 1965, Vol. *1*. P. E10.

Gordon, E. B. and Sim, M. The E.E.G. in Pre-senile Dementia. *J. Neurol. Neurosurg. Psychiatry*, *30*, 285, 1967.

Grahmann, H. and Ule, G. Dementia Pugilistica: Traumatische Boxer-Encephalopathie. *Psychiat. et Neurol.*, Basel, *30*, 285, 1957.

Holbourn, A. H. S. Mechanics of Head Injuries. *Lancet*, *2*, 438, 1943.

Hughes, R. P., Kernohan. J. M. and Craig, W. M. Caves and Cysts of the Septum Pellucidum. *Arch. Neurol. Psychiat.*, *74*, 259, 1955.

Isherwood, I., Mawdsley, C. and Ferguson, F. R. Pneumoencephalographic Changes in Boxers. *Acta Radiologica*, *5*, 654, 1966.

Johnson, J. Organic Psychosyndromes Due to Boxing. *Br. J. Psychiat.*, *115*, 45, 1969.

Jokl, E. and Guttmann, E. Neurologische-Psychiatrische Untersuchung On Boxern. *Münch. med. Woch.*, *15*, 560, 1933.

Kaplan, H. A. and Browder, J. Observations on the Clinical and Brain Wave Patterns of Professional Boxers. *J.A.M.A.*, *156*, 1138, 1954.

Lindgren, S. O. Studies in Head Injuries. Intracranial Pressure Pattern during Impact. *Lancet*, *1*, 1251, 1964.

Martland, H. S. Punch Drunk, *J.A.M.A.*, *91*, 1103, 1928.

Mawdsley, C. Personal Communication, 1969.

Mawdsley, C. and Ferguson, F. R. Neurological Disease in Boxers. *Lancet*, *2*, 795, 1963.

McCown, I. A. Protecting the Boxer. *J.A.M.A.*, *169*, 1409, 1959 a.

McCown, I. A. Boxing Injuries. *Am. J. Surg.*, *98*, 509, 1959 b.

Neuberger, K. T., Sinton, D. W. and Denst, J. Cerebral Atrophy Associated with Boxing. *Arch. Neurol. Psychiat.*, *81*, 403, 1959.

Parker, H. L. Traumatic Encephalopathy of Professional Pugilists. *J. Neurol. Psychopath.*, *15*, 20, 1934.

Pudenz, R. H. and Shelden, C. H. The Lucite Calvarium. A Method for Direct Observation of the Brain. *J. Neurosurg.*, *3*, 487, 1946.

Ravina, A. L'encéphalite traumatique ou "Punch Drunk." *Presse Med.*, *45*, 1362, 1937.

Roberts, A. H. Brain Damage in Boxers. A. Study of the Prevalence of Traumatic Encephalopathy Among Ex-Professional Boxers. Pitman, London, 1969.

Schunk, H. Congenital Dilatations of the Septum Pellucidum. *Radiology*, *81*, 610, 1963.

Schwidde, J. T. Incidence of Cavum Septum Pellucidi and Cavum Vergae in 1032 Human Brains. *Arch. Neurol. Psychiat.*, *67*, 625, 1952.

Spillane, J. D. Five Boxers. *Br. Med. J.*, *2*, 1205, 1962.

Spillane, J. D. The Septum Pellucidum in the "Punch-Drunk" Syndrome. *Proc. 8th Internat. Cong. Neurol.*, 1965, *Vol. 1.* P. 249.

Van Wagenen, W. P. and Aird, R. B. Dilatation of Cavity of Septum Pellucidum and Cavum Vergae; Report of Cases. *Am. J. Cancer*, *20*, 539, 1934.

Winterstein, C. E. Head Injuries Attributable to Boxing. *Lancet*, *2*, 719, 1937.

543

CHAPTER 17

POSTTRAUMATIC EPILEPSY

THEODORE RASMUSSEN, M. D.

INTRODUCTION

Any insult to the brain of any significance leaves behind some degree of scarring, gross or microscopic, diffuse or focal. In a variable percentage of patients, the scarred area of the brain produces, in some poorly understood fashion and usually after a latent period of months or years, episodic neuronal hyperexcitability of sufficient intensity to bring about epileptic seizures of some type. If the word trauma is used in its broadest sense, therefore, the great majority of patients with secondary or symptomatic epilepsy would be classified as "posttraumatic," whether the underlying cause is brain tumor, arteriovenous malformation, birth anoxia or compression, inflammatory brain disease, or postnatal brain injury. By custom, however, the term posttraumatic epilepsy refers to the development of epilepsy as a sequel to the postnatal application of a blow or force to the head, of sufficient magnitude to produce some injury to the brain. There is no clear understanding why a brain injury in one individual is followed by the development of recurring epileptic seizures, and an apparently identical injury in another person is not, but there are some hints that the genetic make-up of the individual may play some rôle.

Epileptic seizures caused by postnatal trauma do not differ in character from those due to other types of brain lesions, and the fact must be emphasized that seizures represent a *symptom* of brain dysfunction and not a *disease* per se. The symptom, epilepsy, may be mild and transient, or severe and persistent. The nature of the individual attack or seizure depends primarily on the site of the initial seizure discharge and on the manner of its propagation throughout the brain. Thus, the seizure discharge may produce focal somatomotor, somato-

544

sensory, visual, auditory, or psychic phenomena at the onset of the clinical attack (Penfield and Kristiansen, 1951; Penfield and Jasper, 1954). If the seizure discharge remains localized in the brain, the seizure may stop at this point and the attack is classified as a minor focal seizure. If the attack is so minimal as to produce no disturbance of consciousness or obvious motor manifestation, the attack is usually described as an aura or warning. In many instances, following the focal onset, the seizure discharge spreads more widely throughout the brain, and the initial focal phenomena are followed by a generalized tonic and/or clonic convulsion, often called a major seizure or – in the older literature – a grand mal attack. Seizures due to more diffuse epileptogenic brain lesions, posttraumatic or due to other causes, usually consist of major convulsive seizures, with little or no evidence of a focal onset. Many patients with minor focal seizures also exhibit more or less frequent major non-focal convulsions, due either to the occasional unusually rapid generalization of the focal seizure discharges, or to the presence of a more diffuse epileptogenic tendency or lesion, in addition to the more focal epileptic lesion.

The classification of seizures on the basis of the origin of the discharging cortical lesion is of importance in giving evidence as to the area of the brain that is mainly involved (Penfield and Kristiansen, 1951). The description of the *severity* of the attack – major attack, minor attack, or aura – gives a clue as to the social impact of the seizures on the patient's life and activity, but provides no evidence as to the localization of the epileptogenic process in the brain, or as to the nature of the causative lesion.

A major attack (grand mal) consists of a generalized convulsion, tonic and/or clonic, with loss of consciousness. If it begins with some focal manifestation (numbness in one hand, clonic movement of one side of the face, turning of the head and eyes to one side, etc.), it is called a focal major seizure. If it starts with simultaneous involvement of both sides of the body and without warning, it is classified as a non-focal major seizure.

In attacks quantitatively classified as *minor*, consciousness is not lost but may be disturbed and, if clonic movements occur, they involve only part of the body. Contact with the environment may be lost, but stereotyped or irrelevant behavior often continues. When the loss of awareness is brief and not accompanied by automatic behavior, the attack may mimic true petit mal, but this term should be reserved for the absence attacks of idiopathic, essential, or genetic epilepsy, characterized in the EEG by bilaterally synchronous 3-per-second spike and slow-wave complexes, interrupting normal background activity (Daly, 1968; Gastaut, 1968; Gloor, 1968).

When the epileptic manifestation consists of sensory phenomena only, without associated motor disturbance and with no or minimal disturbance of consciousness, it is classified as an *aura*. The attack may stop at this point, and the patient describe it as a warning, or after a few seconds it may develop into a minor attack. If the seizure discharge spreads more widely, the minor attack more or less rapidly generalizes into a major seizure.

An elaborate classification of the epilepsies has been proposed by the International League Against Epilepsy, based on both clinical and EEG criteria and using four main headings: 1) generalized epilepsies; 2) secondary generalized epilepsies; 3) partial (focal, local) epilepsies; and 4) unclassified epilepsies (Gastaut, 1969 and 1970; Merlis, 1970).

DEFINITION AND CRITERIA OF POSTTRAUMATIC EPILEPSY

In order for a head injury to be incriminated as a potential cause for epileptic attacks, and for a presumptive diagnosis of posttraumatic epilepsy to be entertained, it must be clear that the patient was not subject to seizures prior to the head injury, and that the onset of the seizures, therefore, occurred subsequent to the head injury. The head injury must have been severe enough to have caused some injury to the brain and, in addition, other causes of epilepsy must be absent. Since both head injury and epilepsy from other causes are common, both may exist in a patient and be completely unrelated.

When focal attacks arise from the vicinity of a focal penetrating brain injury, such as a depressed fracture or missile wound, the diagnosis of posttraumatic epilepsy may be considered conclusive, for practical purposes. In other situations, the diagnosis must be considered presumptive only. From time to time, a patient originally considered to have posttraumatic epilepsy is found at operation to have a slowly-growing brain tumor, a vascular malformation, or some other lesion which was responsible for the seizures, and the earlier head injury was thus merely coincidental (Cavanagh, Falconer and Meyer, 1958; Edgar and Baldwin 1960; Perot, Weir, and Rasmussen 1966; Falconer, 1970; Krayenbühl et al, 1970).

EARLY EPILEPSY

Epileptic attacks during the first week after the head injury — early epilepsy — seem to have a different pathophysiological basis than those beginning after a longer interval. Early epilepsy occurs in about 5 percent of patients with head injury, and is more common after severe or complicated injuries (Whitty, 1947; Phillips, 1954; Jennett and Lewin, 1960; Evans, 1963). About one-third of patients with early epilepsy go on, after a latent period as a rule, to develop continuing epileptic seizures, and it is this group, late epilepsy, that constitutes the clinical problem of posttraumatic epilepsy.

Jennett (1969) found that epilepsy was 25 to 30 times more frequent in the first week after injury than in any of the subsequent seven weeks. There is considerable evidence that early epilepsy (first week) differs from epilepsy appearing later. It is less likely to persist, it is more likely to take the form of focal motor attacks, and temporal lobe attacks do not occur. Early epilepsy after non-missile injury is important, since it indicates a considerably increased risk of the later development of continuing epilepsy.

ONSET OF LATE EPILEPSY

Most reports and discussions of posttraumatic epilepsy refer primarily to this group of patients who begin to have seizures after a latent period of weeks, months, or years after the head injury. In about half of the head-injured patients who ultimately develop epilepsy, the first seizure appears during the first year after the head injury. In another quarter of the patients, the seizures begin during the second year. The remaining one-fourth of the patients develop their seizures with decreasing incidence over the ensuing 30-40 years (Symonds, 1935; Watson, 1947; Russell and Whitty, 1952 and 1953; Walker and Jablon, 1959; Evans, 1962; Caviness, Jr., 1966; Paillas, 1969).

In general, the statistics concerning the onset of seizures are similar in a number of well-documented studies of wartime patients with missile wounds of the head (Wagstaffe, 1928; Credner, 1930; Baumm, 1930; Ascroft, 1941; Caveness, Walker, and Ascroft, 1962); and in patients with closed head injuries (Penfield and Shaver, 1945; Walker, 1949; Wilson, 1951; Phillips, 1954; Wertheimer, 1956; Gurdjian and Webster, 1958; Jennett and Lewin, 1960; Kaplan, 1961; Rasmussen, 1969; Paillas, Paillas, and Bureau, 1970).

INCIDENCE OF LATE EPILEPSY

The incidence of posttraumatic epilepsy varies directly with the severity of the injury to the brain and is roughly comparable in civilians sustaining

547

blunt head injuries (Jennett, 1962; Paillas, 1969; Paillas, Paillas, and Bureau, 1970) and in wartime patients sustaining missile wounds of the brain. In the latter category, review of the literature indicates the incidence has remained about the same in the wars of the last hundred years (Rawling, 1922-23; Turner, 1923; Wagstaffe, 1928; Credner, 1930; Ascroft, 1941; Gliddon, 1943; Wilson, 1951; Caveness, Walker, and Ascroft, 1962; Hori, Utumi, and Hahori, 1964; Walker, 1966).

Caveness and Liss (1961) studied 407 adult males with head injuries sustained in the Korean campaign between 1951 and 1953. In those with intact dura the incidence ranged from 8.5 percent in those without significant neurological symptoms, to 26.6 percent in those with persisting objective evidence of brain injury. In those with penetration of the dura the incidence ranged from 17.4 percent in those who had no unconsciousness or neurological deficit, to 50.6 percent in those with objective evidence of severe brain damage. When brain-injured patients from World War II were categorized on the same basis, the incidence of epilepsy followed a similar pattern.

Jennett's (1962) comprehensive studies of epilepsy after blunt head injuries indicate that late traumatic epilepsy (onset after the first week) occurs in about 5 percent of all patients followed for more than four years, but with the risk varying widely in different types of cases. Thus, the risk of epilepsy was about 1 percent for all head injuries uncomplicated by early epilepsy, intracranial hematomata, or depressed fracture, but was over 50 percent in the case of depressed skull fracture with intact dura and with early epilepsy, or with posstraumatic amnesia exceeding 24 hours. In the case of depressed skull fracture with dural penetration, and either early epilepsy or posttraumatic amnesia of more than 24 hours, the risk rose to 80 percent.

Caviness, Jr. (1969) has shown in a study of German veterans of World War I that increasing depth of injury also increases the risk of the development of epilepsy, a finding that is in agreement with the suggestion that deep-lying mechanisms of activation and inhibition, as well as cortical irritability, are important in the establishment of a post-traumatic epileptic tendency (Russell, 1968).

DIAGNOSIS

The investigation of a patient with cerebral seizures is not altered significantly by the suspicion that the seizures are related to earlier mechanical injury to the brain. The physician must attempt to answer the questions, "Where is the lesion that is responsible for the seizures?" and, "What is the nature of the lesion?" Study of the patient's attack pattern or patterns and the EEG give the most important evidence related to the first question, whereas x-ray studies, including pneumo-encephalogram and sometimes angiogram, give the most valuable evidence as to the nature of the lesion.

Attack Pattern

The initial phenomena of a seizure usually give the most valuable evidence as to its site of origin in the brain. Repeated questioning of the patient as to what he feels and does at the onset of the attack, and repeated questioning of the family as to what they see at the beginning of the seizure, usually enable the physician to identify the region of the brain that has given rise to the seizure. Descriptions of attacks witnessed in the hospital by nurses, who are trained to observe seizures and to describe them in objective terms, provide important localizing information, and often indicate that the patient actually has more than one type of attack. Once the attack becomes generalized, detailed description is of little value, but the presence of postictal hemiparesis or postictal dysphasia provides important localizing information.

The localizing evidence of the patient's attack pattern usually identifies quite satisfactorily the general region of the brain with the lowest threshold for epileptogenic discharges, but does not give any good evidence as to the total extent of the epileptogenic areas of the brain.

EEG

The EEG carried out with montages designed to localize the seizure discharges (Jasper and Hawke, 1938; Jasper and Kershman, 1941; Walker, Marshall, and Beresford, 1947, Jasper, 1949), and with anticonvulsant medication reduced or stopped, gives more refined evidence as to the localization of the epileptogenic area of the brain, and gives the only evidence as to its total extent. Special examinations are often required to map out the epileptogenic area satisfactorily. These may include activation studies with sleep (Gibbs and Gibbs, 1947), sodium thiopental (Pentothal) (Lombroso and Erba, 1969), Metrazol or Megimide (Kaufman, Marshall, and Walker, 1947; Cure,

Rasmussen, and Jasper, 1948; Delay, Schulter, Drossopoulo and Verdeux, 1956), the use of pharyngeal, sphenoidal (Pampiglione and Kerridge, 1956; Rovit, Gloor, and Rasmussen, 1961) or chronic implanted intracerebral electrodes (Delgado and Hamlin, 1958); Ajmone-Marsan and Van Buren, 1958; Lichtenstein, Marshall, and Walker 1959; Crandall, Walter and Rand, 1963), intracarotid Amytal-Metrazol EEG studies (Rovit, Gloor, and Rasmussen, 1961; Garretson, Gloor, and Rasmussen, 1966) and, more recently, telemetering of the EEG during daily living activities on the ward (Penry and Dreifuss, 1969; Mark, Erwin, Sweet, and Delgado, 1969).

X-Ray

Skull x-rays are studied with special reference to evidence of old fractures, pathological intracranial calcifications, and asymmetries (Schechter and Zingesser, 1969). The latter often indicate the presence of atrophic areas of the brain, dating from birth or early infancy, since early focal brain injury frequently results in smallness of the related cranial fossa or hemicranium, loss of normal brain markings, or local increased thickness of the skull over the involved area of the brain (McRae and Castorina, 1963). The presence of definite smallness of the right middle fossa in a patient with seizures, arising in the right temporal lobe and beginning at 12 years of age, for example, would strongly suggest that the brain damage responsible for the seizures occurred at birth or in the early months of life, rather than at the time of a head injury, occurring 1 to 2 years before the onset of the seizures, that might otherwise be incriminated as the cause of the seizures.

Pneumoencephalography is the most valuable x-ray contrast study and should be carried out with the injection of enough gas to visualize the subarachnoid spaces as well as the ventricular system. The films are then studied with special reference to asymmetries which might indicate diffuse or focal atrophy, or loss of substance of the brain (McRae, 1948; Lindgren, 1951).

Angiograms are not done routinely unless there is some suspicion that the attacks may be due to a brain tumor, as is always the case when seizures first appear in adult life (Lund, 1952; Rasmussen and Blundell, 1961), even though there may be a history of an earlier head injury as a possible cause for the seizures. Angiograms are also done if the pneumograms show some asymmetry or irregularity of the ventricular wall that might indicate the presence of a space-occupying lesion or an AV malformation.

The radioactive brain scan, when positive, is useful in patients with seizures starting in adult life who must, therefore, be suspected of having a brain tumor or an AV malformation. The scan, however, is nearly always negative in cases of indolent astrocytoma and oligodendroglioma that sometimes cause seizures for many years before producing evidence of neurological deficit or increased intracranial pressure; it is also normal in patients with epilepsy due to brain scarring or cerebral atrophy.

Psychological Testing

Special psychological testing (as developed by Dr. Brenda Milner and her team at the M.N.I.) in the course of investigations of localization and lateralization of certain intellectual functions, often gives useful evidence of focal dysfunction of certain regions of the brain, which correlates well with the EEG abnormality (Milner, 1954, 1958, 1964, 1965, 1968). In addition, these tests sometimes give evidence that the patient's speech functions may not be located in the left cerebral hemisphere as would ordinarily be expected, and would thus indicate the need for identifying the cortical speech area by the intracarotid Amytal speech test, if craniotomy is being considered.

Intracarotid Amytal Speech and Memory Test

This test, devised by Wada, is carried out if operation is being considered in any patient in whom it is suspected that the speech functions may not be located in the left cerebral hemisphere (Wada, 1949; Wada and Rasmussen, 1960). Thus it is carried out in all patients being considered for operation if they are not clearly right-handed, since some left-handed and ambidextrous patients have their speech functions in the right rather than the left hemisphere.

The test is also carried out if operation is being considered for right-handed patients with evidence of injury to the left hemisphere in the early years of life, since this may have resulted in the development of speech functions in the right rather than the left hemisphere. With certain types of localized injury to the left cerebral hemisphere during the first few years of life, speech may develop in the right

551

hemisphere instead of the left, without a corresponding shift in handedness.

This special speech test is also carried out in right-handed patients if the patient's seizure pattern gives some hint that the speech functions may not be located in the left cerebral hemisphere, for example, when there is evidence of postictal dysphasia following seizures arising in the right hemisphere.

During this intracarotid Amytal speech test, memory functions are also tested (Milner, Branch, and Rasmussen, 1962), and the results of these simple memory tests that are carried out when one cerebral hemisphere is inactivated by the carotid Amytal injection, provide considerable safety in avoiding postoperative memory deficit (Penfield and Milner, 1958) when operating on temporal-lobe seizure patients who have some EEG or x-ray evidence of damage to the opposite temporal lobe, or who show some psychological-test abnormalities, that suggest dysfunction of both temporal lobes (Milner, 1958).

COURSE OF POSTTRAUMATIC EPILEPSY

The severity of the seizure tendency that develops after brain injury varies widely. A small percentage of patients may have only one or two attacks, with the tendency to seizure then disappearing spontaneously but, at the other extreme, some patients will continue to have severe daily or weekly attacks, year after year. The usual attack frequency, however, is of the order of one, two, or three per month. With the passage of time, there is a tendency in some patients for the seizures to decrease spontaneously (Walker, 1957; Evans, 1962; Caveness, 1963; Masquin and Courjon, 1963; Caveness, Jr., 1966). Walker and Erculei (1970) found that 15 years after injury, 40 percent of 230 veterans of World War II with posttraumatic epilepsy had had no seizures of any type between the fifth and fifteenth year. The tendency for spontaneous regression of seizures usually occurs during the third to fifth year after injury. After the fifth year, the seizure tendency remains fairly stable in most patients. Statistics for World War I veterans indicate that, after 15 years had elapsed, about 25 percent of patients who developed posttraumatic epilepsy continued to have recurring seizures indefinitely.

Serial EEG studies reveal a tendency for generalized EEG abnormalities to become focal or to disappear with time, but EEG abnormalities may persist even though the clinical seizures disappear. EEG abnormalities may become normalized during the phase of incubation of the seizure tendency, or abnormalities may persist even though the patient never develops epilepsy. Thus the EEG cannot be used to predict the risk of later development of epilepsy, although it is of major importance in the study of the epilepsy after it is well established (Jasper, Kershman, and Elvidge, 1940; Masquin and Courjon 1963; Courjon, 1969 and 1970).

PROPHYLAXIS

In some neurological centers phenobarbital or Dilantin are given routinely for 1 to 2 years after head injuries carrying significant risk of development of posttraumatic epilepsy, but there is no conclusive evidence that this reduces the incidence. Most neurosurgeons follow the practice of starting anticonvulsant medication only after the seizure tendency has manifested itself clinically.

The only effective prophylaxis is prevention of head injury (Kristiansen, Henriksen, and Ringkjob, 1969). Despite the steadily improving surgical management of head wounds, the incidence of posttraumatic epilepsy is essentially the same in head-injured soldiers from World War I, World War II, and the Korean campaign. The area of the brain that is damaged through the force imparted by the missile extends far beyond the track of the wound or the area lacerated by a depressed bone fragment, and the decrease in severity of local scarring — the result of modern neurosurgical management of brain lacerations — has little or no bearing on the more remote effects of the injury. Thus, it is not surprising that the incidence of posttraumatic epilepsy has not lessened with the increasingly effective management of brain wounds and trauma. In addition, the larger percentage of patients with severe brain wounds who survive, as a result of the improvement in neurosurgical care, increases the number of patients with maximum risk of developing posttraumatic epilepsy.

MEDICAL TREATMENT

The general principles of treatment of posttraumatic epilepsy are identical with those pertaining to any patient with seizures whose underlying lesion does not require special attention (Rasmussen and McNaughton, 1959). Once it becomes clear that the patient is subject

553

to recurring attacks, it is important for him and his family to acquire a thorough understanding of the nature and implications of the epileptic disability. Normal activities should be maintained as much as possible, avoiding such obvious hazards as driving a car, working on ladders or scaffolding, working around machinery with exposed moving parts, etc. Regularity of eating and sleeping is important, since chronic fatigue tends to increase the epileptogenic tendency. Alcohol should be avoided, since it also tends to increase the liability to seizures.

Management of the Actual Seizures

Once the attack has begun, it cannot be arrested and bystanders can only help protect the patient from injuring himself. If there is time, the patient can be helped to a chair or couch, or eased to the floor. A blunt object, such as several tongue depressors bound together with adhesive tape, should be put into the mouth between the jaws, to protect the tongue. A finger should *never* be used for this purpose, since it may be badly chewed. Clothing about the neck should be loosened, and the patient turned on one side or into a semiprone position, to avoid aspiration of secretions and to prevent the tongue from falling back and obstructing the airway. If the patient is restless and confused afterwards, it is important to use as little restraint as possible. If the attack lasts for more than 5 to 10 minutes, or if attacks occur repeatedly during the day, intravenous Sodium Amytal, Dilantin or diazepam (Valium) are required, and it is often wise for the patient to be taken to the nearest hospital emergency department.

The Antiepileptic Drugs

The first antiepileptic drug, bromide, is rarely used at present, although for over 50 years following the accidental discovery of its antiepileptic properties in 1857, it was the only effective agent for the patient with seizures. The drugs primarily effective in true petit mal, the diones (Tridione and Paradione) and the suximides (Milontin, Celontin and Zarontin) are rarely of help in posttraumatic and other forms of secondary epilepsy. The newest, Zarontin, is sometimes useful, however, when added to some of the other standard anticonvulsant drugs.

554

The barbiturates (phenobarbital and Mebaral), the hydantoins (Dilantin and Mesantoin) and the primidones (Mysoline) constitute the most effective medications for posttraumatic and other types of secondary epilepsy. Phenylacetylurea (Phenurone) is sometimes quite effective in treating seizures arising in the temporal lobe, but must be used with caution because of its tendency to damage the liver and bone marrow. Carbamazepine (Tegretol), recently introduced for control of tic douloureux, seems to have some useful anticonvulsant action as well, in a small percentage of patients.

Principles of Drug Therapy

Patients vary widely in their responses to these anticonvulsant drugs, and each patient must be managed on a trial-and-error basis. To assist the physician in adjusting the drug dosages, the patient or a relative should keep a record of the attacks.

The simpler and safer drugs should be used before the newer and potentially more toxic ones are tried.

One drug, usually Dilantin, phenobarbital, or Mysoline should be tried first, and the dosage increased gradually as needed and as tolerated. If seizures persist despite maximal doses of the first drug tried, Dilantin for example, it should be reduced gradually over a period of 1 to 2 weeks and replaced by phenobarbital, perhaps, and subsequently by Mysoline, if necessary. If maximal tolerable doses of these drugs given singly do not give satisfactory seizure control, the two most effective and best tolerated drugs should be tried together. If seizure control is still unsatisfactory, the third drug should be added to average doses of the first two, and the dose gradually increased. Should this fail to improve the seizure control, the least effective of the three medications being given should be replaced by one of the second-rank drugs, Mesantoin, Zarontin, Tegretol, etc. In each instance, the initial dose should be small and increases made at intervals of one to two weeks, as needed and as tolerated.

Monthly blood counts are required when Mesantoin, Tridione, Phenurone, or Tegretol are administered, since in a certain percentage of patients these agents are toxic to the bone marrow. Any of these drugs, however, may produce toxic side-effects in a small percentage of patients, so that patients being started on a new drug must be seen at frequent intervals when the dosage is being increased. If signs of toxicity appear (rash, ataxia, somnolence, leukopenia, or hepatitis), the drug should be stopped promptly.

When satisfactory seizure control can be achieved, it is important to keep up the anticonvulsant medication for at least two or three years. Gradual reduction of the medication, one dose at a time at 6-or 12-month intervals, may then be possible. If attacks recur as the medication is reduced, the original dosage should be resumed.

Status Epilepticus

Frequently recurring attacks with continuing unconsciousness are always a major medical emergency and require prompt treatment with intravenous Valium (Gastaut et al, 1965), Dilantin (Murphy and Schwab, 1956), or Sodium Amytal. If the attacks are not quite so continuous and the patient is conscious between the attacks, less rigorous treatment with hypodermic administration of sodium phenobarbital or the administration of paraldehyde (Whitty and Taylor, 1949) by mouth or rectum, may suffice to stop the series of attacks.

A patient in status epilepticus requires constant nursing care. He should be kept in a semiprone position, and a clear airway should be maintained. His position must be changed frequently, and chest physiotherapy used to safeguard against pulmonary atelectasis and aspiration pneumonia. Dehydration and disturbance of electrolyte imbalance must be avoided.

SURGICAL THERAPY

Cortical resection carried out under local anesthesia, and controlled with cortical electrographic recording and stimulation, has stood the test of time as an effective treatment for well-selected patients with focal epilepsy (Penfield and Jasper, 1954; Penfield and Paine, 1955; Rasmussen and Branch, 1962; Rasmussen and Gossman, 1963; Rasmussen, 1963; Rasmussen, 1969 a and b). Thus, if a thorough trial of maximal tolerable doses of the principal anticonvulsant drugs does not keep the attacks under sufficient control so the patient can live a reasonably normal life, investigation into the possibility of surgical therapy may be indicated.

556

Criteria for Surgical Therapy

1. Failure of medical management, as noted above, is the first criterion, since the need to consider surgery ordinarily does not arise if the attacks are well controlled, regardless of how focal and surgically accessible the epileptogenic area of the cortex may be.

2. The attacks must have been present for a long enough period of time for one to be reasonably sure that all potentially epileptogenic areas of the brain have matured and become symptomatic, and to be reasonably sure that a spontaneous regression of the seizure tendency is unlikely. Operation is rarely recommended earlier than 3 to 4 years after the onset of seizures unless the seizure tendency is severe or is becoming progressively worse, despite maximal anticonvulsant medication. Our statistics suggest that cortical resection is just as likely to reduce the seizure tendency satisfactorily when carried out 10, 20, or 30 years after the onset of seizures, as when it is done two, three, or four years after the onset.

3. Clinical and EEG evidence must indicate that the attacks are focal in origin and are arising in an area of the brain that can be excised without producing a significant neurologic deficit, or without increasing one that is already present.

4. The patient himself must be well motivated toward considering a major surgical procedure. The patient's complete and enthusiastic cooperation is essential for some of the more complicated diagnostic procedures and for the operation, when it is carried out under local anesthesia.

Surgical Hypothesis

Continuing follow-up studies of patients operated upon for focal epilepsy at the Montreal Neurological Institute since 1928 have shown that success in stopping the seizures seems to be reasonably well correlated with the completeness of the removal of the epileptogenic cortex (Rasmussen and Branch, 1962; Rasmussen and Gossman, 1963; Rasmussen, 1963; Rasmussen, 1969 a and b). The surgical aim, therefore, is to identify and map out the total epileptogenic area and to remove the involved cortex as completely as possible, without incurring

557

too great a risk of producing a significant neurologic deficit, or of increasing one that is already present.

Surgical Technique

1. The operation is done under local anesthesia as a general rule, except in children under the age of 12 to 13 years, or when a hemispherectomy is planned. The use of local anesthesia enables one to identify and map out the epileptogenic area with maximum accuracy by recording the cortical electrical activity unaltered by any anesthetic agent.

2. Local anesthesia also permits the surgeon to map out the motor, sensory, and speech zones in appropriate detail (Penfield and Rasmussen, 1950), so that maximal removals of the epileptogenic area can be made with the least possible risk of producing a neurologic deficit. Periodic testing of motor, sensory, and speech functions during the cortical excision gives maximal safety in this regard.

3. The cortical excision is made with a small bore suction, in a manner designed to produce the least possible trauma and vascular disturbance in the adjacent remaining convolutions and in the underlying white matter. The removal is planned to follow sulci, whenever possible, and the cortex is gently sucked away from the pial margins of the removal bank, with no retraction or manipulation of the remaining convolutional margins.

4. If the post-excision cortical EEG shows a significant amount of epileptiform abnormality, further excision is carried out providing it can be done without too great a risk of producing a neurologic deficit. One, two, or three further excisions are often done before a satisfactorily clean cortical EEG is obtained, or the attempt to do so is abandoned.

RESULTS OF CORTICAL EXCISION ON THE SEIZURE TENDENCY

Since 1928, continuing follow-up examinations and inquiries have been carried out from the beginning in the series of patients undergoing craniotomy for focal epilepsy at the Montreal Neurological Institute, and complete follow-up data, much of it on a yearly basis, are available for over 80 percent of the patients. By the end of 1970, this surgical seizure series consisted of 1508 patients who had undergone 1751 craniotomies with cortical resection of epileptogenic tissue, including some with tumors and other space-occupying lesions. On the basis of the criteria described earlier, postnatal trauma was considered to be responsible for the brain damage that led to the development of the seizure tendency in 280 patients out of the total series, and these patients are thus classified as having posttraumatic epilepsy.

Analysis of the results in the 274 patients with posttraumatic epilepsy who had been operated upon up to the end of 1968 (to permit a minimum follow-up period of two years) (Table 1), shows that 37 percent have become seizure-free and another 33 percent have had a marked reduction in seizure frequency, so that the residual attacks

TABLE 1

Results of Cortical Excision for Posttraumatic Epilepsy

Patients operated upon from 1928 through 1968

Seizure free since discharge	37 pts. (15%)	92 pts. (37%)	174 pts. (70%)	246 pts. with follow-up data of 2-36 yrs. median 13 yrs.
Became seizure free after some early attacks	55 pts. (22%)			
Marked reduction of seizure tendency	82 pts. (33%)			
Moderate to no reduction of seizure tendency	72 pts. (30%)			
Inadequate follow-up data	23 pts.			
Postoperative deaths	5 pts.			
Total	**274 pts.**			

were of the order of 1 to 2 percent of the preoperative frequency. Thus, a complete or nearly complete reduction in seizure tendency followed the cortical resection in 70 percent of the patients in this series who were classified as having posttraumatic epilepsy. The remaining 30 percent had a less satisfactory reduction in seizure tendency, ranging from a moderate reduction to none. It should be

559

TABLE 2

Epilepsy Due to Birth Trauma, Anoxia or Compression

Results of Surgical Therapy - patients operated upon from 1928 through 1966

Seizure free since discharge	87 pts. (27%)	159 pts. (50%)		320 pts. with follow-up data of 2 yrs. or longer
Became seizure free after some early attacks	72 pts. (23%)		221 pts. (69%)	
Marked reduction of seizure tendency	62 pts. (19%)			
Moderate to no reduction of seizure tendency	99 pts. (31%)			

Inadequate follow-up data	23 pts.	duration of follow-up 2-36 yrs.
Postoperative deaths	2 pts.	median 9 yrs.

Total	345 pts.

Chapter 26, "Surgical Treatment of Posttraumatic Epilepsy," by T. Rasmussen. In *The Late Effects of Head Injury,* edited by A. E. Walker, W. F. Caveness, and M. Critchley. Springfield, Ill.: Charles C Thomas, Publisher, 1969..
Reprinted by permission of the publisher.

emphasized that in all patients in this series, the seizures were refractory to medical anticonvulsant therapy, which had often been carried on for many years.

These results are comparable to those obtained in the other principal etiological categories in the series. Thus, in patients whose epileptogenic lesion seemed to be most likely due to birth anoxia or trauma, 50 percent became seizure-free and a total of 69 percent have shown a complete or nearly complete reduction in seizure tendency (Table 2) (Rasmussen, 1969 b).

In the post-inflammatory group, 49 percent became seizure-free, and a total of 73 percent have shown a complete or nearly complete reduction in seizure tendency (Rasmussen, 1969 b).

In those classified as of unknown etiology, often because there was more than one potential etiological factor present, 38 percent became seizure-free and a total of 58 percent have shown a complete or nearly

When the patients in this series are classified according to the principal complete reduction in seizure tendency (Rasmussen, 1969 b).

cipal anatomical area involved in the seizure process, the results of the cortical excision are also quite comparable to those given above. In the largest of the anatomical groups, those whose epileptogenic area involved mainly the temporal lobe, 46 percent became seizure-free, and a total of 69 percent showed a complete or nearly complete reduction in seizure tendency (Table 3) (Rasmussen, 1969 a). The results in the smaller anatomical groups, frontal, parietal, central, occipital, and those with large destructive brain lesions, were also similar (Rasmussen, 1969 a).

TABLE 3

Temporal Lobe Epilepsy — Results of Surgical Therapy

Patients with non-tumoral lesions operated upon from 1930 through 1966

Seizure free since discharge	126 pts. (25%)	235 pts. (46%)	352 pts. (69%) — 508 pts. with follow-up data of 2 yrs. or longer
Became seizure free after some early attacks	109 pts. (21%)		
Marked reduction of seizure tendency	117 pts. (23%)		
Moderate to no reduction of seizure tendency	156 pts. (31%)		

Inadequate follow-up data	71 pts.	duration of follow-up	2-36 yrs.
Postoperative deaths	4 pts.	median	8 yrs.
Total	**583 pts.**		

From "The Role of Surgery in the Treatment of Focal Epilepsy," by T. Rasmussen in *Clinical Neurosurgery*, vol. 16, 1969. Baltimore: Williams & Wilkins Company. Reprinted by permission of the publisher and the Congress of Neurological Surgeons.

Thus the data from this series indicate that the effectiveness of cortical resection for the treatment of focal epilepsy is correlated with the completeness with which the epileptogenic cortex can be removed, rather than with the nature of the underlying cause of the original brain damage, or the anatomical location of the principal epileptogenic area.

PATHOLOGY OF POSTTRAUMATIC EPILEPSY

The pathologic lesions encountered in this series of patients with posttraumatic epilepsy range across the entire spectrum of the late

561

pathologic residuals of brain trauma. The most minimal lesions consisted of more or less restricted areas of gliosis with preservation of normal-appearing convolutions, and with normal color distinction between gray and white matter, but with a definite increase in consistency. Both the gray and white matter in these areas often exhibited a distinctly yellow tint. Fine filamentous or stout adhesions between the cortex and dura were often present, representing the late residual of blood in the subdural and subarachnoid spaces over the involved area.

More severe lesions showed evidence of gross destruction of brain tissue and replacement by a mesoglial cicatrix of greater or lesser extent. When there had been laceration of the dura by a depressed skull fracture or by a missile, attachment of the mesoglial scar to the meninges resulted in the typical meningo-cerebral cicatrix (Del Rio-Hortega and Penfield, 1927; Penfield and Humphreys, 1940).

In the most extensive lesions, large areas of the hemisphere were destroyed and replaced by multicystic mesoglial scar tissue, or by porencephalic cysts which, in some instances, were separate from the ventricle and in others, communicated with it.

The epileptic activity, as judged by the preoperative scalp EEG and the cortical EEG, is usually less widespread than the total area of damaged brain, but ordinarily the activity does involve sizeable areas of cortex, even if the grossly visible area of brain damage is small and discrete. In the process of carrying out the removal, however, both the gray and the white matter in these adjacent normal-appearing areas are usually found to be definitely, and sometimes markedly, increased in consistency, and are also often slightly yellow in color, as noted above.

These gross and microscopic characteristics have been well summarized by Payan, Toga, and Bérard-Badier (1970). Extensive investigations, however, have failed to show any distinctive histologic characteristics that distinguish between epileptogenic and non-epileptogenic areas of brain scarring, atrophy, or gliosis (Haymaker, Pentschew, Margoles, and Bingham, 1958; Courville, 1958).

PATHOPHYSIOLOGICAL MECHANISMS

The basic mechanisms involved in posttraumatic epilepsy are doubtless the same as those responsible for other types of symptomatic or secondary epilepsy, and may be similar or identical to those responsible for essential, primary, or so-called idiopathic epilepsy. An enormous wealth of clinical and experimental studies have been directed at these mechanisms since the turn of the century. Attention has been directed to acute and chronic changes in cerebral circulation, mechanical effects of gliosis and the meningo-cerebral cicatrix, effects of alteration of the blood-brain barrier and glial-neuronal relationships, discharge characteristics of individual nerve cells, disruption of inhibitory systems in the brain, etc., to indicate some of the principal lines of investigation (Jasper, Ward, and Pope, 1969; Jasper, 1970). Our understanding of the pathophysiology of the generation of the seizure, however, is still meager (Walker, 1969).

Nevertheless, certain well-established facts provide some guidance. Several lines of clinical evidence indicate that a certain minimum bulk of cortex, or number of neurons, must be recruited into action in order to produce a seizure. Thus, the tiny meningo-cerebral cicatrix that follows a ventricular puncture has probably never produced a clinical seizure, whereas increasing severity of brain injury produces an increasing incidence of epilepsy, up to 50 percent or more.

Since only a certain percentage of patients with brain injury ultimately develop recurring seizures, it seems highly probable that some innate tendency must exist in the brains of those who do develop them. The development of the seizure tendency thus seems to be the result of the synergistic effect of the healed brain damage, plus a preexisting, subclinical vulnerability. The nature of this is obscure, but there are hints that it may be genetically determined (Metrakos and Metrakos, 1961; Andermann and Metrakos, 1969; Sorel, 1969; Metrakos and Metrakos, 1970).

The fact that the great majority of patients who develop posttraumatic epilepsy do so only after a latent period of months or years provides another important, but as yet undecipherable, clue to significant factors in the genesis of the seizure tendency.

The development of the epileptic state in an area of the brain is marked in the EEG by the appearance of random "spiky" high voltage discharges (Jasper and Penfield, 1943; Marshall and Walker, 1961; Courjon, 1969 and 1970) which are assumed to represent evidence of neuronal hyperirritability in the area. When these random interictal discharges become rhythmic, and recruit into synchronized action a larger number of cortical and subcortical neuronal circuits, a clinical seizure develops.

Microelectrode, histochemical, neurochemical, and electron-micros-

563

copic studies are steadily increasing our understanding of the intricacies of the nerve-cell discharge and of the alterations seen in neurons of epileptogenic cortex, but we know little of the factors that lead to the spread and rhythmicity of the discharges, and the resulting clinical seizure. Although these investigations have focused mainly on the excitatory mechanisms, inhibitory mechanisms may be of equal, or even greater importance, and are now receiving increasing investigative attention.

Until these basic investigations permit the development of a truly definitive therapy for the convulsive state, empirical medical and surgical methods must continue to be refined. However, as with many other great scourges, such as smallpox and polio, mankind would benefit most from the prevention of head trauma and, as a consequence, the elimination of its sequelae.

BIBLIOGRAPHY

Andermann, E. and Metrakos, J. D. EEG Studies of Relatives of Probands with Focal Epilepsy Who Have Been Treated Surgically. *Epilepsia, 16*, 415, 1969.

Ajmone-Marsan, C. and Van Buren, J. M. Epileptiform Activity in Cortical and Subcortical Structures in the Temporal Lobe of Man. *Temporal Lobe Epilepsy.* Springfield, Ill.: Charles C Thomas, 1958.

Ascroft, P. B. Traumatic Epilepsy after Gunshot Wounds of the Head. *Br. Med. J., 1,* 739, 1941.

Baumm, H. Erfahrungen Über Epilepsie Bei Hirnverletzten. *Z. Ges. Neurol. Psychiat., 127,* 279, 1930.

Cavanagh, J. B., Falconer, M. A. and Meyer, A. Some Pathogenic Problems of Temporal Lobe Epilepsy. *Temporal Lobe Epilepsy.* Springfield, Ill.: Charles C Thomas, 1958.

Caveness, W. F. and Liss, H. R. Incidence of Post-Traumatic Epilepsy. *Epilepsia, 2,* 123, 1961.

Caveness, W. F., Walker, A. E. and Ascroft, P. B. Incidence of Post-Traumatic Epilepsy in Korean Veterans as Compared with Those from World War II. *J. Neurosurg., 19,* 122, 1962.

Caveness, W. F. Onset and Cessation of Fits Following Craniocerebral Trauma. *J. Neurosurg., 20,* 570, 1963.

Caviness, V. S., Jr., Variable Features of Chronic Post-Traumatic Epilepsy. *Trans. Amer. Neurol. Assn., 91,* 204, 1966.

Caviness, V. S., Jr., Epilepsy: A Late Effect of Head Injury. Chap. 21, *The Late Effects of Head Injury.* Springfield, Ill.: Charles C Thomas, 1969.

Courjon, J. A. Post-Traumatic Epilepsy in Electroclinical Practice. Chap. 23, *The Late Effects of Head Injury.* Springfield, Ill.: Charles C Thomas, 1969.

Courjon, J. A. A Longitudinal Electro-clinical Study of 80 Cases of Post Traumatic Epilepsy Observed from the Time of the Original Injury. *Epilepsia, 11, .29, 1970.*

Courville, C. B. Traumatic Lesions of the Temporal Lobe as the Essential Cause of Psychomotor Epilepsy. *Temporal Lobe Epilepsy.* Springfield, Ill.: Charles C Thomas, 1958.

Crandall, P. H., Walter, R. D. and Rand, R. W. Clinical Applications of Studies on Stereotactically Implanted Electrodes in Temporal Lobe Epilepsy. *J. Neurosurg., 20, 827, 1963.*

Credner, L. Klinische Und Soziale Auswirkungen Von Hirnschädigungen. *Z. Ges. Neurol. Psychiat., 126, 721, 1930.*

Cure, C., Rasmussen, T., and Jasper, H. Activation of Seizures and Electroencephalic Disturbances in Epileptic and Control Subjects with "Metrazol." *Arch. Neurol. Psychiat., 59, 691, 1948.*

Daly, D. D. Reflections in the Concept of Petit Mal. *Epilepsia, 9, 175, 1968.*

Delay, J., Schulter, E., Drossopoulu, S., and Verdeux, J. Un Nouvel Activant des Electroencéphalogrammes: l'Imide de l'acide éthyl-méthyl Glutamique (NP 13), ou Mégimide. *Rev. Neurol., 94, 315, 1956.*

Delgado, J. M. R. and Hamlin, H. Direct Recording of Spontaneous and Evoked Seizures in Epileptics. *Electroenceph. Clin Neurophysiol., 10, 463, 1958.*

Edgar, R. and Baldwin, M. Vascular Malformations Associated with Temporal Lobe Epilepsy. *J. Neurosurg., 17, 638, 1960.*

Evans, J. H. Post-Traumatic Epilepsy. *Neurology, 12, 665, 1962.*

Evans, J. H. The Significance of Early Post-Traumatic Epilepsy. *Neurology, 13, 207, 1963.*

Falconer, M. A. The Pathological Substrate of Temporal Lobe Epilepsy. *Guy's Hosp. Rep., 119, 47, 1970.*

Garretson, H., Gloor, P. and Rasmussen, T. Intracarotid Amobarbital and Metrazol Test for the Study of Epileptiform Discharges in Man: A Note on Its Technique. *Electroenceph. Clin Neurophysiol., 21, 607, 1966.*

Gastaut, H., Naquet, R., Poire, R. and Tassinari, C. A. Treatment of Status Epilepticus with Diazepam (Valium). *Epilepsia, 6, 167, 1965.*

Gastaut, H. Clinical and Electroencephalographic Correlates of Generalized Spike and Wave Bursts Occurring Spontaneously in Man. *Epilepsia, 9, 179, 1968.*

Gastaut, H. Seizures, Epileptic, Clinical and Electroencephalographic Classification. *Epilepsia, 10,* Supplement 2, 1969.

Gastaut, H. Clinical and Electroencephalographic Classification of Epileptic Seizures. *Epilepsia, 11, 102, 1970.*

Gibbs, E. L. and Gibbs, F. A. Diagnostic and Localizing Value of Electroencephalographic Studies in Sleep. *Proc. Ass. Res. Nerv. Ment. Dis., 26, 366, 1947.*

Gliddon, W. D. Gunshot Wounds of the Head. (A Review of the After Effects in 500 Canadian Prisoners from the Great War, 1914-1918.) *Can. Med. Ass. J., 49, 373, 1943.*

Gloor, P. Generalized Cortico-reticular Epilepsies; Some Considerations on the Pathophysiology of Generalized Bilaterally Synchronous Spike and Wave Discharge, *Epilepsia, 9, 249, 1968.*

Gurdjian, E. S. and Webster, J. E. *Head Injuries.* London: Churchill, 1958. P. 482.

Haymaker, W., Pentschew, A., Margoles, C. and Bingham, W. G. Occurrence of Lesions in the Temporal Lobe in the Absence of Convulsive Seizures. In *Temporal Lobe Epilepsy*. Springfield, Ill.: Charles C Thomas, 1958.

Hori, Y., Utumi, S. and Hahori, Y. The Clinico-Statistical Studies on the Traumatic Epilepsy in Civil Life. *J. Nara. Med. Assn.*, 15, 319, 1964.

Jasper, H. and Hawke, W. A. Localization of Seizure Waves in Epilepsy. *Arch. Neurol. Psychiat.*, 39, 885, 1938.

Jasper, H., Kershman, J. and Elvidge, A. R. Electroencephalographic Studies of Injury to the Head. *Arch. Neurol. Psychiat.*, 44, 328, 1940.

Jasper, H. and Kershman, J. Electroencephalographic Classification of the Epilepsies. *Arch. Neurol. Psychiat.*, 45, 903, 1941.

Jasper, H. and Penfield, W. Electroencephalograms in Post-Traumatic Epilepsy: Pre-operative and Post-operative Studies. *Amer. J. Psychiatry*, 100, 365, 1943.

Jasper, H. Electrical Signs of Epileptic Discharge. *Electroenceph. Clin. Neurophysiol.*, 1, 11, 1949.

Jasper, H. H., Ward, A. A., Jr., and Pope, A. L. (Eds.) *Basic Mechanisms of the Epilepsies*. Boston: Little, Brown & Co., 1969.

Jasper, H. H. Physiopathological Mechanisms of Post-Traumatic Epilepsy. *Epilepsia*, 11, 73, 1970.

Jennett, W. B. and Lewin, W. Traumatic Epilepsy after Closed Head Injuries. *J. Neurol. Neurosurg. Psychiatry*, 23, 295, 1960.

Jennett, W. B. *Epilepsy After Blunt Head Injury*. Springfield, Ill.: Charles C Thomas, 1962.

Jennett, W. B. Epilepsy after Blunt (Nonmissile) Head Injuries. Chap. 22 in *The Late Effects of Head Injury*. Springfield, Ill.: Charles C Thomas, 1969.

Kaplan, H. Management of Craniocerebral Trauma and Its Relation to Subsequent Seizures. *Epilepsia*, 2, 111, 1961.

Kaufman, I. C., Marshall, C., and Walker, A. E. Activated Electroencephalography. *Arch. Neurol. Psychiat.*, 58, 533, 1947.

Krayenbühl, H., Hess, R., Weber, G. and Siegfried, J. Pseudo-traumatic Epilepsy. *Epilepsia*, 11, 59, 1970.

Kristiansen, K., Henriksen, G. F., and Ringkjob, R. Traumatic Epilepsy, Prophylaxis. Chap. 25 in *The Late Effects of Head Injury*. Springfield, Ill.: Charles C Thomas, 1969.

Lindgren, E. Encephalography in Cerebral Atrophy. *Acta Radiol.*, 35, 277, 1951.

Lichtenstein R. S., Marshall, C., and Walker, A. E. Subcortical Recording in Temporal Lobe Epilepsy. *Arch. Neurol.*, 1, 288, 1959.

Lombroso, C. T. and Erba, G. A Test for Separating Secondary from Primary Bilateral Synchrony in Epileptic Subjects. *Epilepsia*, 10, 415, 1969.

Lund, M. Epilepsy in Association with Intracranial Tumor. *Acta Psychiat.*, 81, 149, 1952.

Mark, V. H., Erwin, F. R., Sweet, W. H., and Delgado, J. Remote Telemeter Stimulation and Recording from Implanted Temporal Lobe Electrodes. *Confin. Neurol.*, 31, 86, 1969.

Marshall, C. and Walker, A. E. The Value of Electroencephalography in the Prognostication and Prognosis of Post-Traumatic Epilepsy. *Epilepsia*, 2, 138, 1961.

Masquin, A. and Courjon, J. Prognostic Factors in Post-Traumatic Epilepsy. *Epilepsia*, 4, 285, 1963.

McRae, D. Focal Epilepsy. Correlation of the Pathological and Radiological Findings. *Radiology, 50,* 439, 1948.

McRae, D. and Castorina, G. Radiological Findings in Temporal Lobe Eilepsy of Non-tumoral Origin. *Acta Radiol., 1,* 541, 1963.

Merlis, J. K. Proposal for an International Classification of the Epilepsies. *Epilepsia, 11,* 114, 1970.

Metrakos, K. and Metrakos, J. D. Genetics of Convulsive Disorders. II. Genetic and Electroencephalographic Studies in Centrencephalic Epilepsy. *Neurology, 11,* 474, 1961.

Metrakos, K. and Metrakos, J. D. Genetic Factors in Epilepsy. *Modern Problems in Pharmacopsychiatry,* Vol. 4, Epilepsy, (E. Niedermeyer, Ed.), Basel and New York: S. Karger, 1970.

Milner, B. Intellectual Functions of the Temporal Lobes. *Psychol. Bull., 51,* 42, 1954.

Milner, B. Psychological Defects Produced by Temporal Lobe Excision. *Res. Publ. Ass. Res. Nerv. Ment. Dis., 36,* 244, 1958.

Milner, B., Branch, C., and Rasmussen, T. Study of Short-Term Memory After Intracarotid Injection of Sodium Amytal. *Trans. Amer. Neurol. Ass., 87,* 224, 1962.

Milner, B. Some Effects of Frontal Lobectomy in Man. In J. M. Warren and K. Akert (Eds.) *The Frontal Granular Cortex and Behaviour.* New York: McGraw-Hill, 1964.

Milner, B. Visually-Guided Maze Learning in Man: Effects of Bilateral Hippocampal, Bilateral Frontal and Unilateral Cerebral Lesions. *Neuropsychologia, 3,* 317, 1965.

Milner, B. Visual Recognition and Recall after Right Temporal Lobe Excision in Man. *Neuropsychologia, 6,* 191, 1968.

Murphy, J. T. and Schwab, R. S. Diphenylhydantoin (Dilantin) Sodium Used Parenterally in Control of Convulsions. *J.A.M.A., 160,* 385, 1956.

Paillas, J. E. Post-Traumatic Epilepsy. *Marseille Med., 106,* 999, 1969.

Paillas, J. E., Paillas, N. and Bureau, M. Post-Traumatic Epilepsy. *Epilepsia, 11,* 5, 1970.

Pampiglione, G. and Kerridge, J. EEG Abnormalities from the Temporal Lobe Studied with Sphenoidal Electrodes. *J. Neurol. Neurosurg. Psychiatry, 19,* 117, 1956.

Payan, H., Toga, M. and Bérard-Badier, M. The Pathology of Post-Traumatic Epilepsies. *Epilepsia, 11,* 81, 1970.

Penfield, W. and Humphreys, S. Epileptogenic Lesions of the Brain. A Histologic Study. *Arch. Neurol. Psychiat., 43,* 240, 1940.

Penfield, W. and Shaver, M. The Incidence of Traumatic Epilepsy and Headache after Head Injury in Civil Practice. *Res. Publ. Ass. Nerv. Ment. Dis., 24,* 620, 1945.

Penfield, W. and Rasmussen, T. *The Cerebral Cortex of Man.* New York: Macmillan, 1950.

Penfield, W. and Kristiansen, K. *Epileptic Seizure Patterns.* Springfield, Ill.: Charles C Thomas, 1951.

Penfield, W. and Jasper, H. *Epilepsy and the Functional Anatomy of the Human Brain.* Boston: Little, Brown & Company, 1954.

567

Penfield, W. and Paine, K. Results of Surgical Treatment of Epileptic Seizures. *Can. Med. Ass. J.*, *73*, 515, 1955.

Penfield, W. and Milner, B. Memory Deficit Produced by Bilateral Lesions in the Hippocampal Zone. *Arch. Neurol. & Psychiatry*, *79*, 475, 1958.

Penry, J. K. and Dreifuss, F. E. Automatisms Associated with the Absence of Petit Mal Epilepsy. *Arch. Neurol.*, *21*, 142, 1969.

Perot, P., Weir, B, and Rasmussen, T. Tuberous Sclerosis: Surgical Therapy for Seizures. *Arch. Neurol.*, *15*, 498, 1966.

Phillips, G. Traumatic Epilepsy after Closed Head Injury. *J. Neurol. Neurosurg. Psychiatry*, *17*, 1, 1954.

Rasmussen, T. and MacNaughton, F. L. Epilepsy. Long-Term Illness. In *Management of the Chronically Ill Patient*. Philadelphia: W. B. Saunders, 1959.

Rasmussen, T. and Blundell, J. Epilepsy and Brain Tumor. Chap. 10 in *Clinical Neurosurgery*. Baltimore: Williams and Wilkins, 1961.

Rasmussen, T. and Branch C. Temporal Lobe Epilepsy: Indications for and Results of Surgical Therapy. *Postgrad. Med. J.*, *31*, 9, 1962.

Rasmussen, T. and Gossman, H. Epilepsy Due to Gross Destructive Brain Lesions. *Neurology*, *13*, 659, 1963.

Rasmussen, T. Surgical Therapy of Frontal Lobe Epilepsy. *Epilepsia*, *4*, 181, 1963.

Rasmussen, T. The Role of Surgery in the Treatment of Focal Epilepsy. Chap. 15 in *Clinical Neurosurg.*, Vol. 16, 1969(a).

Rasmussen, T. Surgical Therapy of Post-Traumatic Epilepsy. Chap. 26 in *The Late Effects of Head Injury*. Springfield, Ill.: Charles C Thomas, 1969(b).

Rawling, L. B. The Remote Effects of Gunshot Wounds of the Head. *Brit. J. Surg.*, *10*, 93, 1922-23.

Rio-Hortega, P. Del and Penfield, W. Cerebral Cicatrix. *Bull. Johns Hopkins Hosp.*, *14*, 278, 1927.

Rovit, R., Gloor, P. and Rasmussen, T. Sphenoidal Electrodes in the Electroencephalographic Study of Patients with Temporal Lobe Epilepsy. *J. Neurosurg.*, *18*, 151, 1961.

Rovit, R., Gloor, P. and Rasmussen, T. Intracarotid Amytal in Epileptic Patients. *Arch. Neurol*, *5*, 606, 1961.

Russell, W. R. and Whitty, C. M. M. Studies in Traumatic Epilepsy; Factors Influencing the Incidence of Epilepsy after Brain Wounds. *J. Neurol. Neurosurg. Psychiatry*, *15*, 93, 1952.

Russell, W. R. and Whitty, C. M. M. Studies in Traumatic Epilepsy; Focal Motor and Somatic Sensory Fits: Study of 85 Cases. *J. Neurol. Neurosurg. Psychiatry*, *16*, 73, 1953.

Russell, W. R. The Development of Grand Mal After Missile Wounds of the Brain. *Johns Hopkins Med. J.*, *122*, 250, 1968.

Schechter, M. M. and Zingesser, L. H. Neuroradiologic Aspects of the Post-Traumatic Syndrome and of Post-Traumatic Epilepsy. Chap. 24 in *The Late Effects of Head Injury*. Springfield, Ill.: Charles C Thomas, 1969.

Sorel, L. The Descendents of Epileptic Patients. *Epilepsia*, *10*, 91, 1969.

Symonds, C. P. Traumatic Epilepsy. *Lancet*, *2*, 1217, 1935.

Turner, W. A. Epilepsy and Gunshot Wounds of the Head. *J. Neur. Psychopath.*, *3*, 309, 1923.

Wada, J. A New Method for the Determination of the Side of Cerebral Speech Dominance - A Preliminary Report on the Intracarotid Injection of Sodium Amytal in Man. *Med. Biol. Tokyo, 14,* 221, 1949.

Wada, J. and Rasmussen, T. Intracarotid Injection of Sodium Amytal for the Lateralization of Cerebral Speech Dominance: Experimental and Clinical Observations. *J. Neurosurg., 17,* 266, 1960.

Wagstaffe, W. The Incidence of Traumatic Epilepsy after Gunshot Wounds of the Head. *Lancet, 2,* 861, 1928.

Walker, A. E., Marshall, C., and Beresford, E. N. Electrocorticographic Characteristics of the Cerebrum in Post-Traumatic Epilepsy. *Res. Publ. Ass. Nerv. Ment. Dis., 26,* 502, 1947.

Walker, A. E. *Post-Traumatic Epilepsy.* Springfield, Ill.: Charles C Thomas, 1949.

Walker, A. E. Prognosis in Post-Traumatic Epilepsy: A Ten-Year Follow Up of Craniocerebral Injuries of World War II. *J.A.M.A., 164,* 1636, 1957.

Walker, A. E. and Jablon, S. A Follow-Up of Head Injured Men of World War II. *J. Neurosurg., 16,* 600, 1959.

Walker, A. E. Post-Traumatic Epilepsy. *Proc. Austr. Assn. Neurol., 4,* 1, 1966.

Walker, A. E. Pathogenesis and Pathophysiology of Post-Traumatic Epilepsy. Chap. 27 in *The Late Effects of Head Injury.* Springfield, Ill.: Charles C Thomas, 1969.

Walker, A. E. and Erculei, F. Post-Traumatic Epilepsy 15 Years Later. *Epilepsia, 11,* 17, 1970.

Watson, C. W. The Incidence of Epilepsy Following Craniocerebral Injury. *Res. Publ. Ass. Nerv. Ment. Dis., 26,* 516, 1947.

Wertheimer, P. L'Epilepsie Traumatique. Réflexions à Propos De 108 Observations. *Lyons Chir., 52,* 130, 1956.

Whitty, C. M. M. Early Traumatic Epilepsy *Brain, 70,* 416, 1947.

Whitty, C. M. M. and Taylor, M. Treatment of Status Epilepticus. *Lancet, 2,* 591, 1949.

Wilson, D. M. Head Injuries in Service Men of the 1939-45 War. *N. Z. Med. J., 50,* 383, 1951.

CHAPTER 18

PSYCHIATRIC STATES FOLLOWING HEAD INJURY IN ADULTS AND CHILDREN

KARL MURDOCK BOWMAN, M. D.,
ABRAM BLAU, M. D. AND ROBERT REICH, M. D.

INTRODUCTION

The relation of head injury to psychiatric illness is often controversial. While in many cases it is obvious that a particular mental disorder is the result of a head injury, in other cases the causal relationship is less clear and divergent opinions may be held by physicians equally experienced and competent in this field. The lay public tends to overemphasize head injuries as a cause of mental illness. It does so because a head injury appears to provide a simple and intelligible explanation for an otherwise mysterious disorder, and also because it is sometimes felt that it removes the stigma attached to having mental disease in one's family. The common tendency to resort to the "post hoc ergo propter hoc" type of reasoning is misleading. If one event follows another, it is often assumed that the first event was causally related to the second. Obviously, this is not invariably true and one must guard against such erroneous conclusions.

With the increase in number of accidents and with the introduction of industrial compensation, this whole subject has become one of great practical importance. A medical expert is frequently called upon to render an opinion concerning the role of head injury in the etiology of various diseases including certain mental disorders. Large sums of money are often involved. It therefore is important to consider the relationship of head trauma to the development of mental disorders. An accurate diagnosis in such cases depends upon a careful history and detailed neurologic and psychiatric examinations. Knowledge of the premorbid mental status of the patient is important in determining the exact effect of a particular trauma. Unfortunately, this is often lacking and must be estimated from the accounts of the

570

family and associates and from the employment history. One must keep in mind the possibility of deliberate misstatements or denial of a preexisting derangement in order to improve the chances of compensation. If new employees were subject to careful medical examination including a neurologic and psychiatric survey and if all employees in industry were routinely checked periodically, it would be possible to evaluate the facts in cases of injury with greater certainty and to render more accurate opinions. From the standpoint of both employer and employee, this would result in a more equitable award for compensation injuries.

Mixed clinical pictures are extremely common. Frequently psychogenic symptoms are superimposed on a truly organic syndrome. The mere presence of psychogenic symptoms does not necessarily disprove the organic basis of the condition. Every individual reacts in a different fashion to organic disease; some people always tend to exaggerate while others tend to minimize their complaints. The question of simulation or conscious malingering must also be taken into account and here again it is well to point out that it is perfectly possible for an individual to exaggerate consciously a condition which is truly organic.

On the other hand, one occasionally sees cases in which the clinical picture is colored by obvious malingering or simulation. This subject is discussed in detail in Chapter 20, and will be dealt with only briefly here. Considerable controversy exists among psychiatrists with regard to posttraumatic malingering. Inexperienced physicians tend to make this diagnosis all too readily. It is probable that truly uncomplicated malingering is rare, and that when it occurs, it is in itself a pathological symptom, usually of an underlying sociopathic personality. Wechsler's comprehensive definition states that "the individual becomes a malingerer only when he consciously and purposely, in order to deceive, to evade responsibility, or to derive gain, feigns illness and voluntarily tries to reproduce signs and symptoms which he really does not have, or extravagantly exaggerates minor ones which he has." In accordance with this definition, one must differentiate malingering from the unconscious mechanisms of the neuroses and the mild or even severe exaggeration of symptoms which often occurs in some truly sick persons.

True malingering is often easy to recognize. To the experienced observer, there are obvious inconsistencies in behavior and contradictions among symptom complexes. In some cases, however, prolonged observation may be necessary and differential diagnosis may be extremely difficult. It requires extraordinary histrionic ability and presence of mind to malinger consistently over any length of time and almost invariably the patient overreaches himself in his efforts to convince the physician.

GENERAL CONSIDERATIONS

Historical Background

The older writers were greatly interested in the influence of head trauma in the production of mental and neurologic disease and made many significant observations. Modern psychiatric literature on the subject had its inception over a hundred years ago in the writings of Esquirol (1837) in France and Prichard (1837), in the United States. Many comprehensive monographs have since appeared. Experience gained from gunshot and other head injuries in both World Wars contributed a great deal to our knowledge and the more recent growth of industrial compensation legislation has led to many important studies.

The literature dealing with the effects of head trauma is extensive. Among the more significant contributions are those of Ajuriaguerra and Hécaen (1960), Denny-Brown (1942, 1945), Faust (1955, 1960), Goldstein (1919, 1942, 1952), Heygster (1949), Hillbom (1949, 1960), Hohiesel and Walch (1952), Kleist (1934), Kretschmer (1949, 1956), Lindenberg (1951), Lishman (1968), London (1967), Mutschler (1956), Puech and Mallett (1946), Russell (1932, 1951, 1959, 1971), Russell and Espir (1961), Schilder (1934), Symonds (1937, 1937, 1962), Teuber (1959, 1962), Walch (1956), Walker and Erculei (1969), and Walker and Jablon (1961).

Frequency

In recent years the number of cases of severe head injuries has increased markedly due to the increased number of automobile accidents. In 1967 in the United States there were three-quarters of a million patients with head injuries, of whom 18,000 died and 13,000 suffered a permanent disability. Critchley, in "The Late Effects of Head Injury" (1969), remarks that "the introduction of forensic considerations adds to the complexity and maintenance of the disability." With the courts granting ever increasing amounts of money for the very severe

572

emotional sequelae of car accidents, amounts often larger than the individual could earn in his lifetime, there is a great temptation for such disability to persist at least until the case comes to court.

Because of variations in terminology, diagnostic criteria, and type of case material, it is difficult to compare the findings and conclusions reported by different authors. The connotation of the word "psychosis" as used by different observers is not uniform. Some authors use this designation for even a mild transient organic state, others only for a very severe organic mental syndrome, while still others reserve the word for a schizophrenic-like picture.

A report by Ota (1969) surveys 1168 cases of closed head injuries seen by the author between 1956 and 1961. In this series the incidence of epilepsy was 3.3 percent, a figure much lower than after wartime open head injury (44.2 percent according to Hillbom, 1960). Disorders due to such localized cerebral lesions as apraxia and agnosia were found in only 1.3 percent of cases. General impairment of intellectual function occurred in 1.9 percent, character changes in 5.8 percent, and neurotic symptoms were present in 21.8 percent of cases. The data suggested that there was little, if any, relationship between head trauma and the endogenous psychoses.

Achté, Hillbom, and Aalberg (1967) reviewed 3,552 cases of severe wartime head injury. A "psychosis" developed in 346 cases some time subsequent to injury. Psychiatric symptoms not sufficiently severe to be classified as psychotic were observed in an additional 503 patients. A conspicuous change of character occurred in still another 440 cases. Thus a total of 37 percent showed "fairly severe mental disturbances." While it might be a contributory factor, trauma did not appear to be causally related to the occurrence of an endogenous psychosis.

Mental disability, mostly involving intellect or mood, occurred in 51 of 230 survivors of severe head injury studied by London (1967).

Lishman (1968) reported the psychiatric sequelae observed in a series of 670 patients with dural penetrating injuries followed 5 years or longer. The degree of psychiatric disability was considered mild in 433 cases and severe in 144. Severe psychiatric disability was characterized by persistent symptoms — usually in several areas of mental function; however, in 17 it was restricted to impairment of intellect, and in 12 to affective disorders. Only 5 patients developed unequivocal psychoses.

Available statistics generally refer to patients with severe head injuries treated in hospitals. However, very many head-injured patients with mild psychiatric sequelae are treated on an ambulatory basis and these cases are usually not reported.

Age

Age is probably an important predisposing factor in the development of posttraumatic mental sequelae. The effects of cerebral trauma have been generally recognized to be more severe with advancing age. The presence of arteriosclerosis in older persons would seem to predispose to more serious damage. It is perhaps worthwhile to point out that exactly the opposite holds with regard to epidemic encephalitis, since in these cases personality changes occur more frequently in children than in adults. In most studies of head injury the more serious after-effects with deterioration are seen in the older age groups. This contrasts with the age incidence of head injury in general which reaches its maximum between the ages of 20 and 30 years (Russell, 1932).

Pathogenesis

Mental sequelae may develop after slight or severe degrees of head injury. A skull fracture is not always present even in the most severe cases. A traumatic mental disorder may also occur when the major lesion is essentially extracerebral as in subdural or epidural hemorrhage. The development of organic mental symptoms following brain injury is attributable partly to local, but in all probability mostly to general, cerebral damage. Local injury is of relatively negligible significance in comparison with the widespread diffuse effects, generally referred to as commotio cerebri or cerebral concussion. Still it may be difficult to determine the effects of diffuse brain damage over and above a focal cerebral lesion. Strauss and Savitsky (1934) reviewed the various opinions regarding the intracranial changes that occur in concussion and presented an extensive list, including compression of the cerebral cortex, cerebral anemia, "shaking up" of the cerebral centers, mass movements of the brain and spinal fluid, disturbances of the intracellular equilibrium, molecular disorganization of the ganglion cells, vasomotor changes, and many others. As indicated in Chapter 4 there is reason to believe that concussion is the result of generalized neuronal injury. Such injury to nerve cells and fibers is of varying severity and is not invariably reversible. The occurrence of permanent sequelae would appear to depend on the severity of the injury and the extent of irreversible damage to neurons (Symonds, 1962).

Experimental and pathological studies (Webster and Gurdjian, 1943; Loken, 1959) show that diffuse effects following penetrating injuries may be considerable, but these are almost certainly less than in the case of closed head injuries. Concussion occurs much less often after penetrating wounds than after closed head injuries (Denny-Brown, 1945).

Bloomquist and Courville (1947), in a study of the lesions found post mortem in 350 cases of cerebral trauma, observed that when the head had been in motion at the time of injury (e.g., falls, traffic accidents) there was much contrecoup effect; 18 patients in whom the head was stationary at the time of injury (e.g., assault, blows, bullet wounds) showed chiefly a local lesion at the site of impact.

In his analysis of penetrating injuries Lishman (1968) stressed that the *quantity* of brain tissue destroyed and the depth of brain damage appeared to be related to the extent of psychiatric disability defined in terms of intellectual, emotional, and behavioral disturbance.

Cerebral Localization

The idea of the brain as an organ functioning as a whole is generally accepted. The concept of "centers" has undergone change and the tendency now is to less rigidly restrict a given function to a particular area. Nevertheless, there is evidence that injuries to certain areas of the brain are more likely to result in various forms of psychiatric disability. Many neurologists consider that the prefrontal area of the brain possesses a special influence over behavior and intelligence. Bianchi (1922) reviewed work on this subject and found that removal of the frontal lobes in monkeys is followed by a considerable falling off in spontaneity and general organization of behavior. In man, it has been customary to suppose that frontal lesions tend especially to be associated with deterioration of the personality which shows itself in loss of finer feelings, childishness, and intellectual and emotional decay. The famous "crowbar case" is usually quoted. In 1848, a man had an iron bar driven through the frontal region of his skull, and lived for 12 years afterwards. Autopsy showed that only the prefrontal lobe was involved. He had been a most efficient workman, but after the accident his disposition was so changed that he could not hold his former position. In a series of 200 gunshot wounds of the head, Frazier and Ingham (1920) found that four patients had suffered serious mental deterioration — both frontal lobes were involved in three and the right frontal and left parietal lobes in the other. Feuchtwanger (1923) concluded from extensive study of cases of injury of the frontal lobe that emotional and temperamental changes occur but that intelligence is affected only insofar as it seems to be conditioned by emotional factors. Duret's treatise (1919) on cranial injury noted the remarkable incidence of changes in character, together with impulsiveness and irritability, in cases of trauma of the frontal region. Some observers in the past have emphasized the importance of mental symptoms in cases of tumor of the frontal lobe, but such symptoms by themselves have little localizing value. The most significant observations in humans relative to injuries of the frontal lobes were made in patients who had undergone lobectomy. The sequelae of frontal lobectomy in man (Brickner, 1936; German and Fox, 1932; and Spurling, 1934) consist of changes in personality and disturbances of behavior, comparable in many respects to those observed experimentally in animals.

Kleist (1934), drew a distinction between the effect of wounds of the lateral convexity and those of the orbital aspect of the frontal lobe. The former produced mainly psychomotor and intellectual abnormalities, the latter mostly changes in the emotional sphere.

Heygster (1949) stressed the special psychiatric difficulties of patients with bifrontal wounds. Lindenberg (1951) reported that frontal injuries were particularly likely to produce changes of character. Mutschler (1956) contrasted the frequency of criminal behavior with the rarity of occurrence of the neuroses after frontal injuries and suggested that in some way frontal injury interfered with the development of a neurotic pattern.

Walch (1956), in a study of 340 cases of frontal brain injuries, confirmed Kleist's observations concerning the difference in the effects of orbital and convexity lesions. In the case of convexity lesions the picture was mainly one of lack of drive or loss of inhibition. In many cases there were no psychic changes whatever. Few among the patients with orbital lesions were without striking psychological symptoms, and a very high proportion showed changes in "the more highly developed qualities of personality."

Faust (1955, 1960), in a study of 80 frontal wounds and an extensive review of the literature, arrived at conclusions very similar to those of Kleist. In cases of convexity lesions he stressed the lack of productive thinking, indifference, euphoria, and incapacity for decisions. Patients with orbital lesions, while failing to show defects on formal intelligence tests, exhibited radical personality changes. They failed to maintain satisfactory human relationships, lacked perseverance, were demanding, uninhibited, interfering, and aggressive. Their sexual life was often marked by increased libido, coupled with disregard for their partner. Criminal behavior was especially marked in the orbital group and often took the form of sexual offense.

Injury to the basal parts of the brain has also attracted special attention. Kretschmer (1949, 1956) described a "basal syndrome" which has found wide support in the German literature. This syndrome results from lesions of the midbrain, hypothalamus, and orbital frontal cortex. Along with marked sluggishness and apathy there is a disturbance of fundamental drives and instincts — appetite, thirst, sleep — and varied sexual abnormalities. Fluctuations of mood and aggressive outbursts are seen along with specific vegetative and endocrine abnormalities. Hohiesel and Walch (1952) have described five patients with marked fluctuations of mood persisting for a long time after head injury. One such case had a shell splinter in the hypothalamus, and the other four showed clinical signs which indicated diencephalic injury.

For a more detailed account of the functions of the frontal lobe and of the symptomatology of frontal lobe lesions, the publication of the Association for Research in Nervous and Mental Disease (1948) and the writings of Denny-Brown (1951) and of Luria (1969) are recommended. Luria suggests that the frontal lobes may play a "decisive role in the regulation of human activity." For example, in cases in which frontal lobe function is severely affected, patients lie in bed, indifferent and disinterested in themselves and their environment. Additional components of the frontal lobe syndrome are listed by Luria as follows: disturbed regulation of voluntary actions in that "movements cease to be controlled by the program assigned and fall under the influence of irrelevant factors"; defective perception, described as being "fragmentary and impulsive"; memory disturbances evident during "active learning by heart and selective reproduction of material"; impairment of constructive intellectual activity involving analysis of a problem and formulation of a program; and emotional and personality changes.

Little has been written of distinctive psychiatric pictures after injury to other parts of the brain. Teuber et al (1959, 1962) have extensively investigated the defects resulting from regional brain damage in a large series of penetrating injuries. Patients with left parietotemporal lesions showed significant impairment of general intelligence. No such defects

577

were found after lesions elsewhere. The differences persisted after excluding patients with dysphasia. Those with left parietotemporal lesions showed maximal impairment on a nonverbal task (a visual conditioning reaction). The evidence, therefore, suggests that lesions of this region of the brain especially may be associated with intellectual deficits that are, to a considerable extent, independent of language loss.

Ajuriaguerra and Hécaen (1960) mention the frequency of personality difficulties and atypical psychoses after temporal lobe injury. Hillbom (1949, 1960) is in agreement, especially with regard to the occurrence of "schizophreniform" psychoses.

In 1960 Hillbom surveyed a large number of wartime head injuries, of which 415 (188 with penetrating injuries) were randomly selected for special study. In cases of unilateral wounds those with left-sided lesions exhibited more psychiatric disturbances than those in whom the right half of the brain was involved, particularly with regard to the occurrence of dementia and psychosis. Bilateral and midline wounds in particular were apt to produce dementia, and psychiatric disturbances were especially frequent in frontal injuries. By contrast, patients with parietal, occipital, or cerebellar lesions were relatively free of gross psychiatric disorders.

With regard to the specific symptomatology and derangement of function resulting from lesions in locations other than the frontal region, the temporal lobes are of considerable interest in connection with disturbances of feeling and behavior. Patients with temporal lobe epilepsy experience intense emotions including anxiety and fear, complex sensations involving vision, sound, taste, and smell, disorders of spatial and temporal perception, depersonalization, and disturbances of memory, consciousness, and behavior (Williams, 1968). Profound loss of memory for recent events follows bilateral hippocampal lesions (Scoville and Milner, 1957). The temporal neocortex is intimately related to the rhinencephalon and limbic lobe, structures concerned with visceral, instinctual and emotional activity. The relation of the limbic system to emotions was first suggested by Papez (1937). A permanent dampening of drive and affectivity results from bilateral lesions of the limbic system (Poeck, 1969). Pathologic rage has been observed in patients with lesions of the septal region, hypothalamus and medial temporal lobe. It would appear that the neocortex controls the activity of the limbic system and that loss of cortical control may lead to violent behavior (Mark and Ervin, 1970). Anxiety and fear are experienced after stimulation of parts of the limbic system. The Klüver-

Bucy syndrome manifested by oral tendencies, placidity, abnormal sexual behavior, and severe memory impairment results from bilateral lesions of the medial temporal lobes. There is evidence to indicate that the left temporal lobe "contributes to the rapid understanding and subsequent retention of verbally expressed ideas," whereas the right temporal lobe "facilitates rapid visual identification" (Milner, 1958).

Aside from language disturbances and disorders of tactile function and vision, parietal lobe lesions give rise to various apraxias, the Gerstmann syndrome, and abnormalities referable to body image and spatial perception (Critchley, 1953). Patients are often unaware of their disabilities and indifferent to their deficits.

Lesions of the occipital lobe result primarily in disturbances of visual perception though elements of parietal lobe dysfunction may also be evident.

The above data would make it appear that psychiatric disability after head injury may, in fact, vary according to the location of the brain damage and that lesions in some areas pose a greater psychiatric hazard than others.

Symptomatology

There are no symptoms that are specific for the primary traumatic mental disorders. The picture is the same as that observed in the whole group of psychoses associated with organic lesions, and to which the term *organic mental syndrome* is applied. The mental picture in such cases is characterized by confusion, disorientation, poor attention span, and defective memory; elements of aphasia and apraxia may also be evident. The differential diagnosis at times is extremely difficult, particularly when the history is inadequate and/or there are multiple etiologic factors. The most frequent combination is that of alcoholism with head trauma. It may also be very difficult to determine the effect of head injury in a person already suffering from an organic brain disease. At times it is difficult to distinguish between a psychoneurosis and a truly organic mental syndrome. In general, the functional psychoses present less of a problem in differential diagnosis, the clinical picture usually being sufficiently distinctive.

CLASSIFICATION

The different mental syndromes that may occur in association with head injury are listed in the table. They may be divided into two main categories: A) primary traumatic disorders in which there is a fairly clear relationship between trauma and the resulting mental symptoms, and B) secondary traumatic disorders in which the part the brain injury played in their etiology is less clear. The primary disorders may be further classified, on the basis of symptomatology, as acute, subacute, and chronic. What is considered an acute condition may, at a later time, be listed as subacute or chronic. The chronic states may be thought of roughly as comprising two categories: 1) posttraumatic personality disorders, and 2) posttraumatic defect conditions. In the traumatic personality disorders, the qualities of the personality which are mainly affected are those not thought of as purely intellectual; whereas in the

Classification of Mental Sequelae of Trauma

A. *Primary Traumatic Mental Disorders* (Mental disorders due to head trauma)

    I. *Acute and Subacute*
      Concussion syndrome
      Traumatic coma (and subsequent stupor)
      Traumatic delirium
      Confusion
      Automatism (including the Korsakoff or amnesic-confabulatory psychosis)
      Other types: stuporous, apathetic, twilight states
    II. *Chronic*
      Posttraumatic personality disorders
      a. Of adults
      b. Of children
      Posttraumatic defect conditions
      a. Focal
      b. Generalized
    III. Other types
      Traumatic encephalopathy of pugilists ("punch drunk")
      Traumatic convulsive disorders (traumatic epilepsy)

B. *Secondary Traumatic Mental Disorders* (Mental disorders associated with, or precipitated or complicated by, but not due primarily to head trauma)

    I. Psychoneurosis with head trauma
    II. Psychosis with head trauma (e.g., psychoses due to alcohol, psychoses with cerebral arteriosclerosis, endogenous psychoses, etc.)
    III. Mental deficiency with head trauma

defect conditions, the involvement is chiefly one of intellectual function. Since the effect of head trauma seems to be quite different in children than in adults, the traumatic personality disorders in this age group may be considered separately.

The traumatic psychoneuroses are included with the secondary traumatic mental disorders. This subject is discussed in another chapter, but perhaps it is important to point out here that differences of opinion exist regarding the validity of the term, traumatic psychoneurosis. If psychoneuroses are regarded as being of purely psychogenic origin then those that follow head injury are not different from those that follow trauma elsewhere, and the mechanism is the same as that of the psychoneuroses generally.

PRIMARY TRAUMATIC MENTAL DISORDERS (SYNONYMS: PSYCHOSES DUE TO TRAUMA, POSTTRAUMATIC PSYCHOSES)

Primary traumatic mental disorders are those which are exclusively the result of brain injury caused by direct or indirect physical force to the head. It is considered that the mental condition is specifically related to organic alterations within the brain induced directly by the head injury.

Acute and Subacute Primary Traumatic Mental Disorders

The acute and subacute reactions which follow head trauma include the following organic mental states: concussion; coma; delirium; stupor; confusion; automatism; apathetic, twilight or dream states; and the amnesic-confabulatory syndrome. In the more severely injured patients a more or less regular sequence of stages, manifested by coma, stupor, delirium, confusion, automatism, and finally recovery, may be observed. In mild cases consciousness may be briefly lost, or the patients appear dazed and subsequently have no recollection of events for a period of time (posttraumatic amnesia).

Occurrence

In all cases of head trauma other than very minor ones, acute mental symptoms occur to varying degrees, depending on the severity of the injury. Profound coma terminating in death, may occur following severe trauma; in severely injured though nonfatal cases, the period of unconsciousness may be of long duration. Patients with minor injuries may be merely stunned or dazed for a few minutes or seconds. Between these two extremes one may find a great variety of acute and subacute conditions, marked by stupor, delirium, and protracted confusion along with amnesia, paramnesia, and occasionally confabulation.

The outstanding feature of cerebral concussion has been generally assumed to be the reversibility of the process. As already indicated, however, there is reason to believe that diffuse neuronal injury is responsible for this condition and that the more severe the injury the more prolonged the duration of the state of unconsciousness. Symptoms of acute traumatic mental disorders appear also in cases that cannot be characterized solely as concussion, there being evidence of other types of cerebral pathology such as contusion, laceration, and hemorrhage. From a pathological standpoint, therefore, the acute traumatic mental disorders occur in association with heterogeneous lesions.

Symptomatology

The *concussion syndrome* as commonly understood, is one which follows mild head injuries and is characterized by momentary loss of consciousness. Delirium does not occur. Difficulties in perception and thinking may appear for a short time, and may be accompanied by mild confusion and disorientation. Many patients who suffer concussion show a peculiar lack of insight into their need for medical attention and make light of their illness. Emotional changes in the form of euphoria or irritability may accompany the other symptoms. The prognosis is usually favorable in these mild cases and they recover completely in a short time. Occasionally, however, chronic mental symptoms may be noted later.

The more severe acute and subacute posttraumatic mental disorders may persist for weeks or months. In such cases the sequence of events which marks the transition from coma to full consciousness and normal behavior follows a pattern that may be divided into stages: a) coma, b) stupor, c) excitement or delirium, d) confusion, e) automatism, and f) recovery. The different stages may vary in length, depending on the severity of the injury. Some may be of short duration or relatively inconspicuous. Usually there is a gradual transition from one stage to another, with fluctuations in some cases. Amnesia for events which occurred between the time of injury and full return of consciousness is a characteristic phenomenon (posttraumatic amnesia). The loss of memory also includes those events which occurred just prior to the injury (retrograde amnesia). During the period of recovery the Korsakoff syndrome may be in evidence.

The period of *coma* may be short or prolonged, depending on the severity of the injury. In mild cases the patient can get up after a few minutes and proceed unaided. The more severe degrees of trauma are associated with unconsciousness of prolonged duration lasting from hours to days and sometimes even for weeks. The stage of coma is followed by *stupor,* the depth of which gradually lessens until the patient is fully awake. In occasional instances the initial period of unconsciousness that follows injury is succeeded by a lucid interval of several hours or even days, after which stupor and coma again supervene. This sequence of events is characteristic of extracerebral hemorrhage. Recovery of consciousness ushers in the stage of *delirium* which is marked by acute excitement and confusion combined with restlessness and heightened motor activity. Patients jump out of bed, pull at their shirts, throw off the bed covers, tear at their bandages, wander aimlessly about the ward, fail to recognize people, and are unaware of their surroundings. Sometimes they believe that they are at home with friends, or in their places of work. Patients with war injuries may act as if they are on the battlefield, vividly describe dangerous or threatening situations, and exhibit considerable anxiety and excitement. In general, most patients display an affect of extreme anxiety, fear, or bewilderment. Hallucinations are common and these are mainly of a visual or tactile nature. The delirium may continue unabated for many days or even weeks with only short remissions. In some cases, the delirious behavior becomes aggravated at night and subsides during the day. The severity of the delirium may vary considerably with periods of relatively quiet behavior interrupting the marked psychomotor hyperactivity. In rare instances, the patient's state of activity may attain such a degree that he is continually restless and thrashing about.

Various other reaction types that have been described include: *twilight or dream states; negativistic states* (Schilder, 1934); *stuporous states* (Pfeifer, 1928); and the *apathetic syndrome* (Allers, 1916). The *twilight, fugue* or *dream* states resemble similar conditions that occur in epileptics. They are characterized by the performance of purposeful activities in a half-conscious dreamlike state very much like somnambulism. Some patients may appear entirely rational and behave appropriately and yet there is a complete amnesia for events during this period. Others act and talk in a senseless manner, and wander around aimlessly. States of extreme furor with violence have also been described.

Gene Tunney's subjective account of a twilight state is interesting: "One day while boxing with a sparring partner, Frank Muskie, we bumped heads.... I was terribly dazed. As I straightened up a long, hard right swing landed on my jaw. Without going down or staggering, I lost all consciousness of what I was doing and instinctively proceeded to knock Muskie out. Another sparring partner, Eddie Eagen, entered the ring; we boxed three rounds. I have no recollection of this, nor have I any recollection of anything that occurred until the next morning when I was awakened in my little cabin by the water's edge, wondering who I was and what I was doing there. . . . Gradually my name came to me.... I arose and asked guarded questions.... For three days I could not remember the names of my most intimate acquaintances.... On these occasions all seemed queer. I was unable to orient myself."

Pfeifer (1928) described a *stuporous* state which is in many ways the opposite of the delirious type. Patients in this condition show a lack of spontaneity accompanied by inhibition and slowing of motor and speech function. They lie quietly in bed, make few movements and do not respond to outside stimuli. Lassitude and marked lack of interest are characteristic features. In the severe cases of this type of reaction, a *catatonic stupor* may be mistakenly suspected. Schilder (1934) reported *negativistic resistance* in association with clouding of consciousness. A special type of disturbance which he called the *apathetic syndrome* was described by Allers (1916). The outstanding characteristic of this syndrome, which appears in the early weeks after injury, is a lack of interest. This is not associated with clouding of consciousness, disorientation, perceptual weakness, or intellectual defects. Patients express no wishes, offer no complaints, and react to all situations with the same lack of interest. The *Korsakoff syndrome* is characterized by disorientation for time and place, marked impairment of recent memory, confabulation, retrograde amnesia, and poor perception, the patient being conscious and remote memory good.

After consciousness is regained, there is a period of time for which the patient has no recollection. Symonds (Chapter 4) states: "As a permanent sequel of the injury there is loss of memory which is almost always complete for the events immediately preceding the accident and for the accident itself (*retrograde amnesia*) and for a variable period after the accident (*posttraumatic amnesia*). The duration of the retrograde amnesia after the patient has had full time to recover from

584

the injury is usually brief" (a few seconds). A longer retrograde amnesia is generally indicative of more severe brain trauma; it tends to diminish during recovery. The duration of the posttraumatic amnesia, as measured by the time required for the patient to recover continuous memory, varies from minutes to days, or even weeks. There may be no amnesia in cases of mild head injury and, not uncommonly, in gunshot wounds. On the other hand, in some cases amnesia may be the only posttraumatic symptom. During an athletic contest, for instance, a player who has sustained a head injury may continue playing after a few moments and subsequently be found to have no recollection of what happened in the interim. The amnesia may partially account for the remarkably little concern which these patients frequently show in regard to their head injuries. For a comprehensive discussion of amnesia, the reader is referred to the monographs of Whitty and Zangwill (1966) and of Russell (1971).

During the stage of *confusion* which follows the delirious phase, the patient is no longer agitated, but relatively quiet and amenable. Nevertheless, his thinking remains incoherent and confused. Further improvement marks the stage of *automatism*. The patient is now aware of his environment and capable of some purposeful activity, although judgment, insight, and memory remain grossly defective. Impulsive behavior commonly occurs owing to lack of inhibition.

Difficulties in perception and in the synthesis of perception are found to varying degrees during the stages of confusion and automatism and in patients exhibiting the Korsakoff syndrome. The most obvious defects are found in vision and hearing, although they can be demonstrated in the tactile, olfactory, and gustatory fields when these are examined carefully. The derangement in perception is particularly striking in view of the otherwise seemingly natural behavior of many of these patients (automatism, Korsakoff state). Their conduct is usually orderly, they seem to be well aware of their surroundings and their ability to grasp questions directed to them is not obviously impaired. Yet immediately after a meal they do not know what they have eaten. They are unable to recall the names of physicians and attendants whom they see daily. On formal tests, they forget — within a few seconds or minutes — objects shown to them, or a number they have been asked to remember. They cannot perform simple tasks in the usual intelligence tests even though these are well within their normal intellectual abilities.

Disorientation for place and time persists until the final stage of

585

recovery when the ability to remember is restored. Until such time patients do not know where they are, they cannot find their places on the ward and walk past their beds. They have no idea how long they have been in the hospital and do not know the date, including even the year.

The tendency to *confabulation* is a specific characteristic of the Korsakoff complex which is related to the disturbances in perception, orientation, and recent memory. If the patient is asked where he is, what the date is, what he did that morning or the day before, he will rarely answer that he does not know or cannot remember. He will fill in the gaps in orientation and memory with falsehoods which generally fall within the realm of possibility. He will not have the slightest doubt about their reality no matter how absurd they may be in the light of the known facts. The confabulations are not consistent and contradictions may be easily suggested.

Contrary to the statements of some writers that the Korsakoff state is a constant feature of the later stage of every prolonged traumatic psychosis (Pfeifer, 1928; Schilder, 1934), not all patients with gross memory defects confabulate (Symonds, 1937). In fact, Whitty and Zangwill (1966) state that "a florid confabulatory syndrome, as opposed to the brief and isolated paramnesias, is rare in traumatic amnesia. Of 1931 cases of closed head injury observed at a special centre during World War II, only 38 cases were recorded. Of these only six showed confabulation persisting for more than two or three days. However, all did offer some pseudo-reminiscence either spontaneously or in reply to questions, for a period for which they were, on objective evidence, quite amnesic; and this occurred at a time when there was no evidence from their general behavior of any drowsiness or confusion."

The *emotional reactions* in the acute traumatic mental disorders show considerable variation. Changes of mood may occur during the course of a particular patient's illness. In the earlier periods when there is clouding of consciousness, patients appear dazed and show an apathetic demeanor which should not be interpreted as depression. In the delirious states, there is bewilderment, anxiety, and apprehensiveness. The Korsakoff cases may exhibit a euphoric, cheerful mood with a tendency to facetiousness, singing, and groundless laughter. In many of these cases such behavior may be misinterpreted as manic. Not infrequently, patients manifest irritability, especially when they are disturbed, examined, or questioned. They then become annoyed, sullen, angry, and complain a great deal. In general, they lack insight into their condition, demand discharge and threaten legal measures against the physician or hospital on account of their confinement. In the later stages when improvement occurs and they regain insight, some patients develop a reactive depression due to a realization of the financial and personal problems created by the traumatic situation.

Several other aspects of the symptomatology of acute traumatic mental disorders deserve brief comment. The mistaken impression of mental retardation may be suggested during the transitional phase of clouded consciousness, and also during the Korsakoff stage when there is difficulty in perception and association, and general ineffectiveness. Furthermore, aphasic and other types of focal deficits may lead to mistakes in diagnosis. Illusions may be experienced during the stage of delirium or occasionally thereafter at night. Hallucinations do not occur in the Korsakoff state, and the confabulations must not be misinterpreted as such; the confabulations have an entirely different mechanism; they are often produced in response to suggestive questions, are inconsistent, and are commonly forgotten. Although delusions are not part of this clinical picture, the patients may become suspicious of mistreatment and persecution because of their basic lack of insight. In the euphoric moods, delusions of grandeur and expansive ideas may be expressed to substantiate the affect.

The acute traumatic mental disorders of children have some special characteristics. Blau (1936) reported a group of these cases. After regaining consciousness the children exhibited marked impulsiveness and restlessness. They were noisy, cried and screamed continually, and made constant demands on the nursing staff.

Superficially, these children resemble severe behavior problems, and one's first impression may be that they are merely reacting as poorly trained children. This view is reinforced by their clear consciousness and good contact. However, closer study shows that their behavior is impulsive and beyond their control. The emotional accompaniments are mainly irritability, fear and anxiety. They lack the ability to exercise self-restraint and inhibition, and continually manifest infantile behavior to attract attention. Children do not generally experience hallucinations, nor do they confabulate. Retrograde amnesia occurs but otherwise their memory is quite good. The children are able to recognize parents, physicians and attendants, and readily recall facts regarding their personal history. A complete lack of insight, similar to what is seen in adults, may cause them to attempt to induce their parents to take them home from the hospital.

587

Prognosis

The duration of the acute and subacute traumatic mental disorders varies considerably, as has been stated previously, from a few days to weeks or months, depending on the severity of the lesion. The prognosis in general is favorable with a tendency towards complete recovery. Following recovery from the acute traumatic psychosis, patients who have been severely injured may exhibit residual defects referable to memory, judgment, and behavior which usually improve slowly but in some cases persist indefinitely. As a rule, the shorter the initial disturbance of consciousness, the better the prognosis. The association of alcoholism or arteriosclerosis aggravates the course and makes the prognosis graver. In children complete recovery is more frequent, and younger adults generally do better than older individuals. As a rule, an unfavorable outcome is attributable to severe trauma, to complications resulting therefrom, or to associated systemic conditions.

Treatment

During the immediate posttraumatic period treatment is primarily concerned with the care of wounds and conditions of a surgical nature. Expert nursing care, desirable at all times, is especially important as long as the patient remains comatose. Nutrition and fluid balance must be maintained and appropriate measures taken to avoid decubiti, pneumonia, and other complications. Later, as the coma recedes and delirium develops, it may be expedient to transfer the patient to a separate room or special psychiatric ward. The aim of therapy at this point is to quiet the patient and to protect him from further injury and from complications until the period of excitement has run its course. Careful temporary mechanical restraint with proper attention to padding of vulnerable parts may be necessary.

In some cases the delirium may be the result of metabolic changes associated with restriction of fluids and salt in an attempt to prevent cerebral edema. As indicated in Chapter 6, various derangements of water and electrolyte balance (including cerebral salt retention believed to be caused by dehydration and cerebral salt wasting due to an inappropriate secretion of antidiuretic hormone causing water retention) may occur after head trauma. Hypertonic dehydration or hypotonic water intoxication may produce neurologic signs and symptoms. Acid-base disturbances may also cause mental changes and profound neurologic dysfunction. The diagnosis in such cases depends upon the results of specific laboratory tests. Appropriate therapy is then instituted to correct the underlying abnormality. In cases in which the mental disturbance is prolonged it is important that an adequate food and vitamin intake be maintained since mental symptoms may develop as a result of nutritional deficiency. Sedative drugs should be kept at a minimum. Paraldehyde, chloral hydrate, chlordiazepoxide hydrochloride (Librium), haloperidol (Haldol), diazepam (Valium), chlorpromazine (Thorazine), and the barbiturates may be helpful.

Morphine is contraindicated because of its depressant effect and its tendency to increase intracranial pressure.

If the phenothiazine drugs (e.g., Thorazine or Sparine) are utilized, one must be alert to the possible development of a parkinsonism-like syndrome, akathesia, or dyskinesia which may complicate the clinical picture. The above symptoms may respond to decreased dosage of the drug or the use of antiparkinson medication.

The phenothiazines lower the seizure threshold, but in our experience this has not presented a major problem in their utilization. Chlorpromazine (Thorazine) is probably the most useful drug in the treatment of the acutely agitated patient. Large doses of more than a gram a day in divided doses may be required in some cases. It is wise, however, to begin with a small dose and gradually increase the amount as required.

It goes without saying that when phenothiazine compounds are employed the patient must be carefully observed for such adverse reactions as hepatitis, blood dyscrasias, etc.

The possible danger of masking ensuing complications such as intracranial hemorrhage should be kept in mind when using sedative or tranquilizing drugs.

Chronic Primary Traumatic Mental Disorders

The majority of cases of severe head injury are not fully recovered when the acute symptoms recede and they continue to show residual neurologic and mental disturbances which persist for a variable time. Many of the residual symptoms improve, but a number of patients are chronically incapacitated.

Chronic symptoms may immediately follow the acute phase of the injury, or they may occur after a shorter or longer latent period. The connection between the trauma and the mental syndrome is obvious in the acute cases; it may be more difficult to establish a causal rela-

589

tionship in the chronic cases, especially when the sequelae are late in onset.

The chronic or late traumatic sequelae include diverse syndromes, many of which have a relatively short and mild course while a lesser number are serious and prolonged. These are best divided roughly into posttraumatic personality disorders and posttraumatic defect conditions. In many instances there is a mixture of both.

Posttraumatic Personality Disorders

The posttraumatic personality disorders of adults and children are sufficiently distinctive to merit separate discussions.

Post-Concussion Syndrome and Posttraumatic Personality Disorders of Adults

Definition. The post-concussion syndrome and posttraumatic personality disorder are late chronic sequelae of head injury. The two designations are used to differentiate the common milder form (postconcussion) syndrome from the less frequent severe disorder (posttraumatic personality disorder). Both conditions are characterized by a predominance of psychiatric rather than neurologic symptoms. Neurasthenic-like complaints are commonly outstanding, and these are accompanied by emotional disturbances and defects in mental functioning, with actual character changes in the more severe cases. Neurologic examination as a rule discloses little, if any, abnormality.

Significance and Nomenclature. The so-called post-concussion syndrome represents one of the most common problems in traumatic medicolegal practice. The influence of compensation factors, the differentiation of psychogenic or functional disorders, and the question of simulation all complicate the issue. Resolution of the problem may be extremely difficult and it is not surprising that considerable difference of opinion and much confusion concerning this condition have arisen.

Differences in the literature concerning nomenclature add to the complexity of the problem. Some clinicians employ different terms when referring to this condition, and others use one designation for this as well as for other syndromes which are only remotely related. Writers use varying terms such as traumatic constitution, traumatic psychopathic constitution, traumatic encephalopathy, and even trau-

590

matic neurosis — among others — as synonyms for this condition. The term "traumatic constitution," introduced by Meyer in 1904, has been discontinued because of its hereditary or congenital connotation; a similar criticism applies to "traumatic psychopathic constitution." "Traumatic encephalopathy" is not specific enough and has a generic significance applicable to other traumatic cerebral conditions. "Traumatic neurosis," a term formulated originally by Oppenheim in 1889, is the least acceptable and has contributed to much of the confusion. The designations "neurosis" and "psychoneurosis" are now generally considered to be synonymous and applicable only to psychogenic or functional disorders — not to organic conditions of the brain.

Pathology. The structural basis of these conditions, if any, is unknown. It is generally agreed that the likelihood of occurrence of these sequelae is not directly proportional to the severity of the blow or the extent of the damage. A history of actual fracture of the skull is not essential. Symptoms may appear after injuries that are unassociated with a period of unconsciousness.

Symptomatology. The symptomatology of the posttraumatic personality disorders is quite uniform.

In the post-concussion syndrome, headache is a common complaint. Other sensations referable to the head and located, more or less, at the site of the injury include a "feeling of pressure," of "crawling," or of dullness. Dizziness occurs frequently and the patient may feel faint, especially after sudden movements of the body and head as when getting up in the morning or after bending over; the blood seems to rush to the head, dizziness becomes aggravated and headache increases. There is an oversensitivity to strong sensory stimuli as noise, brilliant sunlight or excessive heat or cold. Alcohol is tolerated less well. Insomnia is common and patients claim to be aroused by slight noises and disturbances. Occasionally, such cardiac symptoms as tachycardia, palpitation, and a crushing sensation in the chest occur. Often the patient experiences feelings of nervousness and anxiety, of diminished physical and mental capacity, and of easy fatigability. Impairment of memory is a frequent complaint, though formal tests may show no defect.

Superficially these patients may appear fairly normal, the clinical manifestations being essentially subjective. However, it is obvious that they are not functioning normally. They are often unable to concentrate even when engaged in such recreational activities as reading and playing cards. They often prefer to be alone, avoid conversation, and

591

will sit around doing little or nothing, apparently brooding over their condition. Exacerbation of symptoms may occur following ingestion of alcohol, or on physical exertion or emotional stimulation.

In severe cases (posttraumatic personality disorder), emotional and character changes are usually very definite. The most outstanding changes in affect are irritability and impulsiveness. Individuals who were formerly good-natured and even-tempered become irascible and hard to get along with. Relatives and friends see a complete change in the patient's personality. Conscientious fathers and husbands cease to care for their family and their irritability may reach such a degree that living with them becomes impossible. They become quarrelsome, get into fights, and exhibit sudden outbreaks of rage. Some patients, however, show a very different reaction characterized by a diminution of emotional expression. They appear dull, apathetic and withdrawn, and show little interest in engaging in any activity. Emotional lability is marked so that rage, tears, and laughter may follow in rapid sequence. A common feature, especially of the more protracted cases, is the complete lack of initiative. Patients are satisfied if their bodily needs are cared for and show no desire to make an occupational adjustment or to plan for the future.

As mentioned previously, neurologic signs are infrequent in these patients. Retention, recall, and speed and accuracy of apperception should be tested using digits, pictures, objects, etc. The results of a battery of psychological tests – particularly the WAIS, the Bender-Gestalt, and Rorschach – may be very helpful in arriving at a diagnosis.

Because of the compensation motive and the fact that a pretraumatic personality disorder may frequently color the posttraumatic syndrome with superimposed psychogenic symptoms, differentiation from psychoneurosis and malingering is often difficult. Kozol (1945, 1946) and Miller (1961, 1966) have emphasized the role of psychological, compensational, and litigatory factors. According to Kozol, "there is a significant correlation between the incidence of posttraumatic mental symptoms and the existence of complicating psychosocial factors such as the persistence of associated bodily injuries, occupational stresses, marital difficulties and pending litigation or continuing compensation." Miller believes that compensation is often the determining factor in such cases and has stated (1966): "I cannot believe that the clinical features of this disorder justify its speculative attribution to cellular damage." (See Chapters 19 and 20.)

Prognosis. The course and prognosis in cases of posttraumatic personality disorder are variable. Many patients recover completely and improvement may continue for as long as two to three years after the injury. The physician is justified, therefore, in withholding a completely unfavorable prognosis until a reasonably sufficient period of time has elapsed. A few cases, however, fail to improve or even get worse, and a number of these have to be institutionalized. As in other conditions, the age of the patient and the presence of such complicating factors as arteriosclerosis or. alcoholism may affect the ultimate issue.

Treatment should be directed not only to the specific physical complaints but also towards helping the individual readjust to the situation. It may be important that the individual become reconciled to the idea of a mild degree of invalidism for a short period and learn to accept his temporary limitations. Care should be taken not to overestimate the severity of the injury and make the patient more of an invalid than is necessary, because certain individuals welcome an excuse for giving up activity and playing this role. The psychiatrist must be on his guard against either extreme.

Most authorities agree that when compensation is involved, a prompt settlement of all financial controversy by payment of a lump sum is important. The patient who continues to receive compensation owing to the persistence of neurotic symptoms usually finds it difficult to rid himself of them. He should return to work and be occupied to the greatest extent possible. If he cannot resume his previous occupation, attempts should be made to fit him into some other type of work to which he can adapt. If necessary, he should start out working a limited number of hours and gradually build up to his regular schedule. In selected cases, psychotherapy may help by giving the patient insight into the nature of his disability, the degree to which he is psychologically incapacitated, and the extent to which he can help himself. The patient should be reassured and encouraged in his efforts to adjust.

Posttraumatic Personality Disorders of Children

The organic mental disorders that occasionally follow head injury in children are characterized by a distinctive personality change. They are usually not accompanied by focal neurologic signs, and correspond to the posttraumatic personality disorders of adults. Personality changes and psychologic phenomena were the outstanding post-concussion features in 47 of 50 children studied by Dillon and

Leopold (1961). There were 35 boys and 15 girls in this series. Behavioral changes included increased aggressiveness, regression, withdrawal, and antisocial behavior in 31. Sleep disturbances were common and enuresis developed in eight. In a series of 105 cases of head-injured children, Black et al (1969) found behavioral manifestations in 22 percent.

The causal head injury may be an apparently simple trauma or a very severe injury. Some children have a history of repeated injuries. The syndrome is more frequent in boys than in girls, probably because of the greater exposure of boys to accidents. In general, children can withstand head injury better than adults and it is the impression of experienced observers that serious neurologic after-effects are not common (Black et al, 1969).

All psychiatric observers who are familiar with this posttraumatic syndrome of children have remarked upon its similarity to the common postencephalitic behavior disorders of this age group.

The onset of the personality change is noted shortly after convalescence from the acute injury. In most instances, however, the case does not come to the attention of the physician, especially the psychiatrist, until many years later. In Blau's series, (1936), the ages of the patient at the time of trauma varied from 3 to 10 years; but the ages on admission to the psychiatric hospital ranged from 7 to 14 years. While the child is young and at home, the family seems able to tolerate his misbehavior. However, when he becomes older and is thrown into greater contact with the outside world, the difficulty becomes accentuated and the family is no longer able to cope with the situation. Puberty aggravates the personality difficulties in many cases and increases the likelihood of misbehavior in the sexual field.

The *symptomatology* of the syndrome may be characterized briefly as a complete reversal of personality. The previously normal child becomes asocial, unmanageable, and unyielding to any form of training. Hyperkinesis is an outstanding symptom. Such children become disobedient and disrespectful towards their parents and may run away from home. Emotional upsets, temper tantrums, and marked irritability are of frequent occurrence. Patients are usually exceedingly impulsive and even explosive in their activities. Common antisocial trends are unrestrained aggressiveness, destructiveness, quarrelsomeness, cruelty to younger children and to animals, lying, and stealing. In school these children are unable to concentrate, have a short at-

594

tention span, and are often truants. They are disruptive in the classroom so that suspension is unavoidable. As they grow older, their school grades and accomplishments become poorer and they may be considered mentally retarded. However, when careful psychological tests are patiently applied, the defect is readily demonstrated to be one of performance rather than of formal intelligence, even though the children's attention and cooperation are poor. Under observation, transient periods of cooperation with moderate self-control may be noted. The usual methods of training and discipline are often unsuccessful. What to do with these children becomes a special problem since they do not fit into available public institutions. Psychiatric treatment should be attempted. For the younger children, Ritalin or Dexedrine may be helpful. Thorazine or Mellaril in fairly large doses may control some of these patients' more aggressive behavioral actions and thus make it possible for them to remain in the community. Special schooling, preferably in a therapeutically oriented setting, is generally required. Psychotherapy, group therapy, and vocational guidance may prove useful. If the patient becomes a serious danger to himself or others he should, of course, be hospitalized. Occasionally, long-term institutional care is required.

Posttraumatic Defect Conditions

Focal Posttraumatic Defects. Cases of head injury in which there are various defects of a psychologic and neurologic nature are included in this group. These patients differ from those who have personality disorders and in whom subjective symptoms are the most prominent feature. Manifestations of posttraumatic defect conditions are the result of organic lesions of the brain caused by destruction and loss of tissue. Many of the defects are on the borderline between neurology and psychiatry; they include the aphasic, agnostic, anomic, apractic, and visual disturbances such as spatial-perceptual disorders. Frequently, as in cases of motor or sensory loss, the neurologic abnormality is readily apparent. Some deficits, however, are evident only upon examinations that utilize psychological tests. For example, tachistoscopic analysis may be required to bring out alexia which may not be immediately apparent on ordinary reading tests (Goldstein, 1948). In addition to the valuable information yielded by these examinations, the data frequently suggest practical methods for the rehabilitation of the injured person. We would, however, caution strongly against depending only on the results of psychological tests, especially isolated studies, in arriving at a final assessment. As always, the psychological tests must be evaluated in the context of the overall clinical picture. In children one is sometimes able to determine the presence of a defect condition by comparing the child's scholastic and intellectual development before and after injury.

Detailed discussion of the various posttraumatic defects may be found in other sections of this book and in the publications of Bryden (1960), Newcombe (1969), Russell (1951), Russell and Espir (1961), Semmes et al (1960), Teuber et al (1949, 1960), Walker and Erculei (1969), and Walker and Jablon (1961).

The course of the acute focal manifestations of brain trauma is frequently one of gradual improvement. In general, the prognosis is better in children and young adults. Treatment in such cases involves the use of rehabilitation techniques adapted to the individual's needs, e.g., speech therapy.

Generalized Posttraumatic Defects. Persistent intellectual impairment following severe trauma, manifested by defective memory and judgment, and personality changes, is not unusual. According to Russell (1959), slight degrees of traumatic dementia are very common after head trauma, and it is usually the most highly developed and complex mental mechanisms that are affected. Improvement may occur slowly, but in some instances both physical and mental capacity are permanently impaired.

Persistent disability due to posttraumatic dementia is rare according to Symonds (1937). Referring to severe head injuries, Maciver et al (1958) wrote that "the majority who recovered have developed little in the way of intellectual deterioration or severe mental symptoms. Most of the patients will be fit to return to productive work and will not remain a burden on their family or the community"; 16 of their series of 26 intensively treated severe head injuries survived and, of these, two showed "fairly pronounced mental changes for some time." Miller and Stern (1965) found that 10 out of 92 severely injured adults were to some extent demented, and of these five were unemployable, after an average interval of 11 years following trauma. A less optimistic note was sounded by Fahy et al (1967), who reported persistent dementia in 50 percent of 26 cases of severe head trauma six years after injury.

References to primary traumatic generalized deterioration of a progressive nature by older writers are now thought to be undiagnosed cases of arteriosclerosis or other forms of degenerative disease. It is significant that such progressive generalized deterioration following cerebral trauma is usually observed in older individuals and that definite evidence of preexisting cerebral pathology as arteriosclerosis, etc., is very common.

Parents of retarded children not infrequently attribute the condition to head trauma. Potter (1933) estimated that about one percent of institutionalized cases of mental deficiency are due to brain injury sustained after birth. It must be kept in mind that mental retardates often suffer head and other injuries as a result of their poor judgment. Head injuries may complicate or exaggerate an already existing mental deficiency. When children require institutional care after serious head injury it is generally because of behavioral difficulties rather than generalized severe intellectual deficits.

Traumatic dementia may be improperly diagnosed in individuals suffering from head injury on the basis of impairment of their work record and of poor scores in intelligence tests. In such cases, lessened ability is often due merely to a lack of interest and initiative, and inability to concentrate.

Varying degrees of dementia may be encountered. If slight, the mental defect may become evident only when the patient attempts to resume his occupation, or is otherwise subjected to environmental stress. In the more severe cases the intellectual impairment is more readily apparent. Tasks formerly accomplished with ease require greater effort or become insurmountable. Failure of memory is a prominent feature, involving especially recent events and not uncommonly, events which antedated the injury. Sometimes memory gaps are filled in with confabulations. Efficiency, judgment, initiative, the ability to deal with unfamiliar situations or abstract ideas, and comprehension all suffer. Patients tire readily. They neglect their duties and display a general loss of interest. Emotional instability, irritability, restlessness, insomnia, headache, dizziness, tinnitus, and paresthesiae are common symptoms. Periods of clouding of consciousness, sudden rages, and episodes of violence may occur. Insight may be fairly well preserved in some cases but in the more markedly demented, it is poor.

Patients who remain severely handicapped present a serious problem and may require institutional care. Some caution is indicated in the more acute and subacute cases because a considerable number make a remarkable recovery after a period of time. Patients handicapped by lack of motivation and interest may be helped by educational and psychotherapeutic methods.

Other Types of Posttraumatic Disorder

Traumatic Encepholopathy of Pugilists ("Punch Drunk" State). This type of mental deterioration is due to repeated and frequent head injuries received by professional pugilists (see Chapter 16). It is noteworthy that this condition was known to the lay public for a long time before medical men recognized it as an authentic sequel. It was first described by Martland (1928) who retained the lay designation "punch drunk" as being most appropriate and descriptive of this condition. Since then studies on boxing injuries have been published by Blaustein and Clarke (1954), Critchley (1957), Spillane (1962), Ferguson and Mawdsley (1965), and Johnson (1969), among others. Cerebral atrophy is believed to be responsible for the mental changes. There is frequently evidence of injury to the septum pellucidum.

The "punch drunk" state is especially common in second-rate fighters who are used for training purposes and are knocked out several times a day. The more skillful pugilists who use their speed, coordination, and ability defensively, are exempt from this condition, except after very long careers in boxing. The decline of the better boxer, when it finally comes, is often abrupt and a single severe beating may result in a marked decrease in his efficiency. It has been estimated that the "punch drunk" state is seen in at least a mild form, in 60 percent of men who remain in the professional ranks for five years or longer. About 5 percent have a fairly advanced condition and a few deteriorate to the extent that institutionalization is necessary. The prominence of objective mental changes and the relative freedom from subjective symptoms is in striking contrast with the traumatic personality disorders. The clinical picture may show considerable variation from case to case but there is invariably evidence of diffuse involvement of the brain.

The earliest signs of the condition usually appear after a period of approximately four years when the professional boxer has engaged in about 30 to 60 bouts. He begins to show a diminished tolerance to head blows and his defensive ability becomes less effective, so that the formerly unmarked pugilist now begins to develop a flat nose and "cauliflower" ears.

Although the fighter still boasts of feeling fine and capable, he begins to lose engagements which previously he could have won with ease. At the same time, people in close contact with the man begin to notice mental changes. They note that certain of his faculties have begun to deteriorate, particularly concentration and memory. In the midst of a conversation he may go into a reverie, and suddenly change the subject or ask the same question several times. He is apt to become excessively sociable and voluble. He usually develops some degree of dysarthria and his eyes become slightly glazed or have a staring expression. Thus, the overall impression may be that of a person who is mildly intoxicated.

In the more severe cases, the voice may become thick, hesitant, and gutteral. Features reminiscent of parkinsonism may appear — poverty of movement, tremor of the hands, nodding of the head, and unsteadiness of gait. In a few instances, vision may begin to fail or some degree of deafness may occur. Headache, dizziness, and tinnitus are often present for a few hours or days following a fight, but they rarely persist as a part of the syndrome. Fits may occur.

Intellectual and personality changes may become very marked and memory grossly defective. Emotional instability is prominent and an euphoric mood common. Involuntary purposeful movements such as those that occur during a prize fight are frequently displayed when the person is preoccupied or under emotional stress. Such patients are completely lacking in insight regarding their mental state or behavior, and resent any implication that these are not normal.

Once the symptoms of the "punch drunk" state have appeared, they persist and usually progress for a period of a year or more when, as a rule, the condition becomes stationary. The more intelligent pugilists recognize its early manifestations and plan to retire from active competition before more ominous evidence appears. However, the majority of boxers seem to lack insight and they continue to fight until they become so ineffective that they cannot obtain further engagements. Some fighters, usually from economic necessity, will then enlist as sparring partners and receive further punishment while assisting in the training of others. The degree of deterioration in this type of traumatic encephalopathy varies depending on the amount of trauma sustained. Advanced cases may require institutionalization.

Posttraumatic Convulsive Disorders (Epilepsy)

Posttraumatic Convulsive Disorders are dealt with in detail elsewhere in this book and will be considered only briefly in this section. Epilepsy is an important sequel of head injury reaching its highest incidence, about 40 percent, in cases of missile wounds with dural penetration. Fits may be focal or generalized, motor or sensory, psychic or somatic. Wounds of the parietal region are most likely to be associated with seizures. While focal manifestations frequently initiate an attack, in most cases the seizures are generalized. Convulsive attacks may occur soon after trauma or be delayed for years. According to Caviness (1969) depth of injury and infection are the most important factors relating to the occurrence of fits. His study indicated that "an injury which combines cortical injury with damage to deep-lying systems is potentially more epileptogenic than an injury characterized by cortical damage alone." Epilepsy after blunt injuries was the subject of an extensive review by Jennett (1962). He found that: a) early epilepsy (in the first week after injury) occurred in less than 5 percent of hospitalized cases and that between a quarter and a third of such patients develop late epilepsy; b) late traumatic epilepsy (after the first week) occurs in about 5 percent of all blunt injuries followed for over 4 years; c) depressed fractures increase the risk of epilepsy only in adults, and then only if the dura has been penetrated, if there has been early epilepsy, or if the period of post-traumatic amnesia has exceeded 24 hours; d) the risk of epilepsy is about 1 percent for all injuries uncomplicated by early epilepsy, intracranial hematoma, or depressed fracture even when the duration of the posttraumatic amnesia is over 24 hours; e) although just over half the cases of late epilepsy have the first fit within a year of injury, this is delayed beyond the fourth year in more than 25 percent of cases; and f) a normal or an abnormal but nonepileptic electroencephalogram is common at any time in patients who develop late epilepsy.

Genetic or constitutional factors have been assumed by many writers to play a part in the development of posttraumatic epilepsy.

Psychomotor seizures (temporal lobe epilepsy) characterized by paroxysmal abnormal behavior of which the patient has no recollection is of particular interest from the psychiatric standpoint. The bizarre behavior is of relatively short duration and may be accompanied by motor phenomena such as smacking movements of the lips. Violence or destructiveness may be exhibited during an attack and permanent psychotic behavior may ensue.

There has been much controversy concerning the personality in epilepsy. One view has been that because of his disorder, the epileptic feels set apart and handicapped, and therefore becomes egocentric, irritable and antisocial. Some epileptics, including those in the traumatic category, show this type of personality. Depressive states are not infrequent in the interictal phase of epilepsy. Usually patients whose seizures are well controlled and who are able to participate in all ordinary activities exhibit no behavorial abnormality.

Mental deterioration has been reported in epileptics having frequent seizures over a long period of time; this too is a controversial point.

SECONDARY TRAUMATIC MENTAL DISORDERS

In this section, we will discuss the possible relationship between head injury and a number of the more common psychiatric disorders. Ordinarily, head injury plays no role in the etiology of these illnesses, other factors generally being held responsible. Head trauma is never considered as the sole cause and the question that arises is whether the injury is a precipitating, aggravating, or contributing agent. In some cases there appears to be no relationship whatsoever. In others, it is very remote or doubtful and the question seems to come up when there is a desire to erase possible familial stigmata or to benefit financially through compensation for the accident. The practical demands of civil courts for expert medical opinions in cases of compensation litigation have made this problem one of considerable importance.

It is generally agreed that a patient is entitled to compensation when the relationship of head trauma to the development or exaggeration of the disorder has been proven. From this viewpoint, it is often necessary to venture opinions as to the proportional influence of a trauma. Sometimes this plays a relatively minor but nevertheless definite role in the causation of disease. At other times it is not at all causally related, in which case this must be clearly stated. It is unfortunate that our knowledge is often deficient in this respect, and in many cases it is impossible to assert definitely that head injury has or has not played a role.

It is not the province of this chapter to describe the symptomatology of what we have designated the secondary traumatic mental disorders; this information is available in the standard texts on psychiatry. We shall discuss only certain points with regard to the factor of trauma. We would emphasize again that most authors do not acknowledge a cause and effect relationship between head trauma and the endogenous or functional psychoses.

Psychoses Due to Alcohol and Head Trauma

Alcoholism and head injury frequently occur together; this results in considerable confusion and difficulty in diagnosis and prognosis. Recurrent head injuries are common in alcoholics. Therefore, it may be difficult to decide whether the resultant condition is a true primary traumatic mental disorder of organic origin, precipitated or aggravated by alcoholism, or an alcoholic psychosis coincident with, precipitated, or aggravated by head trauma. The distinction is often important in compensation cases, since both conditions may present essentially similar symptoms. The most that can be said in many cases is that the patient shows a combination of both traumatic and alcoholic sequelae. In attempting a differential diagnosis, it should be kept in mind that alcoholism and its after-effects are of frequent occurrence, and that chronic alcoholics often display characteristic physical features.

An acute attack of delirium tremens may be precipitated by head trauma as well as by other injuries, surgical procedures, or febrile illnesses. The fact remains however, that delirium tremens occurs only in individuals who have consumed large amounts of alcohol over a long period of time. Alcoholics are more prone to develop psychotic manifestations following head trauma and the prognosis for recovery in such cases is less good. In evaluating a particular case one must consider the pretraumatic personality, the duration and degree of excessive alcoholic intake, the evidence indicative of preexisting deterioration, the severity of the head injury, including the period of unconsciousness, and the extent of the neurologic deficits. In many cases, alcoholism or arteriosclerosis, or both, probably play the major role rather than head trauma. The possibility of a chronic subdural hematoma must be kept in mind and appropriate diagnostic studies performed in all suspected cases.

Psychoses with Cerebral Arteriosclerosis and Head Trauma

It is generally agreed that head trauma may precipitate or accentuate symptoms in patients with organic psychoses associated with cerebral arteriosclerosis. Many individuals with cerebral arteriosclerosis are not seriously handicapped and are able to continue at their work for a number of years. Changes in personality and decline of intellectual function may be slight and hardly perceptible. In such patients, however, deterioration following head trauma may become

602

much more rapid and devastating. Cerebral arteriosclerosis and alcoholism are frequently complicating factors in traumatic dementia.

One must always be alert to the possibility that a cerebral vascular accident has caused the patient to fall and sustain a head injury.

Psychoses with Idiopathic Epilepsy and Head Trauma

The relationship of trauma to the production of convulsive disorders has been discussed earlier in this chapter. We now turn to the question of head trauma as a precipitating or aggravating factor in true idiopathic epilepsy. Head injuries may aggravate idiopathic epilepsy and, since the epileptic sometimes injures his head when falling during attacks, it is possible that an increase in the frequency of seizures and changed behavior may at times be due to head trauma. It would appear reasonable to assume that head trauma is responsible for the occurrence of a seizure in a well-controlled known epileptic when the convulsion follows the injury immediately or within a few days. In such cases there should be other evidence of brain injury such as impairment of consciousness, amnesia, or demonstrable neurologic disturbances. Obviously the resolution of such problems may be difficult and every case must be decided on its own merits.

Mental Retardation with Head Trauma

Despite the idea commonly held by the laity that head injury in childhood frequently plays a role in the causation of mental conditions, there is very little evidence in favor of this view. True mental deficiency resulting from head injury in childhood is probably comparatively rare. It is also quite likely that the role of perinatal trauma as a causative factor has been exaggerated in the past.

Functional Psychoses (Manic-Depressive, Schizophrenia) and Head Trauma

The etiology of these disorders is not well understood. It would seem that constitutional and hereditary factors play a significant role, and later that psychogenic and physiological conditions are also of great importance in the production or precipitation of the endogenous psychoses. Most authorities today agree that the etiology of these psychoses bears no direct relationship to trauma. The opinion is held

603

that if head trauma does precipitate such a psychosis, it is due mainly to the emotional disturbance and the effect is the same as injury elsewhere. It is probable that in most of these cases the individual would ultimately have developed a psychosis in any event.

Mental symptoms due to head trauma may occur in the course of these psychoses, when suicide attempts, accidents, or fights lead to head injury. One must differentiate between certain of the syndromes described under the acute traumatic mental disorders and the excitements and depressions of the manic-depressive; and also between the states of acute confusion and the disorganized language of the schizophrenic. Schizophrenic-like syndromes are occasionally seen in toxic and other organic psychoses, including the traumatic ones. The usual interpretation of this phenomenon is that the organic disease has mobilized the schizophrenic mechanisms, not that the lesion, as such, has caused the specific schizophrenic symptoms.

Head injury may aggravate an existing functional psychosis. One must not, however, be misled by the "post hoc" reasoning fallacy. If typical schizophrenic deterioration occurs following a head injury in a well-developed case of schizophrenia, there is no ground for saying that the head injury per se produced the deterioration. On the other hand, if the head injury produced a definite posttraumatic mental disorder, and if later schizophrenic deterioration with *definite organic factors* occurred, one would be entitled to assume that the head injury had aggravated the schizophrenic psychosis. In some cases it may be impossible to make an absolute statement about the relationship of trauma to the psychosis.

MINIMAL BRAIN DAMAGE IN CHILDREN

The term minimal brain damage as currently used does not refer to a specific disease entity but is descriptive of a certain behavioral constellation. No specific anatomic, electrophysiologic, or biochemical changes are seen in patients with this condition.

The manifestations of this condition are generally: 1) hyperkinesis — the child is constantly in motion and there is no particular external stimulus responsible for this activity; 2) decreased attention span — the child has great difficulty in concentrating even on things he enjoys; he moves from one activity to another in rapid succession, is given to inappropriate focusing on trivial aspects of the environment, and is generally completely unpredictable; 3) temper tantrums and impulsive acts — again, generally without apparent precipitating cause and often directed against people toward whom the child showed affection a few minutes earlier; 4) poor frustration tolerance — reprimands, changes in routine, or unfamiliar demands may produce violent outbursts of rage; 5) intellectual deficits — these may be specific and selective, involving, for example, reading or arithmetic, in the face of excellent intellectual skills in other areas, or they may be generalized, with the patient's overall intellectual level being in the borderline or defective range. In addition, there may be difficulties with regard to memory, speech, understanding, and the ability to generalize or classify. In some children, however, the IQ may be normal or even in the superior range. Studies such as those performed by Baumann et al (1962) suggest that the IQ is in the borderline range in about half the cases studied.

Because of the nature of the symptoms, the problem is most evident in school. These children often are referred for evaluation by the school authorities when they exhibit inability to learn or to remain in class for any period of time.

Diagnosis

The diagnosis rests in part upon evidence of previous organic insult. Pasamanick and Knobloch (1960) in keeping with their concept that minimal cerebral dysfunction is part of a "continuum of reproductive casualty" related this syndrome to perinatal brain damage; the most severe damage, they contended, results in fetal or neonatal death or cerebral palsy; the less severe results in a variety of learning and behavioral disorders depending on the location of the lesion.

A clear-cut history of prenatal hemorrhage, toxemia, or prematurity is alleged to be of significance in arriving at the diagnosis. Such other factors as difficult labor, abnormal presentation, or anoxia at birth are believed to be important. Of some interest in this connection is the fact that Apgar et al, using standard tests at 26 and 47 months of age (1955) found no correlation between the degree of intellectual function and the level of oxygenation at birth. A good developmental history is essential in trying to determine whether the child had trouble from birth.

The role of drugs and viral infections during pregnancy is not well defined. Nevertheless, it is important to question the mother concerning a history of viral infection or drug ingestion during pregnancy.

Reference to the postencephalitic syndrome was made in a previous

605

section of this chapter dealing with posttraumatic disorders in children. A history of a viral exanthema followed by serious neurological symptoms or an abnormal electroencephalogram is suggestive but not conclusive evidence of organic pathology which might subsequently manifest itself in the "minimal brain damage" behavior pattern.

Other organic factors which must be considered are lead poisoning, arrested hydrocephalus, meningitis, and head injury. The diagnosis in such cases is generally clear on the basis of the history and neurologic examination. In children from ghetto areas especially, a history of pica should suggest the possibility of lead intoxication.

The presence of a seizure disorder is presumptive evidence of an organic background in children with disturbed behavior. Grand and petit mal seizures generally present no difficulty in diagnosis. Psychomotor epilepsy, by virtue of its protean manifestations, may offer more of a diagnostic problem. Common to all of these seizure disorders is an alteration in the state of consciousness during the episode and amnesia for the events of the seizure.

Children with major neurologic deficits such as hemiplegia may present behavioral difficulties. This does not necessarily mean that the cerebral lesion is responsible for the behavioral deviation. The presence of abnormal neurologic signs does however increase the likelihood that the behavioral deviations may be related to organic factors.

The relationship between minimal cerebral dysfunction and disturbance of language is a complex one. Dyslexia, dysgraphia, or dysphasia may exist as a nearly pure entity but many patients with language problems exhibit other abnormalities including those of minimal cerebral dysfunction. In our judgment these specific disorders of language in pure form represent developmental problems and not the effects of brain damage as the term is usually understood.

The electroencephalogram is sometimes important in arriving at a proper diagnosis of minimal brain damage. It is especially important in cases where the possibility of a seizure disorder is being considered. The problems of EEG diagnosis, particularly in children, are well known. Nevertheless, it is generally indicated in the neurologic evaluation of behavioral symptoms, especially in cases in which seizures are being considered as a possible etiologic factor.

Psychologic evaluation of intelligence (Wechsler, Stanford-Binet), perceptual (Bender, Gestalt), and projective (Rorschach) test results provide useful diagnostic data. The most valuable diagnostic criteria are discrepancies between verbal and nonverbal functions, and the wide range of variability with regard to ability in different areas, disturbed spatial relations, problems in motor coordination, and distractible behavior. Repeated psychological testing may provide objective evidence of the efficacy of treatment.

In addition to electroencephalographic and psychologic studies, such children should have a complete neurologic examination, including skull x-rays and special tests (e.g., audiometric, visual), when indicated. When there appears to be progressive deterioration or when focal lesions are suspected, further neurologic investigation may be required.

Therapy

Pharmacotherapy has been very beneficial to some children. At times, the resulting improvement can be measured by repeated psychological tests. Dextroamphetamine (Dexedrine), beginning with 2.5 mg/day and gradually increasing the dosage to as much as 30 mg/day has been shown to be helpful. Methylphenidate (Ritalin) has been reported to have similar beneficial effects in doses of as much as 80 mg/day. Some children who do not respond to these drugs improve dramatically when the major tranquilizers, chlorpromazine (Thorazine) or thioridazine (Mellaril), are administered. Some younger children are relieved greatly by diphenhydramine (Benadryl). Other minor tranquilizers appear to be of little value.

Anticonvulsant medication is, of course, prescribed as indicated.

Environmental manipulation, special schooling and family counselling all appear to be helpful. Sometimes changes in parental attitudes result in surprising alterations in the child's behavior. In our own experience, a total approach which combines psychotherapy, pharmacotherapy, special school placement, and family counselling has proved most beneficial.

BIBLIOGRAPHY

Achté, K. A., Hillbom, E., and Aalberg, V. Post-Traumatic Psychoses Following War Brain Injuries - Reports from the Rehabilitation Institute for Brain Injured Veterans in Finland. Helsinki, 1967.

Ajuriaguerra, J. De, and Hécaen, H. *Le Cortex Cérébral*, 2nd ed. Paris: 1960.

Allers, R. *Über Schädelschusse*. Berlin: J. Springer, 1916.

Anderson, W. W. Hyperkinetic Child: Neurological Appraisal. *Neurology, 13,* 968. 1963.

Apgar, V., Girdany, B. R., McIntosh, R., and Taylor, H. C., Jr. Neonatal Anoxia. I. Study of Relation of Oxygenation at Birth to Intellectual Development. *Pediatrics, 15,* 653, 1955.

Baumann, M. C., Ludwig, F., Alexander, R. H., Bergin, T. C., and Rauch, A. E. *A Five-Year Study of Brain Damaged Children.* Springfield: Mental Health Center, 1962.

Bianchi, L. *The Mechanism of the Brain and the Function of the Frontal Lobes.* New York: William Wood & Co., 1922.

Birch, H. G. *Brain Damage in Children: The Biological and Social Aspects.* Baltimore: Williams & Wilkins, 1964.

Black, P., Jeffries, J. J., Blumer, D., Wellner, A., and Walker, A. E. The Post-traumatic Syndrome in Children. In A. E. Walker, W. F. Caveness, and M. Critchley (Eds.), *The Late Effects of Head Injury.* Springfield, Ill.: Charles C Thomas, 1969. Pp. 142-149.

Blau, A. Mental Changes Following Head Trauma in Children. *Arch. Neurol. & Psychiat., 35,* 723, 1936 (comprehensive bibliography).

Blaustein, J. L., and Clarke, E. Further Observations on the Medical Aspects of Amateur Boxing. *Br. Med. J., 2,* 1523, 1954.

Bloomquist, E. R., and Courville, C. B. The Nature and Incidence of Traumatic Lesions of the Brain. *Bull. Los Angeles Neurol. Soc., 12,* 174, 1947.

Bowman, K. M., and Keiser, S. Treatment of Disturbed Patients with Sodium Chloride Orally and Intravenously in Hypertonic Solutions. *Arch. Neurol. & Psychiat., 41,* 702, 1939.

Bradley, C. Behavior Disturbances in Epileptic Children. *J.A.M.A., 146,* 436, 1951.

Brickner, R. M. *The Intellectual Functions of the Frontal Lobes.* New York: Macmillan, 1936.

Bryden, M. P. Tachistoscopic Recognition of Non-Alphabetical Material. *Canad. J. Psychol., 14,* 78, 1960.

Busch, A. Über die Ausfallserscheinungen nach Sehhirnverletzungen und einige Vorrichtungen zur Prüfung der optischen Orientierung und der Arbeitsanpassung. *Ztschr. f. ang. Psychol., 19,* 156, 1921.

Byers, R. K. and Lord, E. E. Late Effects of Lead Poisoning on Mental Development. *Am. J. Dis. Child., 66,* 471, 1943.

Caviness, V. S., Jr. Epilepsy: A Late Effect of Head Injury. In A. E. Walker, W. F. Caveness, and M. Critchley (Eds.), *The Late Effects of Head Injury.* Springfield, Ill.: Charles C Thomas, 1969. Pp. 193-201.

Chapman, L. F., and Wolff, H. G. The Cerebral Hemispheres and the Highest Integrative Functions of Man. *Arch. Neurol., 1,* 357, 1959.

Cohn, R. Delayed Acquisition of Reading and Writing Abilities in Children: Neurological Study. *Arch. Neurol., 4,* 153, 1961.

Critchley, M. *The Parietal Lobes.* London: Edward Arnold, 1953.

Critchley, M. Medical Aspects of Boxing. *Br. Med. J., 1,* 357, 1957.

Critchley, M. Introduction. In A. E. Walker, W. F. Caveness, and M. Critchley (Eds.), *The Late Effects of Head Injury.* Springfield, Ill.: Charles C Thomas, 1969.

Dencker, S. J. A Follow-up Study of 128 Closed Head Injuries in Twins Using Co-twins as Controls. *Acta psychiat. Scand.,* Suppl. 123, 1958.

Dencker, S. J. Closed Head Injury in Twins. *Arch. Gen. Psychiat., 2,* 569, 1960.

608

Denny-Brown, D. E. The Sequelae of War Head Injuries. *New Engl. J. Med.*, *227*, 771 and 813, 1942.

Denny-Brown, D. E. Disability Arising from Closed Head Injury. *J.A.M.A.*, *127*, 429, 1945.

Denny-Brown, D. E. Cerebral Concussion. *Physiol. Rev.*, *25*, 296, 1945.

Denny-Brown, D. E. The Frontal Lobes and Their Functions. In A. Feiling (Ed.), *Modern Trends in Neurology*. New York: Paul B. Hoeber, 1951.

Dillon, H. and Leopold, R. L. Children and the Post Concussion Syndrome. *J.A.M.A.*, *175*, 86, 1961.

Duret, H. *Traumatismes Cranio-Cérébraux*. Paris: Felix Alcon, 1919.

Eager, R. Head Injuries in Relation to the Psychoses and Psychoneuroses. *J. Ment. Sc.*, *66*, 111, 1920.

Ebaugh, F. G. and Benjamin, J. D.: Trauma and Mental Disorders. Chapter VIII in L. Brahdy and S. Kahn (Eds.), *Trauma and Disease*. Philadephia: Lea and Febiger, 1937 (comprehensive bibliography). Pp. 231.

Eisenberg, L. Psychiatric Implications of Brain Damage in Children. *Psychiat. Quart.*, *31*, 72, 1958.

Esquirol, E. *Des Maladies Mentales*, Tomes I, II. Paris: J. B. Balliere, 1837.

Fahy, T. J., Irving, M. H., and Millac, P. Severe Head Injuries. *Lancet*, *2*, 475, 1967.

Faust, C. Zur Symptomatik frischer und alter Stirnhirnverletzungen. *Arch. Psychiat. Nervenkr.*, *193*, 78, 1955.

Faust, C. Die psychischen Störungen nach Hirntraumen. In Gruhle (Ed.), *Psychiatrie der Gegenwart, Band II*. Berlin, 1960.

Ferguson, E. R., and Mawdsley, C. Neurological Disease in Boxers. *Eighth International Congress of Neurology Proceedings*, *1*, E10, 1965.

Feuchtwanger, E. *Die Funktionen des Stirnhirns*. Monogr. a. d. Gesamtgebiete d. Neurol. u. Psychiat., Heft 38. Berlin: Julius Springer, 1923.

Frazier, C. H., and Ingham, S. D. A Review of the Effects of Gunshot Wounds of the Head. *Arch. Neurol & Psychiat.*, *3*, 17, 1920.

Frontal Lobes. *Proceedings of the Association for Research in Nervous and Mental Disease*, Dec. 12-13, 1947. Baltimore: Williams and Wilkins, 1948.

German, W. G., and Fox, J. C. Observations Following Unilateral Lobectomies. Chapter 13 in *Localization of Function in the Cerebral Cortex*. Baltimore: Williams and Wilkins, 1932.

Glaser, M. A., and Shafer, F. P. Skull and Brain Traumas: Their Sequelae. *J.A.M.A.*, *98*, 272, 1932.

Goddard, H. H. *Feeblemindedness — Its Causes and Consequences*. New York: Macmillan, 1914.

Goldstein, K. *Die Behandlung, Fürsorge und Begutachtung der Hirnverletzten*. Leipzig: F. C. W. Vogel, 1919.

Goldstein, K. *The Organism: A Holistic Approach to Biology*. New York: American Book Co., 1939.

Goldstein, K. *After Effects of Brain Injuries in War*. New York: Grune and Stratton, 1942.

Goldstein, K. The Mental Changes Due to Frontal Lobe Damage. *J. Psychol.*, *17*, 187, 1944.

Goldstein, K. The Effect of Brain Damage on the Personality. *Psychiatry, 15,* 245, 1952.

Gordon, N., and Taylor, I. G. The Assessment of Children with Difficulties of Communication. *Brain, 87,* 121, 1964.

Gruvstad, M., Kebbon, L., and Gruvstad, S. Social and Psychiatric Aspects of Pre-traumatic Personality and Post-traumatic Insufficiency Reactions in Traumatic Head Injuries. *Acta Soc. Med. Upsalien, 63,* 101, 1958.

Guttmann, E. Late Effects of Closed Head Injuries: Psychiatric Observations. *J. Ment. Sci., 92,* 1, 1946.

Hagsberg, B. Sequelae of Spontaneously Arrested Infantile Hydrocephalus. *Develop. Med. & Child Neurol., 4,* 583, 1962.

Healy W. A Review of Some Studies of Delinquents and Delinquency. *Arch. Neurol. & Psychiat., 14,* 25, 1925.

Heygster, H. Über doppelseitige Stirnhirnverletzungen. *Psychiat. Neurol. Med. Psychol.* (Lpz.) *1,* 114, 1949.

Hillbom, E. Schizophrenia-like Psychoses after Brain Trauma. *Acta Psychiat. Scand.,* Suppl. 60, 36, 1949.

Hillbom, E. After-Effects of Brain Injuries. *Acta Psychiat. Neurol. Scand.,* Suppl. 34, 142, 1960.

Hohiesel, H. P., and Walch, R. Über manisch-depressive und verwandte Verstimmungszustände nach Hirnverletzung. *Arch. Psychiat. Nervenkr., 188,* 1, 1952.

Huddleson, J. H. *Accidents, Neuroses and Compensation.* Baltimore: Williams & Wilkins, 1932.

Isserlin, M. Über Störungen des Gedächtnisses bei Hirngeschädigten. *Ztschr. f. d. ges. Neurol. u. Psychiat., 85,* 84, 1923.

Jennett, W. B. *Epilepsy After Blunt Head Injuries.* Springfield, Ill.: Charles C Thomas, 1962.

Johnson, J. Organic Psychosyndrome Due to Boxing. *Br. J. Psychiat., 115,* 45, 1969.

Kalberlah, F. Über die acute Commotionpsychose zugleich ein Beitrag zur Aetiologie des Korsakowschen Symptomencomplexes. *Arch. f. Psychiat., 38,* 402, 1904.

Kennedy, F. Head Injuries: Effects and their Appraisal. IV. Evaluation of Evidence. *Arch. Neurol. & Psychiat., 27,* 811, 1932.

Kleist, K. Kriegsverletzungen des Gehirns. Leipzig, 1934. Quoted by P. M. Tow, in *Personality Changes Following Frontal Leucotomy.* London, 1955.

Knobel, M., Wolman, M. G., and Mason, E. Hyperkinesis and Organicity in Children. *Arch. Gen. Psychiat., 1,* 310, 1959.

Knobloch, H., and Pasamanick, B. Syndrome of Minimal Cerebral Damage in Infancy. *J.A.M.A., 170,* 1384, 1959.

Kozol, H. L. Pretraumatic Personality and Psychiatric Sequelae of Head Injury. *Arch. Neurol. Psychiat., 53,* 358, 1945 and *56,* 245, 1946.

Kretschmer, E. Die Orbitalhirn — und Zwischenhirnsyndrome nach Schädelbasisfrakturen. *Allg. Z. Psychiat., 124,* 358, 1949.

Kretschmer, E. Lokalisation und Beurteilung psychophysischer Syndrome bei Hirnverletzten. In E. Rehwald (Ed.), *Das Hirntrauma,* Stuttgart, 1956.

Lashley, K. S. *Brain Mechanisms and Intelligence.* Chicago: University of Chicago Press, 1929.

Laufer, M. W., and Denhoff, E. Hyperkinetic Behavior Syndrome in Children. *J. Pediatr.*, *50*, 463, 1957.

Lindenberg, W. Hirnverletzung, organische Wesensänderung, Neurose. *Nervenarzt*, *22*, 254, 1951.

Lishman, W. A. Brain Damage in Relation to Psychiatric Disability After Head Injury. *Br. J. Psychiat.*, *114*, 373, 1968.

Loken, A. C. The Pathologic-Anatomical Basis for Late Symptoms After Brain Injuries in Adults. *Acta Psychiat. Scand.*, Suppl. 137, 30, 1959.

London, P. S. Some Observations on the Course of Events after Severe Injury of the Head. *Ann. Roy. Coll. Surg. Eng.*, *41*, 460, 1967.

Luria, A. R. Frontal Lobe Syndromes. In P. J. Vinken and G. W. Bruyn, (Eds.), *Handbook of Clinical Neurology*. Vol. 2. Localization in Clinical Neurology. Amsterdam: North Holland Publishing Co., 1969. Pp. 725-757.

Maciver, I. N., Lassman, L. P., Thomson, G. W., and McLeod, I. Treatment of Severe Head Injuries. *Lancet*, *2*, 544, 1958.

Marks, V. H. and Ervin, F. R. *Violence and the Brain*. New York: Harper & Row, 1970.

Martland, H. S. Punch Drunk. *J.A.M.A.*, *91*, 1103, 1928.

Martland, H. S. and Beling, C. C. Traumatic Cerebral Hemorrhage. *Arch. Neurol. Psychiat.*, *22*, 1001, 1929.

Meyer, A. Anatomical Facts and Clinical Varieties of Traumatic Insanity. *Am. J. Insan.*, *60*, 373, 1904.

Meyerson, A. Relation of Trauma to Mental Diseases. *Am. J. Psychiat.*, *92*, 1031, 1936.

Miller, H. Accident Neurosis. *Br. Med. J.*, *1*, 919 and 992, 1961.

Miller, H. Mental After-effects of Head Injury. *Proc. R. Soc. Med.*, *59*, 257, 1966.

Miller, H., and Stern, G. The Long Term Prognosis of Severe Head Injury. *Lancet*, *1*, 225, 1965.

Milner, B. Psychological Defects Produced by Temporal Lobe Excision. In *The Brain and Human Behavior*. Proc. Assn. Res. Nerv. Ment. Dis., Vol. 36. Baltimore: Williams and Wilkins, 1958. P. 244.

Milner, B., and Teuber, H-L. Alterations in Perception and Memory in Man: Reflections on Method. In L. Wiskrantz (Ed.), *Alterations in Behavior*. New York: Harper & Row, 1968.

Moncrieff, A. A., Koumides, O. P., Clayton, B. E., Patrick, A. D., Renwick, A. G. C., and Roberts, G. E. Lead Poisoning in Children. *Arch. Dis. Childhood*, *39*, 1, 1964.

Mutschler, D. Neurosebildende Faktoren bei Hirnverletzten. In E. Rehwald (Ed.), *Das Hirntrauma*, Stuttgart, 1956.

Newcombe, F. *Missile Wounds of the Brain. A Study of Psychological Defects.* London: Oxford U. Press, 1969.

Oppenheim, H. *Die traumatischen Neurosen nach den in der Nervenklinik der Charité in der 8 Jahren 1883-1891 gesammelten Beobachtungen*, 2nd ed. Berlin: A. Hirschwald, 1892.

Ota, Y. Psychiatric Studies on Civilian Head Injury. In A. E. Walker, W. F. Caveness, and M. Critchley (Eds.), *The Late Effects of Head Injury*. Springfield, Ill.: Charles C Thomas, 1969. P. 110.

611

Paine, R. S. Minimal Chronic Brain Syndromes in Children. *Develop. Med. & Child Neurol.*, 4, 21, 1962.

Pasamanick, B., and Knobloch, H. Brain and Behavior: Symposium, 1959. Brain Damage and Reproductive Casualty. *Am. J. Orthopsychiat.*, 30, 298, 1960.

Paskind, H. A., and Brown, M. Constitutional Differences Between Deteriorated and Nondeteriorated Patients with Epilepsy. *Arch. Neurol. & Psychiat.*, 36, 1037, 1936.

Pfeifer, B. Die Psychischen Störungen nach Hirnverletzungen. *Handb. der Geistenkrankheiten*, Bd. 7 (comprehensive bibliography). Berlin: Springer, 1928.

Piercy, M. F. The Effects of Cerebral Lesions on Intellectual Function: A Review of Current Research Trends. *Br. J. Psychiat.* 110, 310, 1964.

Pincus, J. H., and Glaser, G. C. The Syndrome of "Minimal Brain Damage" in Childhood. *New Engl. J. Med.*, 275, 27, 1966.

Papez, J. W. A Proposed Mechanism of Emotion. *Arch. Neurol. & Psychiat.*, 38, 275, 1937.

Poeck, K. Pathophysiology of Emotional Disorders Associated with Brain Damage. In P. J. Vinken and G. W. Bruyn (Eds.), Disorders of Higher Nervous Activity. *Handbook of Clinical Neurology*, Vol. 3. Amsterdam: North Holland Publishing Co., 1969. P. 343.

Poppelreuter, W. Über Psychische Ausfallserscheinungen nach Hirnverletzungen. *Münch. med. Wchnschr.*, 62, 489, 1915.

Potter, H. W. A Clinical Consideration of Mental Deficiency. *Psychiat. Quart.*, 7, 195, 1933.

Prichard, J. C. *A Treatise on Insanity and other Disorders Affecting the Mind.* Philadephia: Haswell, Barrington and Haswell, 1837.

Puech, P., and Mallett, J. Suites éloignées des traumatismes cérébraux. *Encéphale*, 36, 129, 1946.

Rosenhagen, H. Über postkommotionelle Veränderungen im Gehirn. *Deut. Ztschr. f. Nervenh.*, 114, 29, 1930.

Russell, W. R. Cerebral Involvement in Head Injury. *Brain*, 55, 549, 1932.

Russell, W. R. Disability Caused by Brain Wounds. *J. Neurol. Neurosurg. Psychiatry*, 14, 35, 1951.

Russell, W. R. *Brain; Memory; Learning.* Oxford: Clarendon Press, 1959.

Russell, W. R. *The Traumatic Amnesias.* London: Oxford, 1971.

Russell, W. R., and Espir, M. L. E. *Traumatic Aphasia.* London: Oxford, 1961.

Schilder, P. Psychic Disturbances after Head Injuries. *Am. J. Psychiatry*, 91, 155, 1934.

Scoville, W. B., and Milner, B. Loss of Recent Memory after Bilateral Hippocampal Lesions. *J. Neurol. Neurosurg. Psychiatry*, 20, 11, 1957.

Semmes, J., Weinstein, S., Ghent, L., and Teuber, H-L. *Somatosensory Changes after Penetrating Brain Wounds in Man.* Cambridge: Harvard U. Press, 1960.

Spillane, J. D. Five Boxers. *Br. Med. J.*, 2, 1205, 1962.

Spurling, R. G. Notes on the Functional Activity of the Prefrontal Lobes. *South. Med. J.*, 27, 4, 1934.

Strauss, I., and Savitsky, N. Head Injury: Neurologic and Psychiatric Aspects. *Arch. Neurol. & Psychiat.*, 31, 893, 1934 (comprehensive bibliography).

Symonds, C. P. Mental Disorder Following Head Injury. *Clin. Jour.*, 64, 397, 1937.

612

Symonds, C. P. Mental Disorder Following Head Injury. *Proc. R. Soc. Med., 30,* 1081, 1937.

Symonds, C. P. The Assessment of Symptoms Following Head Injury, *Guy's Hosp. Gaz., 51,* 461, 1937.

Symonds, C. P. Concussion and its Sequelae. *Lancet, 1,* 1, 1962.

Symonds, C. P., and Russell, W. R. Accidental Head Injuries. Prognosis in Service Patients. *Lancet, 1,* 7, 1943.

Teuber, H-L. Some Alterations in Behaviour After Cerebral Lesions in Man. In A. D. Bass (Ed.), *Evolution of Nervous Control.* Washington: American Association for the Advancement of Science, 1959. P. 157.

Teuber, H-L. Effects of Brain Wounds Implicating Right or Left Hemisphere in Man. In V. B. Mountcastle (Ed.), *Interhemispheric Relations and Cerebral Dominance.* Baltimore: Johns Hopkins Press, 1962. P. 131.

Teuber, H-L. Neglected Aspects of the Post Traumatic Syndrome. In A. E. Walker, W. F. Caveness, and M. Critchley (Eds.), *The Late Effects of Head Injury.* Springfield, Ill.: Charles C Thomas, 1969. P. 13.

Teuber, H-L., Battersby, W. S., and Bender, M. B. Alterations in Pattern Vision Following Trauma of Occipital Lobes in Man. *J. Gen. Psychol., 40,* 37, 1949.

Teuber, H-L. Battersby, W. S., and Bender, M. B. *Visual Field Defects after Penetrating Missile Wounds of the Brain.* Cambridge: Harvard U. Press, 1960.

Thelender, H. E., Phelps, J. K., and Kirk, E. W. Learning Disabilities Associated with Lesser Brain Damage. *J. Pediatr., 53,* 405, 1958.

Tunney, E. A Man Must Fight. *Collier's,* Mar. 26, 1932.

Walch, R. Über die Aufgaben der Hirnverletztenheime nach dem Bundesversorgungsgesetz. In E. Rehwald (Ed.), *Das Hirntrauma,* Stuttgart, 1956.

Walker, A. E., and Erculei, F. *Head Injured Men Fifteen Years Later.* Springfield, Ill.: Charles C Thomas, 1969.

Walker, A. E., and Jablon, S. A Follow-up of Head-Injured Men of World War II. *J. Neurosurg., 16* 600, 1959.

Walker, A. E., and Jablon, S. *A Follow-up Study of Head Wounds in World War II. V. A. Medical Monograph.* Washington, D. C.: U. S. Government Printing Office, 1961.

Webster, J. E., and Gurdjian, E. S. Acute Physiological Effects of Gunshot and Other Penetrating Wounds of the Brain. *J. Neurophysiol., 6,* 255, 1943.

Wechsler, I. S. Trauma and the Nervous System. *J.A.M.A., 104,* 519, 1935.

Weinstein, S., and Teuber, H-L. Effects of Penetrating Brain Injury on Intelligence Test Scores. *Science, 125,* 1036, 1957.

Whitty, C. W. M., and Zangwill, O. L. Traumatic Amnesia. In C. M. W. Whitty and O. L. Zangwill (Eds.), *Amnesia.* London: Butterworths, 1966. P. 92.

Williams D. Man's Temporal Lobe. *Brain, 91,* 639, 1968.

Wilson, S. A. K. Role of Trauma in the Etiology of Organic and Functional Nervous Disease. *J.A.M.A., 81,* 2172, 1923.

CHAPTER 19

NEUROSIS FOLLOWING HEAD INJURY

LOUIS LINN, M. D.

INTRODUCTION

When an individual sustains a head injury a variety of psychiatric syndromes may ensue, depending on the site and severity of the injury, the premorbid personality of the victim, and the psychosocial circumstances attending the accident (Weinstein and Kahn, 1955). Thus, the patient with a focal lesion may develop an aphasia with secondary personality changes. Or, he may develop a convulsive disorder with specific ictal disturbances of thought, feeling, and behavior. Generalized severe brain damage with a prolonged period of unconsciousness may result in a reaction of psychotic delirium during the acute recovery phase. Chronic widespread brain damage may result in a spectrum of amnestic-confabulatory states. Milder degrees of diffuse brain damage may cause the post-concussion syndrome characterized by frontal and occipital throbbing headaches (present on waking, accentuated by bending, coughing, or sneezing, and intensified by alcohol intake), "dizzy spells" with transient staggering, tinnitus, irritability, impaired concentration, hypersensitivity to light and noise, and fatigability.

This last symptom sequence leads almost imperceptibly into the problem of neurosis following head injury and, at this point, the issues become less clear. Some believe that neurotic symptoms after even minor head injury are the result of physical damage to the brain; others hold equally firmly to the view that the entire post-concussional symptom complex is of psychogenic origin. The prevailing point of view is that certain limited symptoms, specifically throbbing morning headaches which are accentuated by movement as well as vertigo induced by postural change, are probably organic sequelae of closed head injury and may occasionally follow even minor trauma. On the other hand, many hypothesize that the florid neurotic manifestations that characteristically follow trivial head injury and which are associated with a total loss of the ability to work, represent a clinical syndrome of specifically psychogenic origin. The elucidation of this latter symptom complex is the main theme of this chapter.

The last two decades have witnessed the virtual displacement of the contagious diseases by trauma as the major epidemic scourge of our civilization (Klonoff and Thomson, 1969). The neurotic disturbances following head injury constitute a particularly costly and puzzling segment of this larger problem and merit our special attention.

CLINICAL MANIFESTATIONS OF NEUROSIS FOLLOWING HEAD INJURY

Following either some trifling accident or a more serious one which may or may not have been accompanied by temporary unconsciousness, many individuals develop a characteristic train of neurotic symptoms (Wechsler, 1935). These symptoms may start gradually from the moment of impact, and the fright of that moment may merge imperceptibly into continuing complaints of nervousness, with anxiety and depression. More frequently, however, there is an "incubation period" of a few days, weeks, and occasionally months in which the individual is seemingly well and shows no signs of organic involvement of the nervous system. These symptoms generally follow industrial accidents. They have been observed in soldiers who have been in combat. They may also occur in individuals who have been terrified in an automobile collision or an explosion without having received any demonstrable physical injury.

A word of comment is warranted concerning this so-called "incubation period." With few exceptions, objective signs of organic injury to the brain set in immediately, occasionally within a few hours or more rarely after a few days following the accident. *Grand mal* seizures constitute an outstanding exception and may set in months or years after the receipt of the head injury. For the most part, however, objective signs of injury tend to appear at once and to improve with time, thereby contrasting with the sequence of events when *neurotic* symptoms set in following head injury.

Head pain, a common complaint in the post-concussion syndrome, assumes dramatic intensification in the neurotic symptom complex following head injury. Postural or exertional dizziness seen in the

615

latter is not true vertigo in the sense that there is no objective evidence of abnormal vestibular function. These patients complain of irritability and they are easily provoked into arguments. They are easily startled. They complain of poor memory and inability to concentrate. Specific psychological testing suggests that the memory difficulties of which they speak are a consequence of poor concentration and do not follow patterns characteristic of organic memory defects. Insomnia is a common complaint. This is usually expressed as difficulty in falling asleep because of a fear of nightmares the vivid contents of which often relate to the accident. Sites of physical injury tend to become the focus of complaints of intractable pain. Complaints of motor weaknesses may be vague and frequently respond to simple persuasion or to psychological devices calculated to deceive the patient. Changeable and anatomically incongruous sensory losses are frequent.

The most consistent clinical feature is an unshakable conviction of unfitness to work (Hirschfeld and Behan, 1963a and 1963b; Miller, 1961a, 1961b, and 1966). The equanimity with which these people will accept the tedium of months or even years of idleness, apparently unmitigated by any pleasurable diversion, is remarkable. Another consistent clinical feature is the patient's absolute refusal to admit to any degree of symptomatic improvement. Often the patient claims that pain at the site of injury has become steadily more severe over a period of months or years in spite of every treatment effort. Even more remarkable, perhaps, patients often give a history of months of uninterrupted suffering without having ever attempted to secure interim relief from a physician. Once absence from work has been officially sanctioned, a process has been initiated which may go on indefinitely, with interminable courses of physiotherapy and intervening periods of total idleness. The patient frequently reacts to any promise of effective treatment as if this constituted, in some strange way, a threat.

What is at issue here is not whether the patient does indeed suffer from the symptoms in question, or even whether tissue damage exists in the brain or elsewhere in the body, but whether these symptoms or these injured tissues can by themselves explain the patient's total inability to work.

The Problem of Malingering

In practically every instance of neurotic symptom formation following injury there is a tendency to overestimate the severity of the symptoms, to exaggerate complaints, to be preoccupied with symptoms and a desire to shift responsibility from oneself onto others. Even patients with definite signs of brain injury are apt to show a symptom overlay of psychogenic origin. That is, these two sources of symptom formation — organic brain damage and emotional stress — are by no means mutually exclusive.

By definition, an individual becomes a *true malingerer* when he consciously and purposely feigns illness and voluntarily tries to reproduce signs and symptoms which he does not have, or when he extravagantly exaggerates minor symptoms which he does have in order to deceive, to evade responsibility, or to derive gain. In any given case it may be almost impossible to differentiate symptoms which are hysterical from those which are consciously simulated. More important, even in those instances of provable conscious simulation, the need to maintain the deception is motivationally so complex and is based on factors so irrational and unconscious that they have nothing to do with true malingering as previously defined. This issue will be discussed later.

The Special Importance of Head Injury in Neurosis Following Accidents

In a random sample of patients with injuries involving various parts of the body, such as limbs, abdomen, spine, thorax, and head, injuries to the head are by far most likely to induce incapacitating neurotic sequelae. However, physical injury to any body part can initiate the process as can indeed a simple fright without any physical injury whatsoever. It is usually conceded that the head and brain occupy a place of special importance in an individual's self-estimate. This is largely due to the fact that the head contains the brain and the special sense organs of vision, hearing, taste, and smell. Fear of impairment of brain function with deterioration of mental capacities, and concern over loss of vision or hearing play a conspicuous role in the preoccupations of head-injured neurotic patients. Moreover, organic post-concussion symptoms such as headache or dizziness may provide a specific frame of reference or target for the production and elaboration of neurotic symptoms following head injury.

617

For purposes of completeness it should be mentioned that in addition to the common neurotic syndrome described above, one sometimes encounters episodes of typical endogenous depression following head injury, particularly in patients with a history of previous episodes of depression and, on occasion, an acute traumatic delirium following severe brain injury may merge imperceptibly into a chronic schizophrenic disorder.

TERMINOLOGY

The term "traumatic neurosis" coined by Oppenheim (1889) to give a name to the foregoing neurotic symptom complex is unsatisfactory for two reasons. First, he attributed the condition to organic neuronal damage. While it is true that certain limited components of the post-concussion syndrome may indeed be the result of subtle neuronal injury on a molecular level, by definition we are limiting ourselves in this discussion to those residual neurotic sequelae following head injury which remain when signs and symptoms clearly traceable to organic brain disease have been excluded. There is still another reason why Oppenheim's term is unsatisfactory for the modern clinician. Whereas trauma for Oppenheim meant physical trauma, many present-day psychiatrists have preempted the term "traumatic neurosis" for a disorder of purely psychogenic origin, specifically for an acute anxiety state in a previously intact individual which is precipitated by a terrifying experience as may occur, for instance, in combat. The idea of trauma in this use of the term "traumatic neurosis" relates to psychic or emotional trauma exclusively and has nothing to do with physical trauma per se (Fenichel, 1945).

Among other labels for this symptom complex the terms "compensation neurosis" or "litigation neurosis" have been suggested. These have the advantage of emphasizing that litigation is an almost constant feature of these cases and that early settlement of an outstanding compensation claim is often the single most significant factor contributing to ultimate recovery. On the other hand, these latter terms prejudge the issue of etiology.

Miller (1961a and 1961b) has proposed the more general term "accident neurosis" to emphasize that the entire post-accident neurotic symptom complex may arise quite independently of demonstrable physical injury of any kind. In my opinion this is the most satisfactory designation for this condition. To bring this designation into line with current official terminology of the American Psychiatric Association, I propose that we retain Miller's clear and descriptive term "accident neurosis" but subsume it under the larger category of Transient Situational Disturbances, adjustment reaction of adult life (307.3). According to the APA Diagnostic and Statistical Manual (DSM-11), "This major category is reserved for more or less transient disorders of any severity (including those of psychotic proportions) that occur in individuals without any apparent underlying mental disorders and that represent an acute reaction to overwhelming environmental stress. A diagnosis in this category should specify the cause and manifestations of the disturbance so far as possible. If the patient has good adaptive capacity his symptoms usually recede as the stress diminishes. If, however, the symptoms persist after the stress is removed, the diagnosis of another mental disorder is indicated" (Amer. Psych. Assn., 1968). By placing "accident neurosis" within this rubric we make two points. First, a considerable percentage of these cases seem to be functionally intact prior to the accident. That is to say, the symptoms of accident neurosis, particularly the inability to work, commonly become clinically manifest for the first time during a specific presumably stressful period of life which is highlighted for the patient by the occurrence of an accidental injury. Second, although the overall prognosis in accident neurosis is generally regarded as poor, many cases do return to their previous level of functioning after a time lapse during which the primary stress is presumed to have lessened and during which compensation issues are usually settled.

ADDITIONAL ASPECTS OF ACCIDENT NEUROSIS

Age Incidence of Accident Neurosis

Since the most consistent clinical feature of accident neurosis is an unshakable conviction of unfitness to work, it is not surprising that the age group affected ranges from 20 years to 60 years in over 90 percent of the cases. It is also not surprising that the condition is twice as common in men and that it is encountered practically not at all in childhood (Miller, 1961a and 1961b).

That accident neurosis can affect children on rare occasions is demonstrated by the following case history.

619

The patient, aged five, sustained a head injury when she was three years and ten months old. While at play on an embankment she fell several feet to a tiled path, landing on her head. She was unconscious for 30 seconds after which there were nausea, vomiting, and mental confusion for the next six hours.

On recovery from these symptoms she had a total amnesia for the head injury. However, she was present during many discussions of the incident. She was aware of her parents' anxiety. She was particularly impressed with the fact that her parents even went to her nursery school together to discuss the accident with her teacher.

Several months later the housekeeper, to whom the youngster was closely attached, became ill and had to leave the home. The child grieved for her. She became increasingly irritable and unmanageable as a succession of unsatisfactory housekeepers and baby sitters came and went.

This was the setting which prevailed when the patient sustained a second head injury while in the playground with her parents. This was a minor accident and was not associated with any loss of consciousness. However, the child was lethargic for several hours thereafter. She complained of nausea, and retched for some time. She was manifestly frightened. Physical examination was completely negative for evidence of organic disease.

For several months thereafter the child would complain of nausea during periods of separation from her parents. Associated with the nausea she developed a fear that she would soil herself while vomiting. In contrast with the complete amnesia attending the first head injury, the child frequently spoke of the second accident, recollecting with great accuracy all the details, dwelling especially on her nausea and vomiting. Some time later, with the housekeeper back with the family, these symptoms gradually subsided.

Relationship to Severity of Injury

Miller observed (1966) that "in whatever way the cases are broken down they demonstrate an inverse relationship of accident neurosis to the severity of the injury." This inverse relationship was first observed by the writer in a study of combat casualties during World War II (Linn and Stein, 1945). The data and conclusions of this investigation are reported in some detail at this time because they provide an "experiment in nature" which eliminates fairly conclusively a positive role for organic brain damage in the etiology of accident neurosis.

Blast injuries of the ear afford a unique opportunity to study the psychiatric implications of cerebral concussion. Rupture of the tympanum is objective evidence of physical proximity to an explosion of considerable force, directed toward the head. A peculiar heuristic advantage lies in the fact that this type of injury to the head is not associated with a visible or palpable wound, a factor of considerable psychological importance.

Two groups of patients were studied at a military hospital in North Africa during the Tunisian compaign in 1943. Group A consisted of 40 patients admitted to the ENT Service in whom there was objective evidence of traumatic (blast) rupture of one or both eardrums. Group B consisted of 40 psychiatric battle casualties chosen consecutively from the psychiatric files during the same period. In these, the onset of neurotic symptoms was associated with proximity to blast.

In every case of ruptured eardrum in which inquiry was made, there was some impairment of consciousness at the time of the injury. This varied from momentary stunning to complete loss of consciousness lasting up to two hours.

Not one of this group ever displayed sufficient anxiety to warrant psychiatric referral. It should be mentioned that the ENT Service was alert to the presence of psychiatric complications among their patients. Of this group, 27 men returned to full field duty, 2 were placed on non-combatant status because this admission represented the second episode of ruptured tympanum due to blast, while 11 were transferred to general hospitals for further treatment or reclassification on purely otologic grounds. Not one of this group was reclassified or transferred because of neurotic symptoms.

All of our psychiatric patients stated that they had lost consciousness at the time of their "injury." The duration of this loss of consciousness varied from a few minutes to several hours. Of those patients who complained of impaired hearing not one displayed traumatic rupture of the eardrum.

In striking contrast to the first group is the disposition of soldiers in the neurotic group. Of the latter, only one returned to combat; 37 were placed on a non-combatant status because of neurotic symptoms, and two were transferred to a general hospital.

The absence of psychiatric symptoms in the first group in conjunction with a high rate of return to combat duty is noteworthy. Every member of this group was exposed to blast of considerable severity and it may be safely assumed that some degree of cerebral concussion must have been present in every case. It might have been anticipated on the basis of other studies that at least 10 percent of this group would have developed neurotic symptoms sufficiently severe to prevent return to full duty. If concussion played the special role so often ascribed to it the percentage should have been higher.

What then is the explanation of this phenomenon? We are compelled to conclude that in this first group there was an organically determined amnesia, at least for the injury itself and to some extent for the emotionally charged events occurring at the time. True concussion, in effect, cushions the sensorium against the full impact of a catastrophic situation. The soldiers of this group were actually spared the conscious experience of the terror-inspiring explosion.

In spite of the superficial resemblance to the clinical picture of concussion, the actual sequence of events leading to the disturbance of consciousness in the neurotic group is quite different. It may be inferred from the complete absence of ruptured eardrums in this group that they were further removed from the force of explosion than the first group. If the concussion in the latter was mild to moderate then in the former it must have been extremely mild or absent. The amnesia in the neurotic group is completely reversible. With careful questioning, for example, patients will recall with horror seeing limbs flying in the air,

621

the flash, the sound and the commotion of the earth. Far from the protective dulling or obliteration of the sensorium which occurs in concussion, the neurotic patient has been fully conscious, indeed, hyperacutely aware of the horror of the situation. The result of the inordinate emotional stress may be syncope or a fugue state not to be compared with the alteration of consciousness following true concussion. The organic amnesia of concussion is absent and there is complete retention, conscious or unconscious, of all the dreadful details of the cataclysm.

It may be conjectured, therefore, that individuals in the first group were actually spared the emotional experience associated with the explosion, whereas in the second group it is this very emotional experience which is the element of fundamental importance in the pathogenesis of the battle-incurred neurosis.

Psychological Significance of Work

Hirschfeld and Behan (1963 a and 1963 b) have characterized accident neurosis as a condition which marks "the death of the patient as a worker." The recurrent emphasis on the impairment of the capacity to work in accident neurosis calls for a brief review of the psychology of work.

Ideally, work fulfills a number of positive functions. Nowhere is this more dramatically illustrated than in the case of a retired worker whose unaccustomed freedom may lead to a sense of aimlessness and create serious marital discord. The vast majority of people who occupy middle-class jobs if given the choice choose to continue working at retirement age. For individuals who have failed to cultivate leisure-time interests, a lack of work means a lack of anything else to do and for them idleness breeds boredom and frustration. In addition work fulfills an important social function. It is the basis of friendships, group memberships, outings, etc. Many jobs have the effect of reinforcing one's basic identity. For men in particular it is an important source of self-esteem, particularly in their role as family provider. On a more subtle level many are imbued with what has been called the Protestant ethic, that is, the need to work hard in order to "deserve" the pleasures of leisure. For such people work may be a compulsion, and separation from work may produce severe anxiety, guilt, and depression. Freud (1961) summarized the work role as follows: "No other technique for the conduct of life attaches the individual so firmly to reality as laying emphasis on work, for his work gives him a secure place in at least a portion of reality in the human community." Add to the foregoing the economic factor and we are left with a paradox. The motivations to continue working are clear enough. What is not so clear is the nature of this strange and pathological force which can arise within the mind at times and neutralize the natural impulse to stay on the job. This is the puzzle to which we will address ourselves in the next section.

The Accident Process

In his study of accident neurosis, Miller (1961a and 1961b) found a complete lack of evidence of predisposition to neurosis in over half of his cases. This is particularly baffling since we seem to be dealing with a major neurosis of disabling proportion having its onset suddenly in adult life without apparent warning. However, a clue is offered by Hirschfeld and Behan (1963 a and 1963 b) who suggest that the onset is never really sudden and that if one reads the warning signals properly it is never entirely unexpected. In their study of 300 cases of industrial accidents and injuries, these authors concluded that the accident which supposedly marks the onset of the disorder is only a single event in a continuing psychological process which started in the patient's mind long before the accident itself and continues long thereafter.

For a period of weeks or months preceding the onset of the accident neurosis, the patient shows a characteristic pattern of *premonitory* behavior. During this premonitory period the worker commonly shows a sharp rise in the frequency of sick call. In other instances a previously unobtrusive worker may present himself to a shop foreman or a first aid attendant with minor nuisance complaints which seem on the surface to be so inconsequential that they commonly go unheeded. In current psychiatric parlance these complaints are a "cry for help." As the latter goes unheeded the worker becomes involved next in safety infractions. A worker with an excellent safety record going back many years may break several rules simultaneously. On occasion the worker has sent a safety assistant off on some trivial errand leaving him momentarily unprotected. When asked to explain this behavior his answer may be vague or even silly. Patients often describe premonitions that they are going to incur serious injury. Hirschfeld and Behan describe a patient who became involved in a series of petty thefts carried out so conspicuously and so clumsily that they could hardly be ignored, and yet they were ignored and the patient became a victim shortly thereafter of a serious accident.

One may infer that for the patient who develops an accident neurosis

623

the role of worker or wage-earner has become intolerable. He expresses this in a succession of benign requests to be rescued from the job. When these appeals go unheeded he precipitates a real accident. Even now the worker may not yet have reached the point of no return. He may incur a series of minor accidents following each of which he resumes his work with increasing anxiety and hesitation until the final accident. Thus the final accident which precipitates the neurosis is part of a series of preceding events and others which may follow it over a period of months and even years. Together they constitute what Hirschfeld and Behan have called the "accident process." In its entirety the accident process may be viewed as an ongoing attempt to solve a problem.

These phenomena which are premonitory of accident neurosis shed light on the concept of the "accident-prone" patient. It has been contended that there is an identifiable personality type which is particularly prone to have accidents. While there may indeed be such a personality type it seems much more likely that accident proneness is not so much the expression of an ongoing personality trait as it is an intermittently present state of mind. The latter is commonly associated with a mood of depression, a highly ambivalent attitude toward one's own health and safety, outbursts of rage followed by guilt, and an increased alcohol intake. Many of the accidents which touch off the accident neurosis are thinly veiled suicide attempts which take place, often during a state of inebriation.

Psychodynamics of the Accident Process

Whatever the life problem which the accident process endeavors to solve, it seems clear that the patient arrives at this solution reluctantly, after a great struggle over a period of months, with many vain appeals for help and with much ambivalence. The accident process spells out a struggle between the essentially normal impulse to cling to the job on one hand versus a growing inability to tolerate the work situation on the other.

One could predict on the basis of this formulation that those most likely to succumb to accident neurosis are those for whom the drive to keep working is weakest. Thus it comes as no surprise to learn that unskilled and semiskilled workers constitute the bulk of the accident neurosis caseload. They tend to occupy jobs which are both dangerous and poorly paid. A large impersonal factory complex contributes more

624

cases of accident neurosis than the intimate setting of a small business or farm. When work fails to provide a sense of purpose to one's life, where there are no friendships or shared recreational interests, where the job is dull and dangerous, where the only point of working is the salary and a paltry one at that – in short, when the worker is depressed, isolated, and anomic (Miller and Butler, 1966) he is particularly prone to develop an incapacitating accident neurosis.

That a positive commitment to work protects against incapacitating accident neurosis is illustrated by the following case.

A business executive sustained a head injury in an automobile accident. There was a laceration of the scalp and a brief period of unconsciousness. During the following months he suffered from throbbing morning headaches and episodes of dizziness. In addition he had episodes of panic which descended upon him without warning, particularly while at work and during which times he would relive the moments preceding the car crash.

Although the other vehicle was clearly at fault, the patient was not interested in pursuing active litigation and in fact settled for a relatively inconsequential sum. This man carried major decision making responsibilities in a creative enterprise and his work was a major source of personal satisfaction. Even though he developed clear-cut symptoms of accident neurosis the positive rewards of his job outweighed by far any impulse to withdraw from work because of physical suffering.

While the foregoing deals with the strength of the drive to keep working as a factor in the etiology of accident neurosis, it does not explain why for some individuals the idea of work has come to be absolutely abhorrent and why individuals so affected are apt to look with suspicion and even hatred on physicians trying to "cure" them. This is the issue which we will turn to next.

Following an intensive psychoanalytic study of a series of patients with accident neurosis, Noy (personal communication) concluded that the litigious attitude of the worker toward his employer is a displacement of a conflict within the family. According to Fallik (1960), the patient himself is typically insecure, dependent, and emotionally infantile, and within the family he maintains only a precarious hold on his masculine role. A change within the family balance, occasioned, for example, by the birth of a child or the death of a crucial relative, may compel his wife or others to decrease their emotional investment in the patient. This shift, demanding greater independence, may leave him depressed, impotent, embittered, and helpless. When, out of fear of further rejection, he is unable to express these feelings directly at home he transfers them to his place of work. He projects his feelings of persecution onto his employer. He becomes increasingly resentful and complains of unfair treatment. His sense of personal hurt and retaliatory vindictiveness grow. Anger at a preoccupied wife, for example, may be expressed in inappropriate outbursts of rage at his supervisors. This emotional instability brings with it guilt, anxiety, and a sense of bewilderment (Ostow, 1970). The job which he uses as his scapegoat now seems, inexplicably, to be the source of all his suffering and he is well into the premonitory phase of the accident neurosis.

The following case history is cited to exemplify the number of personal changes that can ensue in the life of a patient with accident neurosis which doubtlessly impinge on the overall clinical picture and which have to be taken into consideration if the case is to be successfully treated.

A 35-year-old man came to the Mount Sinai Hospital outpatient department in August of 1967 with complaints of headache, dizziness, and peculiar sensations in his neck and skull, all of which developed gradually following a head injury sustained at work the preceding January. For 17 years before that the patient had worked steadily in a laundry.

The patient, his wife, his 14-year-old daughter, and his 10-year-old son made up a closely knit family. In 1966, for reasons not at all clear, his wife began insisting that she wanted another child, saying she would adopt one if she did not become pregnant. During the period of these discussions the patient struck his head on a pipe while at work, sustaining a scalp laceration which was sutured in the hospital's emergency room. During the ensuing months his alcohol intake increased and his wifes importunateness continued. In January of 1967, he arrived at work somewhat inebriated, sustained a fall and a minor head injury which went untreated at the time. However, he became increasingly irritable and one day in August of 1967, he was discharged after an argument with his employer. He has not worked a single day since that time (approximately three years to date).

Shortly thereafter his wife became pregnant. The patient now abstained from drinking and developed hyper-religious tendencies. He became estranged from his mother, who lived only a block away and who had previously been a constant visitor in his home. During his wife's pregnancy he gained over 50 pounds. He worried constantly that the baby would be abnormal. The birth of a normal baby gave him little satisfaction. The patient had a large number of physical and laboratory examinations, all negative. He received a variety of treatments, including medications and psychotherapy, in both an outpatient and inpatient setting, all to no avail.

While one cannot document the relationship of these events, clearly his inability to work seemed to start with his wife's determination to have another child.

She got the child she demanded. It seems as if she got herself another child in the process that she did not bargain for, namely, her invalid husband.

We may hypothesize that this passive, dependent, infantile man was threatened by the birth of an infant, was unable to share his wife's attentions with yet another child, and was unable to cope with the additional responsibilities of an enlarged family. He was unable to deal with these increased demands on his limited adult masculinity. For a time, he showed the premonitory symptoms characteristic of the accident process and finally succumbed to total invalidism when his wife actually became pregnant.

To withhold his own contribution at work and yet to continue to collect his wages somehow seems to the patient a way of "getting even" and a technique which promises relief. The formula of an accident which is his employer's fault and for which his employer will make full restitution by now comes to fulfill a deep-rooted uncontrollable desire for vengeance. Only when this matter has been resolved, usually with a financial settlement, can he turn his mind to other issues and resume his work.

According to Noy, any therapeutic approach to accident neurosis which is not family centered and which does not help the victim to deal with his sense of rejection in his own home can at best give only temporary relief. This is the temporary relief of the compensation settlement. The process can start all over again the next time the family balance changes and the subject again feels himself victimized.

Socarides' analytic study of the vengeance motif (1966) has an important bearing on the subject of accident neurosis. Socarides emphasized the role of early infantile emotional deprivation in the character structure of individuals strongly predisposed to vengeance. According to this formulation the sense of injury which the subject experiences as an adult in his own home and which he transfers to his employer has its origin during childhood in relation to parents and siblings. Once the vengeance mechanism has been set in motion it acquires the force of an irresistible impulse. There can be no peace of mind until scores have been settled. The subject is willing to absent himself from the normal pursuits of congenial society, indeed feels compelled to break off all irrelevant relationships, until his aim of vengeance has been fulfilled.

Miller (1961a and 1961b) ascribes accident neurosis to the polarization of interests which exists between worker and employer. "The exploitation of his injury represents one of the few weapons available to the unskilled worker to acquire a larger share — or indeed a share of any kind — in the national capital." In short, Miller sees in the

627

accident neurosis a vengeance motif of a more superficial kind, a process whereby the underdog worker gets even with an affluent society. He hypothesizes that a progressively more successful socialization of industry will reduce the incidence of accident neurosis. He admits, however, that there are no data as yet with which to test the hypothesis. If the revenge motif in accident neurosis is primarily a wish to get even — or, as Socarides says, "to get more than even" — with an exploitive affluent society we would still be left with a puzzle. How can it happen in that case that accident neurosis emerges suddenly? Why, for example, should a worker with a 20-year history of uninterrupted diligence succumb to accident neurosis seemingly without warning? In many of these cases, moreover, there have usually been regular wage increases and the job situation itself has probably improved as a result of union protection and new contract negotiations. It would seem to be an unavoidable conclusion that the adaptational breakdown represented by accident neurosis must be a consequence of extra-vocational stress.

We have focused on the vengeance motif as an illustrative psychological mechanism, perhaps even the chief mechanism underlying accident neurosis. Other mechanisms can undoubtedly be cited. For example, a hazardous job which is tolerable when a worker is young may become a source of unbearable anxiety as he grows older and fears that his powers are failing. In almost every instance, however, an essentially irrational core will be uncovered involving personal family issues and lifelong emotional impairments.

Once we understand the irrational core of accident neurosis, once we comprehend how deeply this irrational core extends into the unconscious, and how far back in time it extends in the developmental history of the patient, we are in a position to comprehend the extraordinary phenomena which comprise the accident neurosis.

Thus the patient may persist in his invalidism until he has exacted his revenge in the form of a financial settlement. Cure without revenge is the last thing he wants. He exaggerates all symptoms in an obvious determination to emphasize the seriousness of his disablement. Treatment is unavailing, and yet the ineffectiveness of therapy notwithstanding, the accident neurosis patient presents himself for treatment conscientiously and even gratefully, provided only that no serious steps are taken to get him back to work before a compensation settlement has been arranged.

Indeed, many patients do not even bother to go for treatment in spite of ostensible suffering and disability. Medications generally prove valueless for the relief of pain and insomnia. Electroshock therapy which is ill-advisedly used at times in a spirit of desperation results only in an entirely new chain of complaints. The accident neurosis patient views the overzealous physician with suspicion regarding him as an arm of the company, that is to say, a member of the enemy camp. Such behavior, which may seem on the surface to be crafty, scheming, and outright dishonest, may be understood in part from a psychoanalytic point of view as a compulsion to fulfill a complex need. Thereby the patient hopes to be relieved of unbearable tension and feelings of impotence and to restore his potency, his self-esteem, his capacity to work, and his ability to function as head of his household.

The primary script of accident neurosis is thus set by unconscious factors which in many cases create an uncontrollable compulsion not to work until a financial settlement has been made. However, secondary factors are swiftly brought into play which complicate matters. The modern worker, in his vengeful quest, does not face his employer-adversary alone. His union steward is always at his side and behind the union representative are many organizational facilities reinforced by batteries of lawyers and even by considerable political pressure at times. Needless to say, these mighty pressures create a backlash both within the insurance company and the employers. The consequence can be a veritable military encounter between opposing armies. Bitter accusations and recriminations on both sides may unnecessarily prolong the process of legal settlement, and regrettably, the entire "war" may be waged in ignorance of the real issues, without awareness of the unconscious factors which gave rise to the problem in the first place.

Perhaps the most bewildered victim of this complex process is the physician who is called on to diagnose, treat, and to mediate in relation to the accident neurosis patient. In his mind's eye the physician sees himself as a healer, friend, and counselor. The accident neurosis patient, on the other hand, sees the physician as an enemy. Unaccustomed to a patient who is hostile, ungrateful, obstructive, and totally unresponsive to every form of treatment, the physician experiences a blow to his self-esteem. It is important at this point to emphasize that the accident neurosis patient can be extraordinarily irritating and provocative. The motivations for this are complex. In addition to his fear that the physician will frustrate his compulsive drive for revenge, the accident neurosis patient suffers much guilt and may be unconsciously driven as a result to provoke punishment from the physician.

Thus far the physician's reaction of irritation and anger is well within the limits of normal expected behavior. However, the physician is often disappointed in himself for losing control of himself in accordance with his own idealized professional self-concept. In response to essentially inappropriate feelings of guilt he leans over backward to be conscientious. In this way there comes to pass the ritual of multiple somatic treatments, the combined effect of which is not only futile but even deleterious to the clinical course of accident neurosis. To complicate matters further, these procedures are often painful and may damage tissues. And so it happens that overt clinical conscientiousness may conceal an unconscious drive to retaliate or punish. At this point we are no longer dealing with angry feelings which are appropriate and therefore essentially normal but with what is called psychoanalytically an attitude of *negative countertransference*. In other words, neurotic mechanisms within the physician have been released. Now not only is a hostile neurotic patient facing a hostile physician but he is also facing a neurotic physician who is no longer able to recognize the extent of his own hostility, destructiveness, and impairment of judgment. Under these circumstances there can be no rapport and the likelihood of making any headway therapeutically is practically nil.

It is necessary to add that the physician's misery in treating these cases by no means goes unrewarded. The average medical bill in these cases is approximately the same as the amount paid to the claimant. Hirschfeld and Behan (1963 a and 1963 b) raise the question whether the physician himself is not by this time enmeshed in a vengeance motif and caught up in a system of unconsciously accepting financial gain for his part in what has become a chronic irrational interaction between himself and his patient.

So far we have described "the accident" as a culminating event in an industrial setting involving behavioral and emotional changes antedating the accident itself by weeks, months, or even years. Most accident neurosis cases are of this category and by and large the clinical documentation of industrial cases is most complete. On the other hand, many accident neurosis cases are precipitated by trauma in other settings. "Concussion" cases arising in combat have already been alluded to. Emotional disturbances, with or without litigation, after automobile accidents are quite common.

The following case history, cited by Hirschfeld and Behan (1963a

630

and 1963b), illustrates how complex the emotional factors in these latter cases can sometimes be.

A woman sustained serious injuries when her husband drove their car into a locomotive on their honeymoon. In this case a severe sexual problem antedated the accident. The resulting chronic invalidism of the wife in the form of a rather typical accident neurosis provided a solution of sorts to their unresolved sexual difficulties. The previously hostile husband was now solicitous and kind. The adaptation which followed, effectively excluding sex from the marriage, was acceptable to her passive, undemanding spouse.

In another instance of young man, aged 22, went into a severe depressive reaction following the death of his grandfather. During the ensuing months he suffered from anorexia with considerable weight loss, a sleep disturbance characterized by early morning insomnia with agitation, and an inability to concentrate. One day, he was a passenger in an automobile which was involved in an accident in which the driver, a considerably older man whom he identified with his grandfather, was killed. At the time the patient was stunned and there was a question of loss of consciousness. No litigation was involved. Thereafter the subject complained of severe headaches, attacks of dizziness, and a fear of leaving the house. Detailed physical examinations and laboratory studies were consistently negative for evidence of organic brain disease. Nevertheless the subject became increasingly fearful. A period of outpatient psychotherapy was of no avail and he was hospitalized for further care. After several months of inpatient treatment he remained depressed, preoccupied with complaints of headaches and dizziness, and unable to venture out of the hospital unaccompanied. It was the staff's opinion that a chronic schizophrenic disorder had set in.

Still another setting for accident neurosis is illustrated by the following case.

A 23-year-old single man joined the Peace Corps upon graduation from college in June of 1966. After a period of preliminary training he was sent to Peru. While there he suffered increasingly from homesickness and depression. One morning on his way to work he fell down a flight of stairs. There was no loss of consciousness and no injuries were found on physical examination. He was not drinking or taking drugs at the time and he attributed the incident to his own carelessness. Shortly after the accident he developed severe headache which he described as a throbbing ache throughout his scalp with lancinating pains shooting from his right eye to his left occipital area. The pains were constant but most severe in mid-afternoon. The patient was returned to the United States for further studies which were entirely negative. He was discharged from the Peace Corps with the recommendation that he get psychiatric help. He broke off treatment after a short time, apparently improved as far as his complaints of headaches were concerned. His life pattern as a rather withdrawn compulsive character persisted.

631

Thus, accident neurosis may have its inception on the battlefield, at work, in automobile accidents, in settings of separation from home, etc. What all these situations have in common as far as the problem of accident neurosis is concerned is a life situation which has become emotionally intolerable. Accident neurosis, like all neurosis, has the adaptational function of providing an essential escape mechanism. Problems may be resolved in various ways, some healthy and others pathologic, the latter including neuroses, psychoses, addictions of one kind or another, and flights into physical illness.

As a corollary of this point of view it is noteworthy that accident neurosis is rarely seen as a sequel to injuries incurred in recreational settings.

PROGNOSIS

It is usually said that most patients with accident neurosis re-cover after the case has been settled. Reporting on a group of his own patients, Miller stated (1966): "Nearly all of these cases recover completely and without treatment after the case is settled — win or lose. Of my own fifty cases this was the indubitable outcome in forty-five. Each of three chronic neurotics was restored to his previous state of lifelong martyrdom after a lucrative interval during which trauma was held responsible for his troubles. Two of the fifty remained to be accounted for and these must represent the minority of cases often invoked by those psychiatrists who claim (without statistics) that compensation neurosis *often* persists after settlement. Both of them were men of low intelligence and morale. In both injury had been trivial. In each there had been diagnostic confusion and dispute. Both were still in receipt of continuing weekly pensions for industrial disablement two years after they had been very generously compen-sated at Common Law. Four years later one — an older man — remains as before, an apparently contented semi-invalid consoled by material comfort. The other had his pension terminated by a hard-hearted medical board shortly after the completion of my study following which his practitioner told me his recovery was rapid and complete."

Fallik (1960) reports a more guarded prognosis. In a three-year follow-up of 38 cases, five patients were unimproved and in the remainder he found persisting albeit milder manifestations of ac-cident neurosis in most cases, in spite of financial settlement. These symptoms consisted of somatic complaints, hypersensitivity to stimuli

632

resulting in social withdrawal, and a pattern of continuing domestic discord. Fallik (personal communication) goes even further and states that no accident neurosis patient ever resumes his former vocational status; in effect, he develops a pattern of phobic avoidance in relation to his previous employment. When he resumes his role as wage earner it is almost without exception in a job that in certain ways is more rewarding, for example, one that is less physically exhausting, less hazardous, or permits more leisure time. While this is commonly achieved by taking a step downward vocationally to a more sheltered work setting, Fallik reports cases in which the patient educated himself during his period of invalidism and actually succeeded thereafter at a higher-paying white-collar job at a time when the idea of returning to his previous job remained completely abhorrent. In short, if the goal of therapy is to remotivate the patient to resume his role as wage earner, this can be achieved only if a properly modified work situation is included in the treatment program. To maintain such improvement, however modest, it is often necessary to provide ongoing supportive psychotherapy to the patient and his family.

In any event, more optimistic figures such as those reported by Miller concern themselves with the resolution of a single attack. They do not take into account the episodic nature of the illness and the fact that patients often return to a changed and possibly less stressful home environment. In short, what almost all the literature omits is the fact that although accident neurosis may seem to arise out of a clear blue sky as far as the work situation is concerned, the situation at home may not be cloudless, a consideration that has been curiously overlooked in the voluminous literature on the subject of accident neurosis.

Certain patients who have gone through a cycle of accident neurosis, compensation payment and return to work, have had subsequent episodes of accident neurosis. What is impressive about these recidivists is the failure to refer to the previous episodes unless specifically questioned. Also, the symptoms presented during the subsequent episode usually differ entirely from those which characterized the earlier ones. For these patients this is not a recurrence, but an entirely new illness. There is a need to study the problem of recidivism in accident neurosis. As of now, definitive information on this subject is lacking.

633

It has been the central theme of this chapter that accident neurosis cannot be properly understood unless one takes into account the irrational core of this condition, the emotional factors which are transferred from childhood into contemporary adult relationships, and which are transferred from one situation, such as one's home life, into an entirely different situation, such as one's place of work. When this global approach to accident neurosis is adopted then certain consequences logically ensue:

1. If the worker's attachment to his job is weak because of undesirable working conditions then social changes backed by government, employers and unions which foster personal concern for the individual worker as a human being, will also tend to reduce the incidence of accident neurosis.

2. During the premonitory phase of accident neurosis any persistent changes of behavior on the job should be viewed as a precursor of accident neurosis. A previously careful worker who becomes slipshod about safety regulations, a formerly uncomplaining person who begins to appear regularly on sick call with minor complaints, a cheerful worker who becomes irritable and argumentative, a sober person who appears at work intoxicated, an honest and straightforward person who becomes involved in petty thievery — one could extend this list considerably on the basis of clinical experience — any such changed individual should be referred to the psychiatrist. The latter should explore in depth the worker's life situation away from the job. Recent changes in family structure, such as illness or the birth of a child, which have reduced the amount of attention which the wife can provide are particularly significant. Psychotherapy should be offered during this premonitory phase and it should be family centered. As previously noted, reassignment to a less hazardous job or one which is less physically demanding should be included if indicated in the treatment program. In this way a catastrophic accident or a chronic incapacitating accident neurosis may be averted.

Careful records of psychiatric study and treatment may be invaluable in settling future claims in the event of accident neurosis. In any case, study of these premonitory phenomena is urgently needed for a better understanding of accident neurosis for purposes of prevention and treatment. Certainly the notion that accident neurosis is understandable as "a disability motivated by hope of financial gain (and) is regularly thus rewarded" (Miller, 1966) is a gross oversimplification of the phenomena involved. Miller states that a strong case could be made for regarding accident neurosis as a non-compensible disability and states that this appears to be the position in France. However, he feels, that such a policy would imply the unconditional rejection of a number of claims which would be generally regarded as perfectly genuine. It would seem that careful documentation of emotional disturbances during the premonitory phase of accident neurosis and vigorous efforts at family centered therapy with opportunity for job reassignment ought to make it possible to separate out many appropriately non-compensible cases of accident neurosis.

TREATMENT OF ACCIDENT NEUROSIS

Many accidents will occur, unfortunately, before adequate prevention can be effected. In these cases the problem becomes one of avoiding chronic disablement. Hirschfeld and Behan (1963a and 1963b) express the opinion that psychotherapy of accident neurosis should be carried out wherever possible by a primary physician who is responsible for the management of the case in its entirety. If an outside psychotherapist must be brought into the picture, then the primary physician should be clearly identified to the patient as the captain of the treatment team. Few patients are more frequently the victim of fragmented care than those with accident neurosis who shuttle from doctor to doctor for multiple diagnostic and therapeutic procedures. To combat the sense of fragmentation and confusion which the accident neurosis patient tends to develop there must be a primary physician to whom the patient can relate. Hirschfeld and Behan urge that such primary physicians be well trained in the technique of psychotherapy. They warn against the dangers of psychotherapeutic improvisations based on "common sense psychiatry." They recommend seminars, readings, and opportunities for supervised treatment over a period of at least a year. The result of such a new orientation, they say, would for one thing be a change in history-taking procedures. Customary cursory interviews would give way to more elaborate data gathering, greater rapport, and understanding in depth of the patient's complaints. In this connection it is well to sound the alarm: beware of anger in managing cases of accident neurosis. We have previously outlined the complications which follow negative countertransference. It is probably not possible to avoid this problem without a sophisticated psychiatric approach.

The therapeutic effect of prompt, lump-sum financial settlement is regularly cited in accident neurosis literature. This point of view has been legislatively implemented in many states and as a result much of the old-time courtroom melodrama has been eliminated. The vast majority of workmen's claims are settled routinely without litigation. The claimant may go to a doctor of his own choice and the insurance company pays his fee. The law provides a fixed value for each category of injury. Hearings are conducted before a legally appointed referee who makes all final decisions, including the fees which may be charged by the physicians and the lawyers involved.

Massachusetts has gone even further with new "no fault" legislation which declares that "negligence" is an outmoded concept and that society must provide workmen's compensation for disability from any cause. Claims not in excess of $3,000, for example, may be paid with little delay after a rather simplified arbitration proceeding. Larger claims are still processed through established channels as described above.

Some cases do go on to courtroom litigation and in these instances prompt action is a desideratum. Unfortunate and thus far unavoidable delays still occur to the detriment of all concerned. Some of these delays may be attributed to negligence lawyers who have lobbied against "no fault" compensation laws and may thereby have contributed to unnecessary crowding of court calendars. Of greater importance however are poor calendar practices, the lethargy of judges, and the use of the jury system in litigations.

Pure depressive reactions which have their onset following an accident, particularly when they occur in individuals with a history of previous episodes of endogenous depression, respond swiftly to antidepressant medication, etc. On the other hand, in many such depressive reactions there is an overlay of accident neurosis. Relief of depression in such instances may intensify the previously less conspicuous features of accident neurosis.

Although the statement has been made that accident neurosis tends to clear up without treatment, provided only that the financial claim has been settled, our understanding of the accident process suggests that we may at best succeed in clearing up a single episode by such an approach but we leave the patient, his family, and society vulnerable

636

to further episodes of disablement if we do not try for a more fundamental approach to the patient's needs.

BIBLIOGRAPHY

American Psychiatric Association. *Diagnostic and Statistic Manual of Mental Dis-
orders.* Washington, D. C.: American Psychiatric Association, 1968.
Fallik, A. The Social Background and Personality Pattern in Patients Developing
Post-Traumatic Compensation Neurosis. *Harefuah: J. Israel Med. Assn.*, 59,
140-143, 1960.
Fallik, A. Personal Communication.
Fenichel, O. *The Psychoanalytic Theory of Neurosis.* New York: W. W. Norton,
1945. Pp. 117-128.
Freud, S. *Civilization and Its Discontents.* Standard Ed., 21:59-145. London:
Hogarth Press, 1961.
Hirschfeld, A. H. and Behan, R. C. The Accident Process. 1: Etological Consider-
ations of Industrial Injuries. *J.A.M.A.*, *186*, 193-199, 1963a.
Hirschfeld, A. H. and Behan, R. C. The Accident Process. II: Toward More
Rational Treatment of Industrial Injuries. *J.A.M.A.*, *186*, 300-306, 1963b.
Klonoff, H. and Thomson, G. B. Epidemiology of Head Injuries in Adults: A
Pilot Study. *Can. Med. Assn. J.*, *100*, 235-241, 1969.
Linn, L. and Stein, M. H. Psychiatric Study of Blast Injuries of the Ear. *War
Med.*, *8*, 32-33, 1945.
Miller, C. R. and Butler, E. W. Anomia and Eunomia: A Methodological Eval-
uation of Srole's Anomia Scale. *Am. Soc. Rev.*, *31*, 400-406, 1966.
Miller, H. Accident Neurosis (Part I). *Br. Med. J.*, *1*, 919-925, 1961a.
Miller, H. Accident Neurosis (Part II), *Br. Med. J.*, *1*, 992-998, 1961b.
Miller, H. Mental Sequelae of Head Injury. *Proc. R. Soc. Med.*, *59*, 257-261, 1966.
Noy, P. Personal Communication, 1970.
Oppenheim, H. *Die Traumatischen Neurosen.* Berlin: Hirschwald, 1889.
Ostow, M. *The Psychology of Melancholy.* New York: Harper & Row, 1970.
Socarides, C. W. On Vengeance: The Desire to "Get Even." *J. Am. Psychoanal.
Assn.*, *14*, 356-375, 1966.
Wechsler, I. S. Trauma and the Nervous System. *J.A.M.A.*, *104*, 519-526, 1935.
Weinstein, E. A. and Kahn, R. L. *Denial of Illness*, Springfield, Ill.: Charles C
Thomas, 1955.

CHAPTER 20

SIMULATION AND MALINGERING IN RELATION TO INJURIES OF THE BRAIN AND SPINAL CORD

HENRY MILLER, M. D.

AND

NIALL CARTLIDGE, M. B.

Like Jones and Llewellyn (1917), we consider malingering to encompass all forms of fraud relating to matters of health. This includes firstly, the simulation of disease or disability which is not present; secondly, the much more common gross exaggeration of minor disability; and thirdly, the conscious and deliberate attribution, for personal advantage, of a disability to an injury or accident that did not in fact cause it. This last occurs more commonly when there is tangible organic disability: Fits from which the patient has knowingly suffered for many years may be attributed to minor head injury sustained in a recent accident.

Simulation and malingering receive remarkably little attention in psychiatric texts. Indeed the headings are omitted from the indices of several standard psychiatric textbooks. In instances in which the occurrence of malingering is accepted, the fact is not infrequently regarded by psychiatrists as evidence of mental illness, a situation which more than one judge has described as paradoxical. But if some psychiatrists deny the existence of malingering in the sense in which we have defined the term above, this is certainly not true of doctors and lawyers who are concerned with the conduct of claims for compensation on account of injury. Admittedly judges are reluctant to use the term 'malingering' in court, since it raises the spectre of perjury and a possibly awe-inspiring complication of the legal issue. In British courts the judge tends to listen to the evidence and, when this indicates simulation or gross exaggeration, to make his opinion clear in an award of derisory damages, rather than through a discussion of the difficult clinical, legal, and philosophical issues involved. The judge himself has probably had many years of common law practice and is well aware of the whole situation. Indeed, appreciation of the existence and frequency of simulation is to a very large extent a function of the particular experience of the observer. The clinician whose work has been exclusively or largely academic tends to be skeptical, while those with considerable medicolegal experience can have no doubt whatever that it frequently complicates injuries where compensation is involved. This situation is epitomized in the discussion which took place at the 1920 meeting of the American Neurological Association (Dana, 1920) where Charles Dana presented an excellent account of what he called *traumatic conduct disorders,* and expressed profound skepticism that they were other than consciously determined. During the subsequent discussion the opposite view was eloquently pleaded by Harvey Cushing, who suggested that despite the absence of physical signs, generalized complaints following head injury must be attributed to brain damage and that this was likely to lead to permanent intellectual and occupational disablement. In reading this fascinating discussion it seems possible that part of the difference of opinion arose from the fact that Dr. Cushing had more serious injuries partly in mind. On the other hand his attitude suggests that the circumstances of his clinical practice were such that he had hardly ever met the problem. The contributions of Francis Dercum, Bernard Sachs, and Foster Kennedy bespeak more personal experience and, in the view of the present writers, more realism. However, it is an interesting aspect of the continuing controversy in this field that exactly the same viewpoints found expression in a lively discussion of the same subject at the 1970 meeting of the Association of British Neurologists.

The first difficulty then is that some medical authorities and some expert witnesses are inclined to question the actual occurrence of medical simulation following head injury.

Secondly, many authors have made much of the distinction between conscious simulation or frank malingering and the unconscious (or semiconscious) simulation that, following Charcot and Freud, is widely supposed to be the basis of hysteria. Since, in the last resort, this distinction rests on the claimant's credibility and on the doctor's affirmation that he knows and understands accurately what is in the claimant's mind, and since the claimant is certainly aware that he is making a claim for financial compensation, it is not easy to know how much weight to attach to the contention or belief that he is utterly unaware of any connection between his claim and his behavior. If, as in most such cases, he is making a substantial claim on account of a minor injury, there is no conceivable reason why he should admit to the knowledge of such a connection, and very little reason for the doctor to accept at its face value his statement or implication that he has no such knowledge. The patient who simulates or grossly exaggerates is unlikely to tell the unvarnished truth about his disability. What is important is the context. Apart from occasional cases of pyschosis, medical simulation occurs only where it is hoped that it will yield personal economic or social gain. This is the nub of the matter, and unless the possibility of gain is clear the doctor should be very chary indeed of suspecting either malingering or hysteria. He should recall the aphorism of a distinguished British psychiatrist: "When the general physician speaks of hysteria send for the undertaker." On the other hand, it is the examiner's duty to search assiduously for the evidence of possible gain. In nearly all instances except those occurring in prisoners or military personnel, this is financial.

HISTORY

One of the earliest recorded references to malingering comes from the Old Testament — to prevent her father from finding a stolen idol hidden under the chair on which she was sitting, Rachel claimed that "the custom of women is upon me" and used this as an excuse from rising when he entered the room. Other historical references to malingering are quoted by Jones and Llewellyn (1917) and Huddleson (1932).

The syndromes following injuries to the brain and spinal column that were described in the early nineteenth century constitute the first serious recorded clinical interest in the simulation of disability in this context. Writing in 1836, Gavin emphasized that this problem rarely arose except in prisoners, sailors, and the military, for whom it clearly offered the only hope of escape from intolerable circumstances. Such cases have come within the armed service experience of many of those currently practicing neurology and neurosurgery, especially in time of war. In these circumstances great demands are made not only on those who were self-selected for a military career, but on many who were conscripted from the organized milieu of a comfortable civil life, not necessarily anywhere near military action, but into an unfamiliar and sometimes unfriendly environment.

The first world war gave rise to an extended literature, most of which

640

was published in the 1920s. As in many other medical and surgical contexts, the lessons had to be relearned by doctors practicing in the second world war, and again there was an extensive literature. However, in ordinary circumstances and in times of peace these military cases are rare, and fall within the experience of only a particular group of doctors. Simulation and accident neurosis following injuries to the head and the spinal cord on a large scale are in fact disorders of the Industrial Revolution. Attention was first directed to them in Prussia, where the introduction of a national railway system evoked the first accident insurance laws in 1871 and 1884. As early as 1879, Regler drew attention to the frequency with which malingering was encountered in civilians claiming severe disablement after minor industrial injury. He emphasized the importance of financial gain in the genesis of these syndromes, and an exactly similar situation arose a little later in Britain following the Employers Liability Act of 1880 and the Workmens Compensation Acts of 1898 and 1906. The epidemic of functional complaints that arose as a byproduct of this socially admirable legislation attracted the attention of many of the most eminent neurologists of the period including Oppenheim, Erb, Putnam, Dana, and Byrom Bramwell. In less sophisticated hands it led to the creation of a group of new syndromes such as "railway spine," which enjoyed a remarkable vogue for a few decades, until the courts tumbled to its nature and it promptly disappeared. The greater vogue of the emotively titled syndrome of "whiplash injury" in the courts of the United States than in those of Britain is perhaps analogous?

The increased mechanization and the consequent increase in industrial accidents in the twentieth century led to a heightened awareness of malingering. The literature of the early part of this century is clearly reviewed by Collie (1913). As a full-time medical examiner not only for the London County Council but also for a number of insurance companies, Collie accumulated a vast experience in the assessment of claims for disability resulting from injury, and his published work on the subject of malingering remains even today the clearest treatise ever published on the assessment of injury cases. Collie himself pointed out how much the introduction of legislation to aid patients injured in accidents had contributed to the apparent increase in the actual number of non-fatal accidents, and he emphasized that all unjust claims should be "sternly repressed," a viewpoint that is still valid.

Occasional short reviews on malingering have appeared since Collie, such as that of Garner (1939), but the literature of the last few years

641

has been more concerned with psychoneurotic reactions after trauma and their psychiatric explanations. Attempts to study experimental models of simulation (Anderson et al, 1959, Fromm et al, 1964) have not lent themselves to practical exploitation.

The Milroy Lectures of 1961 at the Royal College of Physicians of London (Miller, 1961) dealt extensively with the problem of accident neurosis, reviewing the literature and analyzing two groups of cases. The first of these comprised 200 consecutive cases of head injury referred for medicolegal examination, in which an attempt was made to identify factors associated with the incidence of pronounced functional complaints. The second group comprised 50 claimants with florid accident neurosis who were followed up after the settlement of their claims for financial compensation under common law. Accident neurosis was commoner in male than in female claimants, twice as common after industrial as after traffic accidents, and commoner in members of the lower social and occupational groups. It showed no significant age incidence, apart from the fact that it was not encountered in childhood. Its incidence was inversely proportional to the severity of injury sustained: it was very uncommon after severe head injury and frequent after trivial injuries. It bore no relation to any particularly alarming circumstances of the accident, and the earlier histories of patients affected showed an unexpectedly low incidence of predisposition to psychoneurosis. Not unnaturally this point was often claimed in court as evidence of the genuineness of their symptoms, though to the more sophisticated observer it is interpreted in exactly the opposite sense, so uncommon are disabling functional nervous systems in the middle-aged patient with a perfectly clear previous history, except in the presence of psychosis or severe organic disease. Other clinical features of these cases were the usual absence of objective physiological evidence of emotional disturbance; the absence of any change whatever in symptom pattern over many months or even a few years, without remission; and a complete lack of response to any form of treatment. Of the 50 cases of this kind followed up two years after settlement of their claims, only two remained disabled. In nearly all the remainder the symptoms had cleared up without treatment, irrespective of the outcome of the claim. Both claimants who were still incapacitated had received substantial cash awards under common law, but it is significant that both were still drawing weekly payments under the National Industrial Injury scheme. Indeed in one of the two the symptoms cleared up rapidly when a tough doctor terminated the payments.

642

Although the title of the Milroy lectures was Accident Neurosis, and the clinical analysis used objective parameters as far as possible, the writer does not disguise his skepticism about the unconsciousness of motivation in cases of this kind, and the percipient reader will observe he finds it impossible to distinguish the more florid cases from malingering. The belief that in accident neurosis the patient is in fact deceiving himself as well as hoping to deceive the observer seems a tenuous basis for the distinction.

When symptoms are entirely subjective, as is often the case after minor head injury, the distinction between malingering and "neurosis" rests in the last resort on the credibility of the witness. Only occasionally does an opportunity arise of detecting the malingerer in this context *in flagrante delictu*. One such personal case is worth recording.

A 30-year-old dock laborer referred from a distant city had been struck on the head by a piece of iron ore which fell from a ship 30 feet above his head. He remembered the event clearly and was never unconscious, but sustained a vertical scalp laceration which was sutured at a nearby hospital. He was not detained and returned to work the next day. Two hours later he complained of dizziness and left his job to report back to hospital and did not return to work. During the ensuing three weeks he developed symptoms of anxiety and depression and began to stammer. There was no past history of any form of speech difficulty. Three months after the onset of this symptom his general practitioner referred him to a psychiatrist, but his symptoms resisted a battery of psychotropic drugs. After five months' fruitless treatment on these lines he was given a course of electroconvulsive treatment — after which he promptly ceased to speak at all. At the time of examination he had not uttered for nearly two years.

Not only had the patient's loss of speech resisted expert surveillance by a private detective but it had also been investigated in a teaching hospital and by several psychiatrists. Diagnoses of "posttraumatic cerebral thrombosis", "hysteria", and "schizophrenia" had been made. His mutism had resisted Pentothal injection — but at the same time the hospital records revealed that a patient in the next bed had reported that he talked in his sleep! The last psychiatrist to report recommended his referral to "one of the societies for mutes." In not one of many successive psychiatric reports was the possibility of simulation so much as mentioned.

As can be imagined, examination presented considerable difficulty. The case was well-documented and the patient's wife most informative. His own contribution consisted of grimly nodding his head in affirmation or negation of questions put by written notes passed across the table. This he accomplished fluently and accurately. In this manner he registered complaints of frequent and repeated headaches, dizziness on change of posture, forgetfulness, and intermittent severe depression. None of these symptoms had shown the faintest improvement since very shortly after his injury.

643

Physical examination was entirely negative. The patient only once smiled wanly in response to a joke, and when he was asked the reason for his miserable appearance wrote that he couldn't laugh because of the intensity of his headache. He coughed loudly but would neither whisper nor make the faintest attempt to hum a tune.

From the beginning of this remarkable consultation it was difficult to escape the impression that the patient was malingering. He was tense, evasive, suspicious, and defensive — and his wife's attitude was exactly similar. The examiner's conviction that the patient was endeavoring to deceive was so strong that he telephoned a colleague and arranged for him to accompany the claimant unobserved on his main-line train to the Midlands. He exchanged his first remarks with his wife as the express crossed the Tyne bridge and by the time his companion left the train at Durham the whole compartment was engaged in uninhibited and cheerful conversation on matters of the day.

EPIDEMIOLOGY

The prominence of malingering as well as of gross functional complaints following injury is clearly related to the degree of development of the insurance and welfare services in different parts of the world. The British writer on this subject finds that most of his requests for reprints come from West Germany and Israel, and there can be no doubt that in these three countries the comprehensiveness of welfare coverage contributes to the incidence.

Under British conditions the patient's fitness for work is assessed initially by his general practitioner, who may find it impossible as well as unrewarding to afford sufficient time for scrupulous examination in minor cases. If the patient makes a claim for industrial injury to the Ministry of Social Security he is examined by a medical board of two more than averagely experienced practitioners, with access to radiological or specialist opinions when necessary. However, they are concerned solely with the assessment of disablement and its attributability to injury, and have no responsibility in the matter of the patient's return to work, a prerogative that still belongs to his own practitioner. Since the rate of injury and collateral benefits may not be much less than that of the weekly wage paid in low-level employment and may very occasionally be even a little more, it is hardly surprising that a few patients continue to complain of occupational incapacity long after it really exists. However, the termination of injury benefit by a further medical board, again if necessary supported by specialist assessment, often withdraws the financial crutch and the patient asks his doctor to sign him up as fit for work.

644

But where a claim is also made under common law for damages on account of the employer's negligence or failure to observe a statutory obligation, the scene is set for claims of much more long-continued disablement, even if injury benefit under the social security scheme has ceased or, more often, has been reduced to a minimal level. There is an average interval of two years before common law claims on account of industrial or traffic accidents are settled in British courts, and there can be no doubt that during this period a minority of claimants pretend to be much more severely disabled than is in fact the case. It is very difficult to assess the proportion of claimants in this class. However it is probably less than 15 percent of all those injured, or 30 percent of those who pursue extended common law claims.

Discussion with colleagues suggests that despite the absence of state industrial injury insurance in the United States, the situation is probably not much different, and that the high level of damages awarded by American courts is probably a contributory factor in this connection. The situation in Australia is if anything worse than in Britain, and one important reason for this is that Australian compensation claims are decided by a jury and not as in Britain by an experienced judge sitting alone. The West German situation is comparable with that in Britain. The French have had a reputation for greater realism in the medicolegal assessment of subjective claims and a greater reluctance to award damages unless objective evidence of disablement was present; however, the situation in France now seems little different from that in Britain and Germany. In Luxembourg (Muller, 1970) a rather unique situation prevails in that accident insurance furnishes what appears to be quixotically generous compensation – during the early months after his injury the claimant may receive compensation substantially in excess of his normal wages.

For obvious reasons the condition is less prominent in the underdeveloped countries. However, this is probably only a question of time. For example, the pursuit of exaggerated claims for compensation is a popular sport in the Middle East amongst the minority of Arabs who work for the great oil companies, and also amongst government employees in Indonesia who are the only members of the population of that country covered by sickness or injury insurance.

Simulation after injury to the nervous system is not encountered in children (though their parents sometimes try to persuade them into it) and is less common in women than in men. This applies even in comparable employment and even after traffic accidents. Although it is quite familiar in the young male it is even more conspicuous in the middle-aged man who has decided that it is no longer worthwhile to work, especially in jobs in which the outlook for advancement is bleak.

GENERAL CONSIDERATIONS

More often than not it is impossible to prove simulation even when it is strongly suspected. Confrontation rarely pays dividends in the form of an admission of pretence, and is hardly ever advisable. Nor is it often practicable to verify the disappearance of a visible disability when the claimant does not know he is under observation. In any case, much simulated disablement is entirely subjective.

The extreme difficulty of sustaining some fabricated disabilities is often quoted as an instance of the uniqueness of hysteria. But such disabilities are not always sustained even during the time the patient is under examination: the claimant stripped and instructed to walk will sometimes parade bizarre difficulties quite incompatible with the unremarkable gait that was evident as he entered the room. And the claimant with a severe limp or ataxic gait in the consulting room is sometimes seen walking firmly and normally in the street a few moments later. Is the grotesquely contorted hand that sometimes follows local injury sustained outside the examination room? The intensity of the muscle spasm that maintains this caricature of a peripheral nerve injury might persuade one to think so — except for the nicotine staining on the firmly approximated surfaces of the index and middle fingers — and a follow-up study (Miller, 1961) which shows that even this rather dramatic and extremely "hysteriform" contracture melts away after settlement of the case.

Why are unequivocal simulation, probable malingering, exaggeration of disablement, and "psychoneurotic" elaboration (the "functional overlay" so firmly ensconced in legal jargon), all so very much commoner after head injury — especially minor head injury — than after spinal injury? We believe that there are two main reasons. The first is that the layman has a pretty clear idea about his head and its contents, and some general information about head injury and its sequelae. Headaches, dizziness, and "blackouts," at least, come within his purview. By comparison he knows little or nothing about his spinal cord. He certainly does not know the neurological significance of precipitancy or hesitancy of micturition (or that they are usually associated with constipation), or of the sensation of a string tied round the great toe or the ankle, or of the unsteadiness in the dark that bespeaks posterior column damage. The most the patient with a back injury can manage is entire disappearance of forward flexion in the lumbar region, or painful limitation of movement in every direction in the cervical: occasionally the picture is enlivened by a wildly improbable ataxia inexplicably dissociated from other evidence of either cerebellar or proprioceptive dysfunction. But of course it is to Babinski that we really owe our relative immunity to faked spinal cord disability. The ease with which physical examination will detect a pre-symptomatic spinal lesion in early demyelinating disease is a fair index of its sensitivity, and there is rarely any difficulty in distinguishing between organic and bogus paraplegia in the very rare case of the latter that is encountered. Regrettably, the plantar response affords less help in the evaluation of post-concussional complaints or pseudo-dementia.

What are the factors that raise the examiner's index of suspicion in the matter of simulation? First, of course, the context must be appropriate and in this sense the context implies the claimant's hope of financial gain. Secondly, suspicion is aroused when severe, continued, and disproportionate disablement is claimed to follow trivial injury. Thirdly, the disability must be one that *can* be simulated. It is within our experience for a litigious physician to simulate an extensor plantar response, but this would be unlikely to apply in any other class of claimant. Fourthly, the simulated complaint rarely follows any organic pattern. The deep reflexes of the totally flaccid limb are normal, and the margin of pretended loss of sensation has a sharpness of definition quite incompatible with the overlap of dermatomes or peripheral sensory nerve distribution areas.

The claimant's attitude during examination is also often significant. A few are negativistic and some frankly hostile, but most show a defensive evasiveness that is rather characteristic. Sometimes a claimant asked to describe the accident will state that his lawyer advised him to give no information on this subject at all. Without a clinical history, examination of a case of this kind is a complete waste of time, and if the claimant maintains this attitude the fact should be recorded and the consultation terminated immediately. Very occasionally a patient is encountered of the kind described by Drews (1967) who sits down with a cheerful smirk on his face which is an open challenge to the examiner to try and outwit him. Unfortunately, an appearance of gloom so sustained and inspissated that it is clearly simulated is much more frequent.

One very common feature is a period of delay between the accident or injury and the onset of symptoms or of a neurological deficit. This was referred to by Charcot as the "period of meditation." He was of course referring to hysterical disability, but in our experience exactly the same applies in the case of frank simulation.

There are certain rules that are important to follow in the examination and assessment of these difficult cases. The first is that history-taking and physical examination must be thorough and scrupulously careful. It is not unknown for claimants of this kind to make accusations in court that the physician's examination was incomplete, and every finding should be carefully recorded in the case notes, which can be produced in court if need be. Furthermore, the examination must be conducted with complete detachment. It is not easy for the physician to escape some sense of irritation with a patient who is clearly attempting to deceive him, but any expression of such a feeling must be rigorously suppressed. Given a polite hearing a claimant will often press on until the evidence of faking is inescapable, whereas the faintest display of hostility or incredulity in the examiner's manner will put the patient on his guard and render further examination a waste of time. In all cases of this kind it is imperative to make every effort to obtain all the patient's previous medical records. Sometimes these will indicate that the disability long preceded the relevant accident, and that the patient who is claiming traumatic epilepsy, for example, had suffered fits for years before the accident, or that multiple psychiatric complaints were of similarly long duration. It is sound practice to keep printed forms in the examination room so that the claimant can sign an agreement that his records should be made available to the examiner. The occasional claimant's refusal to grant such permission may in itself be an important piece of evidence, and if the matter is considered sufficiently important the judge can usually subpoena the records when the case comes to court.

Over the course of years, a large number of elaborate tests have been evolved to detect medical fraud, perhaps especially in relation to the special senses. In our experience these are not particularly useful. Often they lead to fruitless technical argument between experts, and present the judge with insuperable difficulties of assessment. Wherever possible the methods used should be simple. It is more impressive to record that the patient whose legs had carried him into the consulting room claimed to be unable to raise his foot from the couch against the weight of the examiner's little finger (a very common sign in these cases) than to enter into a prolonged discussion about synergists and antagonists; or to describe the powerful grip that could be induced in a flaccid hand by strong persuasion, or by persuading the patient to grip with both hands with his forearms crossed.

It was stated at the beginning of this section that it is exceptional to be able to prove that the patient is malingering. It is also well known that there are genuine differences of opinion about the relation between malingering and hysteria. When the physician comes to formulate his considered opinion before the court these difficulties should be accepted, and the wise expert witness is one who can tell the judge first, that there is no physical disability remaining as a result of the relevant injury, and secondly that in his opinion any disability claimed is due either to hysteria or malingering. The honest witness must often admit that he cannot distinguish between these two conditions with certainty, but he can also add that he regards the difference as not very important since experience shows that whichever label is attached to the condition it is almost certain to clear up after settlement.

The remainder of this chapter will be devoted to a systematic account of clinical simulation as it is seen by the neurologist. We would stress that some of the conditions described are numerically rare, and that in our experience simulation, exaggeration, and wilfully false attribution of symptoms are most commonly encountered in certain familiar clinical syndromes – the post-concussional syndrome and its variants; blackouts; abnormal gaits; visual complaints of various kinds, amongst which asthenopia is the most prominent; speech disturbances; and anosmia. Commonest of all of course are subjective psychiatric complaints and here the decision of the court, like the opinion of the physician, rests in the last resort on the claimant's credibility.

CLINICAL FEATURES

Symptoms

Like pain at the site of any other trauma, headache of some degree is almost invariable after a scalp or head injury. Chronic persisting headache however poses difficult and sometimes insoluble diagnostic problems, and this is evident in the number of theories that have been proposed to account for headache of this kind following head injury (Jacobson, 1963). The organic nature of some posttraumatic headache is evident, such as that exacerbated by cold or tension in the neighbourhood of a painful scalp injury. However, tangible intracranial or extracranial pathology is hard to find in cases of chronic persistent headache unresponsive to analgesics, present throughout the working day, and claimed to be occupationally disabling. In some instances it may be related to tension in the muscles of the scalp and posterior cervical region, and such attribution is strengthened by a convincing history of emotional tension or depression, and by the presence of physiological concomitants of tension and anxiety.

Dizziness is another common symptom following head injury. True vertigo, probably labyrinthine in origin, is a common finding in the early days after cranial trauma and is accompanied by positional nystagmus of peripheral type. It rarely lasts for more than a matter of months at the most, and then disappears. On the other hand claimants for compensation examined months or years after head injury frequently complain of dizziness that is difficult to define or assess. It rarely has the characteristics of true vertigo. For example, the patient hardly ever complains of sudden dizziness immediately on turning over in bed. In most of these cases the symptoms are related to movements in the vertical plane. The patient will state that he feels dizzy on standing up after sitting, on bending down to tie his shoelaces, or on rising after doing so. The condition is one of 'swimminess' rather than of vertigo and is more suggestive of orthostatic hypotension than of any other physiological disturbance. Curiously enough, extensive studies have consistently failed to demonstrate any abnormality in the vasomotor control in such patients. In a large personal series of cases the response of blood pressure to the Valsalva maneuver has been consistently normal, and we have no real evidence as to whether this syndrome has any objective reality or any physiological basis. In our view the same applies to its more sophisticated variants which have been described by certain authors, e.g., the posterior sympathetic syndrome of Barré (see Hyslop, 1952). Although nystagmus can be produced experimentally by cutting upper cervical roots in animals (Biemond and De Jong, 1969), the clinical relevance of such observations remains uncertain. The cervical syndrome continues to excite interest in certain quarters (Compere,

1968), though the hypothesis that a syndrome of vestibular dysfunction can be caused by irritation of the sympathetic vertebral plexus remains entirely speculative. These patients are highly suggestible and one must be on one's guard not to persuade them by a series of leading questions into complaints that would never have occurred to them spontaneously.

Amongst other common complaints after head injury are lack of concentration, failure of memory, and emotional irritability. It is common experience that most patients who genuinely suffer intellectual impairment and emotional instability following serious brain damage make no such complaint spontaneously, and are indeed often prone to deny its existence in reply to direct questioning. However, the patient who is attempting to build up a case will promote symptoms that are common to all of us, such as being startled by a banging door or irritated by our children, to the status of a significant disability. Such complaints are again especially unconvincing in the absence of evidence of emotional disturbance and when, as often happens, the injury has been trivial. In our experience the situation in patients of this kind is often clarified by a transparent tendency to exaggerate other symptoms and dramatize trivialities.

The whole question of the post-concussional syndrome remains controversial. This syndrome of headache, postural dizziness, irritability, and failure of concentration is still regarded by some eminent authorities, following in the footsteps of Cushing, as a sign of organic brain damage. Such authors quote the massive cerebral demyelination that has been reported to follow very severe head injuries as a pointer to the kind of changes that might be found in milder forms after less severe trauma — though why demyelination should cause headache and postural dizziness rather than focal signs or definable intellectual impairment and emotional disinhibition is difficult to understand. What seems to us to cast doubt on the pathological basis of this syndrome is the fact that it is rarely prominent in the symptomatology of the patient who has had a serious head injury, and is often seen in its most florid and persistent form following trivial injury, sometimes without even transient loss of consciousness. It is a strange organic syndrome that is more frequent and more severe after minor than after major injury, so common in the medicolegal context and so very rare after injuries sustained in pursuit of sport.

Physical examination plays little part in the assessment of these symptomatic cases. Neither the lack of physical signs nor the presence

651

of minor findings is likely to sway the issue, nor are special investigations contributory. Evaluation depends on the clinical history and the patient's credibility, initially to the examining doctor and ultimately to the court of law. We must admit to a tendency to accept as real symptoms — however strange — that have followed serious injury, and to regard with some suspicion even banal symptoms that have persisted after injury so trivial that general experience suggests that the patient should have long since recovered.

Cranial Nerve Disorders

Disorders of Taste and Smell

Anosmia is well-known as a common sequel of head injury, and consequently is sometimes simulated. Such simulation is usually easy to detect. The patient who cannot smell oil of cloves and also claims to be unable to "smell" a strong ammonia solution despite lacrimation and facial grimacing is obviously bogus. However the view sometimes put forward in court that retention of taste in the presence of anosmia indicates simulation does not hold water. Especially the patient whose palate is unsophisticated may regard retention of the basic tastes of salt, sour, sweet and bitter as entirely adequate.

On the other hand, loss of sense of taste without anosmia immediately suggests simulation, and inconsistent results will usually be apparent on careful testing of various parts of the tongue with sugar, salt and vinegar solutions. Parosmia and similar qualitative changes in the sense of taste are subjective and inaccessible to examination. The best pointer to simulation in this connection is a histrionic over-reaction to testing and an emotionally loaded description of the complaints in striking contrast to the puzzlement that usually characterizes the subject of an organic defect of this kind.

Disorders of Vision

Visual disturbances are by far the commonest simulated syndromes related to the cranial nerves. A pretence of complete blindness is difficult to maintain and extremely rare. Unilateral blindness is somewhat more common especially in relation to injuries in the vicinity of the eye. When the optic fundus is normal and the pupillary reactions brisk in the "blind" eye, simulation is virtually certain. The determined malingerer may use mydriatics to dilate the pupil in the eye claimed to be blind, but a clue to this may be found in the tell-tale conjunctival injection that follows their use. The failure of such a dilated pupil to dilate further in a darkened room also strengthens the suspicion of artificial mydriasis.

A much commoner complaint is variable blurring of vision or asthenopia. It is claimed that print becomes blurred after reading a few lines, and this is accepted by the patient as a severe disablement. Often it probably represents inattention rather than visual defect and does not constitute a significant disability. It is of course a common complaint in psychoneurotic subjects without any history of injury at all. Another problem often encountered is that of the middle-aged patient who claims deterioration of vision after an injury but who requires nothing more than stronger glasses for a defect that has been brought to his notice during his search for symptoms. This is a common instance of false imputation.

The number of ingenious techniques that have been evolved for detecting simulated visual impairment illustrates the difficulties that can arise in this connection, but for the examiner without special training in ophthalmology simple tests are the best. If the patient's attitude suggests simulation, the simplest maneuver is to test the defective eye with a series of different test types, when even the determined simulator will find it difficult to maintain a consistent performance. More elaborate procedures should be left to the ophthalmologist. The tests used in such circumstances are well reviewed by Lasky (1941).

Complaints of visual field restriction are more uncommon in malingerers, and unlikely to be encountered except in those with some special knowledge. They are usually easily revealed by the patient's inability to vary his field defect appropriately in relation to the size or color of the object used. Simulated hemianopia is exceedingly rare, though an interesting case is recorded by Stewart, Randall, and Rieseman (1943). On the other hand, many patients who are trying to build up a case yield bizarre results on perimetry. Except for occasional cases of migraine, tubular vision is rarely, if ever, due to organic disease, and a gradual contraction of the field during testing indicates simulation which will be interpreted by the examiner either as hysteria or malingering, according to taste. The problems of ring scotomata after head injury (Strauss and Savitsky, 1934) have now been resolved and these are generally regarded as being due to fatigue.

Complaints of multiple visual images may be difficult to resolve.

Provided abnormality of the lens or retina can be definitively excluded, monocular diplopia is highly suggestive of simulation. The detection of simulated double vision in general is made easy by the fact that diplopia due to extraocular muscle paresis follows a distinct pattern to the extent that the images become further apart as the eyes move in the direction of the pull of the weak muscle. Patients who are simulating double vision can rarely fulfil this criterion and usually claim that diplopia is present in all directions.

A long-standing phoria may break down after any kind of stress and is not infrequently claimed as a sequel of injury. In the absence of gross cosmetic disorganisation of the orbit we regard claims concerning concomitant squints after head injury as cases of false imputation. We do not believe that paralysis of extraocular muscles can be simulated. Faked ptosis is most simply exposed by suddenly and without warning asking the patient to look at the ceiling. Involuntarily the lid rises with the upward gaze.

Other clinical problems arise from continuous pain in the eye, photophobia, and especially blepharospasm. Where expert opinion reveals no ophthalmic abnormality these symptoms are in our opinion usually simulated.

For further reviews and illustrative cases the reader is referred to Agatson (1944), McAlpine (1944), and Stefel (1964).

Disorders of Hearing

Tinnitus being entirely subjective is difficult to assess, and the disability it causes is determined more by the patient's reaction to it than by the condition itself. Even outside the medicolegal context, many patients find tinnitus extremely distressing and it sometimes seems to be a causal factor in endogenous depression. However, in our experience it rarely renders the patient unfit for work outside the medicolegal context. Whether or not deafness is present, it is impossible to sustain the view that tinnitus in a particular case is simulated. The most that can be said is that in some instances it leads to disproportionate claims of disablement.

It is very uncommon for total deafness to be simulated, and any such condition is usually easy to detect by simple means. A genuinely deaf patient watches the speaker's face carefully, usually turns his better ear towards him, and talks in a monotonous voice. It should be remembered that a clearly articulated whisper is more easily heard than loud but indistinct shouting, and that vowels are usually better heard than consonants. In only a very clever or practiced patient will careful testing yield findings of this kind in simulated deafness.

Unilateral deafness or impairment of hearing is much more commonly simulated, and it is important to remember that conductive as well as nerve deafness may be encountered after head injury. There seems to be no doubt that middle-ear deafness of long standing may be significantly exacerbated by a not very severe head injury. In some such cases the patient claims perfect hearing before the accident and although examination reveals chronic disease and the virtual certainty of some antecedent deafness, his false imputation may be entirely innocent. Organic nerve deafness is unilateral and a sequel of severe injury, but exacerbated conductive deafness is usually asymmetrically bilateral.

Thorough examination is extremely important. The external ear should be inspected to exclude an external meatus full of wax or a perforated drum. Although the Rinne and Weber tests do not rate high with otologists, if the results of these rough and ready tests are inconsistent the question of simulation arises, and such cases should be referred to an otologist for more sophisticated examination.

A proportion of malingerers are naive and of low intelligence. In these cases simulated deafness may sometimes be detected simply by distracting the patient's attention, e.g., by taking his pulse and then asking him in a low voice to put out his tongue.

Other tests are discussed at some length by Fowler and Altman (1966).

We find the most useful test to uncover simulated unilateral deafness to be the use of a double stethoscope with two bells and two earpieces into which the examiner can speak alternately and give commands to the patient. When blindfolded, most malingering patients will eventually make a mistake and answer a question put to the deaf ear.

The problems of conscious false imputation of long-standing ear symptoms are discussed by Collie, who stresses that the subject of long-standing deafness reacts very differently during interview from a person recently deafened.

Psychiatric Disorders

The simulation of gross psychiatric disorder is difficult to sustain except in those with special experience, since the layman's concept of insanity is very different from the true facts of mental illness. The simulated disorder is invariably bizarre, conforms to none of the familiar patterns of psychiatric illness, and is rarely encountered outside the context of serious crime.

The naivete of the claimant without psychiatric experience is almost equally evident in the patient whose post-concussional state is overloaded with florid psychoneurotic complaints. As already stated, these are banal and, although they represent an ignorant layman's idea of a nervous breakdown, they rarely add up to significant disablement.

On the strength of hospital records that describe coherent behavior on admission to hospital, patients are sometimes subsequently unjustly accused of exaggerating the duration of posttraumatic amnesia (PTA) in order to exaggerate the severity of their injury. In this connection two points should be borne in mind. The atmosphere of a casualty or admission department is not compatible with studious examination, and the minor disorders of behavior which bespeak posttraumatic automatism may easily be overlooked in the patient who can speak at all. Secondly, PTA shrinks with the passage of time and inconsistencies in the patient's assessment of it on successive visits is not incompatible with an honest story. In our view it is fairly uncommon for patients to simulate or to exaggerate posttraumatic amnesia. For some reason it is much commoner for them to suggest retrograde amnesia of a duration that strains credibility in view of the short duration of PTA. The extent to which a claimant is prepared to go is exemplified by the case of Dillon and Masani (1937), in which a patient claimed amnesia for an accident which in fact never took place.

Both amnesic fugue states and the Ganser syndrome (in which the patient answers simple questions in a manner that betrays knowledge of the true facts, e.g., that a cow has five legs) may be simulated after head injury in terms of the definition we have applied, but they are perhaps more appropriately treated in the chapter of this book that deals with psychiatric disorders. In our view the Ganser syndrome is undoubtedly an instance of simulation, but we would also suggest that it is often difficult to believe that the fugue is as genuinely amnesic as the patient claims. Its purpose is usually transparently obvious.

In other contexts the distinction between malingering and neurosis is usually easier than in the field under discussion, and indeed malingering is very uncommon in ordinary medical practice. Furthermore, in a neutral situation the patient's previous history of psychoneurosis, predisposition to neurosis, personal inadequacy, or a tendency to seek escape from situational difficulties by medical means is usually clearly apparent and lends force to the genuineness of the present psychoneurotic complaint. Unfortunately these considerations do not apply in accident neurosis, where many patients, even in middle life, claim disabling psychoneurotic disorder without the faintest hint of predisposition in their previous history (Miller 1961). This is often quoted by counsel for the claimant as evidence of the disastrous result of an injury sustained in a previously flawless and well-integrated personality. It has already been pointed out that to the physician with psychiatric experience it more often carries the opposite significance. However, the lack of clues in the past history makes distinction between psychoneurosis and malingering more difficult and sometimes frankly impossible.

The problems of false attribution of psychiatric syndromes are discussed at some length by Collie (1913). Here we would merely say that the attribution of general paresis, presenile dementia, or schizophrenia to head injury is usually bogus. Sometimes it may result from nothing more than a naive application of the *post hoc propter hoc* argument, but on other occasions careful enquiry including an examination of all the patient's previous medical records leaves no doubt whatever as to the preexistence of psychiatric disorder and little doubt that the claim represents a conscious attempt to defraud on the part of the patient, his family or his lawyers. When the head injury is severe it is easy to credit that it has made a real contribution to the provocation of one or other of these illnesses, but it does not cause them. With the possible exception of "normal-pressure" hydrocephalus (Adams, 1966), cerebral trauma – however severe – does not cause a progressive dementia, and in most such cases the injury has happened to a patient already the subject of early organic mental deterioration, which may indeed have been a factor in causing the accident. We have seen one case of frank schizophrenia which followed immediately and inexplicably on the traumatic delirium of a severe cerebral injury, but the situation was made clearer when we found the patient's brother was already a schizophrenic inmate of the mental hospital to which the injured boy was in due course admitted. Nor do we propose to discuss the issues raised by claims of precipitation of organic nervous disease by head injury and the sometimes fraudulent claims that can result. It is enough to say that trauma has been implicated at one time

657

or another in the pathogenesis of practically every organic neurological disorder, and that although there may be room for doubt about the contribution of material injury affecting the nervous system to the provocation of clinically latent nervous disease in some cases, hard evidence in this connection is difficult to come by, and judgment must depend on the assessment of the individual case. In multiple sclerosis, for example, evidence in a handful of cases suggests the possibility that trauma may provoke the onset of the chronic nervous disease (Miller 1964). However, the relationship is in the last resort speculative rather than established, and even in the writer's view is not one that could confidently be expected to hold water in a court of law. Much the same applies to many instances in which a stroke is claimed to have resulted from a previous head injury, and most instances in which organic nervous disease is attributed to trauma are even less likely. Whether the false imputation represents nothing more than a wish to believe what would be convenient for the claimant or his advocate, or whether it is truly fraudulent, must depend on all the circumstances in the particular case but, since neither the claimant nor his advocate posseesses the expert knowledge that would permit a truly critical assessment of the situation, it is our belief that the former is more frequently the case than the latter.

Blackouts

Outside neurological and neurosurgical circles it is insufficiently appreciated that traumatic epilepsy is the result of severe cerebral trauma and most often of open head injury with penetration of the dura. Some of the arguments that take place in courts of law on this subject indicate a profound ignorance of these facts even by those purporting to give expert evidence, and the simulation of epilepsy after minor head injury is not uncommon. Most often it is the *grand mal* seizure that is simulated. The occasional claimant is accommodating enough to demonstrate his attack in court, when the characteristic sequence of aura, cry, tonic, clonic, and comatose stages is conspicuous by its absence, the patient sinking to the floor theatrically and without injury, and then thrashing about moaning and groaning throughout the supposed clonic stage. The process is easily arrested by pressure on a supraorbital nerve, and the plantar and other reflexes of course remain normal. More often however the claim of blackouts is made without the examiner being given an opportunity to witness an attack and sometimes with the claim that there have at no time been witnesses. This is the common situation in simulated epilepsy. Fortunately, such claims are most often made by patients whose injury was so minor that it could not possibly have caused traumatic epilepsy. In cases in which injury has been more severe, diagnosis may be difficult, especially since the interval EEG is usually normal even in well-established traumatic epilepsy. Everything depends on the frequency and circumstances of the attacks and on the manner in which the patient presents his story. Difficulties arise especially where this presentation is unemotional. However, in simulated attacks sleep is rarely disturbed, injury virtually unknown, the time relationship irregular, the attacks unnaturally frequent and, except after repeated leading questions from a succession of examiners, sphincter control is unimpaired.

To the experienced observer simulated *grand mal* can usually be disentangled, and it is fortunate that few claimants are sufficiently expert to simulate minor temporal lobe epilepsy, the differentiation of which from primarily emotional disturbances may baffle even the trained observer who witnesses an attack. Fortunately, minor temporal lobe attacks are not very common after head injury, and true traumatic epilepsy most often comprises a major convulsion even if there is a focal onset.

The false attribution of epilepsy to head injury is almost certainly commoner than we imagine. No less than two out of the first 100 of a consecutive series of head injury subjected to prospective study in Newcastle suffered their injury during a first epileptic fit. Epilepsy is a common disorder. It predisposes the patient to injury of all kinds amongst which head injury is conspicuous. It is not surprising that some such patients seize the opportunity to dishonestly attribute the fits that follow their injury to this rather than to the known pre-existing condition.

The patient who claims that the frequency of his attacks has been increased by head injury presents a more difficult problem, particularly since he (or at the best other interested parties) is the only source of evidence with regard to the frequency with which the fits have occurred. There can be no doubt that the head injury is sometimes followed by a temporary increase or by a reduction in their frequency. Such random variations may well be entirely coincidental. In our experience there are only two situations in which a genuine increase in the frequency of fits seems to be authenticated. The first occurs when there has been severe injury, e.g., when there has been a posttraumatic amnesia of more than 12 hours, the second when there are genuine complicating emotional problems, especially of a depressive nature. Unless one or other of these criteria is fulfilled we are highly suspicious that such a claim is fraudulent.

Finally, we would refer the interested reader to an intriguing case of simulated status epilepticus described by Rowbotham (1964).

Involuntary Movements

Involuntary movements of organic origin following brain injury are extremely uncommon. Intention tremor is a rare sequel of severe head injury, and a parkinsonian state, usually without very conspicuous tremor, sometimes follows repeated head injuries as in the "punch drunk" syndrome. One clinical problem we have several times encountered is the attribution to hysteria or simulation of choreiform movements that have followed a not very severe head injury and which were in fact early manifestations of Huntington's chorea, and the cause of the clumsiness which resulted in the accident. In our experience this has been a not uncommon way in which the disease came to light and, unless careful past and family histories are obtained, the true nature of the lesion may be overlooked or regarded either as a hysterical or simulated sequel of the injury.

Except for the instances mentioned above, involuntary movements following head injury usually present little difficulty in diagnosis and attribution. Such movements usually comprise gross tremor, markedly accentuated by voluntary movements on command, but usually intermittent and, paradoxically, permitting the sufferer to light his cigarette without trouble and often even to pick up a small object from the examiner's desk with a steady hand. More bizarre movements such as those of chorea have occasionally been simulated (Sturton 1932) but such cases are very exceptional.

The onset of Parkinson's disease is practically always insidious, and the claim that it is a sequel of minor head injury is often made. A recent review (Sigwald and Jamet 1966) emphasizes the frequency and medicolegal importance of false imputation in this context.

Disturbances of Motor and Sensory
Function and Coordination

The simulation of gross deficits such as hemiplegia is uncommon, but minor complaints of localized weakness are frequent. It is an interesting instance of the naiveté of most claimants that their complaints of weakness after head injury are usually referred to the site of some coincidental local injury: the patient will attribute weakness in an injured arm or hand to brain damage.

Some clue to the simulated nature of motor weakness will be given by the absence of wasting, altered reflexes, or trophic changes, but the most important evidence is the marked variation in muscular power that occurs when attention is distracted. In many instances this is obvious, but on some occasions it may be necessary closely to observe muscle contraction during the testing of critical movements. When weakness of flexion of the elbow is simulated, simultaneous contraction of the triceps can be seen and felt when the movement is tested. This principle was described by Erben in 1930 and we have found it extremely valuable.

Clumsiness and unsteadiness of gait are frequently simulated. Sometimes this can be recognized by the patient's histrionic manner, and by the contrast between the remarkable clumsiness of his hands during examination and the ease with which he has removed his clothes while apparently unobserved. Routine testing of cerebellar function is equally informative. Few patients can produce an intention tremor that passes muster as organic, and when repeated alternating movements are tested they either perform remarkably well or produce a display so wild that if it were genuine it would make them unable to feed themselves.

Except in the occasional patient who can continuously sustain a caricature of gross cerebellar ataxia (significantly without any disturbance of speech or other compatible sign of cerebellar damage), simulated unsteadiness of gait is usually profound and unconvincing. Asked to walk once he is undressed such a patient who has entered the office with an almost normal stride will stagger wildly, roll about the room, clutch the examiner's coat, and sink threatrically to the ground. Some psychiatrists accept such behavior as hysterical, but its striking variation during examination hardly fulfils the criteria usually put forward for hysterical disability, and we consider that this syndrome is usually consciously simulated, a view that is supported by the frequency with which the patient is to be seen striding down the road unobserved at the end of the interview.

Except for the common complaint of pain, simulation of isolated

661

sensory disturbance is rare. As in the case of visual field changes, sensory defects are more often simulated on examination than the subject of spontaneous complaint. This often applies in the case of a limb claimed to be weak, and the common features of bogus loss of sensation – a sharply defined margin usually at the midline, total hemianesthesia involving the face as well as the trunk and limbs, or impairment of vibration sense on only one side of the skull are too familiar to require further discussion.

Speech Defects

The recrudescence of childhood stammer as a result of emotional stress is well known and was often encountered under military conditions. In our experience stammering or stuttering which is claimed to result from head injury without a previous history of a similar speech defect is rarely genuine. The simulated stammer usually disappears completely when conversation is animated or attention distracted, and the malingerer is also usually unaware that a genuine stammer disappears on singing, reciting, or whispering.

Simulated mutism is rare, though an example has been described earlier in this chapter. It is usually stated that dysphasia is hardly ever simulated, being too subtle a disability. However, the senior author has twice been deceived in this connection. In one instance a prosperous and intensely respectable middle-class woman presented a very good imitation dysphasia with which she had awakened three days after a minor head injury in a traffic accident, and which had been diagnosed by a very experienced neurologist as due to a cortical thrombosis probably provoked by the injury. The minimal lalling and variable hesitancy of speech was so convincing that it seemed quite impossible to exclude this contingency – until a private detective heard the patient's clarion call for tea and muffins ring out across a crowded tea-room within half an hour of the inconclusive consultation.

Simulated deaf-mutism has been described by Yealland (1918) and one bizarre case has been recorded in which the patient claimed inability to sing but had no associated disturbance of spoken speech (Smith & Solomon 1944).

Malingering and the Spinal Column

The relative infrequency with which spinal cord disability is simulated has already been discussed. Backache however is not only one of the most difficult and frustrating problems of clinical assessment in all circumstances, but it is easily simulated and very often exaggerated. Furthermore, minor degenerative x-ray changes are so common after middle life that the definitive exclusion of an organic origin for such symptoms is always difficult and sometimes impossible. Assessment demands a scrupulously careful case history and a meticulous technique of examination.

As with simulation in general, the patient's attitude to his disability and the willingness with which he accepts it as unquestionably incapacitating, the loaded account of his symptoms, his reaction to leading questions, and his impassioned denial of improvement or intervals of freedom may all arouse suspicion. The pain is often described with deliberate vagueness and overlaid with emotive adjectives. It rarely shows anything approaching an organic pattern. The malingerer's back pain, unlike that of disc prolapse, is provoked by spinal movement in any and every direction and not merely on flexion, and it is interesting that his leg pain never even approximates that of true sciatica. The bogus pain radiates down the whole of the limb and not down the hamstrings to the knees or the outer side of the foot. Physical examination is usually very informative. The patient who cannot bend forward more than 15° from the waist when standing will practically touch his toes when the examiner politely asks him to bend forward on the examination couch in the cause of pointless auscultation of the back of the chest. Unilateral spasm of the spinal muscles is rarely simulated. Passive straight leg raising is wildly variable, and often the patient claims inability to lift the outstretched leg against the weight of the examiner's little finger. Turning the patient on to his face may even shift the symptoms from one leg to the other.

Sphincter disturbance is rarely simulated. On the other hand impotence — about which the claimant is the only witness — is a common complaint. This is often loosely regarded as "psychogenic," but the philoprogenitive prowess of some of these patients even at the very time they are bitterly complaining of loss of sexual powers casts some doubt on the reality of the complaint. Strangely enough, the claimant himself rarely feels that the importance of his complaint is jeopardized by the fact that his wife has had two further children since its onset.

One recently established happy hunting ground for the seeker of financial compensation concerns the aggravation of preexisting cervical spondylosis. Since this condition is all but universal in the middle-aged and elderly male, since all of us are subject to minor injury from time to time, and since spondylosis can undoubtedly be aggravated by such injury, the frequency of such claims is hardly surprising. However the fact that most of us recover from such pain within a few days or a few weeks of such injury is bound to raise doubts as to the genuineness of those who confidently attribute years of disablement to the effect of fairly insignificant trauma. There can be no doubt that a severe flexion injury can cause rupture and prolapse of an intervertebral disc in the cervical region. It is inconceivable, however, that a single injury could actually cause generalized cervical spondylosis, and unlikely that minor trauma can do more than evoke temporary provocation or exacerbation of symptoms.

Other Defects

Scrutiny of the enormous literature reveals few syndromes that have not at one time or another been malingered in the cause of financial compensation. Even before the recent interest in so-called whiplash injuries, examples of simulated wryneck had been described by Gill (1929) and Schuttermayer (1938), while Vallet, Storme, and Guille (1961) described a unique case of prolonged simulated coma after head injury.

MALINGERING IN RELATION TO THE ACCIDENT

Most claimants who pretend or exaggerate disablement also exaggerate the severity of their accidents. They are usually unaware that the details are likely to be ventilated in court, and they often tell a blood-curdling story to the medical examiner. If he is wise he will invariably make it clear in his report that the account related is based entirely on the patient's description. Otherwise he may find that the credibility of the rest of his findings is jeopardized by his uncritical acceptance of the claimant's account of the accident itself. Sometimes the facts can be clarified by examination of the hospital case notes, but often judgment must be deferred until witnesses' statements are available. Occasional patients such as the one of Dillon and Masani (1937) have gone so far as to claim compensation for a fabricated accident for which they claim total amnesia, while a Munchausen patient familiar to many British neurologists has secured hospital admission on at least one occasion with an entirely simulated head injury (Blackwell, 1965).

FALSE ATTRIBUTION

In several sections of this chapter we have discussed some of the problems that may arise when patients attempt to relate long-standing disability to a recent injury. In some such instances this clearly falls into the category of malingering, as when a patient knowingly attributes preexisting epilepsy or deafness to recent head injury. On the other hand the universal tendency of patients to seek some kind of explanation for their symptoms must be remembered, and many quite honestly ascribe a multiplicity of unconnected symptoms to a recent accident even when no question of gain arises, and without any element of malingering. In such a case the continued pursuit of a claim after the patient has been competently informed that there can be no relation between his injury and his symptoms raises reservations about motivation. On the other hand, the adversary system of British justice at any rate is such that the claimant's lawyer often encourages him to press his case even in the face of medical evidence to the contrary, feeling that he must make out the strongest possible case for his client and often either shopping around in search of some sort of medical support for the dubious relationship, or endeavoring to trap the expert witness at the hearing into an admission that he cannot positively exclude such a possibility.

It is not easy to formulate rules to deal with situations of this kind, but one point should be remembered. There are no such words as "never" or "always" in medicine, and the expert witness is in court to give a carefully considered and reasoned opinion on the medical aspects of the case. In this connection the term "the balance of probabilities" is a useful one well understood by the judge, who is likely to be more impressed by an honest professional opinion couched in such terms than by the cocksure dogmatism of the more biased and usually less experienced "expert."

BIBLIOGRAPHY

Adams, R. D. Further Observations on Normal Pressure Hydrocephalus. *Proc. R. Soc. Med.*, *59*, 1135-1140, 1966.

Agatson, H. Ocular Malingering. *Arch. Ophthal.*, *31*, 223-231, 1944.

Anderson, E. W., Trethowan, W. H., Kenna, J. C. An Experimental Investigation of Simulation and Pseudo Dementia. *Acta. Psychiat. Neurol. Scand.*, Supp. *132*, 34, 1959.

Biemond, A., De Jong, J. M. B. V. On Cervical Nystagmus and Related Disorders. *Brain*, *92*, 437-458, 1969.

Blackwell, B. Malingering at Guy's. *Guy's Hosp. Rep.*, *114*, 257-277, 1965.

Collie, J. *Malingering and Feigned Sickness*. London: Edward Arnold, 1913.

Compere, W. E. Electronystagmographic Findings in Patients with "Whiplash" Injuries. *Laryngoscope*, *78*, 1226-1233, 1968.

Dana, C. L. Wounds of the Head and Compensation Law. *Arch. Neurol. Psych.*, *4*, 479-483, 1920.

Dillon, F., Masani, K. R. Psychosis or Malingering. *J. Ment. Sci.*, *83*, 15-24, 1937.

Drews, R. C. Organic Versus Functional Ocular Problems. International Opthalmology Clinics; *Annual Concepts in Neuro-opthalmology*, *7*, 665-705, 1967.

Fowler, E. P., Altman, F. Auditory and Vestibular Effects of Trauma to the Head. *J. Trauma*, *6*, 20-42, 1966.

Fromm, E., Sawyer, J., Rosenthal, V. Hypnotic Simulation of Organic Brain Damage. *J. Soc. Abnorm. Psychol.*, *69*, 482-492, 1964.

Garner, J. R. Malingering. *Am. J. Med. Jurisprud.*, *2*, 173-177, 1939.

Gill, A. W. Hysteria and the Workmans Compensation Act. *Lancet*, *1*, 811-814, 1929.

Huddleson, J. H. *Accidents, Neurosis and Compensation*. London: Baillière, Tindall and Cox, 1932.

Hyslop, G. Intra-cranial Circulatory Complications of Injuries to the Neck. *Bull. N.Y. Acad. Med.*, *28*, 729-738, 1952.

Jacobson, S. A. *The Post-traumatic Syndrome Following Head Jnjury*. Springfield. Ill.: Charles C Thomas, 1963.

Jones, A. B., Llewellyn, L. J. *Malingering or the Simulation of Disease*. London: W. Heinmann, 1917.

Lasky, M. A. Simulated Blindness. *Arch. Ophthal.*, *25*, 1038-1049, 1941.

McAlpine, P. T. Hysterical Visual Defects. *War Med.*, *6*, 129-132, 1944.

Miller, H. Accident Neurosis. *Br. Med. J.*, *1*, 919-925, 992-998, 1961.

Miller, H. Trauma and Multiple Sclerosis. *Lancet*, *1*, 848-850, 1964.

Muller G. E. Clinical Data, Electroencephalographic Study and Socio-economic Evolvement of 1925 Head Injury Cases. *Bull. Soc. Sci. Med. Lux.*, *107*, 7-39, 1970.

Rowbotham, G. F. *Acute Injuries of the Head,* 4th ed. Edinburgh and London: E. & S. Livingstone, 1964.

Schuttermayer, F. Psychogenic Torticollis Following Cranial Fracture. *Monatschr. F. Unfallh., 45,* 177-194, 1938.

Sigwald, J., Jamet, F. Injury and Parkinson's Syndrome. Nosological and Medico-legal Implications. *Ann. Med. Leg.* (Paris) *46,* 239-249, 1966.

Smith, H. W., Solomon, H. C. Traumatic Neuroses in Court. *Ann. Int. Med., 21,* 367-401, 1944.

Stefel, J. R. Monocular Hysterical Blindness. *Am. J. Psychiat., 121,* 393-395, 1964.

Stewart, S. G., Randall, G. C., Rieseman, F. R. Hysterical Homonymous Hemianopia with Hemiplegia and Hemianaesthesia. *War Med., 4,* 606-609, 1943.

Strauss, I., Savitsky, N. Head Injury - Neurologic and Psychiatric Aspects. *Arch. Neurol. Psychiat., 31,* 893-955, 1934.

Sturton, S. D. Hysterical Chorea and Catalepsy Following Trauma. *Clin. Med. J., 46,* 313-317, 1932.

Vallet, R., Storme, J. P.., Guille, M. C. A propos d'une grave névrose hystérique post traumatique. *Presse Med., 69,* 845-848, 1961.

Yealland, L. R. *Hysterical Disorders of Warfare.* London: Macmillan & Co., 1918.

CHAPTER 21

PATHOLOGY OF SPINAL CORD DAMAGE IN SPINAL INJURIES

J. TREVOR HUGHES, M. D.

INTRODUCTION

Our knowledge of spinal trauma extends back to the medical records of antiquity. In one of the earliest medical documents, the *Edwin Smith Surgical Papyrus*, dated 3000-2500 B.C., several "case reports" describe the clinical syndrome of spinal cord injury (Hughes, 1966). The works of Hippocrates, Celsus, and Paré all refer to the special significance of injury to the spinal cord. In the published literature throughout the following centuries isolated accounts were abundant but the study of the subject has always been stimulated by the battle casualties of major wars. The account of Otis (1870) made reference to 642 cases that occurred during the American Civil War. Following World War I the medical literature dealing with spinal injuries was extensive. There were British (Holmes, 1915; Thorburn, 1920-1921), French (Roussy and Lhermitte, 1918; Claude and Lhermitte, 1914-1915) and German (Foerster, 1929) accounts. World War II brought a spectacular change in the prognosis of spinal cord injuries (Guttmann, 1953) and in the postwar period the management of these cases continued to improve. Significant reports in the American literature concerning World War II injuries are those of Pool (1945) and Haynes (1946). Reference to spinal cord injuries incurred during the Korean War is included in a paper by Boshes, Zivin, and Tigay (1954).

The recent war in Vietnam further emphasized the problem of spinal injuries which constituted a significant proportion of serious battle casualties.

Three factors account for the need to care for an increasing number of civilian traumatic paraplegics in all developed countries.

Increased Trauma of Civilian Accidents

Hitherto, injuries involving the spinal cord were common only during wars and these were mainly caused by the trauma of high-velocity missiles. Only small numbers of this type of injury were sustained in civilian accidents and only in a few special occupations, such as mining, was there a particular hazard of spinal trauma. But today the increase in travel and also the speed of modern transport has resulted in an appalling rise in the number of road accidents associated with a degree of trauma formerly seen only on the battlefield. Despite attempts to reduce the number of road accidents, this rising trend is likely to continue.

Improved Prognosis of Severe Multiple Injuries

The results of the immediate treatment of casualties in severe traffic and other accidents have so improved during the past few years that today there are many survivors who have incurred multiple injuries involving the limbs, thorax, or abdomen which formerly would have been fatal. A notable advance is the speed with which an injured person is brought to a hospital with an accident service alerted to render emergency treatment of a high order. One consequence of this is that persons who have suffered spinal trauma together with other serious injuries now survive and the neurologic deficit eventually represents the most important residual disability.

Improved Prognosis of Spinal Injuries

World War II brought a spectacular improvement in the prognosis of patients with spinal cord injuries. This was due to experience gained with large numbers of cases and the successful policy of concentrating these cases in specialized paraplegic units. The change in the outlook of these patients has been remarkable. From the prospect of a lingering death after months of pressure sores and ascending urinary infection, the survival of paraplegics for several years is not only possible but expected in the large majority of cases. These patients may resume work, live a reasonably complete home and family life and participate in such sports as are permitted by their handicap. Paraplegics form a group, the general pathology of which still requires elucidation for the further understanding of their management. This study of the total body disturbance in chronic paraplegia presents a problem in addition to that of the local injury to the spinal cord.

Whilst many pathological features are common, irrespective of the nature of the injury, certain types of trauma recur and merit separate consideration.

Gross Trauma to the Spine and to the Spinal Cord

In many cases of spinal cord injury, there is a considerable degree of damage to the spine. Comminuted fractures are often combined with dislocation of vertebrae, resulting frequently in an unstable spine with a malaligned spinal canal. In this group of injuries the damage to the spinal cord may be very extensive; usually the spinal cord has been completely transected. The patient often has associated injuries that involve the thorax or abdomen and overshadow the spinal trauma in the initial period of treatment. Injuries from high-velocity missiles are frequently of this type.

Discrete Penetrating Wounds

Discrete lesions of the spinal cord are a feature of stab wounds which are usually inflicted with a knife or a similar type of weapon. As a rule the knife enters from behind and the spinal laminae deflect the blade so that the weapon penetrates the spinal canal lateral to the midline. Hemisection of the spinal cord is common but there may be a localized lesion of another variety, or there may be a complete cord transection. These cases have attracted considerable interest because the clear-cut nature of the lesion makes it possible to relate the neurologic deficit to the underlying pathology. The pathologic examination is easier than in the other categories of spinal trauma because there are no fractures or dislocations to explore and a conventional histologic examination of the spinal cord will yield a clear picture of the damage sustained.

Flexion Injury

Injuries in which there is forcible flexion of the spine are usually sustained in the cervical region and, as a clinical problem, are seen in young patients involved in severely traumatic accidents. There is often a wedge compression fracture of the vertebral body with an accompanying dislocation which may be bilateral and is usually associated with tearing of the capsular ligaments and of one or the other of the

670

longitudinal ligaments. Often one or more of the articular processes is fractured, giving rise to the familiar but not easily pictured fracture-dislocation. The upper part of the spine tends to move forward in relation to the lower component, the resulting malalignment narrowing the spinal canal. The spinal cord is pinched or crushed between the lower vertebral body and the neural arch of the vertebra above. These injuries are quite difficult to examine at necropsy and their demonstration by careful dissection is important when deciding which type of trauma has been sustained by the spine.

Rotational Injuries

Injuries of the spine commonly result from a combination of flexion and rotational forces. This type of injury usually occurs in the cervical region, giving rise to a unilateral dislocation or fracture-dislocation with rotational displacement of the two separated portions of the spine. This rotation occurs suddenly at the time of the injury, damaging the spinal cord severely, though subsequent roentgenograms of the spinal canal may disclose a fairly normal anatomical appearance. Identification of this type of rotational injury requires some experience with dissection of the spine. As in cases of flexion injury, the pathologist is interested in deducing the type of trauma sustained by the spine.

Compression Injuries

Injuries resulting from compression give rise to a different type of vertebral fracture or disc protrusion. Such lesions may occur in the cervical region (Fig. 1) but are more common in the lumbar area. The compressive force is exerted downward on the whole spine but its effect is often localized in the lumbar region. As a result of the downward force, the vertebral body bursts and bone fragments and disc material are suddenly extruded backwards into the spinal canal, damaging the spinal cord. The reason the bodies of the vertebrae are selectively affected may lie in the fact that in the lumbar region of the spine, the articular facets are deep and strong and less likely to fracture. These compression injuries are rare compared with other types of spinal trauma and require careful exposure of the spinal cord at necropsy for their demonstration. Frequently the pathological examination is made long after the occurrence of the trauma and then the mechanism of the damage must be assessed retrospectively.

671

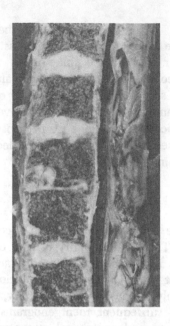

Fɪɢ. 1. Compression injury of the spine. Sagittal section of lower cervical spine. There has been backward herniation of disc material from the C6-C7 intervertebral disc space. The C6-C7 interspace is narrowed and some of the disc material has been displaced upwards as a Schmorl's node into the anterior part of C6 body.

Extension Injuries

The cervical spine is particularly liable to trauma from sudden forcible hyperextension (Fig. 2). This common type of injury may arise in various circumstances. An example is a motor car accident in which the driver or passenger strikes his forehead on the windshield. In some of these extension injuries the degree of damage suffered by the spine and the spinal cord seems out of proportion to the severity of the trauma (Fig. 3). One type of accident (Hughes and Brownell, 1963 a) involves a forward fall sustained by an elderly person with cervical spondylosis. This type of injury can occur with slight trauma and has also happened during the positioning of the patient's head in the course of certain operations (e.g., dental surgery) under general anesthesia. It has little in common with the other types of injury which are associated with much more severe trauma.

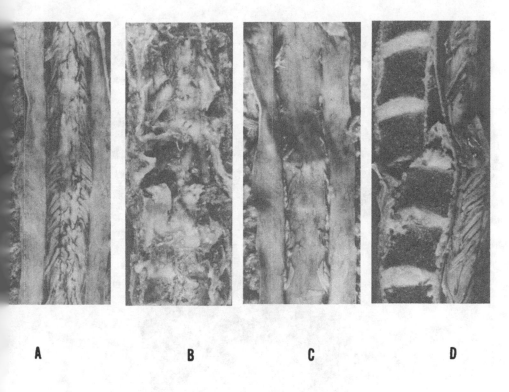

A   B   C   D

FIG. 2. Fracture-dislocation caused by acute hyper-extension of the cervical spine from a diving accident into a swimming pool. The four pictures (Figs. 2A, B, C, D) show the findings during dissection of the pathological specimen.

FIG. 2A. Cervical part of the spinal canal revealed by a posterior laminectomy and midline opening of the dura mater. The spinal cord is bruised at C5 segmental level where it has been pushed backwards (compare with Fig. 2D).

FIG. 2B. The undersurface of the cervical spinous processes and laminae removed at laminectomy *post morten*. Several fractures are present.

FIG. 2C. Cervical part of the spinal canal seen from the posterior aspect after opening of the dura mater and removal of the spinal cord. There is severe deformity caused by backward displacement of the spine below C3-4 intervertebral disc.

FIG. 2D. Sagittally sawn specimen with the spinal cord replaced in position. Note the disc tear at C3-4 and the displacement backwards of the lower part of the cervical spine. The spinal cord is crushed by the backward displacement of both the C3-4 disc material and the C4 vertebral body.

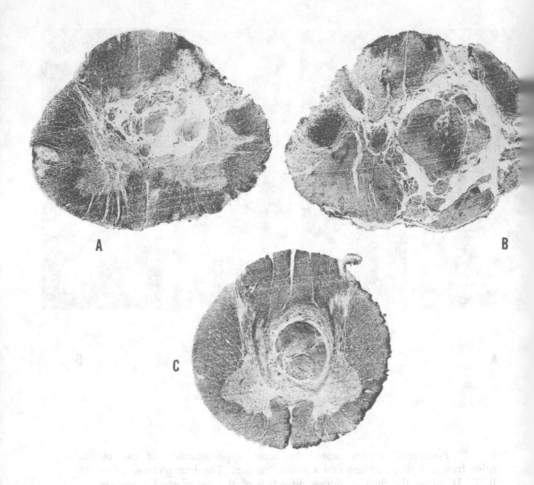

Fig. 3. Photomicrographs of transverse sections of spinal cord from case illustrated in Fig. 2. The three pictures show a region of cord damage in the form of a spindle ending above and below as round area in the posterior columns.
Fig. 3A. Transverse section at C6 segmental level. The upper tapering region of damage is seen as an irregular round area in the posterior columns (Weil, x 7).
Fig. 3B. Transverse section at C7 segmental level showing the segment which received the maximum damage (Weil, x 7).
Fig. 3C. Transverse section at C8 segmental level. Note the gap between the round plug of tissue and the cavity in the posterior columns (Weil, x 7).

PATHOLOGICAL CHANGES

Injury to the spinal cord involves simultaneously the meninges, the blood vessels, and the neural tissues. It is instructive to consider separately the effects of trauma on these different tissues.

674

Spinal Meninges

There is an important anatomical difference between the cerebral and the spinal meninges. The cerebral arachnoid is fairly closely applied to the pia to which it is attached by large numbers of trabeculae. The arachnoid does not pass into the cerebral sulci as does the pia mater but, over the surface of a cerebral gyrus, the two membranes are closely apposed. Because of this intimate contact, injuries of the cerebrum usually cause tearing of the arachnoid and of the pia simultaneously. Injuries of the cerebral dura mater may occur without disruption of the other two membranes.

The disposition of the meninges around the spinal cord is different. The arachnoid forms a loose investment with a capacious subarachnoid space separating it from the pia mater. Only a few arachnoidal trabeculae traverse this relatively large subarachnoid space. Because of this anatomical arrangement, trauma involving the spinal canal may damage the dura mater and the arachnoid simultaneously. Damage to the spinal pia mater usually coexists with damage to the spinal cord itself (Fig. 4).

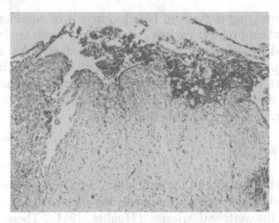

Fig. 4. Photomicrograph of a transverse section of the spinal cord from a case of acute cervical cord injury. The picture shows the posterior aspect where the pia mater is torn with bleeding into the peripheral part of the spinal cord (hematoxylin and eosin x 50).

Both the spinal dura mater and the arachnoid are very strong connective tissue membranes which resist anything less than severe trauma. In many spinal injuries in which one or more segments of the spinal cord are utterly destroyed and a complete transection is clinically evident, the dura and arachnoid remain intact. These membranes are

675

of course pierced by penetrating wounds made by a sharp instrument such as a knife, but even in this circumstance the weapon often penetrates the dura but is deflected from the arachnoid. Tearing of the dura will occur when there is gross trauma and particularly when there is a fracture dislocation and disruption of the intervertebral disc with extensive separation of the two parts of the spine. In this type of injury the arachnoid may also be torn but even here the mobility of the spinal cord in the canal may preserve its integrity.

There is a particular example of trauma to the spine which emphasizes the strength of the dura. Injury to the spine may occur at birth in the course of a breech extraction involving considerable traction and hyperextension of the cervical spine of the infant (Leventhal, 1960). This type of trauma has been studied in newborn cadaver specimens and it has been found that traction will lengthen the spinal column by 5 cm before the dura mater tears.

Spinal Vessels

The accompanying damage to blood vessels is of considerable importance in spinal cord injury. Various categories of vessels are involved and, to understand the effects of trauma, we must distinguish and consider the effects on four separate vascular elements: 1) the extra-spinal arteries such as the vertebral arteries and intercostal or lumbar spinal arteries; 2) the anterior and posterior spinal arteries; 3) the intramedullary arteries; and 4) the spinal veins.

Extra-spinal Arteries

Trauma to the aorta or to the subclavian artery can cause spinal cord infarction, but most cases of trauma to the blood supply of the spinal cord involve the vertebral arteries (Hughes, 1964). These arteries, ascending as they do in the vertebral foramina of the transverse processes of the upper six cervical vertebrae, are vulnerable to trauma. In my experience there has to be bilateral vertebral artery damage before there is spinal cord infarction. There may be effects on the brain stem and cerebellum and even the cerebrum, depending on the efficiency of the circle of Willis. Bilateral vertebral artery injury is often part of a much more extensive traumatic lesion affecting the spine and spinal cord. In these cases the effects of infarction are obscured by those referable to direct injury of the spinal cord.

676

Anterior and Posterior Spinal Arteries

Next to be considered are the three longitudinal vessels on which the detailed arterial supply to the spinal cord is based. The anterior spinal artery and, to a lesser extent, the two posterior spinal arteries are themselves dependent on a number of radicular tributaries, and obstruction of a major tributary may have an effect similar to that resulting from occlusion of the anterior spinal artery (Hughes and Macintyre, 1963). In this respect the largest tributary, called the artery of Adamkiewicz and usually accompanying the left ninth thoracic anterior nerve root, is the most important one. These remarks refer to damage to the spinal arteries with consequent infarction of the spinal cord. In cases of trauma to the spinal cord it is surprising how infrequently these particular arteries appear to be damaged. Even in gross spinal cord injury they are usually preserved, and in many of the pathological examinations at necropsy the anterior spinal artery and vein are the only anatomical structures that can be clearly recognized (Fig. 5). They are present and functioning to supply the scar tissue that is replacing a totally destroyed portion of spinal cord.

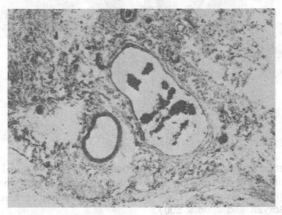

Fig. 5. Photomicrograph of transverse section (T1) of the spinal cord at the site of an old injury. The anterior spinal artery (left) and vein (right) can be recognized although no neurological structures have survived (Hematoxylin and eosin x 50).

Small Intramedullary Vessels

The arrangement of the small intramedullary vessels is complex and may best be understood when they are divided into two groups. Those

677

derived from the anterior spinal artery and entering by sulcal branches via the anterior median sulcus are called the centrifugal group of arteries. They supply the center of the cord except for the posterior columns. The second group arises from the small coronal vessels encircling the spinal cord and these penetrate radially into the cord for a short distance on its anterior and lateral aspects and for a longer distance posteriorly (Fig. 6). These vessels constitute the centripetal group of arteries. Mild grades of trauma to the spinal cord cause slight damage to these intramedullary arteries and capillaries with consequent bruising and swelling. Severe trauma tears these vessels and there is immediate extensive bleeding, disruption of tissue, and the formation of large hematomata. Organization of the hematomata is effected through the formation of new vessels and the appearance of fibroblasts. The vessels and fibroblasts form the connective tissue scar which is the late sequel of spinal cord injury.

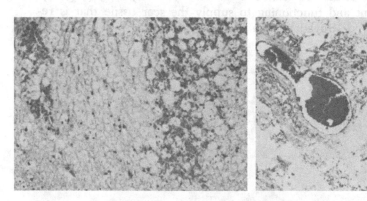

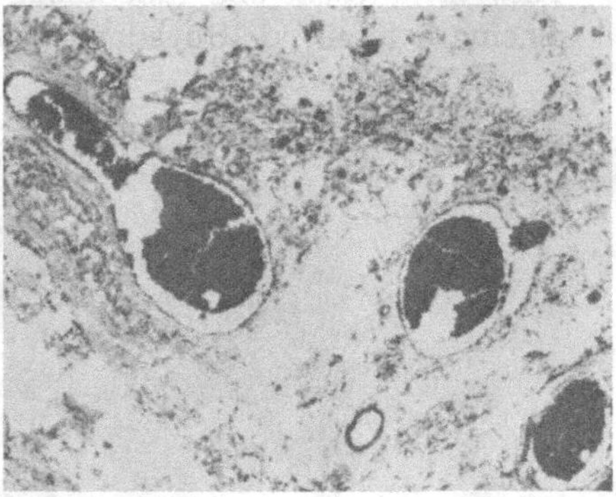

FIG. 6. Photomicrograph of transverse section (C7) of the spinal cord at the site of a recent injury. The picture shows the posterior columns where the penetrating vessels run downwards. There is bruising, perivascular hemorrhage, and edema (hematoxylin and eosin x 200).

FIG. 7. Photomicrograph of transverse section (T1) of the spinal cord at the site of an old injury. The picture shows the posterior spinal veins which are dilated and increased in number (hematoxylin and eosin x 50).

Spinal Veins

Any spinal cord trauma is accompanied by distention of the spinal veins. In slight contusion this may be only a distention of the normally existing venous plexus. But in severe trauma there is usually a great enlargement of the vascular channels of venous return (Fig. 7). The single posterior spinal vein normally present is frequently reduplicated several times by the opening of many longitudinal venous channels often placed posteriorly. The spinal cord injury is associated with venous stasis which is an important factor in the acute swelling of the spinal cord of which more will be said later.

Neural Tissues

The pathological state resulting from the effects of trauma on the various neural components of the spinal cord will depend on the time that has elapsed since the injury, and we shall consider the changes found in three stages — early, intermediate, and late.

Early Pathological Changes

We shall first consider the effects of injury on the spinal cord white matter and particularly on the long tracts. When mildly contused the axons show beading (Fig. 8), but following more severe trauma one finds lines of droplets of axonic material occupying the former position of the axon. If one examines the edge of the traumatized region, one may, in appropriate longitudinal sections, see terminal swellings on the ends of the torn axons (Fig. 9). These changes are present in cases of mild spinal cord trauma or on the edge of a severely traumatized cord. In cases of gross spinal cord contusion, using a silver stain, one can see only an amorphous collection of axonic fragments (Fig. 10). Accompanying the axonic damage are changes in the myelin. The alterations affecting the myelin range from mild swelling which can be seen only under high power magnification to complete fragmentation with abundant fatty droplets scattered throughout the axonic material.

In the grey matter, the cell bodies of the neurons show changes ranging in severity from complete disruption to central chromatolysis, the latter resulting from damage to axons (axonal reaction). This axonal reaction is uncommon and, when it is found, the case is usually one of mild spinal cord injury with severe damage to the anterior nerve roots. The common fracture-dislocation is very likely to damage nerve roots in this way.

The exudative changes that occur in the acute stage of spinal cord

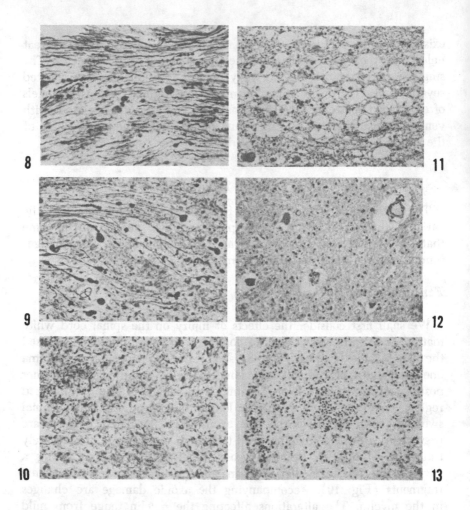

FIG. 8. Axon contusion during the acute phase of spinal cord injury. The photomicrograph is from a longitudinal section (stained by silver) of the posterior columns. Many of the axons show beading (Holmes, x 200).

FIG. 9. End bulbs of torn axons. Picture from longitudinal section of same case as in Fig. 8 (Holmes x 200).

FIG. 10. Axonic fragments seen in region of severe contusion of the spinal cord (Holmes x 200).

Fig. 11. Edema in spinal cord white matter during acute phase of spinal cord trauma (hematoxylin and eosin x 200).

Fig. 12. Edema in grey matter during acute phase of spinal cord trauma. Note the perivascular and perineuronal spaces (hematoxylin and eosin x 200).

FIG. 13. Polymorphonuclear leucocyte exudation during acute phase of spinal cord trauma (hematoxylin and eosin x 200).

injury are of considerable importance because it might be possible with treatment to modify them to some extent. These exudative changes consist of edema (Fig. 11, 12), extravasation of blood, and a cellular inflammatory reaction consisting mainly of polymorphonuclear leukocytes (Fig. 13) but with some lymphocytes and monocytes.

The edema is often very conspicuous. At the light microscope level it is revealed by the round spaces filled with fluid (Fig. 11) which appear in the grey matter as perineuronal spaces (Fig. 12). In mild trauma the edema is confined to the perineuronal and perivascular spaces. But more often we see a more severe state with huge round spaces, filled with fluid. From experimental studies we have learned a good deal about the ultrastructure of edema in the spinal cord. In this state of edema the myelinated fibres become widely separated by the fluid and there is a greatly distended extracellular space. The expansion of the extracellular space separates the myelinated fibres, the nonmyelinated fibres, and the glial processes. The fluid also forces the astrocytic processes away from their normal position around the blood vessels. The basement membranes become swollen with fluid and appear thickened and indistinct. This is the early stage of the edema phenomenon when the various membranes are still intact. Later, with the rupture of the membranes, the edema fluid becomes both intracellular and extracellular in location and, by this time, the glial cells have been irreversibly damaged and are degenerating. What happens to the myelin sheath in edema is extremely interesting. We know the structure of the central myelin sheath to be similar to the familiar myelin wrapping of peripheral nerve fibres. In some cases of edema the myelin sheath shows separation of the outer loop from the outer myelin lamella. The space between the major dense lines becomes widened and filled with fluid.

This edematous state of the acutely damaged spinal cord (Fig. 14) is of the greatest importance. The swelling enlarges the traumatized segment of cord which finally assumes the shape of a spindle. This spindle consists of a fusiform region of cord softening that affects several segments tapering above and below to end in a small round area usually situated in the posterior columns. This round area is a core of damaged tissue which has often been forced upwards and downwards by pressure. The fact that this is displaced tissue may be confirmed in histological sections which show a gap between the round plug of material and the surrounding structures. Such spindle formation always occurs following spinal cord trauma. The upper and lower limits are often precisely in the midline but they can be

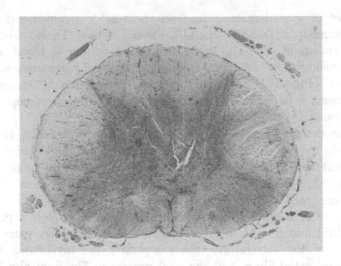

Fig. 14. Transverse section of spinal cord (C5) at site of acute injury where there is severe edematous swelling (hematoxylin and eosin x 7).

asymmetrically placed in one posterior column and are occasionally seen in the lateral white columns.

One of the lines of investigation directed to improve the prognosis of spinal cord injury is concerned with the problem of swelling of the spinal cord in the acute stage of injury. The cerebral shrinking methods using urea, mannitol, etc., have been tried without success. The majority opinion is not to decompress by a laminectomy and not to open the dura because this results in the violent extrusion of part of the softened cord.

Intermediate Pathological Changes

The intermediate changes begin after two or three weeks and proceed for two or more years. The pathological changes in this intermediate phase are sufficiently different from those in the early and late stages to merit separate description. The edema has now subsided and the smaller hemorrhages have been absorbed. The larger hemorrhages form cysts and these, if of any considerable longitudinal extent, have the configuration of a syrinx. This syrinx often forms a cavity replacing the hemorrhagic necrosis previously situated in the posterior columns. In the earlier stages the syrinx has no particular lining other that of damaged cord tissue but later there is often a glial and connective

682

tissue lining which sometimes forms a thick wall (Fig. 15). The interest in these syringes lies in the occasional development of posttraumatic syringomelia (Fig. 16), a complication which develops in a proportion

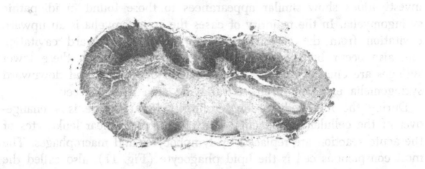

FIG. 15. Photomicrograph of transverse section of spinal cord (stained for myelin) at C3 segmental level above a spinal cord injury sustained several months earlier. Two thick-walled syringes are present (Weil x 7).

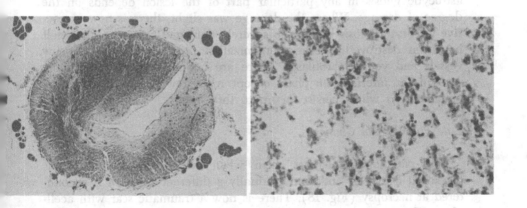

FIG. 16. Posttraumatic syringomyelia. Transverse section of spinal cord several segments above the site of an old injury. A posttraumatic syrinx has developed and in this case extended to the medulla (Weil x 6).

FIG. 17. Intermediate phase after spinal cord injury. Lipid phagocytes form the bulk of the cells present (hematoxylin and eosin x 200).

of cases of spinal cord injury. Long after the initial injury, and at a time when the neurologic deficit has been stable for many months, there are signs of an elevation of the level of cord damage. This can progress quite rapidly with an ascent of neurologic signs even to the medulla. The central part of the spinal cord is most affected and investigations show similar appearances to those found in idiopathic syringomyelia. In the majority of cases the syringomyelia is an upward cavitation from the original traumatic lesion. Downward cavitation can also occur but because of the existing cord lesion these lower syringes are clinically silent. A combination of upward and downward syringomelia extending from a traumatic area may be seen.

During the intermediate stage following injury there is a change-over of the cellular components. The polymorphonuclear leukocytes of the acute reaction are replaced by lymphocytes and macrophages. The most conspicuous cell is the lipid phagocyte (Fig. 17), also called the compound granular corpuscle, and these cells are seen wherever spinal cord necrosis has created breakdown products. They will cluster around small vessels forming rosette-like structures. In grossly damaged areas there are countless numbers of these cells but if the damage was slight there are only scattered lipid phagocytes. The presence of astrocytic gliosis in any particular part of the lesion depends on the degree of damage. Where the damage was slight, there is now a reactive astrocytic gliosis but in the severely damaged areas the glia itself has been destroyed and here organization proceeds by way of new vessels and young fibroblasts. There are no neuronal changes to be seen in the intermediate phase except for a few examples of central chromatolysis which persist for up to three years.

Late Pathological Changes

Late pathological changes occur when the survival period begins to exceed five years and then gradually a different situation is encountered at necropsy (Fig. 18). There is now a traumatic scar with acellular collagenous connective tissue uniting the meninges to the spinal canal and to the spinal cord. In this connective tissue scar the anatomical planes are often quite indistinct. The histological features can be demonstrated best by a connective tissue stain which will show that the grossly damaged part of the spinal cord has now been replaced by connective tissue. In place of what was once blood clot and necrotic spinal cord, there is now scar tissue. The less damaged portions of the spinal cord and invariably the region above and below the main

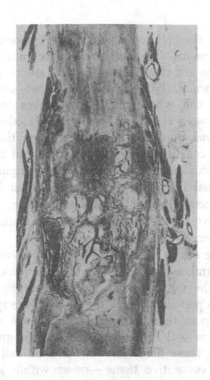

FIG. 18. Longitudinal section of a traumatic scar in the thoracic region of the spinal cord. The spinal injury was sustained many years before death. The center of the scar consists of connective tissue in which are ramifying peripheral-type nerve fibres growing from the posterior roots (hematoxylin and Van Gieson x 6).

site of damage show an intense astrocytic fibrous gliosis. The spindle-shaped region of cord damage is now filled with spongy glia; sometimes a syrinx has been formed. We also now see Wallerian degeneration in the long tracts of the spinal cord.

REGENERATION IN THE SPINAL CORD

An important aspect of the subject of spinal cord trauma concerns the controversial question of regeneration in the spinal cord (Windle, 1955). In discussing regeneration we must define precisely the neural structures we are considering. There is no evidence that a neuron cell body in the adult mammal can be replaced by a similar structure. There is also no evidence that a neuron originating in the central nervous system and terminating in the central nervous system (an

685

example would be the cell concerned in the spinocerebellar tracts) is regenerated after trauma. But there are two neurons which are susceptible to regeneration and these belong to a different anatomical category (Hughes and Brownell, 1963 b). Of these two neurons, the first is the anterior horn cell whose main axon leaves the spinal cord in the anterior spinal nerve root and then becomes clothed with peripheral nerve myelin derived from Schwann cells. When this axon is severed the parent neuron cell body still remains alive and the axon naturally will regrow. The situation is similar to that of peripheral nerve trauma except that in spinal injury the site of the trauma is near the spinal cord. When one discovers regrowth phenomena after spinal cord injury near the spinal nerve roots this should cause no more surprise than the regrowth of a severed peripheral nerve.

The second nerve cell to be considered is the posterior spinal ganglion neuron whose central and peripheral processes possessing a Schwann cell sheath have the same capacity of regenerating after trauma as have the axons in a peripheral nerve trunk. In severe spinal cord trauma it quite often happens that the spinal ganglia are not damaged and the central processes will regrow and may often grow into the scar of the spinal cord. These fibres have a Schwann cell sheath and they grow only within connective tissue — never within glia. This growth must not be confused with regeneration occurring within the spinal cord. These axons will grow into any area of connective tissue and it is not surprising that we find them within the connective tissue scar which has replaced the damaged spinal cord. They do not make any useful connections and they never merge into the central nervous fibres of the spinal cord.

The explanation of the failure of regeneration of the central nervous system is to be found in the sheath around the axon. If the axon has a Schwann cell sheath, regeneration can be expected. In axons without a Schwann cell sheath no regeneration has ever been proven histologically in any human necropsy specimen and the confusing findings that have been reported can be explained along the lines indicated here. Regeneration of central nervous fibres has not been proven in any experimental adult mammal but, again, the difficulties of interpretation referred to in descriptions of human pathology apply.

BIBLIOGRAPHY

Boshes, B., Zivin, L., and Tigay, E. L. Recent Methods of Management of Spinal Cord and Cauda Equina Injuries. Comparative Study of World War II and Korean Experiences. *Neurology*, 4, 690-704, 1954.

Claude, H. and Lhermitte, J. Etude clinique et anatome-pathologique de la commotion médullaire direct par projectiles de guerre. *Ann. Méd.*, 2, 479-506, 1914-1915.

Foerster, O. *Handbuch der Neurologie*. Ergänzungsband. Berlin: Springer, 1929.

Guttmann, L. *British History of the Second World War. Vol. Surgery.* London: H.M.S.O., 1953.

Haynes, W. G. Acute War Wounds of Spinal Cord; Analysis of 184 Cases. *Amer. J. Surg.*, 72, 424-433, 1946.

Holmes, G. The Goulstonian Lectures on Spinal Injuries of Warfare. *Br. Med. J.*, 2, 769-774, 1915.

Hughes, J. T. Vertebral Artery Insufficiency in Acute Cervical Spine Trauma. *Paraplegia*, 2, 2-14, 1964.

Hughes, J. T. *Pathology of the Spinal Cord.* London: Lloyd-Luke, 1966.

Hughes, J. T. and Brownell, B. Spinal-cord Damage from Hyperextension Injury in Cervical Spondylosis. *Lancet*, 1, 687-690, 1963 a.

Hughes, J. T. and Brownell, B. Aberrant Nerve Fibres Within the Spinal Cord. *J. Neurol. Neurosurg. Psychiat.*, 26, 528-534, 1963 b.

Hughes, J. T. and Macintyre, A. G. Spinal Cord Infarction Occurring during Thoraco-lumbar Sympathectomy. *J. Neurol. Neurosurg. Psychiat.*, 26, 418-421, 1963.

Leventhal, H. R. Birth Injuries of the Spinal Cord. *J. Paediat.*, 56, 447-453, 1960.

Otis, A. *Medical and Surgical History of the War of the Rebellion (1861-1865) Vol. 2.* Washington, D.C., U.S. Govt. Printing Office, 1870. P. 452.

Pool, J. L. Gunshot Wounds of Spine. Observations from an Evacuation Hospital. *Surg. Gynec. Obstet.*, 81, 617-622, 1945.

Roussy, J. and Lhermitte, J. *Blessures de la moelle et de la queue de cheval.* Paris: Masson, 1918.

Thornburn, W. The Pathology of Gunshot Wounds of the Spinal Cord. *Br. J. Surg.*, 8, 202-218, 1920-1921.

Windle, W. F. *Regeneration in the Central Nervous System.* Springfield, Ill.: Charles C Thomas, 1955.

687

CHAPTER 22

INJURIES OF THE VERTEBRAL COLUMN
AND SPINAL CORD

DAVID YASHON, M. D. AND ROBERT J. WHITE, M. D.

INTRODUCTION

Permanent paralysis as a result of accidental spinal injury during the prime of life is one of the most devastating occurrences which may befall a human being. In addition to its tragic effect on the patient, the resultant physical, psychologic, and financial burden severely taxes the resources of the family and the community. Spinal injuries result from accidents that are largely preventable and efforts to reduce their frequency and severity should be unremitting.

The automobile is a prime target with respect to prevention. Thus far, measures designed to lower the incidence of serious automobile injuries, do not, unfortunately, seem to have reduced the number of victims. In our experience, alcoholism is a major factor in many automobile accidents. More stringent laws, including more severe penalties, are required to cope with this problem. Rapid deceleration collisions that result in sudden flexion of the neck followed by hyperextension may cause severe spine injury irrespective of mechanical body restraints and cushioning of impact areas. In fact some observers are inclined to think that in this type of accident, chest and shoulder restraints increase the possibilities for cervical spine injury by allowing greater stress on the freely movable cervical spine and head. Properly positioned posterior head rests do limit hyperextension to some degree. Accidents involving motorcycles driven at high speeds on defective roads have frequently resulted in spinal injuries. Diving accidents are another common cause of spinal trauma. With proper precautions such mishaps could be minimized, if not altogether avoided. Unfortunately, however, the tempo of our modern mechanically minded and impatient society is such that these accidents will continue to occur and, very likely, even increase in frequency. No accurate figures reflecting the overall incidence of the increasing number of spinal injuries in the United States are available. Neither are there any hard statistics concerning the number of persons who develop neurologic dysfunction following spinal cord trauma, although it has been estimated that each year approximately 10,000 spinal cord injuries of sufficient severity to render one half of the victims paraplegic and the other half quadriplegic occur in this country. This appalling figure indicates the magnitude of the problem.

Because of the complexity of the problems presented by patients with spinal injuries, physicians responsible for their care must have an understanding of all facets of management. In recent decades advances in therapy have markedly increased the life expectancy of paraplegics. This chapter deals with the history, basic anatomy and physiology, diagnosis, therapy, complications and prognosis of spinal trauma for the purpose of presenting a broad perspective on the subject.

HISTORY

The earliest known medical writings include descriptions of trauma to the human spinal cord. In the famed Edwin Smith papyrus, a treatise on surgical therapy written about four thousand years ago, an unknown scribe faithfully set forth the symptomatology resulting from injuries of the cervical spinal cord (Breasted, 1930; Elsberg, 1931). Hippocrates discussed the nature of dislocation of vertebrae and its relation to paralysis of limbs but it is not clear that he was aware of the importance of the spinal cord in this respect (Markham, 1951). Celsus noted in his *De Medicina* that death follows quickly when the injury involves the spinal cord within the cervical vertebrae, indicating that by then some knowledge concerning the role of the spinal cord had been gained. A notable advance in the understanding of spinal injury was made by Galen who showed experimentally that transection of the spinal cord caused paralysis of motor and sensory function.

Although operative treatment of some spinal injuries was apparently advised and perhaps practiced in the early centuries, it is likely that the surgical procedures were merely superficial explorations. Manipulation of cervical vertebrae was not performed until

689

the middle of the 16th century when de l'Argelata [1531] described the reduction of a cervical fracture-dislocation by pressure applied to the point of angulation (Loeser, 1970). Paré undertook operations for the removal of depressed splinters of bone impinging on the spinal cord and nerve roots as early as 1549. In some dislocations he accomplished reduction by traction and manipulation through the use of a wooden frame. Thereafter the cause of operation upon the spine for traumatic disorders was advanced by other pioneer surgeons (Markham, 1951). Beginning in 1933, Crutchfield popularized the use of tongs for skeletal traction and this has remained an integral part of therapy in cervical spinal injury (Crutchfield, 1936). The history of skeletal traction in the treatment of cervical spine injuries is recounted in an article by Loeser (1970).

ANATOMY AND PHYSIOLOGY

A detailed account of the anatomy of the spinal cord is available in most neuroanatomy textbooks. In this chapter we will concentrate on the anatomic facts that are relevant to a consideration of spinal injury from a clinical standpoint.

The following data are useful in determining the level of cord damage. Significant disruption of cord segments C3-C5 invariably destroys the phrenic innervation, causing diaphragmatic paralysis and respiratory difficulty. Injury to the cervical or upper thoracic cord also affects respiration by abolishing intercostal muscular function. The C5 and C6 nerve roots supply the muscles concerned with abduction (deltoid, supraspinatus), external rotation (infraspinatus, teres minor), flexion of the elbow (biceps, brachialis), and supination of the forearm (biceps, brachioradialis). The C6-C7 roots serve the muscles that extend the elbow and wrist (triceps, wrist extensors) and pronate the forearm. Flexion of the wrist is a function of C7 and C8; C8 and T1 supply the small muscles of the hand (Table 1).

In general, a lesion between T10 and T12 will abolish the lower abdominal reflexes; in such a case Beevor's sign will be demonstrable because of contraction of the upper abdominal muscles and paralysis of the lower ones. A lesion of L1 is revealed by absence of the cremasteric reflex. Hip flexion is mediated by L1-L3 roots (Table 2), extension by L5-S2, while abduction is controlled by the L4-S1 motor segments. Extension of the knee (quadriceps) is mediated by L2-L4 roots; the patellar reflex is absent in lesions involving these segments

690

TABLE 1

Segmental Innervation of Muscles of the Upper Extremity
(modified after Bing, 1940)

MUSCLES	C-1	C-2	C-3	C-4	C-5	C-6	C-7	C-8	T-1
Sternomastoid	x	x	x	x					
Trapezius		x	x	x					
Levator Scapulae			x	x	x				
Diaphragm			x	x					
Teres Minor				x	x				
Supraspinatus				x	x				
Rhomboids				x	x				
Infraspinatus				x	x				
Deltoid					x	x			
Teres Major					x	x			
Biceps					x	x			
Brachialis					x	x			
Serratus Anterior					x	x	x		
Subscapularis					x	x	x	x	
Pectoralis Major					x	x	x	x	x
Pectoralis Minor						x	x	x	
Coracobrachialis					x	x			
Latissimus Dorsi						x	x	x	
Anconeus						x	x		
Triceps						x	x	x	
Brachioradialis					x	x			
Supinator					x	x			
Pronator Teres						x	x		
Ext. Carpi Radialis long. and brev.						x	x		
Flexor Carpi Ulnaris							x	x	x
Flexor Carpi Radialis						x	x	x	
Extensor Digitorum						x	x	x	
Extensor Carpi Ulnaris						x	x	x	
Extensor Indices						x	x	x	
Ext. Digiti Quinti						x	x	x	
Ext. Pollicis Longus						x	x	x	
Ext. Pollicis Brevis						x	x	x	
Abductor Pollicis Longus						x	x	x	
Palmaris Longus							x	x	x
Pronator Quadratus							x	x	x
Flexor Digitorum Sublimis							x	x	x
Flexor Digitorum Profundus							x	x	x
Flexor Pollicis Longus							x	x	x
Opponens Pollicis								x	x
Abductor Pollicis Brevis								x	x
Flexor Pollicis Brevis								x	x
Palmaris Brevis								x	x
Adductor Pollicis								x	x
Flexor Digiti Quinti								x	x
Abductor Digiti Quinti								x	x
Opponens Digiti Quinti								x	x
Interossei								x	x
Lumbricales							x	x	x

TABLE 2

Segmental Innervation of Muscles of the Lower Extremity
(modified after Bing, 1940)

MUSCLES	SEGMENTS OR ROOTS						
	L-1	L-2	L-3	L-4	L-5	S-1	S-2
Iliopsoas	x	x	x	x			
Gracilis		x	x	x			
Sartorius		x	x	x			
Pectineus		x	x	x			
Adductor Longus		x	x	x			
Adductor Brevis		x	x	x			
Adductor Minimus		x	x	x			
Quadratus Femoris		x	x	x			
Adductor Magnus		x	x	x	x		
Obdurator Externus		x	x	x			
Tensor Fasciae Latae				x	x	x	
Gluteus Medius				x	x	x	
Gluteus Minimus				x	x	x	
Quadriceps Femoris				x	x	x	x
Gemelli				x	x	x	x
Semitendinosus				x	x	x	x
Semimembranosus				x	x	x	x
Piriformis					x	x	x
Obdurator Internis					x	x	x
Biceps Femoris					x	x	x
Gluteus Maximus					x	x	x
Tibialis Anterior				x	x		
Popliteus				x	x	x	
Plantaris				x	x	x	
Peroneus Tertius				x	x	x	
Extensor Digitorum Longus				x	x	x	x
Abductor Hallucis				x	x		
Flexor Digitorum Brevis				x	x		
Flexor Hallucis Brevis				x	x		
Extensor Hallucis Brevis				x	x		
Flexor Digitorum Longus				x	x	x	
Peroneus Longus				x	x	x	
Peroneus Brevis				x	x	x	
Tibialis Posterior				x	x	x	
Flexor Hallucis Longus				x	x	x	
Extensor Hallucis Longus				x	x	x	
Soleus				x	x	x	
Gastrocnemius						x	x
Extensor Digitorum Brevis						x	x
Flexor Digitorum Accessorius						x	x
Adductor Hallucis						x	x
Abductor Digiti Quinti						x	x
Flexor Digiti Quinti Brevis						x	x
Interossei						x	x
Lumbricales				x	x	x	x

or roots. The flexors of the knee are controlled by L4-S2. Adduction of the hip is mediated by L2-L4. Dorsiflexion and eversion of the foot and extension of the toes are dependent on L5-S1. Inversion of the foot is a function of L4-L5. Plantar flexion of the ankle, flexion of the toes, as well as contraction of the small muscles of the foot, are mediated by S1 and S2. The perianal muscles are innervated by S3-S5. A lesion of S1 or S2 will depress or abolish the ipsilateral Achilles reflex. Lesions of the conus medullaris and cauda equina cause a flaccid paralysis. Since the cauda equina hangs loosely in the thecal

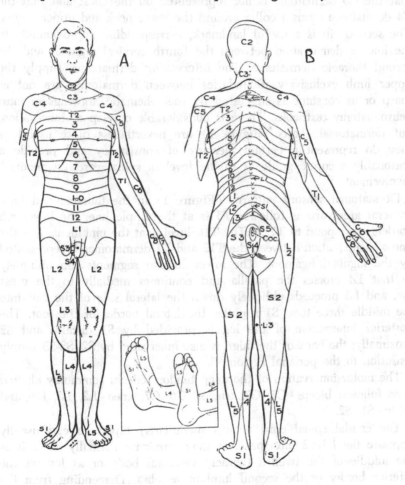

Fig. 1. Segmental innervation of the skin. (Scarff, 1960, after O. Foerster).

693

sac, a lesion at this level by sparing some roots while involving others may be manifested clinically by an erratic anatomic distribution.

With regard to sensory innervation (Figure 1), the shoulder and upper arm are supplied by C5 and C6, the radial side of the arm and hand by C6, the index and middle fingers by C7, and the ulnar portion of the hand by C8. The medial aspect of the upper limb above the hand is innervated distally by the T1 segment and proximally (including the axilla) by T1 and T2. It is important to remember that the C5 dermatome is not represented on the chest and that the C4 dermatome forms a collar around the lower neck and upper thorax. The second rib is a useful landmark, corresponding approximately to the line of demarcation between the fourth cervical segment and the second thoracic dermatome. The intervening dermatomes supply the upper limb exclusively. Boundaries between dermatomes are not as sharp or as constant as suggested by the schematic drawings in most neuroanatomy textbooks. There is considerable overlap of innervation, but dermatomal charts (Figure 1) are nevertheless quite useful as they do represent a certain measure of consistency and provide a reasonably accurate guide as to the level of spinal cord (segmental) involvement.

Dermatomal sensory patterns (Figure 1) in the thoracic and lumbosacral areas are as follows: T5 is at the nipple line; the lower rib borders correspond to T7, 8. The T10 level is at the umbilicus; and the line of demarcation between the T12 and L1 dermatomes is represented by the inguinal ligament. The lower lumbar segments run obliquely so that L4 crosses the patella and continues medially to the great toe, and L5 proceeds obliquely down the lateral side of the calf into the middle three toes. S1 supplies the lateral border of the foot. The posterior innervation of the leg is provided by S1 distally and S2 proximally; the back of the thigh is also innervated by S2. S3-S5 supply sensation to the perianal region.

The motor innervation of the deep tendon reflexes commonly elicited is as follows: biceps - C5, C6; triceps - C6, C7; knee - L2, L3, L4; and ankle - S1, S2.

The caudal spinal cord (conus medullaris) tapers to end usually opposite the L1-L2 interspace. It may terminate normally as high as the middle of the twelfth thoracic vertebral body or as low as the inferior border of the second lumbar vertebra. Descending from the tapered end of the conus medullaris is the filum terminale. This fibrous non-neural structure attaches to the dorsum of the coccyx after

694

penetrating the dura. The anterior and posterior roots of the cauda equina are derived from the conus and lie loosely in the thecal sac.

The relation of the spinal cord segments to the vertebral bodies is of some practical importance (Figure 2). The eighth cervical cord segment is located between the bodies of C6 and C7. The T12 spinal segment is usually located at a level corresponding approximately to the body of the tenth thoracic vertebra. In the thoracic spine a given spinal cord segment is generally located one and one-half to two vertebral bodies higher than its numerically equivalent vertebral

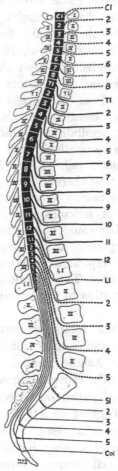

FIG. 2. Alignment of spinal cord segments, vertebral bodies, and spinous processes. The body and spinous processes are indicated by Roman numerals, the spinal segments and nerves by Arabic. (From Scarff, 1960).

695

bony counterpart. In the clinical diagnosis of a thoracic lesion this should be taken into account for anatomic localization. Below L1 the spinal segments of the conus are in close apposition and it is impractical to attempt to relate them to their corresponding vertebral levels. The L1 vertebra can be differentiated from that of T12 by the sharp tip of the spinous process of the latter as opposed to the blunt spinous process of the former.

A surgical landmark of value in most patients is the lowest dentate ligament which is crossed by the posterior root of L1 (Elsberg, 1912). This may be employed as a guide when it is necessary to identify roots of the cauda equina. Another useful anatomic structure is the first sacral anterior root which is usually the largest one arising from the conus medullaris (MacDonald et al, 1946).

Regarding sensory transmission within the spinal cord, the anterolateral tracts convey pain and temperature sensation and, to a lesser extent, impulses perceived as pressure and touch. The posterior columns transmit gnostic sensation — touch, pressure, vibration and muscle, tendon and joint sensibility (position sense).

Serious disturbances in respiration result from lesions of segments C3-C5 that involve the motor cells of the phrenic nerves. Destruction of these cells or their outgoing fibers leads to paralysis of the diaphragm while irritation induced by nearby lesions results in hiccough, dyspnea, and coughing. Affection of reticulospinal fibers from the medullary respiratory center is another cause of respiratory distress. These fibers constitute the major component of the respiratory pathway and are concerned with automatic respiration. Voluntary respiration is mediated by the lateral pyramidal tract. The reticulospinal pathway is probably a diffuse one, medial in location to the lateral spinothalamic and lateral corticospinal tracts.

In our experience, earliest return of sensation is signalled by the interpretation as touch of stimuli that ordinarily cause deep pain. For example, pressure on the Achilles tendon, great toe, or tibia of a degree that would ordinarily cause disagreeable deep pain is experienced by the cord-injured patient as a feeling of touch or pressure, which he tolerates well. Tugging on a Foley catheter inserted into the bladder causes deep pain or at least a sensation of touch and, on occasion, is the only sign of sensory function that remains following injury. Early motor fuctional return is revealed by barely discernible muscle contractions best palpated rather than observed. Electromyographic evidence of volitional motor units verifies this impression.

The Brown-Séquard syndrome is caused by a lesion that involves a lateral half of the spinal cord over one or more segments. In cases of trauma it occurs following hemisection of the cord — most commonly as a result of a knife wound (Lipschitz, 1967). At the level of the lesion there is an ipsilateral segmental lower motor neuron paralysis as well as complete sensory loss in the corresponding dermatomic area. Below the level of the lesion, on the same side, destruction of the descending motor fibers causes a variable loss of voluntary motion, increased tone, increase of the deep reflexes, absence of superficial reflexes, and a positive Babinski toe sign. With regard to sensory signs, analgesia and thermoanesthesia are demonstrable a few segments below the lesion on the opposite side. The discrepancy in levels corresponds to the distance that fibers transmitting sensations of pain and temperature ascend on the same side of the cord prior to crossing, which is usually two to four segments. Tactile sensibility is usually, but not always, intact, because of the many crossed as well as uncrossed fibers subserving this modality. Perception of vibration and muscle and joint sensibility are impaired on the ipsilateral side below the lesion. The classic picture of hemisection is rare but partial syndromes are common.

Fibers comprising the corticospinal tract originate in the cerebral cortex, most of them from the precentral area (Jane et al, 1967). The fibers course downward through the brain and brain stem and upon reaching the lower end of the medulla oblongata, 80 percent cross the midline forming the pyramidal tract. At each spinal segmental level, almost to the very end of the spinal cord, fibers from the tract synapse either with interneurons at the base of the posterior horn or with motor neurons of the anterior horn. About 20 percent of corticospinal fibers do not cross in the pyramidal decussation. Instead, they proceed directly down the cord ipsilateral to their site of origin. Some of these fibers course downward in the anterior column of the cord and others descend in the lateral column of the cord. These fibers then cross at approximately the level of the segments they innervate and synapse either with interneurons or anterior horn cells.

In order to distinguish between radicular paralysis of a segmental nature and peripheral nerve paralysis, it is necessary to keep in mind the pattern of peripheral nerve innervation as well as segmental innervation (Tables 1, 2). If muscles supplied by the same peripheral nerve are affected, the site of the lesion must be peripheral in the nerve. On the other hand, if there is partial or complete paralysis of a group of muscles, each with the same radicular innervation, the lesion must then be located at the anterior root level or in the spinal cord. The same kind of reasoning applies when diagnosing the level of brachial plexus injuries.

The anterior spinal artery which supplies the anterior two-thirds of the cord originates from intracranial branches of both vertebral arteries and is fed by anterior radicular branches emanating from the vertebral, subclavian, intercostal, and lumbar arteries as one proceeds caudally. The first four thoracic segments are most vulnerable to ischemic change as a result of damage to either the anterior spinal artery or its tributaries. This is due to poor collateral circulation in this area. The communicating branches which enter the vertebral canal with the anterior spinal roots contribute significantly to the circulation of the spinal cord, especially the artery of Adamkiewicz which accompanies one of the lower thoracic or upper lumbar anterior roots, most often on the left side. The paired posterior spinal arteries, which are actually one plexiform channel, generally supply the posterior (dorsal) one-third of the cord and communicate with the anterior spinal artery by way of numerous arterial coronae. In the cervical cord the posterior spinal arteries are formed by inconstant branches of the posterior inferior cerebellar or vertebral arteries. In the thoracic cord compromise of the spinal arterial supply may give rise to clinical evidence of a level above the actual site of the lesion due to proximal (cephalic) ischemia particularly in the watershed between T1 and T4.

The state of complete motor paralysis, flaccidity, and areflexia below the site of the lesion following acute spinal cord transection is known as "spinal shock." It bears no relation to surgical shock. Spinal shock also occurs temporarily following atraumatic functional dissolution of the continuity of the cord as by cooling or injecting procaine. Following recovery from spinal shock, another transection just below the site of the original lesion produces no flaccidity.

Spinal transection suddenly interrupts all descending pathways which influence spinal reflexes either by facilitation or inhibition. Monosynaptic segmental reflexes are normally influenced to a considerable extent by descending suprasegmental impulses and undergo an abrupt change in reactivity when deprived of these influences. In lower animals the vestibulospinal and reticulospinal tracts are thought to convey "shock preventing" impulses; in man corticospinal connections play a more important role in this respect.

In addition to paralysis and loss of the deep tendon and superficial reflexes, perception of sensation and autonomic function are abolished below the site of transection. The bladder and bowel are paralyzed with resultant urinary retention, ileus, and meteorism. Owing to lack of vasomotor control, the blood pressure falls temporarily. Sweat secretion is absent below the lesion. In man the period of spinal shock varies from days to weeks. It is generally agreed that the intensity and duration of spinal shock increase as one ascends the evolutionary scale, especially in primates. The state of spinal shock may be prolonged as a result of toxic and septic conditions.

The first movements to return following a period of areflexia are withdrawal movements in response to plantar stimulation, dorsiflexion of the big toe (the sign of Babinski), and anal and bulbocavernosus reflexes. In the later stages the withdrawal response becomes more vigorous and can be elicited by a minimal stimulus applied to the lower extremities. In spinal cord transection above T5 both abdominal and cremasteric reflexes are almost always lost. Occasionally in cases of complete lesions these reflexes, although diminished and readily exhaustible, may be elicited during the subacute and chronic stages.

Following recovery from spinal shock, reflex activity returns and, eventually, in many cases withdrawal movements accompanied by excessive visceral autonomic discharge appear. In such cases, plantar stimulation of the foot may evoke violent withdrawal of the lower extremities, profuse sweating, and evacuation of the bladder and bowel. This reaction is termed a mass reflex, and is indicative of automatic activity of the isolated segment of spinal cord. Mass movements of this nature are very distressing to patients and, as will be pointed out later, frequently require neurosurgical intervention. It was formerly believed that extensor hypertonus (paraplegia in extension) as opposed to increased flexor tone (paraplegia in flexion), beginning soon after transection, indicated that the spinal cord was not completely severed and that some degree of functional recovery might occur. This was not borne out by experience gained in World War II when it was found that paraplegia in extension may occur following complete transection. The order of recovery of the spinal reflexes following trauma varies and, in cases of complete transection, extensor movements of the paraplegic limbs may be observed following a period of flexor activity (Kuhn, 1950; Guttmann, 1969). Generally increased tone appears sooner in incomplete than in complete lesions. In the chronic phase of spinal injury, crossed reflexes occur as a result of heightened reflex activity of the isolated spinal cord. Such crossed reflexes may also occur in cases of incomplete lesions. The most common crossed reflex resulting from plantar stimulation of the foot is the extensor thrust of the contralateral leg involving contraction of the adductors, quadriceps, and hip extensors, together with plantar flexion of the foot and toes (Philippson's reflex) (Ruch, 1965).

In addition to hyperreflexia and extensor plantar responses, clonus and other signs indicative of pyramidal tract dysfunction are demonstrable when increased reflex activity supervenes following spinal transection.

Stretch reflexes even at the segmental level are highly complex in their organization. The concept of muscular hypertonus as a release phenomenon from descending inhibition must also take into account the altered function of the gamma efferent (fusimotor) system. There is evidence that, in a large measure, the brain stem influences alpha motor neurons indirectly by altering the rate of discharge of the gamma motor neurons. Spasticity appears to be associated with hyperactivity of the gamma motor neurons of antigravity muscles which presumably occurs as a result of being released from inhibitory influences. Withdrawal of facilitating effects by interference with cerebellar connections concerned with the integration of the gamma and alpha systems may lead to a suppression of gamma motor activity.

Cephalad effects attributed to interference with ascending impulses acting upon antagonistic reflex arcs have also been demonstrated following spinal transection.

Patients with complete spinal cord transection lose sympathetic reflex responses which depend on efferent pathways from medullary centers to the thoracic cord. Disturbances of vasomotor control result in postural hypotension. There is no vasoconstriction in response to cold, nor is there sweating in response to heat following injury. Later, adaptation takes place. Quadriplegic patients are unable to control their body temperature. It is also generally observed that the heart rate of quadriplegics is not increased in response to a variety of systemic pathologic factors as occurs in the non-spinally injured. Thus the vital signs may not reflect the true pathophysiologic systemic status of the patient. Of interest in this connection are the observations of Jennett (1970) who found that following cervical spinal cord transection, the response of the heart rate to hypoxia (breathing 10 percent oxygen for three minutes) was not markedly different from that of a group of normal controls. Jennett concluded that an intact sympathetic pathway from medulla to spinal cord is not essential for the development of tachycardia subsequent to hypoxia.

The vasomotor reflex or reflex erythema may, in some cases, be utilized to help determine the level of a spinal lesion. It is of localizing value only when absent in the region of the radicular field corresponding to a spinal cord lesion and present above and below this segmental field. The absence of a pilomotor reflex in such a radicular field has the same significance.

BIOMECHANICS OF DAMAGE OF THE SPINAL CORD

The extent of damage to the spinal cord is really the core of the problem in spinal injury. Little imagination is required to appreciate the degree of destruction wrought on the soft cord when portions of fractured vertebrae are driven with piston-like force into the spinal canal, compressing and rupturing tissue substance, or when the extent of dislocation is of such magnitude that the continuity of the cord is literally interrupted. It is the less severely traumatized case in which the injury is more subtle that requires careful evaluation of stresses applied and the capability of the cord unit to resist mechanical deformation in order to explain the resultant lesion.

The spinal cord does not move up and down axially in the canal as was formerly believed, but rather adapts itself to variation in canal length through the mechanism of plastic change of its substance. The dentate ligaments are thought to act as tethers that prevent cephalic-caudal motion; they do not influence dorsal or ventral displacement except under extreme circumstances. In flexion the spinal cord actually elongates, while in extension it shortens, developing folds on its external surface. An isolated 20 cm length of cord suspended in physiologic saline elongates 1 cm owing to the weight of the immersed cord itself. Lateral compression of the cord, especially during flexion of the spine, is resisted by the pia mater.

The dentate ligaments, which provide stability to the spinal cord, stretch in response to flexion movements of the trunk, creating a slight tension which is distributed uniformly over the length of the cord. Nerve roots are capable of undergoing physical change involving both elongation and shortening. In extension, the cross-sectional area of the nerve root increases and the nerve as a whole is converted into a series of gentle folds. In flexion the opposite occurs, with elongation and straightening of the root and its sleeves. Cord substance, without its pial coating, acts like a semi-fluid cohesive mass, offering little or no resistance to applied forces. With the tough pia mater intact, the cord is protected from extreme deformation because it is capable of a certain degree of movement within this tissue envelopment. Granting the biophysical properties described above, it is obvious that damage to spinal nervous tissue will occur when its limits of tolerance of mechanical change are exceeded (White and Albin, 1969).

Sequential experimental and pathological evidence suggests that in many cases of spinal cord trauma, the initial and critical injury involves the central sector of the cord and results in an expanding nucleus of gray matter which produces centrifugal pressure on circumferential white matter fibers within the limiting leptomeninges. The tissue damage observed in the long tracts appears to be delayed in onset by comparison with that in the gray matter (White et al, 1969). A progressive central to peripheral spread of the lesion depending on the severity of the trauma has also been observed in experimental animals by Ducker et al (1971).

While it appears that in the normal setting the spinal cord is afforded both mechanical and hydraulic protection, with advancing age the advantages of this protection are seriously reduced by such pathological changes in the supporting tissues as alterations in elasticity of the intervertebral discs, narrowing of the spinal canal, and osteoporosis.

ACCIDENT SITE MANAGEMENT

The proper care of the individual who has sustained a spinal injury must begin at the accident site. Since a physician would not ordinarily be immediately available, the medical profession (neurosurgeons in particular) must assume the initiative in educating paramedical personnel who normally provide emergency care at the scene of an accident in the proper assessment and handling of injuries. The majority of individuals who have incurred spinal trauma are conscious, so that careful questioning with regard to ability to move the limbs and to perceive sensation, and the presence and location of pain will alert the informed layman to the possibility of spinal injury. Unless the patient requires immediate treatment to combat shock or serious respiratory distress, he should not be moved until suitable assistance and proper equipment are available.

In transporting a person who is suspected of having sustained a spinal injury the following precautions should be observed: 1) minimize movement and postural changes; and 2) maintain head-neck-body alignment at all times. The patient should be rolled onto a firmly

702

supported stretcher — or better yet, a plywood board — for transportation to the hospital. It is dangerous to attempt to transfer a patient with a thoracolumbar injury by lifting him under the armpits while another person supports the dangling legs. Irreparable damage may be caused by such maneuvers. A small pad or folded blanket may be placed beneath the lower back to maintain lumbar lordosis. In cases of cervical trauma, efforts should be directed toward stabilizing the head and neck with whatever items are available (e.g., cushions, sandbags, clothing) in the position presented following the accident. While hand traction may be applied to the head in order to immobilize the neck during transportation in cases of suspected cervical injury, we believe that it is more important to secure the head and trunk to a solid flat surface. During the trip to the hospital, trained personnel should be with the patient at all times, particularly in order to provide respiratory assistance if needed. The relief of respiratory distress takes precedence over body positioning. Should vomiting occur, the patient may have to be placed on his side or transported prone for adequate drainage and naso-oral suction employed if available; continued vertebral immobilization is essential. Because of the ever-present danger of shock, particularly in inclement weather, body warmth should be maintained with blankets.

EMERGENCY ROOM MANAGEMENT

All individuals suspected of having sustained spinal trauma should be transported to properly equipped and staffed centers. The location of such facilities should be known in advance. Ideally they should be geographically situated so as to serve areas with a high incidence of trauma. Examination should be carried out prior to transfer from ambulance stretcher to hospital examining table or cart.

Vertebral fracture dislocations occur most frequently in the regions of greatest mobility, that is, between C5 and T1, and between T11 and L2. In all cases, cardiovascular and respiratory function should be promptly assessed. The mental responsiveness of the patient and the color of his skin and nailbeds should be noted, and his blood pressure, pulse, and temperature recorded. Evaluation of respiratory function is especially important in patients suspected of having suffered a cervical spine injury. It is necessary to determine whether the patient has a clear airway and whether the respiratory excursions of the thorax and diaphragm are adequate. In the face of respiratory distress

703

which does not clear with judicious toilet of the nasopharynx (for example, continuous naso-oral hemorrhage), naso-tracheal intubation or tracheostomy should be performed. Active hemorrhage must obviously be controlled. It must be kept in mind that cervical cord transections invariably present with mild hypotension and bradycardia as well as lowered body temperature (in the neighborhood of 35° ± 1°C) and that such a state is not indicative of hemorrhagic shock. Our experience in such cases is that the mean arterial pressure is above 75 mm Hg and easily raised, if it is thought necessary, with vasopressors. Morphine should never be given to patients with cervical cord injury in whom respiratory function may be in jeopardy. Opiates may be administered to patients with lumbar lesions, there being no respiratory problem, as a rule, in such cases.

Having determined that the patient's respiratory and circulatory status is satisfactory, one proceeds with the neurologic examination. Halter traction and/or sandbags may be utilized at this time to stabilize the head-neck-body axis and to limit movement. The patient should be carefully questioned with reference to ability to move his extremities and to perceive sensation, the occurrence of pain or paresthesias, and bladder and bowel function. Details of the accident should be elicited. Fracture of the spine should be suspected whenever an injured person complains of severe pain or stiffness in the neck or back. Radicular pain (indicative of root compression) also suggests fracture.

It is recommended that an established program of examination be implemented in these patients while they are still in the emergency room and that a detailed record employing the "flow sheet" concept be maintained. The following features should be incorporated in such a plan:

1. An initial, thorough neurologic examination should be performed to disclose the extent of neurologic deficit; the data obtained also provides a baseline for comparison with the results of future examinations. The degree and level of sensory and motor dysfunction must be carefully determined. Tests of reflex activity should be performed. Considerable effort must be expended in cases of apparent complete transection to uncover any islands of spared sensation (e.g., retained sensation in the sacral dermatomes, presence of sensation on catheter tug, deep pain interpreted as touch or pressure) or evidence of residual voluntary

704

muscle activity, since the prognosis for improvement is markedly enhanced if some function is retained.

2. Inquiry should be made concerning the patient's past medical history and a general physical examination performed. It is important to be aware of existing diseases and of drug therapy, particularly in older persons. In all cases, a careful examination must be made in search of associated injuries, particularly of abdominal and thoracic structures, which may have been previously overlooked.

3. Baseline laboratory studies, including blood grouping, hematocrit, blood sugar, urea, electrolytes, and urinalysis should be performed.

For patients having respiratory difficulty, it is recommended that Astrup equipment be used to obtain rapid and repeated determinations of arterial Pco_2 Po_2, and pH to aid in the assessment of pulmonary function and its effect on acid-base balance. If necessary, a Foley catheter is introduced into the bladder, and a record of the patient's fluid intake and output kept. A baseline electrocardiogram is obtained on every seriously injured patient when indicated. Whether it is advisable to perform a lumbar puncture and a Queckenstedt test for diagnostic purposes in a patient with a spinal cord injury is a controversial issue. The proponents of this procedure argue that the demonstration of a complete spinal block is indicative of serious spinal cord compression and assists them in arriving at a decision in favor of surgical decompression. On the other hand, others hold no less firmly that the results of spinal manometric studies are of little value in selecting cases for laminectomy (Mayfield and Cazan, 1942; Evans and Rosenauer, 1956). Certainly the absence of a spinal block does not in itself exclude the possibility of there being a fragment of bone or a herniated disc within the spinal canal compressing the cord and making surgical intervention necessary. If a spinal puncture is to be done, great care must be taken in positioning the patient, and the Queckenstedt test should be performed, preferably in a quantitative manner, with a blood pressure cuff around the patient's neck.

In all cases, the possibility of trauma to other parts of the body should be investigated. Associated injuries commonly occur in patients with spinal cord or cauda equina trauma, irrespective of the location of spinal injury. In a study of 252 stab wounds of the spinal cord (Lipschitz, 1967), 86 patients were found to have associated injuries involving the head, major cervical vessels, brachial plexus, trachea,

705

esophagus, thorax, abdomen, and limbs. Patients involved in automobile accidents often incur both head and spinal injuries. Gunshot wounds of the thoracic spine frequently also implicate the chest, and those of the lumbar and lower thoracic spine often penetrate the abdomen. The main point is that associated wounds in severely injured patients are of frequent occurrence and must not be overlooked, especially since an overwhelming spinal injury may mask their presence and interfere with their detection.

Recognition of injuries to the abdomen may be difficult in patients with traumatic lesions of the cervical or upper thoracic cord. Owing to loss of sensation, such patients may complain only of nausea and referred pain of diaphragmatic origin in the supraclavicular area. Abdominal rigidity and tenderness may be absent even when perforation of a viscus has occurred. Ileus may be mistakenly interpreted as a consequence of spinal trauma. By the same token, the occurrence of fever and leucocytosis may be attributed to urinary tract infection resulting from bladder catheterization. The fact that patients with cervical cord injury are subject to disturbances of thermoregulation poses another pitfall in differential diagnosis. A high index of suspicion is essential to the early diagnosis of abdominal trauma. Hypotension associated with tachycardia and a falling hematocrit should lead one to suspect hemorrhage within the abdomen or chest. X-ray films of the abdomen may provide useful information. Examination of the gastric and rectal contents for blood may be of assistance in detecting an abdominal lesion such as a peptic ulcer resulting from stress or steroid therapy. One must also be aware of the fact that abdominal rigidity may occur in association with spinal trauma and lead to an erroneous diagnosis of intra-abdominal disease. In such cases an abdominal tap may be required to substantiate a diagnosis of peritonitis or hemorrhage.

RADIOLOGICAL EXAMINATION

As soon as the condition of the patient warrants, x-rays are taken in order to determine the location, nature, and extent of vertebral derangement. The patient is transported to the x-ray department on a flat, firm stretcher in halter traction if a cervical fracture is suspected, with a physician constantly in attendance. Under careful manual control every effort is made to adequately visualize the spinal lesion. Standard lateral and A-P projections of the appropriate spinal area

706

are sometimes inadequate, particularly in cases of fracture at the cervico-thoracic junction, which may be obscured by the shoulders. In such instances, special views, e.g. lateral projections taken with counter-traction on the arms or with one arm elevated in the swimmer's position, may be necessary. In upper cervical or cranio-cervical trauma, the odontoid process should be visualized. For this purpose open mouth views are extremely valuable. Laminagraphy may be required for adequate visualization of the lesion. In cases of multiple injury, additional films of the skull, chest, and abdomen may be necessary; as a corollary it is important to obtain cervical spine films in head-injured patients whenever there is a possibility of a concomitant vertebral fracture.

In some cases, myelography may be required to resolve a particular problem. Usually this examination may be accomplished by injecting the radiopaque material into the lumbar subarachnoid space. Occasionally in lumbar injuries, because of the local effects caused by trauma, introduction of the contrast medium by cisternal puncture may be preferable. In cases of cervical trauma myelography may be performed by means of a needle inserted between C1 and C2 while the patient remains in the supine position. Postural hypotension and respiratory embarrassment may limit the extent to which the patient may be tilted during the examination.

After completion of the x-ray study, the next step is to formulate a definitive program of management. In the following section the problem of therapy will be considered in relation to the type of injury sustained.

CLASSIFICATION AND TREATMENT OF SPINE INJURIES

Ligamentous, osseous, and neural structures may be affected by injury to the spine. In cases of serious injury it would be unusual for one of these structural entities to be involved exclusively (White and Albin, 1969).

A. Subluxation

Cervical interarticular joint subluxation (Fig. 3) is distinguished from complete dislocation by virtue of the fact that the articular processes have not actually overridden (Watson-Jones, 1955). In some cases the vertebra may have spontaneously returned to its normal posi-

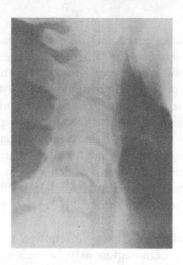

FIG. 3. Lateral view of subluxation of cervical vertebra four on cervical vertebra five. In this case the injury is almost a complete dislocation, but the articular processes are not overriding.

tion by the time the roentgenogram is taken so that the displacement may not be evident on routine x-rays taken in the neutral position. The subluxation may still be demonstrated if x-rays are taken with the neck in moderate flexion. This is a potentially dangerous procedure which should be carried out under a physician's direction. Ideally such stress films should employ lateral view cinefluoroscopy and fluoroscopic image intensification for proper assessment of the degree of subluxation. The hazard of performing this maneuver may be reduced by allowing the patient himself to determine the extent of flexion. From a practical point of view flexion (stress) views are unnecessary during the acute phase in most cases, being required only when routine x-rays disclose normal vertebral alignment. It should be kept in mind that within the pediatric age group a slight degree of anterior subluxation (usually C2-C3) occurring in flexion is a normal variant.

Subluxations may be associated with neurologic deficits of varying severity.

In uncomplicated cases treatment consists of postural reduction with the neck extended, followed by plaster immobilization or the application of a firm brace, maintaining the neck in the position of full extension. Should extension of the neck fail to achieve reduction, skeletal traction is required. In cases of pronounced neurologic deficit, reduction and continued immobilization in skeletal traction are indicated.

708

Laminectomy should be considered in the event the patient is severely paraplegic (see indications for surgical treatment including laminectomy, p. 724). The occurrence of a neurologic deficit in the absence of radiographic evidence of bone injury should lead one to suspect the possibility of an acute retropulsion of an intervertebral disc. X-ray films may reveal narrowing of an intervertebral space. Myelography is indicated for definitive diagnosis.

Early fusion (see page 728) should also be considered in all cases demonstrating persistent bony instability with the attendant hazard of recurrent subluxation.

B. Compression Fracture

Fracture of the vertebral bodies may occur without involvement of the posterior spinal elements. Wedge fractures resulting from compression due to forcible flexion are most common in the thoracolumbar region; they occur less frequently in the cervical and thoracic spine. One or more vertebral bodies may be involved (Fig. 4). Such fractures are regarded as stable since the posterior ligament complex consisting of the interspinous and supraspinous ligaments, the capsules

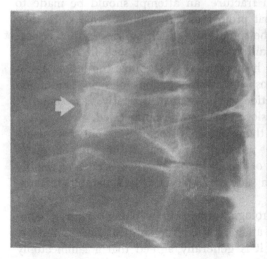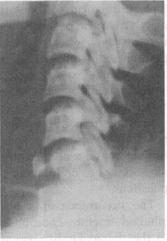

FIG. 4. Lateral view of compression fracture of thoracic spine (arrow). There is osteoporosis of all visualized bone and some compression of vertebral body below.
FIG. 5. Lateral view of bursting fracture of cervical vertebra six with posterior displacement.

of the lateral joints and the ligamenta flava, is intact. They do not as a rule produce cord compression and require only symptomatic treatment. Wedge fractures in the cervical region are uncommon and should be studied by means of flexion x-rays to rule out an element of subluxation. In stable fractures a collar provides symptomatic relief.

Occasionally compression fractures in the cervical area are associated with an intervertebral disc protrusion into the spinal canal, causing neurologic involvement. A myelogram should be promptly performed for confirmation of the diagnosis, and followed by surgical intervention. As an alternative to laminectomy, the herniated disc may be removed through an anterior approach after which an interbody fusion is performed (Cloward, 1961).

Compression injuries may also produce comminuted or "bursting" fractures of the vertebral bodies in the cervical (Fig. 5) and lumbar regions. Neurologic involvement may occur as a consequence of encroachment on the spinal canal. Usually paraplegia produced by compression fractures is incomplete. In the absence of cord compression, the treatment of comminuted fractures in the cervical region consists of immobilization in plaster after reduction by hyperextension or reduction by skeletal traction which is thereafter continued (for six to eight weeks) since many of these lesions fuse spontaneously. In the case of a severe compression fracture, an attempt should be made to replace fragments of bone that project into the spinal canal since they may later cause pressure on the spinal cord. Such injuries in the cervical region may be treated by skull traction with the neck in the neutral position until sufficient union has occurred to stabilize the lesion. Probably internal fixation and posterior spinal fusion following reduction is the preferable course of action in such cases. Recently, early anterior cervical (vertebral body) fusion has been recommended.

Bursting fractures in the thoracolumbar region without paraplegia are treated by plaster-jacket fixation or spinal fusion in the event the anteroposterior diameter of the spinal canal has been appreciably narrowed. Fusion provides a safeguard against late neurologic complications.

The occurrence of a neurologic deficit in a patient with a comminuted fracture constitutes an indication for surgical decompression. In the thoracolumbar region it is generally agreed that a laminectomy followed by a fusion should be performed. Opinions differ, however, regarding the surgical approach in cases of compression fracture with cord compression in the cervical region. Conventional posterior laminectomy permits decompression of the cord and removal of the

710

offending bone and/or disc fragments – at a sacrifice, however, of posterior bony elements. Removal of the compressing fragments may be more readily accomplished through the anterior approach; the cord suffers less trauma, but may not be adequately decompressed. Employing the anterior spinal operation, a fusion is performed after the patency of the spinal canal has been restored. In the event a laminectomy has been performed, a fusion may be done immediately following the decompression or at a later time.

C. Fracture Dislocation

A fracture dislocation is the most pernicious of spinal injuries. As a consequence of a flexion rotation force, the posterior ligament complex and the intervertebral disc rupture and the upper spinal segment is displaced relative to the lower one. The lower cervical and thoracolumbar regions are most commonly affected and neurologic involvement is a frequent occurrence. In the cervical region the articular processes slide off each other and become locked in this position (Fig. 6); the lower vertebral body may be compressed or an anterior marginal fragment may be broken off. There may be associated fractures of the laminae, pedicles, and of the articular and spinous processes. In the lumbar region there may be rotary displacement and locking of the facets together with compression of a vertebral body, but more often one or both articular facets fracture and a fragment of the upper border of the lower vertebral body is sheared off; the laminae or spinous process may fracture.

For reduction and immobilization of fracture dislocations of the cervical spine, skeletal traction is essential and, to accomplish this, we prefer Crutchfield or Vinke tongs. One advantage of Vinke tongs is that they do not slip out readily and can be left in for long periods of time without becoming detached from the skull. They are inserted above the external auditory meatus on each side. Under local anesthesia a stab incision is made down to bone and the outer table penetrated with the Vinke drill. A channel is cut in the diploë between the tables with a special instrument after which a pin with an eccentric flange that locks in the bone is inserted. This enables the tongs to be securely maintained in position.

To accomplish reduction we initially employ 25 pounds of traction in adults. This amount is gradually increased under x-ray guidance until reduction is achieved. As much as 50 pounds or more of traction may be required. Muscle relaxants administered intravenously have

711

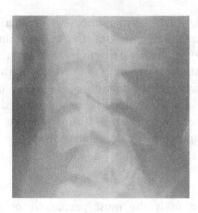

FIG. 6. Lateral view of dislocation of cervical vertebra four on vertebra five. The articular processes are overriding.

been utilized to overcome spasm which may otherwise prevent reduction. For purposes of countertraction head of bed is elevated. During reduction patient's neurologic status should be repeatedly tested.

In most cases normal vertebral alignment is achieved by this form of treatment and traction, reduced to a minimal amount, is thereafter continued for six to eight weeks so as to maintain reduction. Provided there is no serious neurologic dysfunction, early fusion has been recommended to shorten the lengthy period of immobilization required when skeletal traction is employed (Rogers, 1957; Rogers, 1958; Forsyth et al, 1959). An even more important consideration is the stability of the spine following reduction of a dislocation. If the vertebral body is fractured, spontaneous fusion may occur but, if the body is intact, healing of the ligaments alone will not assure stability and redislocation may occur. Internal fixation and fusion enhance the stability of the spine so that the likelihood of a recurrent dislocation with its attendant hazard of late paraplegia is appreciably lessened. Our regimen following anterior or posterior fusion in this type of situation is to maintain the patient in tongs for three to six weeks and in bed without traction for an additional three to six weeks, after which ambulation with a four-poster neck brace is permitted. The brace is worn for three to six months. Stress films are obtained three to four months following fusion.

Should the dislocation prove refractory to skeletal traction, disengagement of the facets by operative means is necessary (Fig. 7). Following open reduction stabilization is achieved by means of internal fixation with wire and a fusion performed.

712

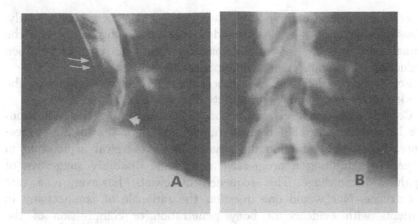

Fig. 7A. Lateral view of fracture dislocation of cervical spine with locked facets (arrow). C1-C2 myelogram revealed complete block (double arrow) due to spinal cord edema one segment above fracture.

B. Lateral view of 7A following laminectomy and open reduction.

Patients with serious neurologic deficits are maintained in skeletal traction on a Stryker or Foster frame.

Open reduction, internal fixation, and posterior fusion is recommended as the treatment of choice in most cases of lumbar dislocation whether or not there is any neurologic deficit (Fig. 8). In the presence of locked facets, attempts to correct the misalignment by manipulative extension alone are hazardous and highly inadvisable since reduction of the dislocation will not be achieved and irreparable injury may be inflicted on the cord or cauda equina.

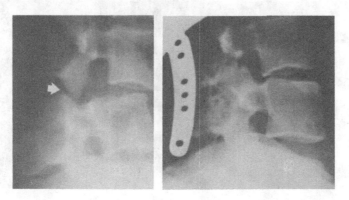

Fig. 8A. Lateral view of jumped facets (arrow) in lumbar region.

B. Lateral view following operative reduction and metallic plate stabilization.

713

Fracture dislocations in the thoracic region occur infrequently. Considerable force must be expended to produce this injury and the spinal cord may be severely damaged. Treatment consists of open reduction and laminectomy combined with fusion.

For technical details of the procedures of operative reduction the reader is referred to the appropriate literature.

Considerable difference of opinion exists concerning the indications for laminectomy in closed spinal injury and the value of this procedure. Few would question the advisability of surgical exploration in a patient exhibiting a progressive neurologic disability suggestive of epidural hemorrhage. This sequence of events, however, is a rare occurrence. Nor would one question the rationale of laminectomy in patients with evidence of bony penetration or compression of the spinal cord, or in whom a herniated disc is suspected. The patient about whom there is most controversy relating to laminectomy is the one with a complete transverse cord lesion, whose vertebral malalignment has been corrected, and who still has a spinal block. Many surgeons hold that operation is futile in this type of case (Scarff, 1960; Barnes, 1961; Harris, 1963). Our inclination is to advise laminectomy if the patient is seen within a few hours of injury and has shown no improvement. It is generally agreed that recovery of function is unlikely if paralysis was immediate and complete, and has persisted unchanged for 24 hours.

D. Special Fractures

A *"tear-drop"* fracture (Fig. 9) is one in which an anterior corner

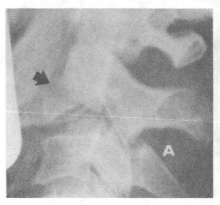 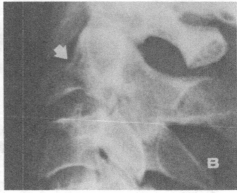

Fig. 9A. Lateral view of tear-drop fracture of anterior inferior body of cervical vertebra 2 (arrow). B. Spontaneous healing one year later (arrow).

714

of bone has been separated from the remainder of the body of a cervical vertebra (Schneider, 1955). It is caused by a flexion injury and is associated with varying degrees of vertebral compression and neurologic deficit. Schneider emphasizes the point that a fragment of bone, detached from the posterior inferior margin of the involved vertebra, may project backward into the spinal canal. Neurologic involvement may be due to protrusion of disc material or bony fragments into the spinal canal. The treatment of this complication was discussed in the section dealing with compression fractures (see page 710).

Flexion-extension films may be indicated to rule out subluxation. The treatment of an uncomplicated "tear-drop" fracture (i.e., one without subluxation, comminution, or neurologic involvement) consists of a short period of bed rest and halter traction followed by ambulation with a supporting collar.

Fracture dislocations of the atlantoaxial region are uncommon. They are usually associated with a fracture through the base of the odontoid (Fig. 10). Anterior dislocation occurs much more frequently than posterior displacement. Fracture of the odontoid process may occur without dislocation of the atlas upon the axis.

In order to adequately demonstrate the odontoid, an "open-mouth" view should be made a routine part of the radiologic examination of the cervical spine in cases of trauma. Laminagraphy is also extremely useful in demonstrating lesions at this level, not well visualized in plain x-rays. In the lateral position the distance between the anterior aspect of the odontoid and the posterior articular surface of the atlas should normally be 3 mm or less in flexion or extension. A distance of more than 3 mm indicates atlantoaxial instability.

An inordinate amount of neck pain and muscle spasm suggests atlantoaxial fracture. There is a surprisingly high incidence of such fractures without neurologic signs. This type of vertebral lesion occurs not infrequently in patients with rheumatoid arthritis (Jackson, 1966), probably due to the weakened ligamentous and bony structures. Spontaneous nontraumatic dislocation of the atlas may also occur in association with nasopharyngeal infection, especially in children.

Reduction by skeletal traction is essential. When undertaken early, treatment by reduction and immobilization may be expected to yield a satisfactory result, i.e., bony or fibrous union of the odontoid, in many cases. Since healing of the odontoid fracture is not altogether reliable, however, early bony fusion of C1, C2, and C3 is recommended to protect the patient from the late neurologic sequelae of recurrent atlantoaxial dislocation (Alexander et al, 1958). In cases in which reduction cannot

715

be achieved, the posterior rim of the atlas should be removed for prevention of angulation and compression of the spinal cord. A few surgeons advise that the occiput be incorporated in the fusion; this may be necessary in cases in which a laminectomy of the atlas has been performed.

Spontaneous atlantoaxial dislocation in children is usually adequately managed by reduction and immobilization in plaster.

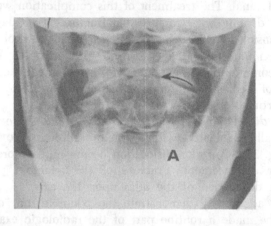

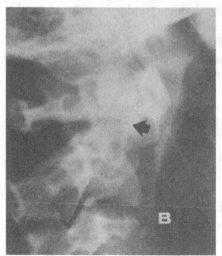
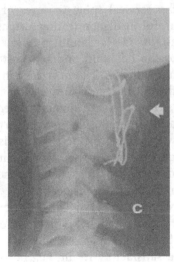

Fig. 10A. Odontoid fracture (arrow) on anterior-posterior x-ray.
    B. Lateral view of instability of atlas on axis with flexion (arrow).
    C. Postoperative lateral x-ray demonstrating excellent position with stabilization and new bone growth (arrow).

716

A *"hangman's" fracture* (Schneider et al, 1965) (Fig. 11) of the cervical spine is one in which the neural arch of the axis is avulsed from its body. The odontoid process is unaffected but the body of the axis may be dislocated upon that of the third cervical vertebra. When

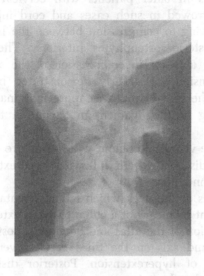

Fig. 11. Lateral view of "hangman's fracture" of cervical spine.

this occurs, the body and odontoid process of the axis remain attached to the atlas while the posterior elements of the axis remain adherent to the third cervical vertebra. This lesion owes its designation to the fact that it is similar to that incurred in a judicial hanging. Among survivors, persistent neurologic deficits are rare. According to DePalma (1970) a severe neurolgic deficit suggests the possibility of a fracture-dislocation at a lower level. Treatment involves realignment of the cervical spine by skeletal traction and immobilization in a cast or brace. DePalma, however, recommends that skeletal traction be followed by a posterior spinal fusion.

Spinal injury may occur as a result of *forcible extension* of a segment of the vertebral column. The cervical region is most commonly affected (Barnes, 1948; Taylor and Blackwood, 1948; Brain et al, 1952). In Burke's series (1971) of 178 cases of cervical spine injury with cord involvement, there were 51 (29 percent) extension injuries. Most frequently this type of force causes the intervertebral disc and anterior longitudinal ligament to rupture while the posterior ligaments remain unaffected. The resultant dislocation usually reduces spontaneously so

717

that x-rays disclose normal vertebral alignment. A clue as to the type of trauma sustained may be provided by the presence of an abrasion or contusion over the face or forehead. This type of hyperextension injury often occurs in older patients with cervical spondylosis. The spinal canal is narrowed in such cases and cord injury is a frequent accompaniment, owing to compression between the ligamentum flavum posteriorly and posterior osteophytes anteriorly. The role of the ligamentum flavum as a factor in compression of the spinal cord during extreme hyperextension was clearly demonstrated by Taylor (1951). He observed that the spinal canal was appreciably narrowed as a result of forward bulging of the ligamentum flavum in the hyperextended position.

Disruption of the vertebral column with a fracture extending through the intervertebral disc may occur following hyperextension in patients with ankylosing spondylitis.

Extension injuries of the neck which reduce spontaneously are stable in flexion. Treatment by means of a collar to avoid extension is adequate.

Fracture dislocation of the atlas and odontoid (posterior dislocation), and of the atlas and axis on the third cervical vertebra, may occur as a consequence of hyperextension. Posterior dislocation involving the lower cervical vertebrae is rare.

Hyperextension fracture dislocation of the lower cervical spine which may simulate a flexion injury has also been described (Forsyth, 1964). The mechanism of injury involves a combination of extension, compression, and rotation forces. In addition to the forward displacement of the affected vertebra, there are multiple small fractures of the posterior bone elements. A small chip of bone may be avulsed from the anterior inferior margin of the body of the displaced vertebra or from the anterior superior margin of the vertebral body below. Reduction by skeletal traction is difficult to achieve so that open reduction and spine fusion have been recommended for patients with neurologic involvement (Forsyth, 1964).

Hyperextension injuries of the thoracolumbar spine are uncommon. When they occur in the lumbar region the vertebral body or neural arch may be affected. Such injuries are treated by immobilization in a plaster jacket in the neutral position. When the thoracic spine is affected complete and permanent paraplegia is apt to occur.

Patients with *ankylosing spondylitis* are susceptible to subluxation and fracture-dislocation of the cervical spine. The occurrence of atlantoaxial dislocation in such cases has already been mentioned.

718

Below this level, owing to loss of flexibility and increased fragility, relatively minor trauma may produce comminuted or transverse vertebral body fractures or transverse intervertebral space fractures, with or without dislocation of the segments (Rand and Stern, 1961; Grisolia et al, 1967). A large proportion of fractures are due to hyperextension. The incidence of neurologic complications is high. The C5-C6 and C6-C7 levels are the most common sites of fracture. Treatment depends on the precise nature of the lesion in a particular case. Immobilization in a brace may be adequate, but skeletal traction may be required to achieve reduction. The indications for laminectomy and/or fusion are the same as those in any case of cervical fracture.

E. Compound Fractures

Compound fractures of the spine are most often caused by penetrating missiles (Matson, 1948; Meirowsky, 1965; Yashon et al, 1970) or knife wounds (Fig. 12). Patients who have sustained gunshot wounds frequently have associated injuries of other parts of the body, the treatment of which may claim priority over that of the spine. Leakage of cerebrospinal fluid from the wound indicates penetration of the meninges. As soon as the patient's general condition warrants, x-rays should be taken to determine the extent of vertebral injury, the path of the missile, and the presence of indriven bone and metallic fragments.

Penetrating wounds should be débrided, and all comminuted and depressed bone fragments and foreign bodies which may be affecting the cord should be removed as early as possible. Dural tears should be repaired after débridement insofar as possible. It may only be possible to cover the dural defect with Gelfoam. Whether an intact dura should be opened to permit intradural exploration is controversial, though many surgeons would prefer to do so (Jacobs and Berg, 1971). In cases of cord contusion it may be preferable to allow the dura to remain open for purposes of decompression. The wound must be meticulously closed in layers in order to avoid leakage of cerebrospinal fluid. Antibiotics should be administered and appropriate measures taken to prevent tetanus.

Obviously the outlook for recovery of function will depend upon the amount of damage to the spinal cord and roots. In our experience (Yashon et al, 1970) the end results in a series of cases of civilian bullet wounds of the cord and cauda equina have been poor. Since

719

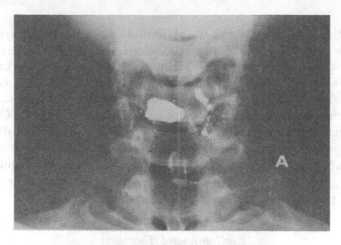

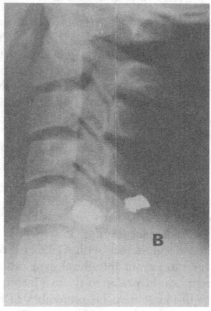

Fig. 12A. Anterior-posterior view of large bullet fragment in midline at cervical vertebra 5.

B. Lateral film verifies the bullet's intraspinal location. A smaller fragment is above the lamina within paraspinal musculature.

surgical treatment did not appear to influence the outcome in these cases, we are reluctant to operate on patients with complete or very severe lesions seen after five or six hours unless the wound is grossly contaminated.

Stab wounds in which the knife blade has not broken off and been retained, and that have not produced fragmentation of bone or resulted in a persistent cerebrospinal fluid leak, do not require operative treatment. The cervical or upper thoracic cord is the usual site of injury. As a rule the cord is incompletely severed and a Brown-Séquard syndrome or variant thereof is the eventual outcome.

F. Spondylosis

That patients with cervical spondylosis are susceptible to hyperextension injury has been pointed out by many authors, including Barnes (1948, 1961), Brain et al (1952, 1967), Symonds (1953) and Hughes and Brownell (1963). Even without the added factor of trauma, spondylosis by itself may damage the spinal cord. When hyperextension occurs in such cases the cord may be severely injured. In fact, hyperextension injury of an arthritic spine is the usual cause of paraglegia in patients over 50 years of age. Usually x-rays show no evidence of fracture or dislocation; avulsion of an anterior osteophyte may be noted.

The vertebral canal is narrowed and the spinal cord compressed between the osteoarthritic protrusion anteriorly and the indented ligamentum flavum posteriorly. Measurements of the sagittal diameter of the cervical canal are useful in patients with spondylosis. Compression of the cord may be expected if the distance measures 10 mm or less at any level. When the minimum diameter measures 14 mm or more, myelopathy due to spondylosis is unlikely.

It has also been suggested that reduction in the blood supply of the anterior half of the cord resulting from compression by cervical spondylosis is a factor in the production of symptoms. Blood flow through the vertebral arteries may be impaired as a consequence of spondylosis or of a fracture dislocation above the level of C-6, the resultant ischemia affecting the brain stem and possibly the cord.

The treatment of cervical spondylosis is discussed elsewhere in this volume. Little information is available as to the value of surgical therapy in the management of the acute manifestations resulting from hyperextension injury. Most of the cases described in the literature were treated conservatively with varying degrees of recovery among those which survived.

721

G. Spinal Cord and Root Lesions

The effects of trauma on the spinal cord vary from complete anatomic transection to temporary dysfunction (concussion) with rapid improvement. The features of complete transection, including spinal shock and the return of reflex activity, have been discussed earlier in this chapter. Incomplete lesions may also be associated with spinal shock at the outset; varying degrees of recovery ensue, extensor hypertonus being predominantly evident. Hemisection of the spinal cord results in a Brown-Séquard syndrome. Injuries involving the cauda equina cause a flaccid paralysis and sensory loss affecting the lower limbs, combined with disturbances of bladder, bowel, and sexual function. Regeneration of the motor roots of the cauda equina is possible provided their neurolemmal sheaths have been preserved.

After injury to the cervical region of the spinal cord, a syndrome characterized by disorientation, stupor, hypotension, bradycardia, and hypothermia sometimes appears. Anoxia (Putnam, 1939) and loss of sympathetic function (Rosenbluth and Meirowsky, 1953) have been suggested as etiologic factors. Possibly the cerebral symptoms may be due to involvement of the vertebral arteries.

In some cases of severe spinal cord injury, especially those that involve the cervical region, priapism occurs following recovery from spinal shock.

Two neurologic syndromes have been described which merit mention here because of their clinical implications. The *syndrome of acute central cervical spinal cord injury* is characterized by disproportionately greater weakness of the upper than the lower extremities, bladder dysfunction, and a variable sensory loss below the level of the lesion. It occurs most frequently as a result of hyperextension injuries in older individuals. Hemorrhage and/or edema or vascular insufficiency due to compression of the anterior spinal artery affect the central region of the cervical cord. The location of the lesion explains the predominant involvement of the upper limbs, the pyramidal fibers supplying the arms being situated most medially. Injury to the anterior horn cells may also explain the selective brachial involvement. Recognition of this syndrome is important because appreciable recovery may occur spontaneously and surgical treatment is contraindicated (Schneider et al, 1954; Schneider, 1969).

The *syndrome of acute anterior spinal cord injury* consists of complete paralysis and sensory loss below the level of the lesion, exclusive

722

of the modalities that are conveyed by the posterior columns — touch, position, and vibratory perception (Schneider, 1955, 1969). It occurs as a consequence of compression by a protruding bone fragment (compression fracture) or herniated disc (alone or in association with a fracture-dislocation) from in front, or actual destruction of the anterior part of the spinal cord resulting from contusion or impaired blood supply via the anterior spinal artery (fracture-dislocation, "recoil" of a herniated disc). The Queckenstedt test is not reliable as a means of differential diagnosis. Since a surgical lesion causing cord compression is not distinguishable clinically from a nonsurgical destructive injury, exploratory laminectomy, possibly preceded by myelography, is indicated; subsequently a spinal fusion may be necessary. An anterior approach combined with a vertebral body fusion has also been advocated (Cloward, 1961).

Concussion of the spinal cord is manifested by transient loss of function which is rarely complete. Usually the vertebrae remain intact (Wolman, 1964). Beginning recovery may be evident within hours. While the physiologic and pathologic basis of this condition in the human is unknown, it is of some interest and perhaps relevant that hemorrhagic changes have been observed primarily in the central gray matter of the spinal cord of monkeys with experimentally induced transitory traumatic paraplegia; edematous alterations occurring in the surrounding white matter were much less marked and presumably accounted for the transient nature of the paraplegia (Wagner et al, 1971). Traumatized animals that were not sacrificed exhibited some degree of recovery from their initial complete sensory and motor paralysis within 12 hours and were able to move about readily in seven to ten days.

Root injuries may accompany spinal cord trauma. In appropriate cases decompression of a lower cervical root has been advocated to improve or preserve some function in the upper extremity. The clinical features resulting from trauma to a single spinal root are similar to those produced by a segmental cord lesion. In addition, however, pressure exerted by a crushed vertebra on a nerve root may cause severe pain in a radicular distribution. Complete severance of a root is not associated with persistent pain.

Brachial plexus injuries occur in the newborn and during adult life most often as a result of traction, and may involve any of its components. There are two varieties of birth injury, one (Erb-Duchenne) involving the roots of C5 and C6, the other implicating the roots of

723

C8 and T1 (Klumpke's paralysis). Lesions of the upper roots affect the deltoid, biceps, brachioradialis, spinati, rhomboids, teres major, and clavicular fibers of the pectoralis major muscle so that the patient is unable to abduct or rotate the arm externally, flex or supinate the forearm, and adduct the scapula; the biceps and radial reflexes are lost, and sensation is impaired over the outer aspect of the shoulder and arm. The lower plexus type of paralysis affects the flexor muscles of the wrist and fingers and the intrinsic hand muscles; sensation is defective over the ulnar aspect of the hand and forearm, the triceps reflex is absent, and a Horner's syndrome may be in evidence. Myelography may show extravasation of contrast medium alongside the main column, indicative of root avulsion.

The muscles innervated by the segment or segments at the level of a transverse spinal cord lesion exhibit a flaccid paralysis owing to destruction of the anterior horn cells and roots. During the acute stage, it is difficult to distinguish the effects of segmental denervation from flaccidity due to spinal shock. Subsequently, recognition is afforded by the persistent flaccidity, atrophy, areflexia, and electromyographic changes referable to the affected segmental level.

It is necessary at times to distinguish between paralysis of organic origin and the functional paralysis of hysterical patients or malingerers. Bona fide paralysis that follows spinal cord trauma is characterized by areflexia, whereas both superficial and deep reflexes are retained in patients with functional disorders. Following the application of a painful stimulus to a supposedly paralyzed limb, the hysterical patient will frequently move it after some delay. In cases of alleged paralysis of one lower extremity, the Hoover test is useful in differential diagnosis. The examiner's hand is placed beneath each heel and the patient requested to attempt to raise the reputedly paralyzed limb. Failure to perceive downward pressure exerted by the unaffected limb indicates that the patient is not attempting to lift the reputedly paralyzed extremity. Loss of sensation in cases of hysteria and simulation does not conform to any anatomic pattern.

INDICATIONS FOR SURGICAL TREATMENT
INCLUDING LAMINECTOMY

In the event that skeletal traction fails to accomplish reduction of a cervical dislocation, operative treatment aimed to unlock the facets

724

is necessary. Open reduction may also be required in cases of fracture-dislocation of the thoracolumbar spine. To assure stability, internal fixation and fusion are performed after reduction has been accomplished.

It is further generally agreed that surgical treatment is indicated 1) in cases of compound fracture or penetrating wound; 2) in the rare instance of progressive neurologic deficit; 3) when there are bone fragments within the spinal canal; 4) in cases of compression caused by an acute protrusion of a disc or a bursting fracture; and 5) when the clinical presentation corresponds to the syndrome of acute anterior cervical cord trauma. Aside from these indications there is a wide difference of opinion concerning the role of decompressive laminectomy. Those opposed to laminectomy argue that traumatic paraplegia is essentially caused by contusion of the cord and that compressive factors are of negligible importance. Divergent opinions have been expressed concerning the significance of a manometric block as an indication for laminectomy. Scarff (1960) believes that edema of the cord is the principal cause of the manometric block in the immediate posttraumatic period and regards the block as a contraindication to laminectomy. Others (Barnes, 1961; Schwartz et al, 1965) advise laminectomy in cases of incomplete paraplegia in which a spinal block persists after reduction of the fracture or dislocation.

The authors advocate a more aggressive policy in the treatment of spinal cord injury based on the concept that the lesion is not instantaneously complete and probably requires at least several hours to become irreversible in many cases (Locke et al, 1971). We perform an immediate posterior decompressive laminectomy whenever patients with complete lesions of the cord or cauda equina and a spinal block reach us within a few hours of injury. In our experience a properly performed laminectomy has not been detrimental. Advanced age and serious injury to other parts of the body are considered to be contraindications to laminectomy in this type of case.

DECOMPRESSIVE LAMINECTOMY

The technical details of a cervical laminectomy will be described. With some modification, the technique is essentially similar in the thoracic and lumbar regions. After the insertion of tongs the patient, preferably awake, is intubated via the nasal route so as to avoid the hazard of hyperextension of the neck. The use of succinylcholine during induction of anesthesia in patients with spinal injury is dangerous because it produces a sudden mobilization of potassium which may lead to cardiac arrythmia (Stone et al, 1970). If necessary, laminectomy may be performed under local anesthesia. Arterial and central venous pressure, body temperature, and electrocardiographic activity are monitored. With careful attention to body-head axial alignment, the patient is positioned on his abdomen while maintaining skeletal traction, and the occiput, neck, and upper thorax are shaved, cleansed, and draped. In thoracic and lumbar injuries the exact level of the lesion is marked on the skin during myelography or x-ray examination.

Since we generally plan to remove the posterior elements of three vertebrae, the skin incision extends over at least four or five spinous processes. Great care is exercised in detaching the muscles from the spinous processes and laminae. Separation of the muscles from the bony elements must proceed in a lateral direction and not downward so as to avoid plunging through a fractured lamina. Sharp subperiosteal dissection is preferable. The laminae immediately above and below the fracture area are exposed before the involved vertebrae are stripped of muscle attachments. Fractures can frequently be palpated prior to actual visualization, permitting the operator to approach the lesion with greater safety. Once the posterior elements are exposed, the laminectomy is begun by first removing the spinous processes and laminae of the vertebrae above and below the involved area. The fracture site is then carefully unroofed exposing the dura. Depressed and in-driven bone fragments are teased free and blood clot gently removed by irrigation and suction. Extradural bleeding is controlled with silver clips, the bipolar cautery, or Gelfoam. We are well aware of the difference of opinion that exists as to the advisability of opening the dura, but have no hesitancy in doing so. The dural incision is started at either end of the laminectomy where the cord is not swollen. The cord is examined for evidence of tissue destruction, swelling, hemorrhage, and topographical deformity. (The use of color photography is very useful for permanent records.) All bone fragments are extracted and blood clot gently washed away. Tiny pledgets of Gelfoam are temporarily applied to control hemorrhage in the cord. We do not recommend incising the pia. The dentate ligaments are sectioned to facilitate inspection of the lateral and anterior aspects of the cord; all loose bone and disc fragments are removed.

If the facets are locked, we attempt to free them by manipulation or, if necessary, by resecting portions of one or more articular processes.

This is undertaken with the cord under direct vision.

For adequate decompression of the cord the dura is left open with silver clips placed at the extremes of the incision. This is useful for postoperative x-ray evaluation. After hemostasis has been achieved the wound is carefully closed in layers without drainage. Considerable attention must be given to wound closure in order to prevent the development of troublesome meningoceles or cerebrospinal fluid leaks. For this reason we employ multilayer, interrupted, silk suture closure.

The indications for decompressive laminectomy in cases of paraplegia due to lumbar and thoracic fracture dislocations are controversial, but the authors believe that regardless of the severity of the deficit, and irrespective of the results of lumbar puncture, these patients should be explored. Laminectomy should be combined with manipulative reduction of the dislocation. Disc extrusion occurs in lumbar fractures and on occasion such lesions must be approached transdurally since many central herniations are not accessible by the ordinary lateral extradural approach.

EXPERIMENTAL HYPOTHERMIA

After intensive laboratory investigation (Albin et al, 1968a), a technique for direct hypothermia of the spinal cord in cases of injury was devised. Clinical application in cases of severe spinal cord trauma is suggested on the basis of laboratory evidence that hypothermia exerts a protective effect on the cord by lowering metabolic demands and limiting the degree of edema and hemorrhage. The authors wish to make clear, however, that this is an experimental procedure, the efficacy of which is yet to be established in humans.

Hypothermia is initiated after the cord is exposed but, if the cord is swollen to the extent that it distends the dura under pressure, cooling is begun before the dura is opened (Albin et al, 1968b). The surgical wound with exposed cord at its depth serves as a reservoir and is filled with ice-cold sterile saline (2°C). Circulation of fluid is accomplished by means of a sterile tygon tubing, the two open ends of which are placed in the wound for delivery and removal of perfusate. A Brown-Harrison pediatric-size heat exchanger is interposed in this circuit and the tubing is placed in a Mark occlusive roller pump to maintain flow of fluid through the heat exchanger and the wound reservoir. A separate cooling circuit is utilized to maintain a low temperature in the heat exchanger. Perfusate at temperatures of 2° to 3° C flowing at a rate of

727

100 to 500 cc per minute is circulated through the sterile tubing and into the reservoir. Cooling is maintained for three hours following which the equipment and fluid are removed and the wound closed in the manner described above. The morbidity associated with this procedure is negligible (Albin et al, 1968c).

ADJUNCTS IN THE TREATMENT OF SPINAL INJURY

Recent innovations in the medical management of spinal cord trauma are the use of steroids and dehydrating agents, an obvious outgrowth of their use in cerebral injuries. While dehydrating agents (urea or mannitol) have enjoyed at best a very limited trial in spinal cord injuries, the steroids (particularly the glucocorticoids) have been employed more extensively. In adults we have followed this regimen: 4 to 6 mgms of dexamethasone are administered parenterally four to six times daily; after three to five days the dose is tapered off and the medication discontinued between the seventh and tenth day. Antacids are currently administered and the patient carefully observed for evidence of adverse gastric effects. Although prescribed empirically there is as yet no conclusive evidence to suggest that steroids are of value in the treatment of spinal cord trauma.

VERTEBRAL FUSION

The indication for spinal fusion in fracture-dislocations is instability (Rogers, 1942, 1958; Alexander et al, 1958; Forsyth et al, 1959; Nicoll, 1962; Holdsworth, 1963; Benes, 1968). Since by definition all fracture-dislocations are unstable, it follows that, generally, a fusion should be performed in all such cases. Surgical fusion is not invariably indicated, however, since there is a higher incidence of spontaneous fusion in cases of dislocation associated with a fracture of the vertebral body than in cases in which the body remains intact. When fracture-dislocations in the atlantooccipital region are treated early by accurate reduction and immobilization, they may heal securely by bony or fibrous union so that stabilization by bone grafting may not be necessary (Blockey and Purser, 1956; Nicoll, 1962).

Fusion is advisable in cases of fracture-dislocation because recurrence of the displacement with resultant pain and delayed paraplegia may occur even after reduction and prolonged immobilization. When not preceded by laminectomy, posterior spinal fusion is performed by se-

728

curely fixing appropriate autogenous bone grafts over the laminae and packing the area with bone chips. Internal metallic fixation (Fig. 8 B, 10 C) is employed to immobilize the injured vertebrae while awaiting bony fusion. Wires, screws and various plates have been utilized for this purpose (Crenshaw, 1971). After a period of 6 to 12 weeks of bed rest, ambulation is permitted in a plaster cast or an appropriate brace which is worn for an additional 6 to 12 weeks. In cervical injuries we utilize a snugly fitting four-poster brace. Some surgeons favor a shorter period of immobilization following fusion.

Because of the unique architecture of the thoracic region, considerable structural stability is inherent in this portion of the spinal column (Howorth and Petrie, 1964). Significant force must be delivered to the thoracic spine to produce a fracture-dislocation and even if this occurs, instability is minimized by the splinting of the rib cage. Unfortunately, however, owing to the narrowness of the spinal canal in this region, the cord is frequently irreparably damaged as a result of shearing injuries or fracture-dislocation. Rarely, an anterior cord syndrome follows a thoracic spinal injury (Schneider, 1955). Shear fractures are invariably associated with complete paraplegia and do not require surgical treatment unless displacement is pronounced. Open reduction with or without laminectomy followed by spine fusion is indicated in cases of fracture-dislocation.

In our experience, nearly all of our patients who suffered a fracture-dislocation of the thoracic or lumbar spine and on whom a spinal fusion was not performed, developed scoliosis over the course of months to years. We have also seen this happen after inadequate or unsuccessful fusion. In general, the younger the patient the greater the likelihood that this deformity will develop. The kyphoscoliosis may be associated with pain and further neurologic dysfunction.

PATHOLOGY OF TRAUMATIC PARAPLEGIA[*]

A. Concussion

Reference has already been made to the pathologic findings in monkeys with experimentally induced transitory traumatic paraplegia (Wagner et al, 1971). Whether these observations have any bearing on spinal cord concussion in the human is of course not known. Concussion of the spinal cord, like its cerebral counterpart, is an evanescent

[*]See also Chapter 21.

729

phenomenon that suggests the likelihood of a similar pathophysiologic basis. Symonds attributes cerebral concussion to diffuse neuronal injury (Chapter 4). Depolarization of nerve cell membranes is regarded by Walker et al (1944) as the physiologic basis of cerebral concussion.

B. Edema

Every major spinal injury that is severe enough to produce neurologic symptoms is associated with at least some degree of edema in addition to whatever other lesions may be present. The cord may swell to twice its normal size. Such an edematous cord may completely fill the dural sac and distend it under considerable pressure. Edema alone is sufficient to induce complete physiologic interruption of spinal cord function (Scarff, 1960). Varying degrees of vacuolation may be observed in light microscopic sections. Edema is usually concentrated in white matter as opposed to gray matter although it is by no means limited exclusively to the former.

C. Epidural Hemorrhage

Epidural hemorrhage alone is rarely a significant cause of physiologic or anatomic disruption of spinal cord function following trauma. The small clots in the epidural space found at operation are clinically insignificant.

D. Subdural Hemorrhage

Subdural hemorrhage is also uncommon in spinal injury but is seen on occasion in cases of severe spinal trauma. The small amount of subdural clot evacuated at operation is of little significance when compared to intrinsic spinal trauma sustained in vertebral fracture-dislocation.

E. Hemorrhage into the Spinal Cord (Hematomyelia)

Parenchymal hemorrhage is an almost invariable consequence of major spinal trauma. It is present to greater or lesser degree whenever the cord has been contused. The term "contusion" refers to the gross ecchymotic appearance of the cord comparable to what may be observed in other organs following trauma. On cross section there are hemorrhages of varying dimensions. Hemorrhage into the subarachnoid space occurs as a result of rupture of small blood vessels. In many cases of spinal cord trauma parenchymal hemorrhage is restricted to the central gray matter. A hemorrhagic lesion is frequently the cause of the acute central cord syndrome previously described.

Osterholm and Mathews (1972) suggest that altered norepinephrine metabolism is responsible for hemorrhagic necrosis and neurologic deficits following experimental spinal injury. Protection against traumatic experimental hemorrhagic necrosis was achieved by norepinephrine synthesis blockade with alpha methyl tyrosine.

F. Microscopic Changes

The cell bodies of the neurons in the gray matter and the nerve fibers in the white matter show varying degrees of degenerative change and disruption. The effects on the nerve fibers involve both axons and myelin. Fluid-filled spaces indicating edema are present.

A predominantly polymorphonuclear leucocytic reaction occurs during the acute stage. Subsequently lymphocytes and macrophages appear.

G. Chronic Stage

The periosteum and dura mater have become densely adherent at the site of trauma. The leptomeninges are often attached to this scar and the subarachnoid space may be partially obliterated. The cord is atrophic and sclerotic and often yellow in color. It may contain cysts representing the residua of old hemorrhage. Demyelination and the presence of glial and connective tissue in damaged areas are prominent histologic features.

ADJUNCTIVE MANAGEMENT OF PARAPLEGIA

From one-third to one-half of all cervical spine injuries are complicated by paralysis; a complete tetraplegia occurs in about half of these (Barnes, 1961). Paraplegia occurring in association with thoracolumbar lesions is mostly caused by rotational fracture-dislocations (Holdsworth, 1963).

To prevent pressure sores, it is essential that the patient be turned every two hours. Erythema that develops over a bony prominence is a danger signal that further pressure at this site must be avoided. Rubber

731

"doughnut" rings, air mattresses, sheepskin and various other devices such as pads and cushions are useful in helping to prevent decubiti. Patients with cervical injuries are managed on a Stryker or Foster frame after skeletal traction has been instituted; this facilitates turning, but only two positions, prone and supine are possible. Also, the patient must be carefully positioned each time he is turned. When in the lateral position, for example, the uppermost leg should be slightly flexed and a pillow placed between it and the limb beneath.

Passive exercises are employed to help counteract the effects of immobility and avoid contractures. All joints, both large and small, of paralyzed limbs should be put through a full range of motion. To prevent deformities appropriate well-padded splints should be applied between exercise periods.

The care of the neurogenic bladder presents a major problem, best handled in conjunction with a urologist. Intermittent sterile catheterization as opposed to the use of an indwelling Foley catheter has been recommended but this is generally impractical. Munro tidal drainage is seldom utilized at present. Our practice is to insert a large Foley catheter (14-18 French) and to tape it so as to avoid traction on the indwelling catheter bag. Constant drainage is permitted for a few days to prevent ureteral reflux. Large amounts of fluid are administered orally or intravenously. After about a week the catheter is clamped off for periods of three to four hours and then released for 15 minutes. Whenever possible this may be accomplished by the patient himself. These "exercises" prevent both overdistention and contracture of the bladder and assist in the development of an automatic catheter-free bladder. A supervised intake of a glass of liquid hourly from 7:00 A.M. to bedtime will ensure an adequate fluid intake, and at the same time permit frequent filling and emptying of the bladder. Daily irrigation with a mild bacteriostatic solution (¼ of 1% acetic acid) is performed and the catheter changed at least once a week. The urine is regularly cultured. Prophylactic antibiotics are not prescribed. Infection is treated with appropriate drugs depending on the sensitivity of the organism cultured from the urine and/or blood. Early mobilization is helpful in preventing the formation of renal and bladder calculi.

Prevention of hypostatic pneumonia also poses a serious problem during the period immediately following injury of the upper thoracic and cervical spine. Respiratory function is impaired owing to varying degrees of paralysis of the musculature involved in breathing. Paralysis and the supine position combine to make it difficult for the patient to

732

cough and clear his mouth and pharynx of secretions. He should be encouraged to cough insofar as possible. Any of the following measures may be employed: turning from side to side with the spinal column splinted (postural drainage); frequent suctioning of the nasopharynx; intermittent positive pressure breathing; the use of antibiotics; and tracheostomy. The abdominal distention which frequently accompanies spinal cord trauma limits diaphragmatic movement, thereby aggravating respiratory distress. Nasogastric tube suction should be instituted in an effort to relieve the distention. Another factor which may influence respiratory function is pain caused by spinal trauma.

Decubitus ulcers, especially those of appreciable size, which have failed to respond to conservative management, are best treated by full thickness skin grafts. Prior to surgery débridement and wet dressings are utilized to cleanse the ulcer in preparation for the graft. Occasionally bone beneath the decubitus must also be removed. Adequate nutrition is an important contributing factor in the healing of skin grafts.

The metabolic changes that follow spinal cord injury and prolonged immobilization bear close observation. A negative nitrogen balance invariably develops, as well as a deficiency of calcium and phosphorus. Anemia, hypoproteinemia, and osteoporosis occur commonly, and virtually all patients lose weight. Appropriate laboratory studies are necessary to follow the patient's progress and to correct any abnormalities that may occur. Careful dietary supervision is essential if a state of adequate nutrition is to be maintained.

Spasms

A significant number of patients rendered permanently paraplegic as a result of spinal cord injury develop involuntary contractions of the lower extremities to such a degree that they interfere with routine management and rehabilitation. Loss of appetite and lack of adequate rest and sleep may seriously debilitate such patients. Decubiti cannot be surgically treated while this condition persists. These motor spasms develop more often in cases of complete transection of the cord but also occur following partial lesions. They represent mass reflex activity of the distal isolated segment of the spinal cord deprived of the inhibiting influences of higher centers. Decubiti, infection, and malnutrition seem to potentiate their severity and frequency.

Simple procedures to control the spasms should be given a trial before resorting to more drastic methods. Removal of such irritating

733

stimuli as pressure sores and urinary calculi, and treatment of infections may provide a measure of relief. In our experience, muscle relaxing drugs have been ineffectual. When paraplegia is complete, anterior rhizotomy (Munro, 1945; Morrison et al, 1969), usually from T10 through S1 employing cystometry with electrical root stimulation (to avoid destruction of the nervous outflow to the bladder), has proved most satisfactory. Identification of the appropriate motor roots to be severed at the lower end of the spinal cord is difficult. According to Elsberg (1912) the dentate ligament ends inferiorly at the general level of the first lumbar vertebra in a fork-shaped extremity which may be used as a surgical landmark for the first lumbar root which rests upon it. Others have since shown that this is not an altogether constant relationship and that the root lying on the lowest slip of the dentate ligament may vary from T12 to L2 (MacDonald et al, 1946). These authors suggested that the relatively large size of the first sacral motor root might provide a means of identification. However the root of S1 is not invariably the largest to emerge from the conus and hence is not a reliable guide (Morrison et al, 1969). We employ electrical stimulation as an aid to root identification. The S3-S5 roots should be preserved so as not to impair reflex control of the bladder. On the other hand, in some of our patients with small spastic bladders that are incapable of holding urine, we have selectively sectioned the anterior roots of S3-S5 to provide a measure of flaccidity. It should be borne in mind that following anterior rhizotomy male patients frequently lose the capacity for erection.

Relief of spasticity may also be achieved by means of Bischof's myelotomy, a longitudinal bilateral incision at the level of the dentate ligaments from T12-S1 with variations in extent depending on bladder function. We prefer anterior rhizotomy because of its more consistently good results.

Obturator nerve section performed bilaterally will relieve scissoring of the legs due to adductor spasm during ambulation. This is the only indication for obturator neurectomy. It is of no value in the nonambulatory patient with paraplegia and severe spasms.

Injection of alcohol (Sheldon and Bors, 1948) has been utilized extensively to control spasticity and in many centers has largely replaced anterior rhizotomy. Relief of spasms is usually not permanent. While it is a simple procedure, alcohol block does not permit the degree of selectivity possible with rhizotomy so that the nerve roots involved in micturition and sexual function are sacrificed. Obviously it is not suit-

734

able for patients who retain some degree of motor or sphincter function. Theoretically subarachnoid phenol block (Nathan, 1959) offers a reasonable degree of selectivity. But unfortunately, even in experienced hands, intrathecal phenol may have a detrimental effect on residual neurologic function, and its salutary effects are of variable duration.

While patients benefit considerably from relief of spasticity the fact remains that to accomplish this, neural structures are permanently destroyed. In general unless the relief of spasticity is necessary as a life-saving measure, it is a good policy to wait a minimum of a year from the time of injury before resorting to any radical procedure. Patients with incomplete paraplegia who are nevertheless incapacitated by spasms present an especially difficult problem. The overall improvement resulting from elimination of the spasms may well outweigh the disadvantages of additional loss of function.

Relief of spasticity of localized distribution may be accomplished in selected cases by injecting dilute phenol into appropriate peripheral nerves.

Pain

Pain is a frequent problem, particularly in cases of cauda equina injury. According to Scarff (1960) it is more common following open trauma. It may be circumscribed, the area involved corresponding to the root distribution at the level of the injury; or it may be diffuse or imperfectly localized below the site of trauma. The physiologic mechanism responsible for the latter type of pain is not known. Pain is more likely to occur in the lower extremities, lower abdomen, or at the level of the lesion. Occasionally phantom sensations are experienced.

In most instances symptomatic treatment, exercises, and increased activity combined with a sympathetic attitude on the part of the physician and hospital personnel will prove effective. Narcotic drugs must be avoided. Occasionally a herniated disc, bony spur, or spinal instability will require operative management.

Severe persistent pain which usually follows thoracolumbar trauma is uncommon. Various forms of treatment, including intrathecal alcohol and phenol, posterior rhizotomy, cordotomy, and sympathectomy have been attempted without noticeable success. Cordotomy is most effective for the relief of radicular pain resulting from cauda equina lesions.

735

Rehabilitation of the paraplegic is a complex problem involving virtually all aspects of human activity — physical, social, vocational, and psychologic. The ultimate aim in cases of injury below the cervical level is complete independence in the activities of daily living, work, and recreation. Achievement of this goal requires the collective effort of a team of medical specialists. A detailed discussion of this subject may be found in Chapter 26. Here we will consider only the principles of physical rehabilitation.

Ideally the objective of physical rehabilitation is ambulation. Unfortunately, this is not always feasible and a wheelchair existence must often be accepted as a substitute goal. Physical therapy should be started during the acute stage as soon as the patient's condition permits. Each immobile joint must be put through a full range of motion daily so as to avoid contractures and deformities. Whether the patient ultimately ambulates with the help of crutches and braces or in a wheelchair, it is essential that the functioning musculature of the upper extremities and shoulder girdles be strengthened to a maximum degree. Patients whose legs are paralyzed must learn to use their upper extremities for such essential activities as changing position, moving from bed to chair, applying braces, ambulation, and propulsion in a wheelchair. Intensive exercise is required to condition the muscles for the additional tasks they must now perform. New skills must be acquired including balancing techniques, ambulation with crutches and braces, various transfer maneuvers, ascending and descending steps, and dexterity in resuming the upright position after an accidental fall. Development of the paravertebral, abdominal, and shoulder girdle muscles is most important for purposes of ambulation.

For purposes of weight bearing, braces are required to splint joints deprived of voluntary function. Adequate muscular development having been achieved and braces fitted, patients with low thoracic or lumbar injuries can be taught to ambulate with the aid of crutches. They must first adapt to the vertical position and learn how to balance. Ambulation is beyond the capacity of patients with cervical or high thoracic injuries and they must depend on a wheelchair for locomotion.

Patients with cervical cord lesions present an especially difficult problem in rehabilitation. The higher the level of the lesion, the greater the degree of disability. A patient with an injury at C7 or C8 still possesses good use of the wrist and some function of the fingers while one with a lesion at C4 or C5 is severely handicapped. Deprived of the use of their hands, patients must resort to various mechanical devices and gadgets to accomplish the activities of daily living. Electronic aids controlled by head and mouth movements have been devised for use by tetraplegics. Exclusive of those with very high cervical lesions, most patients are able to achieve a sitting balance and use a wheelchair. Those with C5-C6 lesions must be assisted into a chair.

MORTALITY AND PROGNOSIS

The long-range mortality figures of patients with traumatic spinal cord lesions vary, but the average is about 15.6 percent (Guttmann, 1967; Nyquist and Bors, 1967; Bors and Comarr, 1971). Nyquist and Bors reported that out of a total of 1851 patients, 86.6 percent were alive more than 10 years after injury; 62.9 percent, 10-19 years after injury; and 23.8 percent, 20 or more years after injury. Of a group of 180 patients of World War II, 132 (73 percent) survived 20 years or more.

Respiratory failure (predominantly in tetraplegic patients), pulmonary embolism, bronchopneumonia, and pyelonephritis are the main causes of death during the acute stage of paraplegia (Tribe, 1963). In the chronic stage, renal failure which encompasses amyloidosis, chronic pyelonephritis, urinary calculi, and associated hypertension is the most frequent cause of death.

With regard to recovery of neurologic function, if paralysis is immediate, complete, and unimproved after 24 hours, the prognosis is extremely poor. Occasionally some degree of recovery may occur at a later stage. Uncommonly we have observed significant recovery but, as a rule, no return of useful function is to be expected. In the event complete transection has been demonstrated at operation, the prognosis is hopeless; on the other hand, a grossly normal spinal cord seen at operation does not necessarily indicate a good prognosis. The outlook in cases of incomplete loss of cord function is infinitely better although the ultimate degree of recovery is unpredictable. Patients with complete paralysis but some sensory preservation may recover an appreciable degree of motor function, but this is not invariably the case (Suwanwela et al, 1962). In civilian spinal injuries caused by bullet wounds, the outlook for significant recovery is poor if a complete or nearly complete lesion has been sustained (Yashon et al, 1970). The same is true of war wounds due to missiles (Jacobs and Berg, 1971).

The various problems which beset the paraplegic patient render him susceptible to many complications. We have already referred to the occurrence of anemia, malnutrition, osteoporosis, spasms, pain, decubiti, respiratory complications, urinary infection, calculi, and amyloidosis. Additional complications include fractures, heterotopic calcification, and autonomic hyperreflexia (see Chaper 26). While the psychologic aspects of spinal cord injury are not dealt with in this presentation, their importance cannot be sufficiently emphasized. Suicide is not uncommon among paraplegics.

A late neurologic complication which may occur following injuries of the thoracic and lumbar spinal cord is a progressive myelopathy involving the cervical region (Barnett et al, 1966). Cystic degeneration, the etiology of which is not clear, appears to be the underlying cause (see Chaper 21).

REGENERATION IN THE SPINAL CORD

Regeneration and even restitution of function has been reported after spinal cord severance in a number of experimental animals (Sugar and Gerard, 1940; Windle, 1955; Freeman, 1962), but there is no convincing evidence of recovery following anatomic transection in mammals. Although there is evidence that regeneration of fibers in the central nervous system of mammals may be initiated, for unknown reasons, continued growth across the site of transection fails to occur. The problem of regeneration in the central nervous system is dealt with at length in the publications of Windle (1955) and Clemente (1964).

Wolman (1966) reported evidence of axon regeneration in 12 of 76 cases of spinal cord injury. The time interval after injury in the cases of reputed regeneration varied from 12 months to 32 years. As possible sources of origin of the regenerating axons the author suggested the posterior roots, anterior horn cells, and perivascular nerve fibers in addition to the descending and ascending pathways of the spinal cord.

The authors are indebted to Dr. John E. Scarff for permission to reproduce Figures 1 and 2, and Tables 1 and 2.

BIBLIOGRAPHY

Albin, M. S., White, R. J., Acosta-Rua, G., and Yashon, D. Study of Functional Recovery Produced by Delayed Localized Cooling After Spinal Cord Injury in Primates. *J. Neurosurg.*, *29*, 113, 1968. (a)

Albin, M. S., White, R. J., Yashon, D., and Massopust, L. C., Jr. Functional and Electrophysiological Limitations of Delayed Spinal Cord Cooling After Impact Injury. *Surg. Forum*, *19*, 423, 1968. (b)

Albin, M. S., Harris, L. S., White, R. J., and Yashon, D. Tolerance of Primate Spinal Cord to Extended Periods of Localized Hypothermia. *Cryobiol.*, *4*, *261*, 1968. (c)

Alexander, E., Forsyth, H. F., Davis, C. H., and Nashold, B. S. Dislocation of the Atlas on the Axis - The Value of Early Fusion of C1, C2, C3. *J. Neurosurg.*, *15*, 353, 1958.

Barnes, R. Paraplegia in Cervical Spine Injuries. *J. Bone Joint Surg.*, *30B*, 234, 1948.

Barnes, R. Paraplegia in Cervical Spine Injuries. *Proc. R. Soc. Med.*, *54*, 365, 1961.

Barnett, H. J. M., Botterell, E. H., Jousse, A. T., and Wynn-Jones, M. Progressive Myelopathy as a Sequel to Traumatic Paraplegia. *Brain*, *89*, 159, 1966.

Benes, V. *Spinal Cord Injury*. London: Baillière, Tindall, and Cassell, 1968.

Bing, R. *Compendium of Regional Diagnosis in Lesions of the Brain and Spinal Cord*. (11th ed.) Ed. by W. Haymaker. St. Louis: C. V. Mosby Co., 1940.

Blockey, N. J. and Purser, D. W. Fractures of the Odontoid Process of the Atlas. *J. Bone Joint Surg.*, *38B*, 794, 1956.

Bors, E. and Comarr, A. E. *Neurological Urology*. Baltimore: University Park Press, 1971. Pp. 454.

Brain, W. R., Northfield, D., and Wilkinson, M. The Neurological Manifestation of Cervical Spondylosis. *Brain*, *75*, 187, 1952.

Brain, W. R. and Wilkinson M. *Cervical Spondylosis*. Philadelphia: W. B. Saunders Co., 1967. Pp. 232.

Breasted, J. H. *The Edwin Smith Surgical Papyrus*. Vol. 1. Chicago: University of Chicago Press, 1930.

Burke, D. C. Hyperextension Injuries of the Spine. *J. Bone Joint Surg.*, *53B*, 3, 1971.

Celsus, A. C. *De Medicina*. Lib. viii Fol. Florent. Nicolaus Laurentii. 3 Vols. Trans. by W. G. Spencer. Cambridge 1935-8: Harvard Univ. Press; London: Wm. Heinemann.

Clemente, C. D. Regeneration in the Vertebrate Central Nervous System. *Internat. Rev. Neurobiol.*, *6*, 257, 1964.

Cloward, R. B. Treatment of Acute Fractures and Fracture-Dislocations of the Cervical Spine by Vertebral Body Fusion. *J. Neurosurg.*, *18*, 201, 1961.

Crenshaw, A. H. *Campbell's Operative Orthopedics*. Vol. 1. St. Louis: C. V. Mosby Co., 1971. Pp. 610-616.

Crutchfield, W. G. Skeletal Traction for Dislocation of the Cervical Spine. Report of a Case. *South. Surg.*, *2*, 156, 1933.

Crutchfield, W. G. Further Observations on the Treatment of Fracture-Dislocations of the Cervical Spine with Skeletal Traction. *Surg Gynec. & Obstet., 63,* 513, 1936.

De Palma, A. F. *The Management of Fractures and Dislocations.* 2nd ed. Vol. 1. Philadelphia: W. B. Saunders Co., 1970.

Duker, T. B., Kindt, G. W., and Kempe, L. G. Pathological Findings in Acute Experimental Spinal Cord Trauma. *J. Neurosurg., 35,* 700, 1971.

Elsberg, C. A. Some Features of the Gross Anatomy of the Spinal Cord and Nerve Roots and Their Bearing on the Symptomatology and Surgical Treatment of Spinal Disease. *Am. J. Med. Sci., 144,* 799, 1912.

Elsberg, C. A. The Edwin Smith Surgical Papyrus. The Diagnosis and Treatment of Injuries to the Skull and Spine 5000 Years Ago. *Ann. Med. Hist., 3,* 271, 1931.

Evans, J. P. and Rosenauer, A. Spinal Cord Injuries. *Arch. Surg., 72,* 812, 1956.

Forsyth, H. F. Extension Injuries of the Cervical Spine. *J. Bone Joint Surg., 46A,* 1792, 1964.

Forsyth, H. F., Alexander, E., Davis, C., and Underdal, R. The Advantages of Early Spine Fusion in Treatment of Fracture-Dislocations of Cervical Spine. *J. Bone Joint Surg., 41-A,* 17, 1959.

Freeman, L. W. Experimental Observations Upon Axonal Regeneration in the Transected Spinal Cord of Mammals. Chapt. XV in *Clin. Neurosurg.* (Proc. Congr. Neurol. Surg., 1960). Pp. 294-319. Baltimore: Williams & Wilkins Co., 1962.

Grisolia, A., Bell, R. L., and Peltier, L. F. Fractures and Dislocations of the Spine Complicating Ankylosing Spondylitis. *J. Bone Joint Surg., 49A,* 339, 1967.

Guttmann, L. History of the National Spinal Injuries Centre, Stoke Mandeville Hospital, Aylesbury. *Paraplegia, 5,* 115, 1967.

Guttmann, L. Chinical Symptomatology of Spinal Cord Lesions. In P. J. Vinken, G. W. Bruyn, and A. Biemond (Eds.) *Handbook of Clinical Neurology,* Vol. 2. Localization in Clinical Neurology. Amsterdam: North Holland Publ. Co., 1969. Pp. 178-216.

Harris, P. Some Neurosurgical Aspects of Traumatic Paraplegia. In P. Harris (Ed.) *Spinal Injuries.* Edinburgh, 1963. Pp. 101-112.

Haymaker, W. *Bing's Local Diagnosis in Neurological Diseases.* St. Louis: C. V. Mosby Co., 1969.

Holdsworth, F. W. Early Orthopedic Treatment of Patients with Spinal Injury. In P. Harris (Ed.) *Spinal Injuries.* Edinburgh, 1963. Pp. 93-101.

Howorth, M. B. and Petrie, F. J. *Injuries of the Spine.* Baltimore: Williams and Wilkins Co., 1964.

Hughes, J. T. and Brownell, B. Spinal Cord Damage from Hyperextension Injury in Cervical Spondylosis. *Lancet, 1,* 687, 1963.

Jackson, R. *The Cervical Syndrome.* 3rd ed. Springfield, Ill.: Charles C Thomas, 1966.

Jacobs, G. and Berg, R. A. The Treatment of Acute Spinal Cord Injuries in a War Zone. *J. Neurosurg., 34,* 1964, 1971.

Jane, J. A., Yashon, D., DeMyer, W. E., and Bucy, P. C. The Contribution of the Precentral Gyrus to the Corticospinal Tract of Man. *J. Neurosurg., 26,* 244, 1967.

jennett, S. The Response of Heart Rate to Hypoxia in Man After Cervical Spinal Cord Transection. *Paraplegia, 8,* 1, 1970.

Kuhn, R. A. Functional Capacity of the Isolated Human Spinal Cord. *Brain, 73,* 1, 1950.

Lipschitz, R. Associated Injuries and Complications of Stab Wounds of the Spinal Cord. *Paraplegia, 5,* 75, 1967.

Locke, G. E., Yashon, D., Feldman, R. A. and Hunt, W. E. Ischemia in Primate Spinal Cord Injury. *J. Neurosurg., 34,* 614, 1971.

Loeser, J. D. History of Skeletal Traction in the Treatment of Cervical Spine Injuries. *J. Neurosurg., 33,* 54, 1970.

MacDonald, I. B., McKenzie, K. G., and Botterell, E. H. Anterior Rhizotomy: The Accurate Identification of Motor Roots at the Lower End of the Spinal Cord. *J. Neurosurg., 3,* 421, 1946.

Markham, J. W. Surgery of the Spinal Cord and Vertebral Column. A *History of Neurological Surgery.* Ed. by A. E. Walker. Baltimore: Williams & Wilkins Co., 1951. Pp. 364-392.

Matson, D. D. *The Treatment of Acute Compound Injuries of the Spinal Cord Due to Missiles.* Springfield, Ill.: Charles C Thomas, 1948.

Mayfield, F. H. and Cazan, G. M. Spinal Cord Injuries: Analysis of Six Cases Show-Subarachnoid Block. *Am. J. Surg., 55,* 317, 1942.

Meirowsky, A. M. Neurosurgical Management. Chapt. 25 in *Neurological Surgery of Trauma.* Washington, D.C.: Office of the Surgeon General, Dept. of the Army. 1965. Pp. 307-332.

Morrison, G., Yashon, D. and White, R. J. Relief of Pain and Spasticity by Anterior Dorsolumbar Rhizotomy in Multiple Sclerosis. *Ohio State Med. J., 65,* 588, 1969.

Munro, D. The Rehabilitation of Patients Totally Paralyzed Below the Waist, with Special Reference to Making them Ambulatory and Capable of Earning Their Living. I. Anterior Rhizotomy for Spastic Paraplegia. *New Engl. J. Med., 233,* 731, 1945.

Nathan, P. W. Intrathecal Phenol to Relieve Spasticity in Paraplegia. *Lancet, 2,* 1099, 1959.

Nicoll, E. A. Fractures and Dislocations of the Spine. Chapt. 6 in J. M. P. Clark (Ed.) *Modern Trends in Orthopaedics.* London: Butterworths, 1962. Pp. 100-129.

Nyquist, R. H. and Bors, E. Mortality and Survival in Traumatic Myelopathy During Nineteen Years from 1946 to 1965. *Paraplegia, 5,* 22, 1967.

Osterholm, J. L., and Mathews, G. J. Altered Norepinephrine Metabolism Following Experimental Spinal Cord Injury. Part 1: Relationship to Hemorrhagic Necrosis and Post-wounding Neurological Deficits. *J. Neurosurg., 36,* 386, 1972.

Osterholm, J. L., and Mathews, G. J. Altered Norepinephrine Metabolism Following Experimental Spinal Cord Injury. Part 2: Protection Against Traumatic Spinal Cord Hemorrhagic Necrosis by Neropinephrine Synthesis Blockade with Alpha Methyl Tyrosine. *J. Neurosurg., 36,* 395, 1972.

Putnam, T. J. Progressive Confusional Syndrome Accompanying Injuries of the Cervical Portion of the Spinal Cord. *Arch. Neurol. & Psychiat., 41,* 298, 1939.

741

Queckenstedt, M. E. Zur Diagnose der Rückenmark-kompression. Deutsche Ztschr. f. *Nervenh.*, 55, 325, 1916.

Rand R. W. and Stern, W. E. Cervical Fractures of the Ankylosed Rheumatoid Spine. *Neurochirurgia*, 4, 137, 1961.

Roberts, J. B. and Curtiss, P. H., Jr., Stability of the Thoracic and Lumbar Spine in Traumatic Paraplegia Following Fracture or Fracture-Dislocation. *J. Bone Joint Surg.*, 52A, 1115, 1970.

Rogers, W. A. Treatment of Fracture-Dislocation of the Cervical Spine. *J. Bone Joint Surg.*, 24, 245, 1942.

Rogers, W. A. Fractures and Dislocations of the Cervical Spine. An End-Result Study. *J. Bone Joint Surg.*, 39-A, 341, 1957.

Rogers, W. A. Fractures and Dislocations of the Spine. In E. F. Cave (Ed.) *Fractures and Other Injuries*. Chicago: Yearbook Medical Publishers, Inc., 1958. Pp. 203-249.

Rosenbluth, P. R. and Meirowsky, A. M. Sympathetic Blockade, An Acute Cervical Cord Syndrome. *J. Neurosurg.*, 10, 107, 1953.

Ruch, T. C. Transection of the Human Spinal Cord: The Nature of Higher Control. In T. C. Ruch, H. D. Patton, J. W. Woodbury, and A. L. Towe (Eds.) *Neurophysiology*. 2nd ed. Philadelphia: W. B. Saunders Co., 1965. Pp. 207-214.

Scarff, J. E. Injuries of the Vertebral Column and Spinal Cord. In S. Brock (Ed.) *Injuries of the Brain and Spinal Cord and Their Coverings*. 4th ed. New York: Springer Publ. Co., 1960. Pp. 530-589.

Schneider, R. C. The Syndrome of Acute Anterior Spinal Cord Injury. *J. Neurosurg.*, 12, 95, 1955.

Schneider, R. C. Trauma to the Spine and Spinal Cord. In E. A. Kahn et al. (Eds.) *Correlative Neurosurgery*. 2nd ed. Springfield, Ill.: Charles C Thomas, 1969. Pp. 597-648.

Schneider, R. C., Cherry, G., and Pantek, H. The Syndrome of Acute Central Cervical Spinal Cord Injury. *J. Neurosurg.*, 11, 546, 1954.

Schneider, R. C., Livingston, K. E., Cave, A. J. E., and Hamilton, G. Hangman's Fracture of the Cervical Spine. *J. Neurosurg.*, 22, 141, 1965.

Schwartz, H. G., Coxe, W. S., and Goldring, S. Trauma of Spinal Cord. In *Neurological Surgery of Trauma*. Washington, D.C.: Office of the Surgeon General, Dept. of the Army, 1965. Pp. 273-286.

Sheldon, C. H. and Bors, E. Subarachnoid Alcohol Block in Paraplegia: Its Beneficial Effect on Mass Reflexes and Bladder Dysfunction. *J. Neurosurg.*, 5, 385, 1948.

Spinal Cord Injury: A Selected Bibliography, 1940-1963. Washington, D.C.: Medical and General Reference Library, Dept. of Medicine and Surgery, Veterans Administration, January, 1965.

Stone, W. A., Beach, T. P., and Hamelberg, W. Succinylcholine — Danger in the Spinal Cord Injured Patient. *Anesthesiol.*, 32, 168, 1970.

Stryker, H. Device for Turning Frame Patient. *J.A.M.A.*, 13, 1731, 1939.

Sugar, O. and Gerard, R. W. Spinal Cord Regeneration In the Rat. *J. Neurophysiol.* 3, 1, 1940.

Suwanwela, C., Alexander, E. Jr., and Davis, C. H., Jr. Prognosis in Spinal Cord

Injury with Special Reference to Patients with Motor Paralysis and Sensory Preservation. *J. Neurosurg., 19,* 220, 1962.

Symonds, C. The Interrelation of Trauma and Cervical Spondylosis in Compression of the Cervical Cord. *Lancet, 264,* 451, 1953.

Taylor, A. R. The Mechanism of Injury to the Spinal Cord and Neck without Damage to the Vertebral Column. *J. Bone Joint Surg., 33B,* 543, 1951.

Taylor, A. R. and Blackwood, W. Paraplegia in Hyperextension Cervical Injuries with Normal Radiographic Appearances. *J. Bone Joint Surg., 30-B,* 245, 1948.

Tribe, C. R. Causes of Death in the Early and Late Stages of Paraplegia. *Paraplegia, 1,* 19, 1963.

Wagner, F. C., Jr., Dohrmann, G. J., and Bucy, P. C. Histopathology of Transitory Traumatic Paraplegia in the Monkey. *J. Neurosurg., 35,* 272, 1971.

Walker, A. E., Kollros, J. J., and Case, T. J. The Physiologic Basis of Concussion. *J. Neurosurg., 1,* 103, 1944.

Watson-Jones, R. *Fractures and Joint Injuries.* 4th ed. Baltimore: Williams and Wilkins, Co., 1955. Pp. 1073.

White, R. J. and Albin, M. S. Spine and Spinal Cord Injury. In E.S. Gurdjian (Ed.) *Impact Injury and Crash Protection.* Springfield, Ill.: Charles C Thomas, 1969. Pp. 63-85.

White, R. J., Albin, M. S., Harris, L. S., and Yashon, D. Spinal Cord Injury: Sequential Morphology and Hypothermic Stabilization. *Surg. Forum, 20,* 432, 1969.

Windle, W. F. *Regeneration In The Central Nervous System.* Springfield, Ill.: Charles C Thomas, 1955.

Wolman, L. The Neuropathology of Traumatic Paraplegia. *Paraplegia, 1,* 233, 1964.

Wolman, L. Axon Regeneration After Spinal Cord Injury. *Paraplegia, 4,* 175, 1966.

Yashon, D., Jane, J. A., and White, R. J. Prognosis and Management of Spinal Cord and Cauda Equina Bullet Injuries in Sixty-Five Civilians. *J. Neurosurg., 32,* 163, 1970.

743

Chapter 23

SPINAL INJURIES: PRINCIPLES OF ORTHOPEDIC MANAGEMENT

EDMOND UHRY, Jr., M.D.

The treatment of spinal trauma is properly the joint responsibility of the neurosurgeon and orthopedic surgeon. In this chapter only the principles of orthopedic management of spinal fractures and dislocations will be discussed. For a more detailed account as is required in handling a particular problem, the reader is referred to the appropriate orthopedic literature. The spinal column has a twofold function. It acts as a support for the body and provides a passageway for the spinal cord and nerve roots. Since the structural changes induced by trauma may seriously interfere with both these functions, the purpose of treatment is to restore normal alignment whenever feasible and necessary, and to facilitate the reversal of neurologic deficits.

The classification of spinal injuries on the basis of stability is most important in any consideration of treatment. The bodies of the vertebrae are united by the intervertebral discs, while the posterior elements are joined by the supraspinous and interspinous ligaments, the capsules of the posterolateral joints, and the ligamenta flava. Stability is dependent on the integrity of this posterior ligament complex.

As indicated by Holdsworth (1970), the spine is generally subjected to one of five types of force: pure flexion, flexion and rotation, extension, vertical compression, and direct shearing force. *Pure flexion* causes a wedge fracture, does not rupture the laminar-spinous ligament complex, and the resulting lesion is stable. *Flexion rotation*, on the other hand, disrupts the laminar-spinous ligamentous structures, causing an unstable fracture dislocation. In the cervical region the articular processes, owing to their disposition, readily slide off one another, the disc ruptures, and a pure dislocation may result. This occurs less often in the lumbar region where the articular processes are large and vertical; here, lateral rotation more often produces a fracture of one or both articular processes and a slice fracture near the upper border of

744

the lower vertebra. This rotational fracture dislocation is especially common in the thoracolumbar region and is the most unstable of all spinal injuries. *Extension* injury of the cervical spine, if severe, may rupture the anterior longitudinal ligament and disc, causing a separation between the cancellous bone of the vertebral body and adjacent cartilaginous end plate or between the disc and end plate, and avulsion of a small fragment of bone anteriorly. This dislocation, which usually does not affect the posterior ligaments, is stable in flexion, and, as a rule, reduces spontaneously (Taylor and Blackwood, 1948). Forsyth et al (1959; 1964) have pointed out that forcible extension combined with compression, or compression and rotation, may result in a hyperextension or rotatory hyperextension fracture dislocation. Hyperextension fracture dislocations are characterized by fractures of the posterior bone elements, the inferior articular processes (in contrast to flexion injuries in which the fracture involves the superior articular process of the vertebra below), pedicles, laminae, or spinous process, all of which tend to be displaced upward, with anterior displacement of the affected vertebra. When a rotatory element is added, there occurs, in addition to the anterior displacement and rotation of the vertebral body, horizontal displacement of the inferior articular process on one side. Hyperextension injuries of the thoracolumbar spine are rare (Burke, 1971). *Vertical compression* injuries which occur in the cervical and lumbar regions fracture the vertebral end plate and force the nucleus of the intervertebral disc into the vertebral body, causing it to burst. Holdsworth classifies this type of vertebral lesion as a stable fracture. *Shearing* produces a displacement of an entire vertebra with fracture of the articular processes or pedicles and disruption of all ligaments.

Stable fractures: Wedge fractures are stable, do not cause paraplegia and require only symptomatic treatment. In the thoracolumbar region this is the commonest type of fracture. After a period of two to three weeks bed rest, ambulation with the aid of a back support is permitted. Wedge fractures without concomitant involvement of the posterior elements are uncommon in the cervical region; a collar provides symptomatic relief. Fractures of the thoracic spine above T-9 occur infrequently. They usually are simple wedge fractures which do not require immobilization.

Bursting fractures are basically stable (Holdsworth, 1970), but painful, and should be immobilized. In the cervical region quadriplegia is a frequent accompaniment; treatment involves the use of skeletal

745

traction in uncomplicated injuries and decompression and fusion in cases of spinal cord involvement.

Extension injuries of the neck which reduce spontaneously are stable in flexion and should be treated by means of a collar to prevent extension. Neurologic damage may be severe, especially in patients with osteoarthritis and a narrowed spinal canal.

Unstable injuries: The unstable fracture dislocations present a much more complex therapeutic problem. Reduction and immobilization are essential in order to achieve stability and avoid damage to the spinal cord and cauda equina. Operative treatment is often required to reduce the lesion and make certain that it remains stable. In view of the tendency of the fracture to displace postoperatively, traction and immobilization must be continued until there is radiologic evidence of healing. Paraplegia is a frequent complication and often necessitates modification of the plan of treatment. Laminectomy, when indicated, must not be unduly delayed.

Emergency treatment: When transporting patients with spinal injuries, it is essential that precautions be taken to avoid damaging or further damaging the cord or cauda equina. The traumatized segment must be immobilized and maintained in the physiologically neutral position. In cases of cervical injury the neck should be held in slight extension with traction applied in a longitudinal direction. Patients with lumbar injuries may be transported either prone or supine provided a mild degree of lordosis is maintained.

CERVICAL SPINE

The stability of the atlantooccipital articulation is entirely dependent on the occipito-atlanto-axial ligaments. Dislocations are rare owing to the strength of these ligaments. Such lesions may cause instantaneous death. Treatment involves the application of skeletal traction followed by cranio-cervical fusion after reduction is achieved.

Fractures of the ring of the atlas (Jefferson) are caused by vertical compression. Unless associated with other injuries of the cervical spine, they are neurologically innocuous; traction and plaster immobilization provide adequate protection.

Rotary atlantoaxial subluxation is characterized radiographically by persistent asymmetry of the odontoid relative to the articular masses of the atlas, the asymmetry not being altered by rotation to either side. Treatment requires traction in the neutral position or in slight extension followed by immobilization after reduction has occurred.

In fracture dislocations affecting the atlantoaxial region there is usually anterior displacement of the atlas, rarely posterior dislocation. Such injuries may be immediately fatal or cause varying degrees of neurologic damage. The dens may be fractured without affecting its relationship to the arch of the atlas, but permit atlantoaxial displacement with narrowing of the spinal canal. Reduction by skeletal traction and immobilization are required in such cases. Fusion may be necessary to achieve stabilization. Failure to recognize this type of injury, or inadequate early treatment, may lead to neurologic complications at a later date due to excessive mobility at this level. Congenital absence of the dens lessens the stability of the atlantoaxial articulation so that moderate trauma may produce a dangerous displacement. Fusion is indicated in such cases. In younger subjects atlantoaxial displacement may occur spontaneously in association with inflammatory lesions in the cervical region.

Fractures of the odontoid process without displacement are treated by plaster fixation in slight flexion.

Below the atlantoaxial region dislocations and fracture dislocations occur most commonly at the C-4-7 levels. They are unstable, often complicated by spinal cord or nerve root involvement and associated with a high mortality in patients with tetraplegia. Reduction by means of skeletal traction is essential. Some surgeons prefer to achieve reduction by manipulation under anesthesia, employing a muscle relaxant, but this is a dangerous maneuver in the presence of severe instability. Traction is continued to maintain reduction. Should the facets remain locked despite an adequate trial of traction, thereby preventing reduction, operative disengagement is necessary. Stability frequently is achieved following reduction by traction and immobilization, but recurrent dislocations occur sufficiently often to lead many surgeons to recommend fusion in such cases (Rogers, 1957; Forsyth et al, 1959; Nicoll, 1962; DePalma, 1970). Skull caliper traction is also employed in cases of cervical fracture dislocation with paraplegia.

Compression fractures of the bodies with fragmentation (bursting) are often associated with displacement of fragments backward into the vertebral canal and neural damage. Treatment by means of traction should be attempted. If this proves ineffectual, operative decompression is indicated. The anterior approach to the cervical spine permitting decompression of the spinal cord and nerve roots and interbody fusion would appear to be most appropiate in such cases. A distinct trend favoring the anterior approach in the surgical treatment of cervical

747

spine fractures and dislocations is evident in the current literature. The lesion responsible for neurologic involvement may be visualized and dealt with directly insofar as possible and vertebral instability corrected by interbody fusion; moreover, postoperative traction is unnecessary and the period of immobilization may be shortened.

Bursting fractures without neurologic involvement are treated by means of skeletal traction for purposes of reduction. Holdsworth considers these to be stable lesions but Rogers (1958) and DePalma (1970) recommend posterior spinal fusion following reduction.

In a discussion of the indications for operative treatment of acute flexion injuries of the cervical spine, Petrie (1964) recommends fusion with or without decompression of the spinal cord under the following circumstances: a dislocation difficult to reduce by traction or one too easily reduced; bilateral dislocation of the articular processes with spinal cord involvement; a fracture dislocation with progressive neurologic deficit; a bursting fracture of the vertebral body with more than 3 mm encroachment on the spinal canal; and a fracture involving two or more elements of a single vertebra.

Unilateral rotary dislocations are usually not amenable to reduction by traction. Open reduction and fusion are required.

Posterior dislocations are produced by shearing forces displacing one vertebra backward upon another. Posterior fracture dislocations result from forcible hyperextension, a backward displacing force being combined with compression in the long axis of the spine. Such injuries occur infrequently and usually produce neurologic deficits. Reduction may be accomplished by traction.

Hyperextension injuries which fail to reduce spontaneously should be treated by means of skull traction.

Fractures of the cervical spine in patients with ankylosing spondylitis may occur following relatively minor trauma owing to loss of flexibility and increased fragility. Reduction by traction should be attempted. Subluxation or dislocation may also occur in patients with rheumatoid arthritis, and atlantoaxial dislocations may result in sudden death.

Subluxations without fracture, in which the facets are not completely disengaged, may be reduced by extension of the neck. Traction and occasionally anesthesia may be necessary to effect reduction. Thereafter the spine is immobilized in plaster in full extension. In the event subluxation recurs following conservative treatment, a fusion should be performed. A mild subluxation may be demonstrable only on a flexion roentgenogram.

Unilateral subluxation occurs infrequently. Reduction is accomplished by hyperextension, or, if necessary, by manipulation, after which the hyperextended position is maintained by means of a collar.

Injuries involving the laminae, pedicles, and articular processes usually occur in association with fracture dislocations. The need for surgical intervention to remove indriven fragments of the neural arch will depend on the neurologic status of the patient. Traction and immobilization are otherwise employed.

Isolated injuries of the spinous processes such as "clay shoveler's" fracture are not uncommon and not neurologically significant. Usually C-6 or 7 or T-1 is affected. Symptomatic relief is all that is required.

THORACIC SPINE

As already noted, fractures of the thoracic spine above T-9 are infrequent and are usually of the simple compression variety. As a rule, neurologic dysfunction does not occur. Such fractures require immobilization but need no reduction. However, when a rotary injury results in an unstable fracture with posterior protrusion of bony elements, the thoracic spinal canal is narrowed and the cord compressed with resultant paraplegia. Decompression is indicated in such cases. Shear injuries, produced by severe violence, are almost always associated with complete paraplegia. According to Holdsworth reduction is necessary only in cases with considerable displacement.

LUMBAR SPINE

Fracture dislocations of the thoracolumbar spine must be reduced and immobilized so as to protect the neural elements. Operative reduction is necessary in patients with intact, locked facets, after which a fusion is performed for stabilization. Thereafter the patient is immobilized in extension. When the facets have been fractured, reduction may be accomplished by extension in the prone position, but fusion is still required to achieve stabilization.

When the dislocation is associated with paraplegia, the use of a plaster jacket, which is hazardous to the skin, must be avoided. To relieve pressure on the underlying conus and/or cauda equina, the dislocation should be reduced. To ensure maintenance of the reduction and immobilization when turning the patient, which is periodically necessary in such cases, internal fixation by means of plates bolted to

749

the spinous processes above and below the lesion has been advocated (Nicoll, 1962; Holdsworth, 1963).

Bursting fractures without paraplegia are treated by immobilization. A fusion may be advisable in such cases, especially when the antero-posterior diameter of the spinal canal has been significantly narrowed. Laminectomy and fusion are indicated in patients in whom this type of lesion has resulted in cord compression.

Fractures of the lumbar transverse and spinous processes require only symptomatic treatment.

BIBLIOGRAPHY

Barnes, R. Paraplegia in Cervical Spine Injuries. *J. Bone Joint Surg.*, *30-B*, 239, 1948.

Braakman, R., and Penning, L. *Injuries of the Cervical Spine*. Amsterdam: Excerpta Medica, 1971.

Burke, D. C. Hyperextension Injuries of the Spine. *J. Bone Joint Surg. 53-B*, 3, 1971.

Cloward, R. B. Treatment of Acute Fractures and Fracture-Dislocations of the Cervical Spine by Vertebral Body Fusion. A Report of Eleven Cases. *J. Neurosurg.*, *18*, 201, 1961.

Cloward, R. B. Surgical Treatment of Dislocations and Compression Fractures of the Cervical Spine by the Anterior Approach. *Proceedings of the Seventeenth Veterans Administration Spinal Cord Injury Conference*, Sept. 29-Oct. 1, 1969. New York, N. Y. Pp. 26-35.

DePalma, A. F. *The Management of Fractures and Dislocations*, 2nd ed. Vol.1. Philadelphia: W. B. Saunders Co., 1970.

Forsyth, H. F. Extension Injuries of the Cervical Spine. *J. Bone Joint Surg.*, *46-A*, 1792, 1964.

Forsyth, H. F., Alexander, E. A., Davis, C. H., and Underdal, R. G. The Advantages of Early Spine Fusion in the Treatment of Fracture-Dislocation of the Cervical Spine. *J. Bone Joint Surg.*, *41-A*, 17, 1959.

Garber, J. N. Fracture and Fracture-Dislocation of the Cervical Spine. American Academy of Orthopaedic Surgeons. *Symposium on the Spine*. St. Louis: C. V. Mosby, 1969. P. 18-53.

Gorgono, B. J. S. Injuries of the Atlas and Axis. *J. Bone Joint Surg.*, *36-B*, 397, 1954.

Holdsworth, F. W. Early Orthopaedic Treatment of Patients with Spinal Injury. In P. Harris (Ed.) *Spinal Injuries*. Edinburgh: Royal Coll. Surg., 1963.

Holdsworth, F. Fractures, Dislocations, and Fracture Dislocations of the Spine. *J. Bone Joint Surg.*, *52-A*, 1534, 1970.

Howorth, M. B., and Petrie, J. G. *Injuries of the Spine*. Baltimore: Williams and Wilkins, 1964.

Nicoll, E. A. Fractures and Dislocations of the Spine. In J. M. P. Clark (Ed.), *Modern Trends in Orthopaedics*. London: Butterworths, 1962. Pp. 100-129.

Petrie, J. G. Flexion Injuries of the Cervical Spine. *J. Bone Joint Surg., 46-A*, 1800, 1964.

Rogers, W. A. Fractures and Dislocations of the Cervical Spine. An End-Result Study. *J. Bone Joint Surg., 39-A*, 341, 1957.

Rogers, W. A. Fractures and Dislocations of the Spine. In E. F. Cave (Ed.), *Fractures and Other Injuries*. Chicago: Year Book Publishers, 1958. Pp. 203-249.

Taylor, A. R., and Blackwood, W. Paraplegia in Hyperextension Cervical Injuries with Normal Radiographic Appearances. *J. Bone Joint Surg., 30-B*, 245, 1948.

Verbiest, H. Anterolateral Operations for Fractures and Dislocations in the Middle and Lower Parts of the Cervical Spine. Report of a Series of 47 Cases. *J. Bone Joint Surg., 51-A*, 1489, 1969.

Watson-Jones, R. *Fractures and Joint Injuries*, 4th ed. Vol. 2. Baltimore: Williams and Wilkins, 1955.

Wortzman, G., and Dewar, F. P. Rotary Fixation of the Atlantoaxial Joint: Rotational Atlantoaxial Subluxation. *Radiology, 90*, 479, 1968.

CHAPTER 24

RADIOLOGY OF SPINAL TRAUMA

BERNARD S. EPSTEIN, M. D.

The oldest known work on the diagnosis and treatment of fractures and dislocations of the spine is to be found in the Edwin Smith Papyrus, presently in the Rare Book Room of the New York Academy of Medicine. Breasted, who translated the papyrus, dates it to about 3000 to 2500 B.C., and suggests that its author might have been Imhotep, the first great Egyptian physician who later was deified. From antiquity to the present time, the management of derangements of the vertebral column has had a long and vivid history of sustained interest and accomplishment.

In evaluating spinal fractures recognition of the effects of trauma requires knowledge of the detailed anatomy of each vertebra as well as of the architecture of the entire spinal column. Consideration must be given to damage incurred by the ligaments, intervertebral discs, muscular attachments, and the contents of the spinal canal. Movements of vertebrae in varying directions are produced by forces of flexion, extension, rotation, and compression. The effects of abnormal forces may be transmitted to successive vertebral segments directly, and can be expressed as the response of the flexible column to a combination of coiling, uncoiling, torsion, compression, or expansion. Direct trauma, such as a blow by a blunt intrument, or a penetrating force such as a gunshot or a knife wound, produces shattering or disrupting effects as well.

Movement at the craniovertebral junction and the atlantoaxial articulation differs from that at other levels of the cervical spine. Similarly, the type and range of movement possible in the lower cervical region are quite different from those which take place at the thoracolumbar and lumbosacral junctions. The structural characteristics of each vertebral element are uniquely suited to these intricate functional patterns.

From the radiological viewpoint, spinal injuries are reflected mainly

752

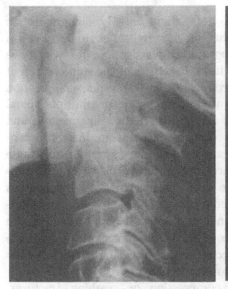
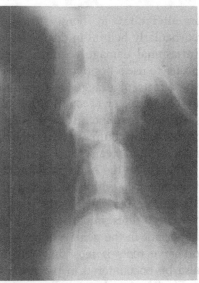
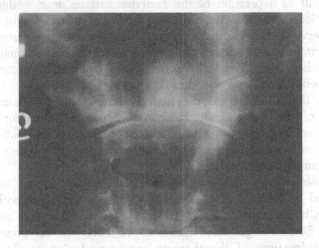

Fig. 1A. Fracture of the base of the dens in an 82-year-old woman who struck her occiput against a concrete floor. Irregularity of the cortex of the midportion of the anterior aspect of the body of the second cervical vertebra is visible just beneath the base of the dens. Soft tissue swelling in the prevertebral area is present.

Fig. 1B. A lateral body section roentgenogram shows the fracture more distinctly.

Fig. 1C. The fracture line is difficult to identify on the anteroposterior laminagram. The left articulation between C-1 and C-2 is narrowed. A faint fracture line passes downward and to the left from the left side of the base of the dens.

753

in alterations in bony structure and alignment. Laminagrams are particularly helpful in displaying changes in vertebral contours (Fig. 1). Intraspinal damage requires myelographic investigation, for which we prefer to use a positive contrast medium. Fractures of the spine represent the effects of exaggerated and forcible flexion, extension, compression and rotation, or a combination of all four on single or multiple spinal elements. Inasmuch as these forces also are exerted on ligamentous and muscular structures, paravertebral damage incident to bleeding, contusions, and tears is a concomitant effect. The extension of these influences to the intraspinal structures may result in bleeding or disruption of tissue within or outside the dura. Displacement of ligamentous structures, particularly the ligamenta flava, and herniation of intervertebral discs into the spinal canal and intervertebral foramina are important in the genesis of spinal cord and nerve root damage. Avulsion of nerve roots is most likely to occur in the cervical region, but may also be encountered in the lower lumbar region.

Flexion injuries usually cause compression or crushing fractures. These result in depression of the superior surface or a wedge-shaped configuration of the affected vertebral bodies, and occur most often in the midcervical, the midthoracic, and the thoracolumbar regions.

Hyperextension injuries are likely to be associated with damage to the neural arches, and often are accompanied by ventral protrusion of the ligamenta flava into the dorsal aspect of the spinal canal. With breaks in the continuity of the neural arches, and particularly with fractures of the laminae, displacement of one vertebra forward on the subjacent segment can take place. Such fracture dislocations may be partial or more or less complete, and associated with severe damage to the ligaments and intervertebral disc.

Rotational injuries can fracture the pedicles and neural arches. A translateral or torsional displacement of one vertebra on another may follow, with associated damage to the adjacent ligaments and intervertebral fibrocartilage. Rib fractures are likely to be present with fracture dislocations of the thoracic spine, producing severe pain as well as pulmonary damage.

Spinal injuries also follow blows to the vertex of the skull. Diving accidents, falls on the head, assaults, and motor car accidents involve a combination of forces. These include *compression* of the long axis of the spine together with rotational and backward or forward propulsion, depending on the angle and intensity of the impact and the position of the body at the moment of the accident. Similarly, a fall in which a patient strikes the ground in an erect or sitting position can produce serious damage to the sacrum, the pelvis, and the lower lumbar spine. In these injuries transmission of forces may affect the remainder of the spine. The spine actually is a unitary structure and, following severe trauma, it is best to examine the entire column if at all in doubt about the extent of the injury.

Cervical spine injuries may affect the cervico-occipital level, the midcervical region, or the cervicothoracic junction, and usually involve one or two vertebrae. With severe injuries multiple vertebrae may be involved. Injuries of the cervico-occipital junction may follow a blow on the head, a fall, a diving accident, or sufficiently intense trauma to the vertex of the skull. One consequence of such trauma is a bursting fracture of the first cervical vertebra, with outward displacement of its lateral masses. Lesser injuries may produce unilateral or bilateral fractures of the anterior or posterior arches, with little or no displacement of fragments. Occasionally the lateral masses of the first cervical vertebra are normally farther apart than might be expected, thereby simulating a bursting fracture.

Avulsion of the cervico-occipital ligaments without a concomitant fracture occasionally occurs after a severe twisting trauma such as may result from an automobile accident in which the patient was restrained by both a lap belt and a cross-chest device. The chief complaint may be excessive pain on motion of the head. The only radiologic change may be a widening of the space between the base of the skull and the first cervical vertebra, exaggerated when the head is flexed. This is admittedly a difficult lesion to diagnose.

Fractures of the second cervical vertebra are encountered more often. The odontoid process is particularly prone to injury (Figs. 1 and 2). When evaluating fractures of the dens it is important to determine whether the transverse atlantal ligament, which retains the dens within the concave notch of the anterior arch of the first cervical vertebra, remains intact. If the dens remains fixed in its normal position, it cannot shift dorsally to compress the medulla oblongata and the upper cervical spinal cord, a complication which can cause sudden death. Dislocation of the first on the second cervical vertebra when the dens is intact is serious because it can then impinge on the cord.

The possibility of a congenital malformation is an important consid-

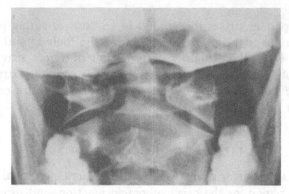

A

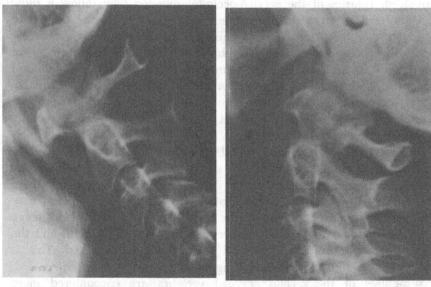

B   C

Fɪɢ. 2A. Anteroposterior roentgenogram of the atlas and axis of a 28-year-old
woman who was in an automobile accident ten months before this examination.
She had struck her head against the dashboard when her car was hit from behind.
The fracture through the base of the dens was identified then and can still be seen.
Fɪɢ. 2B. Flexion lateral film reveals foward movement of the dens. The normal
space between the dens and the anterior arch of the atlas is maintained.
Fɪɢ. 2C. In extension the dens retains its position relative to the anterior arch
of C-1. This gliding movement was best seen on lateral cineroentgenographic
examination. It was decided to fuse the upper cervical segments posteriorly even
though symptoms were mild.

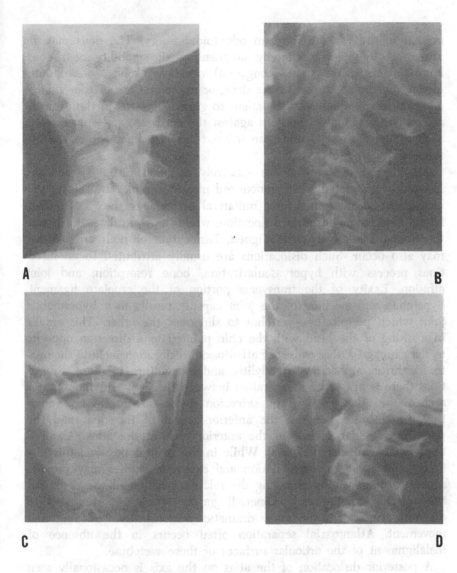

Fig. 3A. Atlantoaxial dislocation in a 9-year-old girl with a retropharyngeal abscess following mumps which had started about four weeks before the onset of neck symptoms. There is a rotary dislocation of C-1 on C-2. The jaw is tilted to the left, the cervical spine to the right.

Fig. 3B. A lateral roentgenogram shows widening of the space between the dens and the anterior arch of the atlas.

Fig. 3C and D. Anteroposterior and lateral roentgenograms eight days later, following conservative treatment, show restoration of the normal relations between C-1 and C-2.

eration in the evaluation of an odontoidal injury. The dens may be absent or hypoplastic, thereby augmenting the mobility of the atlantoaxial structures. Other congenital variations, such as os odontoideum, incomplete fusion of the dens, or malformations of the cervicooccipital junction subject the patient to greater hazard in the event of a fracture. Locking of the dens against the cord may take place when a shortened dens slips under an intact transverse ligament in the absence of a fracture.

Atlantoaxial dislocations are relatively common (Fig. 3) and are frequently associated with pronounced muscle spasm. The rotary type of dislocation may involve a unilateral articular surface, with ipsilateral anterior or posterior dislocation, while the contralateral articulation remains relatively well aligned. Dislocation of both articulations may also occur. Such dislocations are usually attributed to an infectious process with hypervascularization, bone resorption, and joint effusion. Laxity of the transverse portion of the cruciate ligament, hyperemia and swelling of the joint capsule results in a hypermobile joint which permits one vertebra to slip over the other. This results in a tilting of the head with the chin pointed in a direction opposite to the slippage. Other causes of atlantoaxial dislocation include rheumatoid arthritis, ankylosing spondylitis, and mongolism. In these dislocations there is apt to be a separation between the dens and the anterior arch of the atlas. Flexion and extension studies are useful in evaluating the distance between the anterior aspect of the dens and the posterior articular surface of the anterior arch of the atlas. About 3 to 4 mm is considered normal. While in the neutral position, this distance may appear normal, flexion and extension studies may provide a clue to diagnosis by changing the relative position of the dens and the anterior atlantal arch. Cineradiography is an important aid to diagnosis since it provides a dramatic demonstration of abnormal movement. Atlantoaxial separation often occurs in the absence of malalignment of the articular surfaces of these vertebrae.

A posterior dislocation of the atlas on the axis is occasionally seen with fractures or with congenital absence of the dens. Rarely, this may appear following an injury without a fracture.

In radiography of the atlas and axis through the open mouth, a slight lateral displacement is within normal limits, and should not be regarded as indicative of a dislocation. This can be exaggerated in the presence of torticollis, and may be simulated by voluntary sharp lateral bending of the head on the neck.

Spontaneous reduction can take place in subluxations of the cervical spine, particularly those of the atlas and axis. This can occur during examination, as happened in one of our patients recently. This man had a marked torticollis with rotary dislocation of the right side of the first on the second cervical vertebra. While he was being prepared for a second film, he remarked that he suddenly felt better and his neck straightened out. The second roentgenogram of the atlantoaxial articulation showed return of normal alignment.

Spontaneous reduction of cervical dislocations also occurs in the midcervical region as a rebound phenomenon. In such cases the patient may nevertheless suffer cord damage and be rendered immediately quadriparetic or quadriplegic. Some patients suffer delayed consequences and neurologic defects may not appear for some time. It has been suggested that the spinal cord may be damaged as a result of transient retropulsion of the nucleus pulposus. Cord trauma may also occur as a result of an hyperextension injury causing inward bulging of the ligamentum flavum against the posterior aspect of the cord. Patients with narrow cervical canals and spondylotic ridges are especially vulnerable in this respect.

Traumatic spondylolisthesis of the cervical spine requires care in the handling of the patient. If this is suspected clinically, the x-ray examination should proceed with caution under the direct supervision of the responsible physician. It is essential that the entire area be examined (Fig. 4). We limit our initial films to a recumbent anteroposterior and a lateral view, and do not proceed with further studies until these have been reviewed.

Dislocations of the second on the third cervical vertebrae are less frequent than those involving the lower cervical segments. These usually follow trauma but may also occur as a result of metastatic, granulomatous, or inflammatory disease. Pain, stiffness, and limitation of motion are common manifestations. Such dislocations, when slight, are best identified by means of flexion and extension studies of the neck. These should not be undertaken until a lateral film of the cervical spine has been inspected. Normally the second cervical vertebra moves forward to some extent on the third, so that a slightly anterior position of the anteroinferior surface of the second cervical vertebra in flexion should not be misinterpreted. Lower cervical vertebral dislocations are not uncommon, and often are accompanied by fracture of the involved laminae. They may involve one or both of the apophyseal joints. It is possible for such dislocation to occur without visible fracture when

759

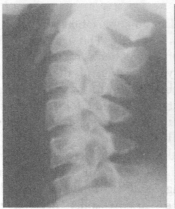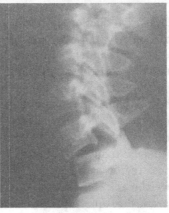

FIG. 4A. This 23-year-old woman had been thrown forward violently in an automobile accident. She had edema over both orbits and tenderness over the cervical spine. Films taken immediately after the accident showed no fracture. Note that the articulation between C-6 and C-7, and the body of C-7, are not visible on this film.

FIG. 4B. The patient continued to have neck pain. Ten days later another lateral cervical spine film clearly reveals a forward dislocation of C-6 on C-7. Forward dislocation of the inferior articular facets of C-6 has occurred so that they are now situated anterior to the tips of the superior facets of C-7.

ligaments binding the spinous processes and laminae are torn. Because of the horizontal disposition of the laminar articular surfaces, loss of ligamentous restraint may be associated with forward subluxations in flexion injuries. Overriding of a superior facet ventral to the infrajacent facet results in locking of the dislocation, a factor which can complicate management of the injury considerably (Fig. 5).

Flexion injuries of the cervical spine also are associated with "teardrop" fractures (Fig. 6) which appear on lateral roentgenograms as a chip of bone separate from the anterior portion of a vertebral body. Such injuries are frequently associated with painful paraspinal hemorrhage. Following resorption of the hematoma, pain subsides and the fracture usually heals. Compression deformities without significant dislocation also are associated with this type of injury, and occur most often in the midcervical region.

More severe fractures may involve multiple segments, often with dislocation of one or more vertebrae. Comminuted fractures with vertical components passing through one (Fig. 7) or more vertebral bodies may be encountered, and may be associated with partial or complete dislocation of one or more vertebrae. Profound damage to the inter-

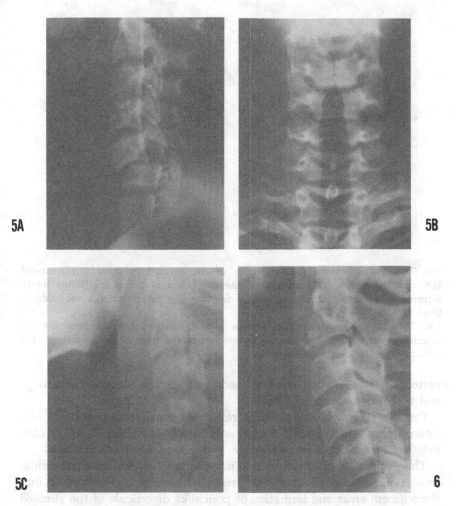

FIG. 5A. Dislocation of C-5 on C-6 incurred during a wrestling match by a 17-year-old boy. The interspace is narrowed. A forward displacement and tilting of the body of C-5 on C-6 is apparent. No demonstrable fracture of the articular facets is visible. The spinous process of C-5 is elevated, that of C-6 is displaced caudad.

FIG. 5B. Anteroposterior cervical roentgenogram shows a narrowing of the silhouette of the body of C-5 due to its anterior displacement and downward tilt. No fracture lines are visible.

FIG. 5C. Another film made three weeks later after traction had reduced the dislocation reveals marked prevertebral soft tissue swelling attributed to hemorrhage.

FIG. 6. Tear-drop fracture of the anteroinferior surface of the body of C-2. Prevertebral soft tissue swelling is visible.

761

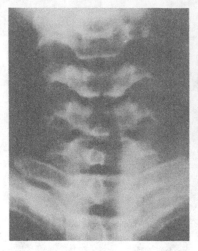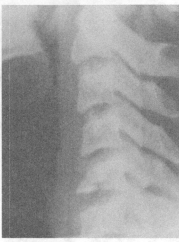

Fig. 7A. Anteroposterior roentgenogram of the cervical spine of a 15-year-old boy who had struck his head against the dashboard in a forward flexion injury incurred in an auto accident. A vertical fracture line passes through the midportion of C-5.

Fig. 7B. Lateral roentgenogram reveals a wedge-shaped fracture involving the anterior aspect of C-5. The vertical component of the fracture passes through the inferior aspect of the vertebral body.

vertebral discs, neural arches, and soft tissues occurs frequently, and such injuries can be fatal.

Posterior spondylolisthesis may result from major disruption of the intervertebral discs and the ligaments which bind the neural arches together. These injuries can occur without concomitant fractures.

The evaluation of nerve root injury requires myelographic examination. Avulsion injuries are characterized by leakage of Pantopaque into the adjacent areas and formation of pouchlike diverticula of the affected nerve sleeves. Intraspinal hematomas can be demonstrated by myelography which may show evidence of an intramedullary expansion causing a cerebrospinal fluid block.

Laminar fissure fractures sometimes cause considerable pain, and are difficult to identify. Special studies, including oblique stereoroentgenograms and laminagrams, may prove helpful. It is important not to mistake congenital variations such as accessory laminar epiphyses or extra articular processes for such fractures.

Fractures limited to the transverse processes of the upper six cervical vertebrae are infrequent. Spinous process fractures, particularly of

762

the seventh cervical vertebra, are more common. Those that occur as stress phenomena have been referred to as "clay-shoveller's fractures." Malnutrition, fatigue, and a sudden strain are important factors in this type of injury. Radiologic identification is readily made on lateral neck films. A clue to such a fracture sometimes can be found on anteroposterior roentgenograms when the tip of a fractured spinous process is displaced downward and approximates the one beneath.

Fractures of the transverse processes of the seventh cervical and the first and second thoracic vertebrae require a special word of comment. These are difficult to demonstrate, and are quite painful. Stereoroentgenograms and laminagrams are helpful. Failure of fusion of the tips of these transverse processes can be distinguished from fractures by the intact cortical periphery of the distal structures.

Repeated examinations are required in order to follow the course of a fracture or dislocation. Evidence of healing is difficult to demonstrate inasmuch as fibrous union takes place and the amount of visible callus formation is small. When incomplete union occurs, excessive mobility may require surgical fixation. Malalignment and spontaneous fusion sometimes follow an untreated injury. The neurologic consequences of spinal trauma are often immediate when there is cord or nerve root damage. However, there may be a considerable delay before neurologic deficits become apparent, and symptoms can appear months or years after the accident. Involvement of vessels supplying the anterior spinal artery may also be responsible for cord damage. Compression of the vertebral artery may lead to vertebrobasilar insufficiency.

Avascular necrosis may follow bony injury, particularly to the dens. Other conditions which augment the effects of trauma include the Klippel-Feil anomaly, fusion of the cervical vertebrae incident to ankylosing spondylitis or rheumatoid arthritis, and congenital malformations of the cervico-occipital junction. When fusion of the vertebrae exists, as for example in ankylosing spondylitis, the fused segments act like a solid bone, and fractures are more likely to be accompanied by cord damage.

FRACTURES OF THE THORACIC SPINE

The thoracic spine is characterized by a gradual increase in the size of the vertebral bodies from above downward. The size and configuration of the respective vertebrae gradually change, becoming less like those of the lower cervical segments and more like those

763

of the upper lumbar vertebrae. The pedicles, which are short and broad in the upper thoracic region, elongate and widen more caudally. Similarly, changes appear in the configuration of the laminae and the spinous processes. The pronounced overlap and downward inclination of these structures in the upper thoracic vertebrae alter perceptibly in the lower thoracic spine.

Fractures of the thoracic spine usually involve the vertebral bodies. For purposes of classification, these may be subdivided into those affecting the upper three segments, the midthoracic fourth to ninth vertebrae, and the distal thoracic tenth to twelfth vertebrae. Because of the anatomic and functional characteristics of the lower thoracic vertebrae, injuries to this region are often associated with upper lumbar vertebral damage.

Fractures of the upper thoracic vertebrae are uncommon, and when present, suggest the possibility of a pathologic fracture. Dislocations of these segments are uncommon except as a result of violent injuries which often are fatal. Laminar fractures occasionally occur in the upper two segments. Spinous process fractures may involve the first or second thoracic vertebrae as stress phenomena, like those which occur in the lower cervical region.

Midthoracic fractures usually involve the fourth, fifth, and sixth vertebrae (Fig. 8). These are mainly hyperflexion injuries resulting from sharp forward bending of the neck on the chest, such as occur with the convulsions of epilepsy, tetany, or electroshock therapy. A wedge-shaped deformity is produced, usually involving two or three segments. The anterosuperior surfaces of the involved vertebrae are compressed but the posterior aspects remain intact, so that there is little effect on the spinal canal and its contents. These fractures, which often appear spontaneously in osteoporotic individuals, are not necessarily painful. They require little in the way of treatment.

Fractures of the lower thoracic vertebrae (Figs. 9 and 10) often are associated with fracture of the first, and sometimes the second lumbar vertebrae. These, too, result most often from hyperflexion injuries. Inasmuch as the thoracolumbar junction is the most flexible segment of the vertebral column, rotational and torsional forces may be brought into play as a result of trauma with concomitant rib fractures and paravertebral soft tissue damage. Shearing injuries may damage the intervertebral discs, producing translateral (Fig. 11) as well as ventrodorsal vertebral displacement. These injuries also involve the pedicles and laminae, so that extensive intraspinal damage may be

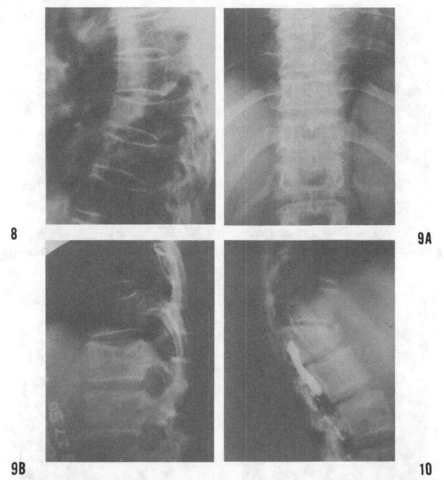

8　　　　　　　　　　　　　　　　　　　　　9A

9B　　　　　　　　　　　　　　　　　　　　10

Fɪɢ. 8. A 63-year-old woman with a compression fracture of the body of T-10 found incidentally during the course of a skeletal survey for neoplastic disease. The sharply localized wedge-like appearance of the midportion of the anterior surface of the vertebral body is unusual.

Fɪɢ. 9A. Old fracture of the superior surface of the body of T-12. A year before this x-ray was taken the patient had been in bed for six weeks because of a "sprain in the back." The superior margin of the vertebral body is demineralized in its posterior portion.

Fɪɢ. 9B. On a lateral film the indentation into the posterosuperior surface of the body is apparent. A rounded radiolucent shadow is seen just beneath the depressed fragment, probably resulting from intrusion of the nucleus pulposus.

Fɪɢ. 10. Complete block at the level of T-12 in a 32-year-old woman who was paraplegic following an automobile accident. Previous laminectomy had disclosed an intraspinal hemorrhage and contusion of the conus and the cauda equina.

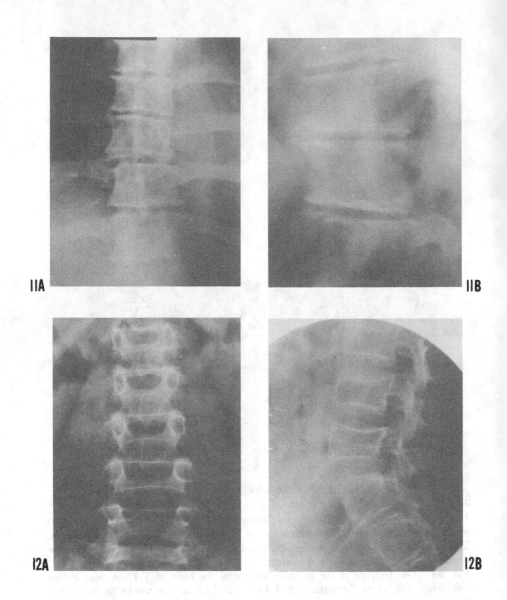

Fig. 11A. Lateral dislocation of the tenth on the eleventh thoracic vertebra.
Fig. 11B. Lateral view also reveals anterior displacement of T-10 on T-11.
Fig. 12A. Intense osteoporosis following prolonged steroid treatment in a 16-year-old boy who had been under care for a skin condition. The vertebral bodies are flattened and the intervertebral discs are widened.
Fig. 12B. Lateral view reveals widened biconvex configuration of the intervertebral discs and partial collapse of the vertebral bodies.

produced. Evidence of cord trauma may be apparent immediately after injury though in some cases it may be delayed. If a compressive as well as a torsional influence is present, such as occurs in falls from a considerable height, automobile accidents, or motorcycle mishaps, the fractures may be comminuted. Fragmentation, vertical displacements, marked disruption of intervertebral discs, and paravertebral soft tissue damage may all be pronounced.

Wedge fractures frequently appear in patients with osteoporosis. The presence of a marked kyphosis of the thoracic spine often is associated with wedging of several segments, notably the fifth to the ninth vertebrae. The dorsal aspects of the bodies usually remain relatively intact. Concomitant symptoms may be minimal except for pain associated with muscular and postural distortions. In other osteoporotic patients without a dorsal kyphosis, the vertebrae become biconvex to varying degrees, due to bulging of the intervertebral discs into the softened vertebral bodies (Fig. 12).

Pathologic fractures are common. While there may be a tendency to wedge-shaped deformities or platyspondyly, destruction of bone more often results in gross compression and distortion of the involved vertebrae. A relatively sharp angulation can occur, and gibbus deformities sometimes are pronounced. Similar changes may appear with granulomatous and inflammatory lesions.

Compression of thoracic vertebrae occurs in other conditions, such as eosinophilic granuloma and spondyloepiphyseal dysplasia. The various osteochondrodystrophies and mucopolysaccharidoses also are associated with vertebral deformities, some of which are characteristic of the underlying condition. Gaucher's disease, vitamin D-resistant rickets, and hypothyroidism are similarly associated with vertebral changes. An interesting type of vertebral compression appears in the thoracic and lumbar vertebrae in patients with sickle cell anemia. This takes the form of a plug-like depression in the articular surfaces of the affected vertebrae, with little or no tendency towards wedge-shaped deformities; it is attributed to alteration in the vascular supply of the vertebral epiphyses. Scheuermann's disease also may be associated with vertebral deformities, sometimes mistaken for granulomatous conditions or fractures.

FRACTURES OF THE LUMBAR SPINE

These fractures occur most often in the upper lumbar segments, are mainly caused by hyperflexion injuries, and are frequently accompanied

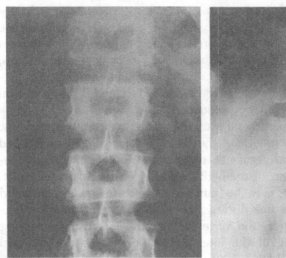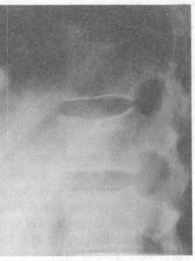

Fig. 13A. This 35-year-old man complained of mid-back pain after falling from a ladder. The anteroposterior roentgenogram of his thoracolumbar junction was unrevealing.

Fig. 13B. The lateral film reveals a tear-drop fracture of the anterosuperior aspect of L-1, with compression of the superior surface of that vertebra.

by similar lesions of the lowermost thoracic vertebrae. Wedging and compression of the anterosuperior aspects of the involved vertebrae are the most frequent structural changes. Similar involvement of the lower surfaces of fractured vertebrae is uncommon, although it can occur with severe injuries. If the anterior portion of a vertebra is affected, and the posterior surface remains intact, only a mild wedge-shaped deformity may be apparent. More extensive injuries can produce gibbus formation. With an added shearing force a portion of bone may be avulsed from the involved body, producing a "teardrop" type of fracture. This fragment may vary in size from a small chip (Fig. 13) to a fairly large piece of bone representing a significant fraction of the anterior vertebral surface. The smaller fractures of this variety are to be distinguished from so-called "limbic bones." These triangular bony structures are not avulsed fragments but rather represent atypical intervertebral disc herniations resulting in marginal osteophytes.

If a torsional component exists when the injury is incurred, only one side of the involved vertebra may be compressed. Here lateral views may not be as informative as the anteroposterior projection. A direct blow either from above or below raises the possibility of a bursting type of lesion. This may result in a comminuted fracture. With less severe damage, the margins of the affected vertebra become blown out and convex in configuration. Vertical linear components are occasionally associated with comminuted fractures. Diminution in the height of affected vertebrae due to compression is frequently observed.

Patients with pronounced osteoporosis tend to have a biconvex configuration of their vertebral bodies caused by the expansile effect of the nucleus pulposus. Osteoporotic spines are further characterized by wide, bulging intervertebral discs. Lesser degrees of osteoporosis may show bone loss only, while the vertebral margins remain sharp and rectangular. Moderate trauma in osteoporotic patients may cause impingement of the intervertebral discs on the opposing surfaces of one or more vertebrae, resulting in compression fractures (Fig. 14). In some such cases, there is increased compactness of bone evidenced by greater density of the upper, and sometimes the lower surfaces of

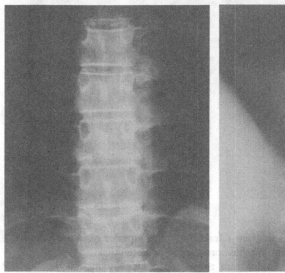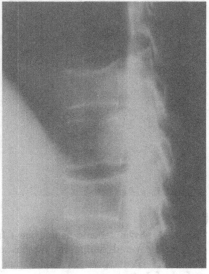

FIG. 14A. Postheparinization osteoporosis (?) in a 24-year-old woman who had been under treatment for multiple pulmonary infarcts for two months, and who was postpartum for about the same length of time. There is diffuse demineralization of the entire vertebral column.

FIG. 14B. Lateral studies, particularly laminagrams, disclose compression fractures of the superior surfaces of multiple vertebrae with irregular widening of the intervertebral discs. Bone loss is conspicuous.

769

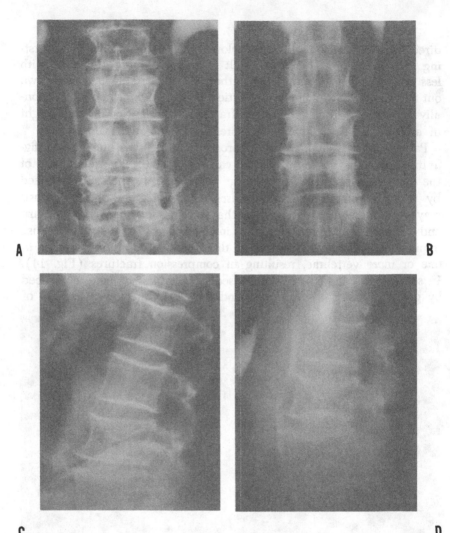

FIG. 15A. Asymptomatic impingement fracture of the superior surface of the body of L-4 discovered during intravenous urographic investigation.

Fig. 15B. Anteroposterior laminagram reveals deep indentation into the superior surface of L-4.

FIG. 15C and D. Lateral roentgenogram and laminagram confirm the deep depression into the superior surface of L-4.

the affected vertebrae. A very similar zone of osseous condensation is occasionally seen in Cushing's disease or in patients who have had steroid therapy with appreciable bone loss. Some reduction of the height of the affected vertebrae is observed in such cases. Similar changes can appear in the thoracic vertebrae, but are infrequent in the cervical and sacral areas. Another change occasionally observed in osteoporotic patients is an impingement of the nucleus pulposus on the superior or inferior surface of a vertebra resulting in a compression fracture involving only the immediately adjacent bone (Fig. 15). Usually such fractures are asymptomatic, are best identified on laminagrams, and are not associated with gross compression of the involved vertebrae.

Severe torsional injuries are associated in some patients with disruption of one or more intervertebral discs (Fig. 16). Lateral, forward, or backward dislocations of one or more lumbar vertebrae may take place. The upper lumbar segments are more likely to be affected in such cases. The spinal cord and paravertebral structures, including ligaments and muscles, are also traumatized to varying degrees. Injuries of the lower lumbar region may be associated with damage to the cauda equina and emerging nerve roots, and adjacent soft tissues.

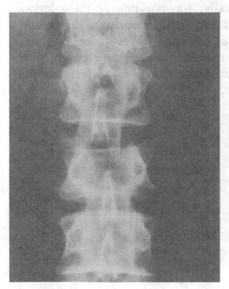 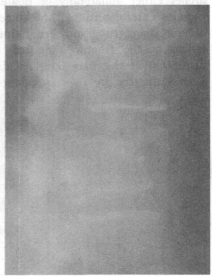

Fɪɢ. 16A.   Seatbelt fracture-dislocation of L-2 on L-3. The intervertebral space is widened and the articular facets are separated.

Fɪɢ. 16B.   A cross-table lateral film reveals a comminuted fracture of the body of L-3 in its anterosuperior aspect, tilting and displacement of the apophyseal joints, and forward displacement of L-2 on L-3.

771

Fractures limited to the pedicles of the lumbar vertebrae are rare. However, the pedicles may be separated from the vertebral body when a particularly violent torsional injury disrupts the neural arch. This type of injury is more likely to be associated with extensive comminuted fractures. Laminar fractures do occur as an isolated phenomenon, but are relatively infrequent. Accessory laminar epiphyses, particularly of the second, third, and fourth lumbar vertebrae are not uncommon, and should not be mistaken for fissure fractures. Fractures through the spinous processes alone are relatively infrequent. Such lesions are likely to be missed unless the examination is so performed that the spinous processes are brought into view. Inspecting the lateral films using a bright light is helpful when such a lesion is suspected, and special films with an appropriately light technic should be obtained when necessary.

The pars interarticularis is particularly subject to injury. While stress fractures may result from a single trauma (Fig. 17), they are more likely to follow repeated injuries. Athletes and ballet dancers are likely to incur such injuries, which may affect one or more vertebral arches either unilaterally or bilaterally. Identification of these lesions requires careful scrutiny, and sometimes laminagrams and stereoscopic oblique roentgenograms are helpful. Healing takes place by bony union, or the fracture line may remain visible. The concept that disruption of the pars interarticularis is a congenital defect has not been supported by recent evidence.

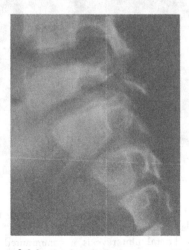

Fig. 17. Traumatic spondylolysis of L-5 in a 6-year-old boy who fell under a roller coaster. A moderate displacement of L-5 on S-1 is present.

Fractures of the transverse processes occur without damage to the vertebral bodies or neural arches. These lesions are best demonstrated by means of anteroposterior stereoroentgenographic projections. When there is some doubt, particularly when the suspected area is obscured by gas or fecal shadows, laminagrams are useful in identifying discontinuity in the transverse processes. As a rule displacement of the distal fragments is relatively slight. However, appreciable separation can occur with severe injuries. While fractures in which there is some degree of separation are readily identified, fissure fractures sometimes are not visible on the initial examination. Should this be suspected on clinical grounds, a repeat examination after a week or ten days may be rewarding.

Spinous process fractures are relatively uncommon. Most occur as a result of a direct trauma or twisting injury, and usually are associated with other fractures of the neural arches. They often are overlooked unless the lateral films are inspected using a bright light or special conedown films are taken. Stress fractures of the lumbar spinous processes are rare. Metastatic tumor involving the spinous processes is infrequent, but may occur in patients with extensive disease. We have seen a few cases in which the lesion was limited to this region.

Metastatic carcinoma (Fig. 18), myeloma, lymphoma, primary sarcoma, and a wide variety of other tumors may produce vertebral deformities and collapse. These are best identified in the context of the clinical picture of the respective diseases. At times there may be difficulty in differential diagnosis as, for instance, in distinguishing between myeloma and severe osteoporosis (Fig. 19). Differentiating metastatic disease from various inflammatory and granulomatous lesions may require considerable acumen, and bone biopsy often is necessary. Identification of various lytic lesions such as aneurysmal bone cysts, giant cell tumors, and rarities such as cystic angiomatosis of bone can be difficult.

Considerable interest exists in fractures associated with automobile accidents in which the subject is confined by a seat belt. This restraint acts as a fulcrum, and produces a curious group of injuries (Fig. 16). In some, the fracture traverses the midportion of the vertebral body in the horizontal plane, and extends through the pedicles and laminae, actually splitting the vertebral body and the spinous process in half. If the injury is limited to the body of a vertebra, a compression type of fracture can result without neurologic sequelae. If, however, the pedicles and the neural arches are involved, injury to the conus or the cauda equina may be incurred. Because of the sudden impact

773

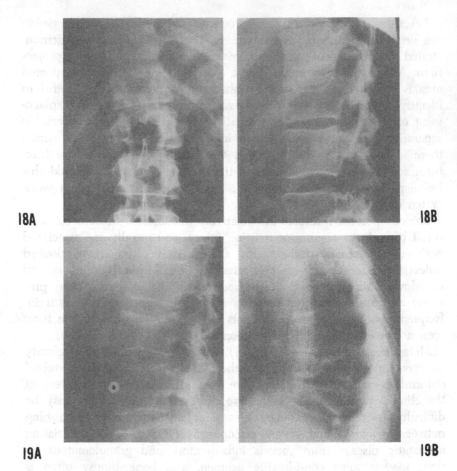

18A

18B

19A

19B

FIG. 18A. Lytic metastasis involves the body of L-1 in a 38-year-old woman who had had a kidney tumor removed three years before.

FIG. 18B. Lateral film reveals partial collapse and diffuse bone loss of the affected vertebra. The pathologic fracture apparently does not involve the pedicle as seen on the anteroposterior film, but definite bone loss is present on the lateral examination.

FIG. 19A. Multiple myeloma in this female patient 62 years old is characterized by severe osteoporosis. A compression fracture has produced osseous condensation in the superior margin of the body of L-1.

FIG. 19B. Multiple fractures are present in the midthoracic segments, with wedging and compression involving T-5, 8 and 9.

and violent forward motion, intervertebral disruption and dislocation may ensue. Visceral injury as part of the seat belt trauma syndrome is also possible. Abdominal contusion and hematoma, rupture of the

774

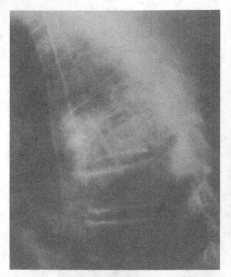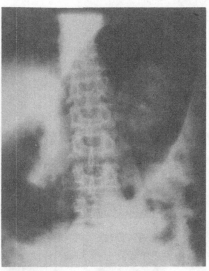

Fig. 20A. Compression fractures of the T-6 and T-7 in a 67-year-old man who fell from a roof.

Fig. 20B. Massive gastrectasia incident to spinal shock.

bowel, and intra-abdominal and retroperitoneal bleeding have been known to occur.

Ileus following severe injury (Fig. 20) may be sufficiently pronounced to mask a concomitant fracture. Retroperitoneal hematomas and fractures of the lower ribs and the upper lumbar transverse processes may simulate laceration of the thoracic or abdominal aorta. Should this problem arise, aortography may become necessary. In one of our cases we were unable, on first examination, to obtain adequate lateral views because the patient was in intense pain and, as a result, slight but quite definite compression fractures of the twelfth thoracic and the upper two lumbar vertebrae were not identified. A flush aortogram was normal. Abdominal exploration was nevertheless deemed necessary because of the severe abdominal symptoms. Only a mild bilateral retroperitoneal hematoma and contused psoas muscles were found. On a film made three days later the compression fractures were readily identified.

Radiologic evidence of healing of vertebral fractures varies from nothing more than a slight increase in the density of the affected bone and blurring of the margins of separated fragments to the for-

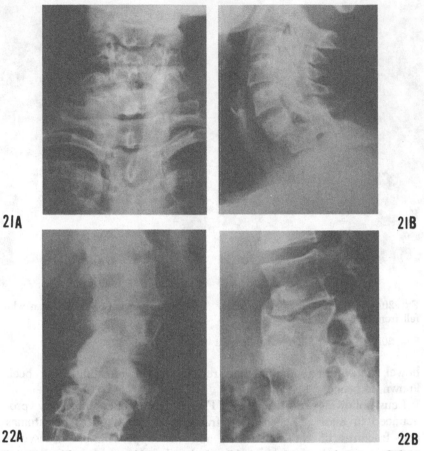

21A

21B

22A

22B

Fig. 21A. This 62-year-old woman had suffered a dislocation of C-6 on C-7 11 years ago. She is presently asymptomatic, but residual symptoms of weakness of the left arm and leg and atrophy of the left hand persist. The spinous processes of C-6 and C-7 are separated, while those of C-4, 5 and 6 are approximated.

Fig. 21B. Lateral roentgenogram reveals the dislocation. The neural arches of C-6 and C-7 are fused.

Fig. 22A and B. Asymptomatic old healed fracture of L-3, found incidentally on abdominal plain film examination.

mation of paravertebral calcareous and ossified bridges (Figs. 21 and 22). Paravertebral calcification incident to an infection or hematoma usually can be identified by the spotty nature of the deposits and their separation from the adjacent, and often intact bone. However, in the case of hematoma associated with spinal fracture, it is quite probable that the calcium deposits will merge and form osseous

776

struts. Compression fractures occurring in association with osteoporosis may remain unchanged over long intervals. The biconvex vertebrae caused by pressure exerted by the intervertebral discs usually do not present evidence of bone condensation. However, in some patients with osteoporosis, following trauma, zones of compact bone at the upper and lower surfaces of the vertebrae may appear with no paravertebral reaction whatsoever. Pathologic fractures which heal under the influence of radiation therapy and chemotherapeutic regimens reossify, but usually a definite deformity of the vertebra persists and the recalcification tends to be irregular. In general, it may be stated that accurate dating of vertebral fractures in the absence of a reliable history and adequate radiographic data often is difficult, at times doubtful, sometimes impossible. It is helpful, whenever possible, to review previous films of the same area. Identification of a vertebral deformity prior to the accident with no change in configuration is strong evidence that the abnormality predated a given injury. However, when no such information is available, the radiologist may have difficulty in attempting to determine the age of a particular lesion.

Corroboration of a diagnosis of epidural hematoma or hematomyelia requires spinal puncture followed by myelography. Avulsion of nerve roots following torsional trauma may be visualized by myelographic examination. Usually such injuries, which are uncommon, involve the roots emerging from the fourth and fifth lumbar intervertebral foramina. As in the case of avulsed cervical nerve roots, myelography characteristically reveals puddling of the Pantopaque and the formation of diverticula.

FRACTURES OF THE SACRUM AND COCCYX

A direct blow such as one incident to a fall, an athletic injury, or an automobile accident are the usual causes of fractures of the sacrum and coccyx. An increasingly frequent cause of violent sacrococcygeal and pelvic injury is trauma resulting from motorcycle accidents. In such cases the sacroiliac joints may be separated forcibly, and fractures of the sacrum with comminution and separation of fragments are apt to occur (Fig. 23). Such trauma is usually not caused merely by the immediate direct force of the fall but probably also by repeated blows and marked rotational stress.

The usual picture of a sacral fracture is that of a linear radiolucent line which passes across the sacrum parallel to the intervertebral

777

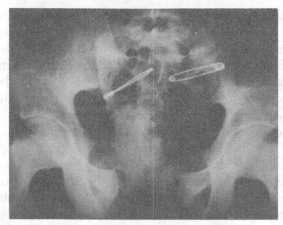

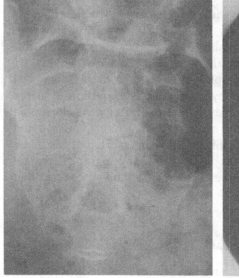
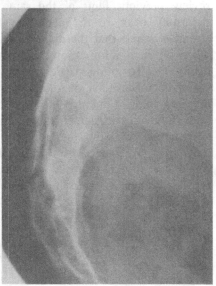

Fig. 23. Pelvic injury in a 24-year-old man whose motorcycle struck a pole. The symphysis pubis is widely separated, and the right sacroiliac joint is dislocated.

Fig. 24A and B. Anteroposterior and lateral roentgenograms of a 47-year-old woman who fell, striking her sacrum. A transverse fracture passes through the 4th sacral segment.

foramina (Fig. 24). Occasionally, particularly after severe injuries, a vertical component also may appear. These fractures can be identified both on frontal and lateral roentgenograms. However, not infrequently the anteroposterior examination is obscured by overlying gas and fecal shadows, so that the fracture line may be missed unless one carefully scrutinizes the lateral films. Oblique films may prove helpful when there is doubt.

Fractures lower in the sacrum and those involving the coccyx usually follow a fall in which the patient strikes the lower spine in a sitting position. These fractures also can be difficult to identify in frontal projections, and often are better seen on lateral and oblique films. At times the patient may have severe local pain with no deformity visible initially. Reexamination after a week or so may then reveal the fracture. Should there be any uncertainty, it is advisable to consider the presence of severe pain on pressure or digital examination as better evidence than a so-called negative x-ray examination, and to reschedule the patient for another investigation before ruling out a fracture.

BIBLIOGRAPHY

Amyes, E. W. and Anderson, F. M. Fractures of the Odontoid Process. *Arch. Surg.*, 72, 377-393, 1956.

Askenasy, H. M., Braham, J. and Kosary, I. Z. Delayed Spinal Myelopathy Following Atlanto-axial Fracture Dislocation. *J. Neurosurg.*, 17, 1100-1104, 1960.

Blaw, M. E. and Langer, L. O. Spinal Cord Compression in Morquio-Braisford's Disease. *J. Pediatr.*, 74, 593-600, 1969.

Blockey, N. J. and Purser, D. W. Fractures of the Odontoid Process of the Axis. *J. Bone Joint Surg.*, 38B, 794-817, 1956.

Budin, E. and Sondheimer, F. Lateral Spread of the Atlas Without Fracture. *Radiology*, 87, 1095-1098, 1966.

Dastur, D. K., Wadia, N. H., Desai, A. D., and Sinh, G. Medullospinal Compression Due to Atlanto-axial Dislocation and Sudden Haematomyelia During Decompression. Pathology, Pathogenesis and Clinical Correlations. *Brain*, 88, 897-924, 1965.

Griffith, G. C., Nichols, G., Jr., Asher, J. D., and Flanagan, B. Heparin Osteoporosis. *J.A.M.A.*, 193, 91-94, 1965.

Griffith, H. B., Gleave, J. R. W. and Taylor, R. G. Changing Patterns of Fracture in the Dorsal and Lumbar Spine. *Br. Med. J.*, 1, 891-894, 1966.

Grisolia, A., Bell, R. L., and Peltier, L. F. Fractures and Dislocations of the Spine Complicating Ankylosing Spondylitis. *J. Bone Joint Surg.*, 49-A, 339-345, 1967.

Howorth, M. B. Fracture of the Spine. *Am. J. Surg.*, 92, 573-593, 1956.

Jacobson, G. and Adler, D. C. Examination of the Atlanto-axial Joint Following Injury. *Am. J. Roentgenol., Rad. Ther & Nucl. Med.*, 86, 1081-1094, 1956.

Jaffe, M. D. and Willis, P. W., III. Multiple Fractures Associated with Long-term Sodium Heparin Therapy. *J.A.M.A.*, 193, 158-160, 1965.

779

Jones, M. D. Cineradiographic Studies of Abnormalities of the High Cervical Spine. *Arch. Surg., 94,* 206-213, 1967.

Newbury, C. L. and Etter, L. E. Clarification of the Problem of Vertebral Fractures from Convulsive Theraphy. *Arch. Neurol.* and *Psychiat., 74,* 479-487, 1955.

Peltier, L. F. and Volz, R. G. Fractures of the Dorsolumbar Spine Uncomplicated by Injury of the Spinal Cord. *Surg. Gynecol. Obstet., 116,* 205-212, 1963.

Rand, W. and Crandall, P. H. Central Spinal Cord Syndrome in Hyperextension Injuries of the Cervical Spine. *J. Bone Joint Surg., 44-A,* 1415-1422, 1962.

Roaf, R. A Study of the Mechanics of Spinal Injuries. *J. Bone Joint Surg., 42 B,* 810-823, 1960.

Schilling, F., Haas, J. P., and Schacherl, M. Die spontane atlanto-axiale Dislocation (Ventralluxation des Atlas) bei chronischer Polyarthritis und Spondylitis ankylopoetica. *Fortschr. Roentgenstr., 99,* 518-538, 1963.

Smith, W. S. and Kaufer, H. Patterns and Mechanisms of Lumbar Injuries Associated with Lap Seat Belts. *J. Bone Joint Surg., 51-A,* 239-254, 1969.

Sujoy, E. Spinal Lesions in Tetanus in Children. *Pediatrics, 29,* 629-635, 1962.

Venable, J. R., Flake, R. E., and Kilian, D. J. Stress Fracture of Spinous Process. *J.A.M.A., 190,* 881-885, 1964.

Wiltse, L. L. The Etiology of Spondylolisthesis. *J. Bone Joint Surg., 44-A,* 532-560, 1962.

CHAPTER 25

THE MANAGEMENT OF THE BLADDER IN TRAUMATIC
SPINAL PARAPLEGIA

PABLO A. MORALES, M.D.

One of the consequences of injury to the spinal cord is disturbance of bladder function. The neurogenic bladder in traumatic spinal paraplegia generally expels its contents involuntarily and incompletely. As a result of urinary incontinence, the paralyzed patient becomes uncomfortable, foul-smelling and socially isolated. Urostasis in the bladder leads to urinary infection, which if not controlled or eradicated, readily spreads to the upper urinary tract and causes irreparable renal damage. Back pressure from the retained urine may eventually cause dilation of the ureter as well as the pelvis and calyces, and consequently further renal destruction. Stagnation of urine, in combination with other factors related to immobilization, promotes the formation of stones, which not only aggravates infection but also destroys kidney function by obstruction. Thus, the paraplegic individual, although no longer doomed to an early death, faces a long-term outlook that remains speculative.

The need for assiduous bladder care from the very beginning of paraplegia is of the utmost importance, and its unremitting continuance throughout the paraplegic's life should be emphasized. Many complications may thus be averted and rehabilitation of the patient greatly accelerated.

NORMAL BLADDER NEUROPHYSIOLOGY

To understand the detrusor dysfunction in paraplegia, it is necessary to review briefly the neuroanatomic features which have a bearing on the physiology of normal micturition (Fig. 1). The center for micturition is located in the second, third, and fourth sacral segments of the cord in the conus medullaris and is linked to the detrusor muscle by parasympathetic sensory and motor fibers which

781

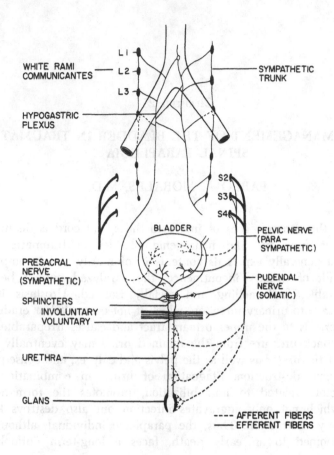

L I
L2
L3

SYMPATHETIC
TRUNK

HYPOGASTRIC
PLEXUS

S2
S3
S4

BLADDER

PELVIC NERVE
(PARA–
SYMPATHETIC)

PRESACRAL
NERVE
(SYMPATHETIC)

PUDENDAL
NERVE
(SOMATIC)

SPHINCTERS
INVOLUNTARY
VOLUNTARY

URETHRA

GLANS

---- AFFERENT FIBERS
—— EFFERENT FIBERS

FIG. 1. DIAGRAMMATIC REPRESENTATION OF BLADDER INNERVATION.

course in the pelvic nerves; together they form the spinal reflex arc
for micturition. Sympathetic motor fibers originating from the eleventh
thoracic to the second lumbar segments in the spinal cord course
through the presacral nerves to reach the trigone and bladder neck.
Somatic lower motor neuron fibers start at the second to fourth
sacral segments (possibly one to two segments higher and lower)
and travel through the internal pudendal nerves to the external urethral
sphincter, external anal sphincter, and perineal muscles. Sensory fibers
accompany the corresponding autonomic and somatic efferents.
Higher medullary and supraspinal centers also exert some influence
on the bladder, but knowledge concerning this is far from complete.
Pathways descend from the higher centers via the corticospinal tract

782

and eventually reach synapses in the lateral and anterior horns of the sacral segments where the functional lower motor neurons start.

The vesical sensations associated with micturition include 1) sensation of a desire to void, 2) sensation that micturition is imminent, and 3) sensation of urine passing through the urethra. The sensation underlying the desire to void originates in the proprioceptors of the detrusor muscle. As bladder filling increases to a certain point, the muscle fibers contract somewhat more vigorously and intravesical pressure increases slightly more steeply, giving rise to a desire to void. The impulses travel via parasympathetic nerve fibers coursing in the pelvic nerves to the second to fourth sacral segments and upward through the spinothalamic tracts to the thalamus, subcortex, and cortex. The sensation that micturition is imminent is different from the desire to void and originates in the urethra; impulses reach the spinal cord via the pudendal nerves and the brain centers via the posterior columns. The sensation that urine is passing through the urethra comprises three components; namely, an awareness of the opening of the sphincter musculature, a feeling of something passing along the urethra, and a thermal sensation. The impulses from the urethra travel via the pudendal nerves; in the spinal cord, the impulses of sphincteric movement and "something passing" ascend via the posterior columns; and the thermal impulses travel over the spinothalamic tracts to the brain.

In patients with total division of the spinal cord, the specific sensations indicating that the bladder needs to be emptied and that urine is passing through the urethra are no longer felt. Many patients, however, experience other sensations related to bladder filling, and they learn to interpret such sensations as an indication that the bladder is full. The most common of the substitute sensations is a vague feeling of abdominal fullness, which results from an increase of intravesical and/or intra-abdominal pressure. Impulses subserving it reach the central nervous system through afferent nerves running in company with the sympathetic nerves and chains; these nerves eventually reach the spinal cord via the posterior roots in the upper thoracic region. The impulses then proceed upward via the posterior columns. Other substitute sensations may be experienced in the form of spontaneous tingling paresthesia in the region of the bladder, urethra, and vagina. A very full bladder may also cause frontal headaches, "goose flesh," chills, sweating in the upper part of the body, or nasal obstruction as a consequence of autonomic hyperreflexia.

Immediately after a spinal-cord injury, in the stage of spinal shock, bladder function is characterized by atonicity and loss of reflex detrusor contractions. The bladder becomes distended and overflow incontinence ensues when the limit of distensibility is reached. Some investigators, however, believe that the bladder in this stage is not really flaccid but retains its inherent smooth-muscle tone.

As the patient gradually recovers from spinal shock, he usual'y acquires either an automatic or an autonomous bladder, depending on the level of the injury. If the spinal cord transection is partial, he develops a voluntary neurogenic bladder although inefficient vesical function may persist.

The *automatic* bladder, sometimes termed "reflex bladder," develops when the injury is located above the undamaged sacral center for micturition. The patient has no control over the act of micturition. Urination occurs reflexly at intervals of up to three or four hours, but sometimes hourly or less. During the intervals between voidings, there is usually no leakage of urine.

The *autonomous* or non-reflex bladder develops when there has been an injury to the sacral spinal segments with destruction of the center for micturition. The reflex arc for micturition is no longer intact and any contraction of the bladder wall is the result of impulses transmitted through an intrinsic nervous mechanism that lies wholly within the bladder wall. Such contractions, however, are of insufficient strength or duration to empty the bladder efficiently. Evacuation of the bladder is accomplished by abdominal straining and manual compression.

Regardless of level, a complete transection of the cord is followed by inability to recognize the normal desire for urination because of interruption of the sensory pathways to the brain. However, vague sensations of fullness may remain in the form of burning or ill-defined painful sensations in the suprapubic area or urethra. These are probably mediated through the sensory sympathetic innervation perhaps originating in the peritoneal reflection over the bladder. In lesions above the sixth and fifth thoracic segments and especially in high cervical injuries, the sensations of fullness completely disappear and are replaced by pathologic autonomic manifestations characterized by flushing of the face, profuse sweats, chilling, headache, "goose pimples," and paroxysmal hypertension.

After partial transection of the spinal cord, there usually is some

784

degree of sensation and voluntary motor power. Bladder function may be normal or almost normal with precipitate micturition or stress incontinence. However, in a considerable percentage of patients with incomplete cord lesions, it is not unusual to encounter a small spastic bladder associated with spasms of the lower extremities.

The urologist is initially called on to determine the extent of nerve damage to the bladder and estimate the subsequent effect of the cord injury on the physiologic status of the urinary tract.

Integrity of the autonomic and somatic activities of the spinal micturition center may be determined by the ice water test, bulbocavernosus reflex, external rectal sphincter test, and the anal reflex test. The ice water test is carried out by instilling 2 to 3 ounces of sterile ice water into the bladder through a urethral catheter. If reflex activity is intact via the pelvic nerves from the bladder to the conus medullaris and back, the bladder will immediately and forcibly contract, expelling the fluid and urethral catheter. The other tests ascertain whether or not reflex actvity is intact via the pudendal nerves. For the bulbocavernosus test, the examiner slowly inserts a finger in the rectum and squeezes on the glans penis or pulls on the Foley bag catheter. If the reflex arc is intact, the sphincter ani should contract briskly. Contraction of the rectal external sphincter around the finger that has been introduced likewise indicates that reflex activity is present (external rectal sphincter test). Visual observation of contraction following pinpricking of the ano-cutaneous line constitutes a positive anal reflex test.

Evaluation of the type and degree of vesical dysfunction and its overall effect on the rest of the urinary tract necessitates a complete survey, which includes cystometry, cystourethrography, cystoscopy, intravenous pyelography, estimation of residual urine, and urinalysis. None of the examinations is sufficient in itself; they must be interpreted in context.

Cystometry

Cystometry is a procedure designed to record graphically vesical activity during the introduction of fluid into the bladder. Of all the varieties of apparatus that have been used, the simple water ma-

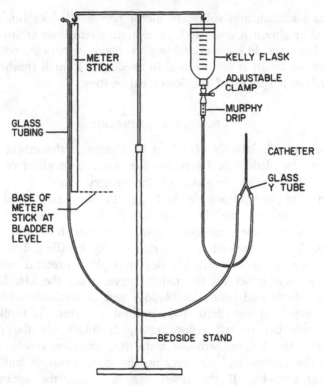

FIG. 2. A SIMPLE WATER CYSTOMETER

nometer is as satisfactory as any (Fig. 2). A graduated reservoir is equipped with a Murphy drip bulb. A manometer consisting of a glass tube is fastened to a meter stick. A catheter, a Y tube, and rubber tubing to connect the tube to the reservoir and manometer complete the equipment. Water is introduced into the previously emptied bladder in a slow continuous flow to simulate physiologic diuresis. Manometric pressure levels are recorded after each 25 cc fluid increment. Reflex contractile waves are noted and recorded in the graph. The points at which the patient first feels the desire to void and the onset of pain from vesical distention are also recorded. If the patient has neither expelled the catheter nor voided around it after instillation of 400 cc fluid, he is asked to strain as in voiding. This final reading is designated as the maximum voluntary pressure.

Representative cystometrograms are illustrated in Figure 3. The atonic bladder in spinal shock is characterized by a low and flat pressure curve, no reflex contractions, increased bladder capacity, and complete

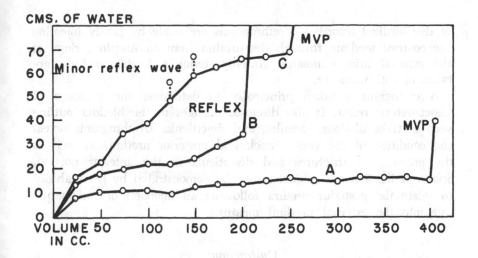

FIG. 3. REPRESENTATIVE CYSTOMETROGRAMS IN TRAUMATIC SPINAL PARAPLEGIA.
A. Atonic Bladder—Flat pressure curve, no reflex contractions, increased bladder capacity, vesical sensations absent. B. Automatic Bladder — Variable pressure curve, forceful detrusor contraction, small to normal capacity, no normal desire to void, vague sensation of fullness, autonomic manifestations. C. Autonomous Bladder — Increased vesical tone, minor reflex contractions, capacity within normal range, no normal urge to void, vague sensation of fullness.
MVP = Maximum voluntary pressure.

absence of vesical sensation. The features of the automatic bladder usually comprise a variable pressure curve, forceful detrusor contractions, failure of recognition of the normal urge to void, vague sensations of bladder fullness and, in high lesions, flushing or a sweating reaction in the upper part of the body when the bladder reflex is imminent. Patients with autonomous bladders exhibit the following characteristics: increased vesical tone, minor reflex detrusor contractions rarely greater than 10 cm water pressure, bladder capacity within normal range, absence of the normal desire to void, and a feeling of discomfort in the suprapubic area when the bladder is full.

Cystourethrography

The cystogram is made by introducing radiopaque dye into the bladder under gravity from a height of 15 cm. When the flow of dye into the bladder ceases or backs up, the bladder is assumed to have reached its capacity. The catheter is then clamped and the amount

787

of dye instilled recorded. Urethrograms are made by gently injecting the contrast medium through the urethra from an Asepto syringe at the external urinary meatus. Anteroposterior and oblique films are taken in both instances.

A cystogram is taken principally to determine the presence of vesicoureteric reflux. It also discloses changes in the bladder outline such as trabeculations, saccules, and diverticula. Urethrograms reveal the condition of the vesical neck and posterior urethra, as well as the presence of strictures and diverticula in the anterior portion. Spasm of the external sphincter may be demonstrated by the inability to dilate the posterior urethra following an injection of radiopaque dye into the external urethral meatus.

Cystoscopy

A cystoscopic examination is of value in ruling out the presence of any organic obstructive lesion, such as prostatic hypertrophy or urethral stricture, which may contribute to an increase in outlet resistance. Sphincteric resistance may be recognized during the insertion of the instrument. Vesical calculi are detected and may be extracted during the examination. An estimate of the degree of bladder infection may also be obtained.

Intravenous Pyelography

Intravenous urograms provide information on the anatomy of the upper portion of the urinary tract and function of the kidney. Back pressure from the bladder is demonstrated by ureteral and renal dilation. Impairment of kidney function is manifested by a delay in the appearance of the dye and diminished concentration.

Estimation of Residual Urine

Urine left in the bladder after voiding is termed residual urine. It is measured by inserting a urethral catheter after the patient has voided by detrusor reflex contraction or by abdominal straining and suprapubic manual compression. The normal bladder empties completely. The presence of residual urine signifies inefficient detrusor action and/or increased outlet resistance. Accurate determination of residual urine in the paraplegic patient with an automatic bladder is difficult to obtain because he generally cannot void effectively on command.

Urinalysis

Microscopic examination of the centrifuged urine specimen provides an approximate indication of the extent of urinary infection. Paraplegic patients invariably show varying degrees of pyuria, ranging from a few white cells to foul, turbid urine loaded with leukocytes. Bacilluria is similarly a common feature and is always present when a catheter is in place. Urine cultures and antibiotic sensitivity tests are advisable.

TREATMENT

Initial Treatment

Immediately following injury of the spinal cord, there is loss of reflex activity below the level of the lesion, and consequently the patient develops urinary retention. Therefore, initial urologic management is directed toward provision of adequate bladder drainage and prevention of bladder distention. Workers in paraplegic centers, however, differ in their advocacy of the most satisfactory method of bladder drainage in early paraplegia.

Continuous indwelling catheter drainage is most widely used and is our procedure of choice. A French 16-18 self-retaining Foley catheter (5-cc bag) is inserted immediately following the onset of paraplegia and connected to a closed drainage system. Scrupulous care and replacement every week with strict aseptic precautions are essential. It should be borne in mind that bacteria can enter the bladder at the junction of the catheter and urethra, at the connection of the catheter to the drainage system, and at the end of the drainage system. Entry of bacteria at the meatus and along the external catheter surface may be lessened by cleansing the urethral meatus and adjacent surface of the catheter with benzalkonium (Zephiran) chloride once daily in the male and twice daily or more often as necessary in the female. Entry at the connecting tube can be avoided by the simple practice of not disconnecting the set. Routine bladder irrigations are not required, provided the patient maintains a high fluid intake. When irrigation has to be performed, it should be done with a completely sterile setup. The junction of the catheter and

789

connecting tube should be bathed in alcohol or other bactericidal agent as it is disconnected. Entry of bacteria at the end of the set is prevented by interrupting continuity with the urine receptacle, thus providing a barrier across which the organisms cannot migrate.

Intermittent catheterization is advocated by Guttmann (1954) who reports that with this method, bladder activity reappears in two to four weeks in contrast to one or six months with other methods. Urine remains sterile in spite of the repeated catheterizations during this period. The patients are catheterized two to three times a day, under aseptic conditions such as those prevailing in a surgical operation. It would, however, seem that such a method can be adopted only in highly specialized centers because it is time-consuming and requires highly trained personnel.

Cutaneous vesicotomy has been favored by Lapides, Ajemian, and Lichtwardt (1960), who recommend the procedure within one to two weeks after injury. A vesicocutaneous fistula is created by means of a tube formed half of bladder and half of full-thickness skin, which remains widely patent and continuously drains the urine from the bladder into a bag. This method may provide excellent drainage of the bladder, does not require a foreign-body catheter in the bladder, and is potentially reversible, should normal vesical function return. Our experience with the procedure has been disappointing (1964). It has been difficult to make the bag adhere because the low position of the stoma prevents effective use of a belt strap. The difficulty is increased when the paralyzed patient slumps in a sitting position causing a deep skin crease in the lower abdomen. Calculi have also formed on the hairs which grow in the skin portion of the tube. Urethral leakage of urine may persist and require closure of the bladder neck; this may be difficult.

Bladder Training

Bladder training has been de-emphasized. It usually consisted of intermittent clamping and opening of the urethral catheter together with a regulated fluid intake of a glass of water hourly from early morning to bedtime. The regimen was supposed to provide near physiologic conditions for the bladder by alternately stretching and emptying it, thus preventing permanent reduction of vesical capacity by fibrosis and accustoming the neurogenic bladder to filling and evacuating in a more-or-less normal manner. However, patients who submitted to bladder training did not become any more continent than the others, and patients not subjected to bladder training did not experience any deleterious effect on their eventual vesical function.

Trials of Voiding

Attempts are made to discontinue the use of the catheter as soon as the patient's general condition is stabilized and satisfactory. Trials of voiding are, therefore, carried out at the earliest possible time and every two weeks thereafter. The patients who have automatic bladders will void reflexly in many instances, but they will be unable to empty their bladders completely and will have uninhibited contractions and wet themselves. Such patients may try to initiate reflex evacuation of the bladder by tapping the suprapubic area, stimulating the rectum digitally, or striking some other trigger area. Patients with autonomous bladders may be able to empty moderately well with straining and Credé's method, but many will be incontinent between voidings. Residual urine is checked frequently during the first few weeks after catheter removal.

The male who achieves urethral voiding is usually incontinent and will require some external appliance to collect the urine. A condom urinary appliance is the most practical. The condom is changed daily and is affixed to the phallus by skin cement. If this alone will not suffice, then Elastoplast is placed around the condom for the entire circumference of the penis. The Elastoplast band must be applied in such a manner as not to constrict the urethra and must allow for possible reflex erection of the penis. No satisfactory appliance has been developed for women. Fortunately, however, the woman has a much shorter urethra and is able to expel the bladder contents more readily by straining and may be able to get along satisfactorily with the use of pads. The woman with a spastic bladder usually needs a permanent catheter.

High Residual Urine

The amount of residual urine is dependent on a balance between the expulsive forces of urination (detrusor contraction, abdominal straining, and suprapubic manual compression) and the outflow resistance (vesical neck, posterior urethra, and external sphincter). If a high residual urine (more than 100 to 150 cc) is present in spite of

791

seemingly adequate expulsive forces, there must be either a mechanical or spastic obstruction which should be relieved.

Transurethral resection of the vesical neck and prostatic urethra can lessen outlet resistance and has been of great benefit to many patients with large amounts of residual urine, irrespective of bladder type and even in the absence of demonstrable bladder neck or prostatic urethral obstruction. The entire circumference of the vesical neck is resected distally to the external sphincter, an attempt being made to remove all prostatic tissue present. This is not a destructive procedure, and if not effective, no harm has been done. Also, if further improvement of cord function occurs, recovery of vesical activity would not have been interfered with in any way. The procedure is generally not performed earlier than six months after injury.

In the patient with an intact sacral reflex arc, a large amount of residual urine may persist in spite of transurethral resections of the bladder neck and prostatic urethra. Further investigation is then indicated to rule out spastic obstruction by the urethral sphincters. Spasm of the sphincters may sometimes be demonstrated by cystourethrographic and sphincterometric studies. Procedures designed to weaken the urethral sphincter may then be carried out. Ross, Damanski, and Gibbon (1958) advocate removing several strips from the posterolateral aspects of the external sphincter with the resectoscope.

More recently, Smythe (1966) accomplished division of the external urinary sphincter by using a knife electrode to make a longitudinal incision at the three-o'clock and nine-o'clock positions from the distal end of the verumontanum to the bulbous urethra. The latter procedure is associated with less bleeding and is as effective as the former. For some time now, we have found no need to resort to such neurosurgical procedures as pudental nerve section, rhizotomy, or subarachnoid alcohol, for the relief of sphincter spasticity.

Urinary Infection

Urinary infection is an almost constant concomitant of the paraplegic state. Use of the indwelling catheter and the presence of residual urine after catheter drainage is no longer necessary are the chief factors in the causation and persistence of urinary infection. Chronic infection has remained uncontrolled in a large number of paraplegic patients and probably is the main factor responsible for the observed high incidence of pyelonephritis and renal insufficiency.

792

Long-term maintenance chemotherapy is ineffective as long as catheter drainage persists. Sterile urine culture is encountered only in the paraplegic patient who has not had a urethral catheter for a while. Persistence of bacilluria after the catheter has been removed is generally treated for a prolonged period with antibacterial agents, preferably nitrofurantoin or long-acting sulfonamides. Broad-spectrum antibiotics are withheld unless bacilluria is associated with clinical evidence of infection, such as fever and chills. Measures should be directed toward eliminating urinary stasis when associated with infection; otherwise, antibiotic therapy becomes a wasted effort.

Vesicoureteric Reflux

Reflux in the paraplegic patient is caused by the combination of obstruction, infection, and possibly neurogenic ureteral dysfunction. Reflux may be associated with or without dilation of the upper urinary tract. At any rate, in whatever form it may appear, reflux is a warning signal of deterioration in the upper urinary tract. It facilitates passage of bacteria from the bladder to the kidney and perpetuates infection in the upper urinary tract.

A patient exhibiting vesicoureteral reflux should be carefully observed and intravenous urograms and cystograms performed every three months. Reflux without upper urinary tract dilation is treated initially with antibiotics if bacilluria is demonstrated. When dilation ensues, efforts are directed toward elimination of high residual urine by transurethral methods. Results with ureteral reimplantation in the bladder to correct reflux have been equivocal. Urinary diversion into an ileal conduit is indicated when reflux is associated with advanced dilation of the upper urinary tract.

Ileal Urinary Diversion

There is a growing tendency among urologists to bypass the bladder and urethra rather than to restore a reasonable vesical function, especially in private practice, where hospital facilities are limited and hospital and medical costs are prohibitive to the patient. Moreover, regardless of the patient's financial status, facilities for care comparable to those available in paraplegic centers are not available at any price for long-term care of private patients. The most common procedure for diversion of urine is the ileal conduit. Both ureters are implanted into an isolated segment of terminal ileum, which empties through the right side of the abdomen and from which urine is collected in a bag. It must be appreciated that creation of an ileal conduit is an irreversible operation. Our indication for urinary diversion is a rapidly deteriorating upper urinary tract in which it is fairly obvious that the lower tract dysfunction and lower tract fibrosis are producing continued obstruction and upper urinary tract destruction.

Electronic Vesical Stimulation

Electronic vesical stimulation in the treatment of neurogenic bladder in experimental animals and in man has been reported by several authors (Hald et al, 1967; Bradley et al, 1963). Among the problems in the clinical application of this technique have been impaired electric excitability and contractility of the detrusor muscle and spread of the stimulus current to the striated muscle of the pelvic floor surrounding the vesical neck. The latter complication produces occlusion of the urethrovesical junction during stimulation. It would seem that if the proper device could be designed, the time for electronic stimulation of the bladder is early in the course of the disease, thus protecting the bladder from the deleterious effects of neurogenic dysfunction.

FOLLOW-UP CARE

The paraplegic patient must be followed with the utmost vigilance for the rest of his life. It should be impressed on him that his future well-being and chance for survival depend to a large extent on his willingness to cooperate fully in the follow-up examinations. Intravenous pyelography and cystography should be performed every year and residual urine measured every six months, even when everything appears to be going well. It should also be borne in mind that dangerous lesions may develop insidiously, and a bladder that empties well is no guarantee of the permanency of good renal function.

BIBLIOGRAPHY

Bradley, W. E., Chou, S. N., and French, L. A. Further Experience with the Radio Transmitter Receiver Unit for the Neurogenic Bladder. *J. Neurosurg.*, 20, 953, 1963.
Guttmann, L. Statistical Survey on One Thousand Paraplegics. *Proc. R. Soc. Med.*, 47, 1099, 1954.

Hald, T., Meier, W., Khalili, A., Girdhar, A., Benton, J., and Kantrowitz, A. Clinical Experience with a Radio-linked Bladder Stimulator. *J. Urol.*, 97, 73, 1967.

Krahn, H., Morales, P., and Hotchkiss, R. Experience with Tubeless Cystostomy. *J. Urol.*, 91, 246, 1964.

Lapides, J., Ajemian, E. P., and Lichtwardt, J. R. Cutaneous Vesicostomy. *J. Urol.*, 84, 609, 1960.

Ross, J. C., Damanski, M., and Gibbon, N. Resection of the External Urethral Sphincter in the Paraplegic; Preliminary Report. *J. Urol.*, 79, 742, 1958.

Smythe, C. A. External Sphincterotomy in the Management of the Neurogenic Bladder: A Preliminary Report. *J. Urol.*, 96, 310, 1966.

CHAPTER 26

REHABILITATION OF THE PATIENT FOLLOWING SPINAL CORD INJURY

ALFRED EBEL, M. D., F.A.C.P.

INTRODUCTION

History

As recently as 30 years ago a chapter dealing with the rehabilitation of the patient following spinal cord injury would have been entirely irrelevant. Survival beyond one year following such an injury was the rare exception. Little progress had been made in the management of this devastating medical problem from ancient Egyptian times until the period of World War II. The hopeless prognosis of this disorder was recognized 5,000 years ago in the Edwin Smith Papyrus (Breasted, 1930) in which it is stated: "Thou shouldst say concerning him, One having a dislocation in the vertebra of his neck while he is unconscious of his two legs and his two arms and his urine dribbles. An ailment not to be treated."

The mortality of spinal cord injuries incurred during the Balkan wars of 1912 and 1913 was 95 percent within a few weeks following injury and rose to 100 percent shortly thereafter (Poer, 1946). Paraplegia aroused the interest of the medical profession as a consequence of World War I when large numbers of military personnel were paralyzed as a result of gunshot wounds. Unfortunately, medical treatment at this time had little to offer these patients. The mortality of World War I British paraplegic casualties was 80 percent; 47 percent of the deaths occurred in the first six to eight weeks following injury (Thompson-Walker, 1937). The American military experience during World War I was considerably worse. A review by Connors and Nash in 1934 indicated that 80 percent of all paraplegic casualties died in the first few weeks following injury. The causes of death were ascending urinary infection and decubitus ulcers. No significant change took place in this bleak situation until the experiences of World War II demonstrated that improved nursing care, early surgical intervention, prevention of decubitus ulcers, and control of urinary infection by means of the newly available antibacterial agents could result in survival and a reasonably good life expectancy for these patients. The mortality rate of 2,000 British paraplegics during and after World War II was only 13.2 percent (Guttmann, 1962). Perhaps the great strides made between the two World Wars are best indicated by the fact that of all Americans rendered paraplegic while overseas during the earlier conflict, only 10 percent returned to the United States, whereas the comparable figure for World War II was 90 percent (Veterans Administration, 1948).

A study conducted by the Veterans Administration (Burke et al, 1960) summarizing a ten-year experience in the care and treatment of paraplegic and tetraplegic veterans sugseted that the life expectancy of these severely disabled individuals was not significantly diminished over that of the normal population of a similar age group.

Common Causes of Spinal Cord Injury

Among military personnel, the most common cause of spinal cord injury during periods of combat is trauma resulting from gunshot wounds, explosive missiles, shrapnel, and other high-velocity objects, with motor vehicle accidents, aircraft accidents, and falls accounting for an additionally significant number of such injuries. In civilian life motor vehicle accidents are by far the principal cause of injury and paralysis, whereas gunshot wounds and diving and other water accidents are the second and third leading causes respectively. An analysis of 423 consecutive admissions for spinal cord injury to Rancho Los Amigos Hospital from January 1964 through December 1967 (Wilcox et al, 1969) revealed that most patients were males between the ages of 15 and 30. Among male automobile accident victims there were two tetraplegics to each paraplegic, whereas among women the ratio was about equal. Gunshot wounds were the second most common cause, while diving and water accidents were the third most frequent cause of injury and paralysis; all patients injured in water accidents were rendered tetraplegic with but one exception. Among males, motorcycle accidents resulted in twice as many paraplegics as tetraplegics, while gunshot wounds produced three times as many paraplegics as tetraplegics.

A subsequent survey of patients admitted to the same hospital during

797

the year 1968 revealed the same pattern of predominant causes, namely auto accidents, gunshot wounds, water mishaps, falls, and motorcycle accidents. But this more recent survey showed a remarkable increase in gunshot victims. Twenty-four percent of the women and 27 percent of the men admitted during 1968 were paralyzed as a result of shooting accidents.

The Spinal Cord Injury Center

The rehabilitative phase of the patient with spinal cord injury must be carried out within the framework of the holistic team approach. One does not deal with trauma to the spinal cord alone, but also with the prevention, and more often the correction, of the many complications resulting therefrom, including changes in protein and calcium metabolism, pain, spasticity, decubitus ulcers, contractures, the various forms of upper and lower motor neuron bladder dysfunction and, finally, the mental and socioeconomic adjustment of the patient as well as his reintegration into society. A narrow, specialistic approach to the care of the patient with spinal cord injury is grossly inadequate and detrimental to the ultimate status of the individual as a member of society. In what has been called a "comprehensive" treatment plan (Abramson, 1964), not only medical personnel, but the patient himself and members of his family participate as a closely-knit therapeutic team.

Because of the complexity of the problem inherent in the rehabilitation of the patient with spinal cord injury, it soon became apparent that the care needed by this type of patient could best be provided in specialized, adequately equipped centers properly staffed with medical and paramedical personnel. The United States Veterans Administration was a leader in setting up a number of specialized spinal cord injury centers in various parts of the country to provide an integrated type of medical care to returning veterans. Unfortunately, these centers are available primarily to veterans and, with few exceptions, the civilian population in this country is still deprived of the expert team approach which is required to restore these patients to a useful and meaningful existence.

Perhaps it may be appropriate to discuss briefly the requirements for the establishment of a spinal cord injury center in terms of personnel, physical plant, and equipment. Of basic importance are the medical specialists including neurologists; neurologic, orthopedic and

798

plastic surgeons; urologists; physiatrists; and internists. It matters little which specialist assumes medical direction of such a center, as long as he is completely familiar with all phases of medical and ancillary care. In addition to the medical specialists, an adequate complement of nurses and dieticians, and physical, occupational, and recreational therapists is essential. The service of a psychologist is of tremendous help to the patient and staff in the management of so devastating a disability as spinal cord injury. An orthotist experienced in the construction of various types of braces and mechanical devices, particularly for upper extremity dysfunction, is a necessity. Social service and vocational counseling must also be available.

The physical facilities which best serve the patient with spinal cord injury during his rehabilitative process include spacious rooms with an adequate distance between beds to permit easy maneuverability of a wheelchair, and storage space for clothing, crutches, braces, and other devices, preferably located adjacent to the bed. Beds should be of the high-low variety, preferably electrically operated, to permit easy transfer from bed to wheelchair and also to facilitate nursing care of the patient confined to bed. Bathroom facilities should be spacious to permit easy entry and full maneuverability of wheelchairs. Adequate numbers of commodes should be provided since the average patient with spinal cord injury requires more time in the toilet than a normal individual. All commodes and urinals should be provided with grab bars to permit easy transfer to and from the chair. Except for the availability of a sink for handwashing, all washing and shaving facilities should be separate from, but adjacent to the bathroom so as to assure privacy. Wash basins should be placed high enough to permit the patient in a wheelchair to come close without striking his knees or thighs. Exposed hot-water pipes beneath the sink must be covered with insulating material to avoid the possibility of the patient being burned on the legs since the skin of the lower extremities of these patients is anesthetic.

Shower facilities should be modified so that the patient in a wheelchair or other contrivance may enter the shower enclosure easily. The controls must be placed low enough so as to be accessible to the patient sitting in a chair or on a bench, and the showerhead should be fitted to a flexible hose that can be held by the patient or an attendant rather than fixed overhead. This arrangement permits the flow of water to be immediately interrupted by dropping the hose should the temperature of the water suddenly rise. In addition, all shower units must have built-in thermostatic controls to prevent the patient from being burned by water that is too hot.

A special well-ventilated room is needed in which enemas may be administered to patients requiring this type of bowel management. The usual dressing and treatment rooms found in nursing units should be spacious enough to provide easy entry of wheelchairs and litters, and should be designed to allow privacy to patients undergoing treatment.

Physical therapy and occupational therapy clinics, a gymnasium outfitted with parallel bars and other exercise equipment, and recreational facilities are essential. An "activities of daily living" clinic is of great help to the patient in mastering the skills required to transform his life from one of complete dependence to one of self-sufficiency.

Since patients with spinal cord injury at the cervical level, especially if the lesion is complete, have lost all vasomotor and sudomotor control, they are unable to conserve heat by vasoconstriction or to dissipate excessive heat through perspiration. Patients with incomplete lesions and those with spinal cord injuries at a lower level are still faced with this problem, though to a lesser extent. To permit these patients to live and function in relative comfort, adequate means of temperature control in the entire unit are a necessity, particularly in geographical regions where extremes of cold or heat are encountered.

Since the ultimate goal is total rehabilitation and complete integration of these patients into society, it is necessary to provide them with adequate means of communication and transportation. Travel by common carrier, except by air when great distances are involved, is most often difficult, if not impossible. Consequently, the automobile becomes the major means of transportation once the patient is ready to resume his place in society. Therefore, an essential part of every spinal cord injury center is a parking area sufficiently spacious to permit easy maneuverability of a wheelchair between two adjacent parked cars. In addition, properly engineered pathways leading to the building entrance which is equipped with a door that opens automatically are highly desirable.

POST-INJURY MANAGEMENT

Immediate Care

Rehabilitation should be started as soon as shock, injury to other

800

parts, conditions requiring early surgical treatment, and any other problems related to the acute trauma have been dealt with. Immediately after the injury the spinal cord is unresponsive to afferent stimuli, with the result that such reflex mechanisms as bladder emptying and bowel evacuation are lost. This period of areflexia — commonly referred to as the period of spinal shock or diaschisis — may be of varying duration, lasting a week or two in some patients and several months in others. The mechanism of shock has never been fully explained. Stewart et al reported in 1940 that following acute spinal cord lesions in monkeys, one could not demonstrate, by electromyographic study, motor unit activity in response to afferent stimuli when either single or multiple volleys were employed; however, when spinal shock subsided, electromyographic evidence of motor activity in response to stimulation appeared. They postulated a depression of anterior horn cell activity during the period of spinal shock, a concept supported by more recent work (Miglietta, 1969).

It has also been found that paralyzed muscles exhibit fibrillation potentials only during the period of spinal shock and not when spasticity supervenes, suggesting that a physiologic depression of anterior horn cell activity results when the neurotrophic influence of upper motor neurons is lost (Rosen et al, 1969). This concept awaits confirmation.

Bladder dysfunction due to loss of detrusor activity and sphincteric control requires the use of an indwelling urethral catheter. The importance of prompt insertion of the catheter cannot be over-emphasized since over-distention of the bladder during spinal shock, if permitted to persist for a prolonged period, may permanently damage the intrinsic neural mechanism within the detrusor muscle and jeopardize the potential for eventual bladder rehabilitation.

Bowel Care

Bowel evacuation during the early post-injury phase is best accomplished through the use of enemas given two or three times a week. One must be alert to recognize impaction of feces in the lower bowel, which is often associated with frequent loose stool leading to the erroneous impression that the patient has diarrhea; a rectal examination will readily disclose the true nature of the problem. Impactions must be removed manually, after which a saline enema

801

is administered; if unsuccessful, an oil retention enema followed by tap water or saline enema is advisable.

Skin Care

Decubitus ulcers constitute one of the most difficult problems that arise in the care of the patient with spinal cord injury. With the loss of motor function below the level of the injury, the paralyzed patient is unable to move about and to change his position in bed, to a greater or lesser degree, depending upon the extent and site of the injury. In addition, there is a variable degree of sensory impairment below the level of the lesion, so that the patient is unable to perceive sensations of discomfort due to pressure on the skin which under normal circumstances, would cause him to shift his position. The mechanism for the maintenance of integrity of the skin is lost and anesthetic areas are subjected to unrelieved pressure. The significance of pressure in the production of decubitus ulcers has been recognized for over a hundred years and led Sir James Paget, in 1873, to suggest placing the patient upon a loose waterproof sheet applied over the surface of a tank filled with water. His advice proved unsuccessful because of technical difficulties, but the concept of the water bed continued to receive intermittent attention and today, modern technology has made it possible to utilize this method frequently in the treatment of decubitus ulcers.

Of far greater importance to the patient is the *prevention* of decubitus ulcers. Sir Thomas Lewis showed (1949) that a pressure of 50 to 60 millimeters of mercury is sufficient to arrest the cutaneous circulation; the maintenance of such pressure for several hours and the resultant ischemia led to necrosis of the skin. Since the average mean capillary pressure is 25 millimeters of mercury, prolonged maintenance of pressure in excess of this degree is likely to lead to permanent damage. The pressure to which the normal skin is ordinarily subjected varies greatly. It has been estimated that a ballet dancer subjects the skin of her toes to pressures of 50 pounds per square inch, while the human body, floating on water, exposes the skin to a pressure of only 20 millimeters of mercury (Weinstein and Davidson, 1965).

A number of other factors tend to favor the development of decubitus ulcers. Probably foremost among these is the decreased blood flow to the muscles of the trunk and limbs resulting from the motor paralysis. While skin blood flow is not directly related to muscle blood flow, the loss of pumping action of muscle in enhancing venous return probably has some deleterious effect. Impairment of venous return may interfere with arterial inflow. Other factors which play a role are edema secondary to hypoproteinemia, and anemia which is frequently present during the early post-injury phase. Anorexia commonly occurs in such cases and results in an inadequate food intake which, in turn, is responsible for the hypoproteinemia, while anemia may be the result of surgery, blood loss due to associated trauma, intercurrent infection, or iron deficiency. The elasticity, resiliency, and vitality of tissues suffer as a consequence of anemia.

Prevention of bedsores depends primarily upon good nursing care and good nutrition. It has frequently been stated that development of decubitus ulcers in spinal cord injured patients is an indictment of the quality of nursing care. There is ample clinical evidence to support this statement. The patient must be turned every two hours day and night, assuming, at different times, not only the prone and supine positions but also both lateral positions, insofar as this is possible from the medical standpoint. A number of devices have been introduced to facilitate this change of position, but none of them are as satisfactory and as effective as manual turning and proper positioning by trained nursing personnel. Stryker frames, Foster frames, and CircOlectric beds have their advocates, but limit the patient to prone and supine positions. They are particularly useful in cases of cervical spine injury that require continued traction during the early phase of treatment. More recently, water beds have become available. In general, these have been found useful in the treatment of decubitus ulcers, their drawback being that nursing care is made more difficult. Various pads and cushions filled with water or water and air, or made of silicone or polyvinyl chloride have come into vogue and are finding limited usefulness in the prevention of bedsores. Sheep skin, either natural or artificial, has also been recommended on the basis of its property of permitting air to circulate in the mesh of wool or synthetic fiber between the bed sheet and the skin.

The most common sites for the development of decubitus ulcers are the sacral region, the greater trochanters, the ischial tuberosities, and less frequently the lateral malleoli. The medial aspects of the knees may become involved in patients with severe adductor spasticity; however, this is rarely encountered in the early post-injury phase while spinal shock prevails. Other less common sites are the anterior superior iliac spines of the pelvis and the elbows and scapular regions in high thoracic or cervical injuries.

803

Nutrition

It is of considerable importance that the patient with spinal cord injury be maintained in a state of adequate nutrition. This is particularly true during the early stage when anorexia — brought on in no small measure by the patient's anxiety, fear, frustration and depression — may lead to a period of starvation and caloric deficiency, resulting in wasting of flesh, and loss of nitrogen, calcium, and phosphorus. These deficiencies must be corrected since continued malnutrition is responsible for anemia and hypoproteinemia, which, as already indicated, are factors in the development of decubitus ulcers. Calcium and phosphorus deficiencies must also be minimized to prevent the development of osteoporosis beyond the degree commonly associated with loss of muscle action upon skeletal structures (Abramson and Delagi, 1961).

Attempts to stimulate the appetite by administration of small doses of insulin prior to meals, or by the use of anabolic agents have, in general, been quite disappointing and these measures have been largely abandoned. There is no substitute for well-balanced, attractively prepared meals that are served while the food is hot. It is essential that an adequate number of sympathetic and cheerful personnel be available to serve patients unable to feed themselves because of immobilization or paralysis of the upper extremities. Rushing the patient through a meal, or displaying impatience will only serve to affect him adversely.

Psychological Support

The emotional impact resulting from an injury to the spinal cord varies with the individual. Some patients whose injuries were self-inflicted frequently express anger and inward hostility for having brought their problems upon themselves. Others appear to accept their disability with equanimity, hopeful that everything will turn out all right. Apparent acceptance may eventually turn into severe agitation or depression, however, when the realization dawns that recovery is not progressing as had been anticipated. Such patients may refuse all attempts at treatment, reject the efforts of physical and occupational therapists, turn away food, and fail to cooperate in every respect — a type of behavior often referred to as "physiological suicide." Nevertheless, efforts must be made to continue to help the patient, and to convey to him the nature of his problem and the need for his cooperation if ultimate rehabilitation is to be achieved. To attain this goal, the assistance of a psychologist who is thoroughly familiar with the problems of patients with spinal cord injury is a most valuable asset. He can play an important role in establishing meaningful avenues of communication between the patient, his family and friends and the hospital staff. His skill may decide whether efforts at rehabilitation will succeed or fail.

Physical Modalities

Injury to the spinal cord may necessitate a prolonged period of immobilization after injury. During this period muscles may waste and joints become stiff, even in areas not directly involved in the neurologic deficit. Faulty positioning of the patient in bed can result in much damage through the action of gravitational force upon the paralyzed musculature. The physical therapist should maintain a full range of motion of all joints made immobile by paralysis to prevent contractures of capsular and ligamentous structures; likewise, muscle and joint function in the uninvolved parts of the body should be supported. As soon as there is evidence of recovery of muscle function, graded exercises are instituted to promote increase in strength. By maintaining full mobility of the hips and knees, it is possible to prevent serious functional limitations which may otherwise develop in some individuals as a result of heterotopic ossification.

Splints are required for joints threatened with contractures due to gravitational force or, later in the course of the disease, as a result of spasticity. Patients with injuries of the cervical cord must be provided with appropriate devices to permit them to engage in such essential activities of daily living as feeding, washing, brushing their teeth, personal grooming, and smoking; otherwise, substitute methods for performing these important activities must be developed. Accomplishing these tasks is of tremendous psychological value not only to the patient, but to his family, since it is an indication that progress is being made.

Respiratory Complications

Patients with cervical or high thoracic injuries may experience considerable distress during periods of upper respiratory infection

805

because of decreased vital capacity and ineffectual cough. They may have great difficulty expelling bronchial or tracheal secretions. It is essential, therefore, that every respiratory infection, no matter how slight, be treated promptly and energetically in order to avoid more serious complications. To assist the patient in expelling bronchial secretions and clearing the airway, postural drainage is performed by the physical therapist. Close observation for early signs of pneumonitis or atelectasis is essential: the former requires prompt treatment with antibacterial agents, while the latter may call for immediate aspiration by means of bronchoscopy. In some spinal cord injury centers, it is standard practice to utilize intermittent positive pressure breathing apparatus for tetraplegics during the winter months or during epidemics of respiratory infection.

MANAGEMENT IN THE LATE POST-INJURY PHASE

Goals of Rehabilitation

Although it may be expedient to divide the rehabilitative aspects of spinal cord injury into an immediate post-injury phase and a late phase, there is no sharp demarcation, since the former phase blends gradually into the latter as the medical status of the patient changes. For practical purposes, one may define the definitive period of rehabilitation as that stage when all acute surgical and medical problems have been brought under control and the patient's overall condition has become fairly stabilized. The major problems which demand attention are those related to the genitourinary tract, the prevention or treatment of decubitus ulcers, spasticity, and the achievement of maximal physical, psychological, and socioeconomic rehabilitation.

Of greatest importance to the paraplegic is the state of his genitourinary tract. Infection, formation of calculi, vesicoureteral reflux, and impairment of renal function due to chronic pyelonephritis, all of which may occur as a consequence of bladder paralysis, constitute a major threat to the patient's life. The help of the urologist is essential in the management of these problems. The treatment of the disturbances of bladder function in traumatic paraplegia and the sequelae resulting therefrom are discussed in Chapter 25.

Bowel Care

The long-term problem of bowel evacuation can usually be managed by one of two means; namely, by enema two or three times a week as necessary, or by the so-called process of bowel training. The latter is by far the preferable method. Once a patient is up and about in a wheelchair he is encouraged to develop a bowel habit pattern by going to the toilet at the same hour every day, preferably early in the morning. Colace by mouth taken the night before, glycerine or Dulcolax suppositories, or digital dilatation of the anal sphincter prior to bowel evacuation, are useful adjuncts. Such training will eventually produce the desired regularity and will free the patient of the danger of accidental soiling.

Skin Care

Vigilant care of the skin is an essential part of the patient's daily life. He must be instructed to examine his skin daily, using a small shaving mirror to inspect areas which are not directly visible. Particularly important are such pressure points as the heels, the malleoli, the trochanteric areas of the femurs, the ischii, and the sacral region. In the tetraplegic patient, inspection of the elbows is also necessary. The patient must be advised to change his position frequently while recumbent; to elevate himself in the wheelchair, if possible; or to shift from side to side and to use proper support whenever necessary to avoid pressure on vulnerable areas. Supporting the calves with a pillow will avoid pressure over the malleoli and the heels; a pillow between the knees in the spastic individual is useful in preventing breakdown of the skin over these sites; foam cushions and pads containing air, water, or synthetic material are also helpful in maintaining the integrity of the skin. The patient must be cautioned against traumatizing the skin of his lower extremities by careless handling of the wheelchair, and the hazard of spilling hot liquid over an anesthetic area must be borne in mind. If redness appears anywhere, pressure over that area must be avoided until the discoloration has subsided.

It is axiomatic that prevention is preferable to treatment. Should a decubitus ulcer nevertheless develop, treatment must be instituted promptly. If the ulcer is shallow, regardless of size, conservative management will usually be effective. The principles of prevention

807

already described are adhered to and further pressure over the ulcerated area avoided. Exposure to air is preferred, though such preparations as scarlet red and brilliant green, and bacitracin and neomycin ointments are recommended by some. Ultraviolet radiation may be of benefit in stimulating formation of granulation tissue. The application of saline, dilute acetic acid, or silver nitrate may be useful in converting a grayish-appearing granulation bed into healthy red tissue. Purulent drainage may be treated with Dakin's solution or 0.2% Clorpactin. Hydrotherapy may also be quite effective.

The contributions of plastic surgery in this area have been most significant. It has been adequately demonstrated that even large, deep-seated ulcers that are associated with extensive necrosis and loss of tissue can be successfully closed by rotation of large regional pedicle flaps of full-thickness skin. The objective in closing decubitus ulcers is to prevent the loss of large quantities of serum which may be equivalent to as much as 50 gms of protein daily. Such ulcers also serve as a portal of entry for many organisms and, on occasion, have been responsible for serious gram-negative sepsis resulting in shock and even death. Chronically infected ulcers that are frequently associated with underlying osteomyelitis, in combination with long-standing pyelonephritis, have resulted in a rather high incidence of secondary amyloidosis leading to renal failure. Successful surgical treatment will permit earlier mobilization of the patient and more rapid rehabilitation.

Preliminary to surgery, the necrotic skin and underlying tissue are debrided and wet dressings applied until the ulcer is clean. Split-thickness skin grafts may be employed at times as a temporary covering to decrease protein loss from the ulcer and thereby improve the patient's general condition. Buried grafts may be used to stimulate islands of epithelialization; these require only small amounts of donor skin. When performing definitive surgery, the ulcer and underlying bursa are excised, bony prominences are removed, dead space is eliminated by mobilizing adjacent muscle tissue, and hemostasis is achieved. Large pedicle flaps of skin and subcutaneous fat are rotated to cover the area and sutured in place. The donor site is covered with split-thickness skin graft secured usually from the thigh. At times, ulcers which are deep, but of smaller size, lend themselves to complete excision and primary closure. Severe spasticity which can interfere with the successful closure of a decubitus ulcer must be corrected prior to operative intervention. Surgical treatment of 1,000 cases of decubitus ulcers over a ten-year period yielded excellent results in 84 percent of the sacral lesions, in 86 percent of the trochanteric ulcers, and in 97 percent of the ischial ulcers (Conway and Griffith, 1956).

Although in prior years radical ischiectomy was frequently performed in conjunction with surgical closure of ischial ulcers, this procedure was often followed by pelvic tilt, scoliosis, and the development of decubitus ulcer over the contralateral ischial tuberosity, necessitating a similar procedure on that side. Removal of both ischial tuberosities led to loss of support of the pelvic floor and posterior urethra, and resulted in a high percentage of perineal fistulae. For these reasons radical ischiectomy has been abandoned and only partial resection of the ischial tuberosity with removal of the overlying bursa is now considered the treatment of choice.

Decubitus ulcers overlying the greater trochanter frequently result in osteomyelitis of the trochanter. This infection must be eradicated before closure of a trochanteric ulcer is undertaken.

Orthopedic Problems and Management

At various times during the course of rehabilitation, the services of an orthopedic surgeon may be required. Because of demineralization, fractures of long bones occur with surprising frequency following mild trauma in paraplegic patients. Such fractures affect the supracondylar portion of the femur, and the tibia. In the femur particularly fracture may occur while passive exercises of the hip or knee are being administered.

Healing of bone is not impaired in paraplegia and fractures usually heal quite readily with proper immobilization. In the ambulatory patient every effort must be made to secure adequate alignment of the fragments before immobilizing the limb, whereas in the non-ambulatory individual less than perfect reduction of the fracture is acceptable, particularly if more vigorous attempts at reduction might jeopardize the limb through damage to vascular structures. Experience has shown that surgical methods of immobilization, such as plates and screws, or intramedullary rods, almost always result in infection and are therefore ill advised in these patients (Eichenholtz, 1963). Immobilization of the limb in a circular plaster cast is equally dangerous unless precautions are taken to guard against pressure effects. Extensive areas of tissue necrosis have been known to occur in patients treated by plaster immobilization, leading at times to amputation. If plaster is deemed necessary to achieve adequate immobilization, the cast must be well padded, particularly over areas of bony prominences, and as soon as practicable the cast must be bi-valved to permit daily inspection of the skin under the plaster. Splints made with pillows and body stockinette, or with several layers of felt, have proven successful in immobilizing the femur or tibia in a non-walking paraplegic patient. Healing of the fracture usually proceeds at a fairly normal pace, not differing significantly from that in a non-paralyzed individual.

Although the views expressed here are held by most orthopedic surgeons with experience in the management of fractures in patients with spinal cord injury, some have employed operative methods, including the use of intramedullary rods, to achieve alignment and immobilization without running into the problem of infection (Meinecke et al, 1967). Operative treatment is not widely utilized, however, and is not recommended.

Certain problems, at times related to spasticity, or to inadequate attention to posture or position, may be encountered which may hinder the progress of rehabilitation. These usually take the form of contractures of joints, particularly of the hips, knees or ankles, or of severe spasticity of muscles which prevent the use of braces and thus hamper standing and ambulation. Such conditions can often be corrected by the surgeon through the use of tenotomy, tendon transfer or tendon lengthening, myotomy, or capsulotomy which, if properly carried out, will often enhance the potential for rehabilitation. It must be stressed that surgery should be undertaken only if function can be improved thereby.

Heterotopic Ossification

Heterotopic (or extraosseous) ossification occurs almost exclusively in patients with spinal cord injury, although it has occasionally been reported in patients with poliomyelitis or hemiplegia. Masses of bone are laid down usually adjacent to joints located below the level of the lesion. Thus in the paraplegic patient heterotopic ossification commonly occurs in proximity to the hip and less often the knee joints, whereas in the tetraplegic it may at times develop about the elbows. Unlike myositis ossificans which is characterized by ossification within muscle, in heterotopic ossification bone is laid down along capsular

810

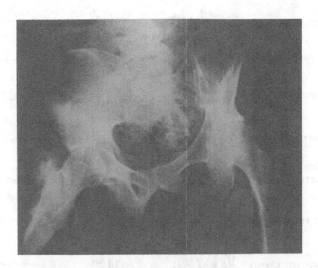

Fɪɢ. 1. Heterotopic bone formation in a patient with paraplegia. Involvement is bilateral and of greater extent on one side. Joint spaces of hips are uninvolved and well preserved.

structures and fascial planes. There is no satisfactory explanation for the occurrence of this condition (Armstrong-Ressy et al, 1959). Trauma has been suggested but in most cases no such history can be elicited. Evidence of heterotopic ossification can frequently be revealed as early as four to six weeks following injury if soft-tissue radiological techniques are used (Rofini, 1970). The process is self-limiting, progressing for a period of six to twelve months and then becoming stable. These bony masses frequently are unilateral, and if present bilaterally, one side is usually involved to a much greater extent than the other (Fig. 1).

Heterotopic ossification may seriously handicap the patient. Following prolonged bed rest in the prone or supine position after injury, severe limitation of motion of the hip joint may develop so that flexion to a degree required to sit up may be impossible. In the past, attempts to remove these lesions surgically have been catastrophic, resulting in such serious complications as osteomyelitis of the remaining osseous tissue with continued purulent drainage and deposition of new bone to an even greater extent. Recently the view has been expressed that removal of heterotopic bone could be performed without danger of infection if operative intervention were delayed until the bone had become completely mature (Freehafer et al, 1966). Too

811

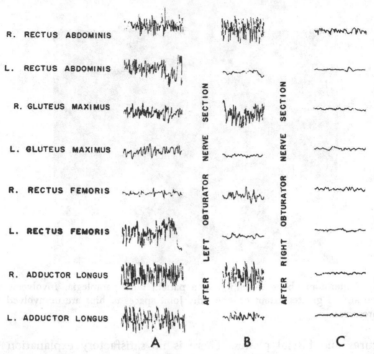

FIG. 2. Simultaneous electromyographic tracings taken from the same four muscles bilaterally in a case of spinal cord injury at D-10 level.

A. Marked spastic contraction occurring in almost all muscles examined, in response to the stimulus of a deep breath.

B. Spasticity greatly reduced on the left side in response to the same stimulus following left obturator section.

C. Spasticity greatly reduced on both sides in response to the same stimulus following bilateral obturator section (Abramson and Hirschberg).

little experience has accumulated thus far to test the validity of this concept.

Since it is not known how the formation of heterotopic ossification can be avoided, it is important to maintain joint mobility by means of physical therapy throughout the post-injury period until the patient has progressed to the wheelchair stage or has begun to ambulate with crutches or braces.

Control of Spasticity

Spasticity results from injuries of the spinal cord above the level of the conus. Its pathophysiology is exceedingly complex and involves

812

a consideration of the gamma motor system with its influence over the proprioceptive discharge of muscle spindles and its central connections including the reticular formation and the cerebellum. For a comprehensive account of current thoughts on this subject the reader is referred to the neurophysiology literature.

For practical purposes, spasticity may be defined as an exaggerated motor response of effector neurons, released from the controlling influence of higher centers, to afferent impulses, both somatic and autonomic. Spasticity of mild degree may be of benefit to the paralyzed patient since it tends to maintain muscle bulk. Moreover, slight contractions of muscle are not disturbing to the patient and will not result in contracture of joints. Severe spasticity, however, may pose a major problem. It may adversely affect nutrition through discomfort and loss of appetite, disturb rest and sleep thereby interfering with the patient's ability to participate in a full rehabilitation program, or produce severe deformities of joints, making proper nursing care and maintenance of good skin hygiene difficult while setting the stage for the development of decubitus ulcers. When spasticity reaches such a stage, steps must be taken to alleviate it.

Despite claims to the contrary, drug therapy has been found wanting. Tranquilizers and antispastic drugs that have been recommended have been found effective only when given in dosages which produce significant sedation bordering on somnolence. Physical therapeutic

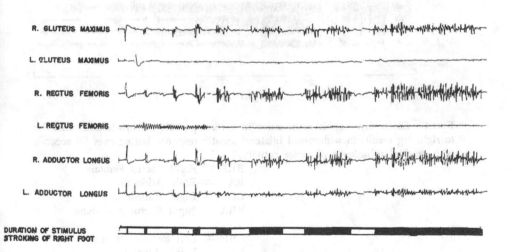

FIG. 3. In mild spasticity, muscle response, although widespread, equals stimulus in duration (Abramson and Hirschberg).

813

measures such as stretching of muscle, electrical stimulation resulting in tetany and fatigue of muscle, or hot baths, may be of value in cases of mild spasticity, but their effects are transient at best and of no consequence in the management of severe spasticity. A number of surgical procedures have been recommended. Anterior rhizotomy, usually from the lower thoracic to upper sacral level, converts a spastic paraplegia into a lower motor neuron paralysis. This procedure results in atrophy of the denervated musculature and is frequently rejected by patients. Rhizotomy of alternate roots has been proposed as a substitute, having the effect of decreasing spasticity and yet maintaining adequate muscle bulk. Injection of absolute alcohol intrathecally has been used extensively in patients with complete loss of motor, sensory, and sphincter function (Sheldon and Bors, 1948). Complete abolition of spasticity is achieved by this relatively simple procedure, its effect being similar to that resulting from surgical rhizotomy. It is not suitable, however, for patients with some preservation of function. In such cases spasticity of a specific segmental distribution

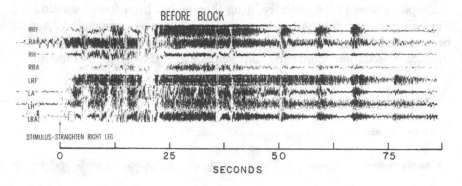

Fig. 4. Electromyographic examination in severe spasticity. Short-duration stimulus to right leg results in widespread bilateral spastic response lasting over 50 seconds with gradual subsidence of motor activity.

RRF = Right Rectus Femoris
RA = Right Adductor
RH = Right Hamstring
RRA = Right Rectus Abdominis

LRF = Left Rectus Femoris
LA = Left Adductor
LH = Left Hamstring
LRA = Left Rectus Abdominis

814

may be controlled by the intrathecal injection of phenol (5 percent) in glycerine at the appropriate level or levels, producing in effect a selective anterior rhizotomy (Nathan, 1959). This procedure is quite simple and in experienced hands has been most gratifying. Unfortunately the duration of the desired effect is unpredictable and the procedure may have to be repeated. Other surgical methods frequently used to achieve reduction of spasticity in specific muscles or muscle groups include peripheral neurectomy (obturator and femoral nerves), myotomy, tenotomy, and tendon transplants. Tenotomy has been useful in correcting equinus deformity of the ankle, and hamstring tendon transplant in reversing flexion deformity of the knee which may result in permanent contracture if not relieved. The injection of aqueous phenol solution (2 percent to 3 percent) directly into peripheral nerves has recently been used successfully to decrease spasticity in muscle groups supplied by a single nerve, e.g., the median nerve in wrist and finger flexion spasticity or the sciatic nerve in knee flexion deformity (Khalili and Betts, 1967). The technique is fairly simple but the long range results have not yet been fully evaluated.

It is advisable that all procedures for the relief of spasticity be accomplished bilaterally so as to avoid asymmetric muscle action which may lead to scoliosis or other serious deformities.

It is frequently desirable to ascertain in advance the effects that

AFTER RT. OBTURATOR BLOCK

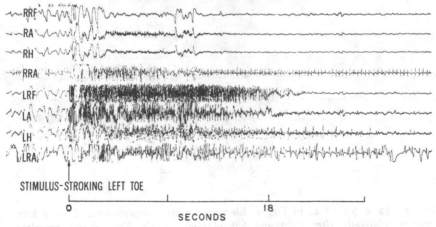

Fig. 5. Same patient as in Fig. 4. Electromyographic examination of same four muscles bilaterally after right obturator block. Note marked reduction in duration of spasticity on left side and complete abolition of spasticity on right.

815

may be expected from certain surgical procedures. This can often be accomplished by means of temporary nerve blocks with procaine or similar agents. One may find that the reduction of spasticity involves a wider distribution than can be accounted for on the basis of the nerve injected (Abramson and Hirschberg, 1952) (Fig. 2). Since clinical estimation of the quantitative reduction of spasticity in individual muscles may at times be difficult, a multi-channel electromyographic examination of a number of muscle groups simultaneously (using an EEG apparatus with eight to sixteen channels) before and after performing a nerve block is often useful in determining which muscles were in a state of greatest spasticity (Ebel, 1966). Bilateral section of the peripheral nerves to these muscles should then produce a fairly predictable beneficial effect (Figs. 3, 4, 5, 6).

One guiding principle must always be kept in mind when considering any permanently destructive type of surgical procedure. No such operation should be performed as long as there is still any likelihood of recovery of function. Practically none of the procedures mentioned above are usually indicated during the first six months following injury. Above, all, no operation should be performed which will deprive the patient of any useful function which has persisted or has been regained.

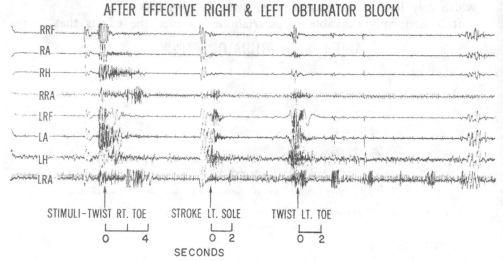

FIG. 6. Same patient as in Fig. 4. Electromyographic examination of same four muscles bilaterally after right and left obturator block. Note almost complete absence of spasticity in all muscles including those not innervated by the obturator nerve, and exceedingly short duration of motor response to stimuli.

816

Autonomic Hyperreflexia

A symptom complex frequently encountered in patients with spinal cord injury at the cervical or high thoracic level, usually above T-5, is autonomic hyperreflexia or sympathetic dysreflexia. It occurs in patients whose peripheral and visceral sympathetic innervation can no longer be regulated by the higher autonomic centers in the midbrain. This syndrome may be thought of as being analogous to spasticity of the somatic neuromuscular system below the level of the lesion, resulting in facilitation of the sympathetic reflex mechanism in the spinal cord below the level of injury. Since sympathetic outflow does not originate above the first thoracic segment, central control is thus completely lost in all complete cervical lesions. In such patients, any stimulus arising from an afferent somatic or afferent sympathetic receptor produces reflexly, through facilitation, increased sympathetic activity in all structures innervated by the efferent sympathetic outflow of the cord distal to the lesion. Such reflex hyperactivity results in marked vasoconstriction of the arterioles in the viscera and skin, reflex sweating in the dermatomes below the level of the lesion (in contradistinction to thermoregulatory sweating, which is absent below the level of the lesion), as well as cutis anserina. The marked peripheral and visceral vasoconstriction results in hypertension of a paroxysmal type which, in turn stimulates the pressure receptors in the carotid and aortic sinuses. Normally afferent impulses from these two pressure-sensitive organs travel via the ninth and tenth cranial nerves to the vasomotor center in the brain stem, which then mediates impulses through the vagus nerve to the cardiac pacemaker, resulting in bradycardia, and also sends impulses via the hypothalamus to the sympathetic outflow in the cord inhibiting vasoconstriction. In cervical and high thoracic injuries, these latter impulses are not transmitted further caudally. Therefore, inhibition of vasoconstriction does not occur and hypertension persists, leading to throbbing headache. To recapitulate, the clinical manifestations of autonomic hyperreflexia consist of bradycardia, paroxysmal hypertension, sweating, cutis anserina, nasal congestion, and headache (Kurnick, 1956) (Fig. 7). The blood pressure may reach systolic levels of 240 to 300 millimeters of mercury and diastolic levels of 110 to 120 millimeters of mercury. The potential for cerebral hemorrhage in patients with sclerotic changes or other abnormalities of the cerebral blood vessels is significantly greater. For this reason, sympathetic dysreflexia calls for prompt treatment. The most effective treatment is blockade of the sympathetic paravertebral ganglia in order

817

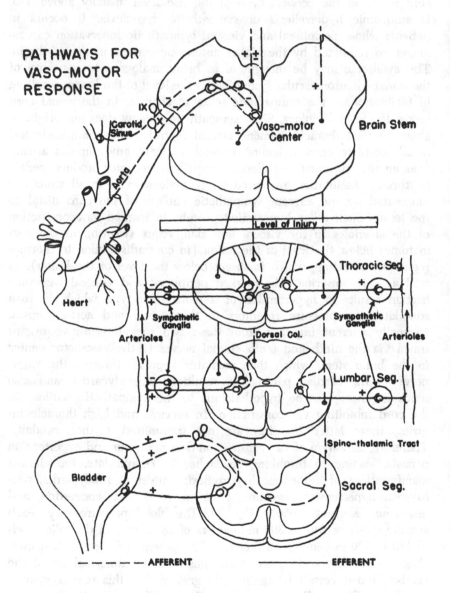

PATHWAYS FOR
VASO-MOTOR
RESPONSE

IX

Carotid
Sinus

X

Aorta

Vaso-motor
Center

Brain Stem

Heart

Level of Injury

Thoracic Seg.

Sympathetic
Ganglia

Arterioles

Dorsal Col.

Sympathetic
Ganglia

Arterioles

Lumbar Seg.

Spino-thalamic Tract

Bladder

Sacral Seg.

——— AFFERENT   ——— EFFERENT

FIG. 7. Pathways for vasomotor response (Kurnick). Mechanism for production
of autonomic hyperreflexia in cervical and high thoracic lesions. Explanation in text.

818

to interrupt the reflex vasoconstrictor mechanism. Since these autonomic crises are frequently initiated by such procedures as bladder irrigation, catheter change, or enemas, or by distention of abdominal viscera, premedication with ganglionic blocking agents is important. Pentolinium tartrate (Ansolysen) orally in doses of 20 mg has been found to be effective and may be repeated in six to eight hours if necessary. For the acute episode, intramuscularly administered pentolinium tartrate in doses of 2.5 to 5 mg will promptly abort an attack.

Prevention and Treatment of Respiratory Infections

Attention to respiratory function and complications is essential throughout the restorative period of the patient with spinal cord injury, particularly one with cervical transection and in whom the ventilatory capacity is markedly impaired as a result of paralysis of intercostal muscles. The methods and procedures previously described for immediate post-injury management are equally applicable at this stage.

Dietary Considerations

Because of the enforced inactivity secondary to paralysis many patients tend toward obesity, a condition to be strenuously avoided since it may interfere with rehabilitation and the ultimate goal of ambulation, or at the least, full mobility in a wheelchair and complete independence.

Physical Restoration

An extensive program in physical reconditioning is undertaken to exploit the patient's limited physical reserves to the maximum. Development and utilization of the muscles of the shoulder girdle and upper extremities is of the utmost importance in patients with injuries at the thoracic level. The muscles of the shoulder girdle, including the latissimus dorsi, are prime factors in permitting the individual with an injury at the lower thoracic level to perform the hip hiking required for successful ambulation with crutches and braces. Development of balancing techniques, transfer activities, and various ambulation skills are accomplished through the medium of physical therapy and occupational therapy, making use of splints, braces, crutches, and other devices as may be required, depending upon the level and extent of spinal cord injury.

Toward the end of World War II and during the post-war period there was tremendous enthusiasm for the "total push" approach in which every patient who possessed even minimal potential for ambulation with crutches and braces was trained in their use. Over the years a somewhat more tempered attitude has developed as it was learned that a paraplegic individual walking with crutches and braces, using a swingthrough gait at a speed of 88 feet per minute, (equivalent to 1 mile per hour) increased his metabolism 5½ to 8 times the basal rate. This level of energy expenditure obviously cannot be maintained for any significant length of time, and attempts to do so are totally unrealistic (Gordon and Vanderwalde, 1956).

Several surveys have also indicated that relatively few paraplegics continue to use their braces for ambulation. While a small number will employ them for the purpose of standing and performing transfer activities from chair to car, the vast majority have found that they can accomplish all the activities of daily living, including travel by automobile, without using braces. The specific needs of the patient and the setting in which he will function following discharge from the hospital will, in the final analysis, decide the issue.

Current experience suggests that training in the use of crutches and braces should be encouraged in individuals with upper and mid-thoracic injuries essentially for the purpose of permitting them to get around in tight places, otherwise inaccessible. Patients with lesions at the level of T9 or below may be able to walk satisfactorily for limited distances with the help of crutches and braces. Ambulation with braces is perfectly practical in cases of lumbar or sacral injury. Patients with cervical or very high thoracic injuries are not candidates for crutch ambulation but should use the wheelchair as a means of transportation (Ebel, 1968).

In a recent study of 91 patients who were provided with bilateral double-bar long leg braces with or without pelvic band and Knight spinal attachments for all types of paraplegia, it was found that less than 20 percent continued the use of braces, and that most of those who did were not paralyzed as a result of spinal cord injury but as a consequence of poliomyelitis (Kaplan et al, 1966).

An early concept that standing and ambulation serve as a means of preventing osteoporosis and renal calculosis is no longer tenable (Abramson, 1948).

820

The table of functional goals (see Table on p. 822) outlines briefly the physical expectations one may anticipate with complete lesions at various levels (Long and Lawton, 1955). A partial lesion will of course increase the potential for functional achievement.

The counseling psychologist plays an important role in helping the patient adjust to a totally new life. Only through his cooperation and that of the clinical psychologist, the vocational counselor, and the social worker is it possible for the many problems that face the disabled individual to be surmounted. Vocational testing and evaluation help clarify the goals still within reach of the patient. Vocational retraining may be required. New areas of education may have to be explored so that, in view of his limited physical capabilities, the patient may use his mental faculties to the best advantage. This is particularly true of the patient with tetraplegia whose only hope for gainful work lies in activities requiring little — if any — use of the upper extremities. Devices such as dictating machines and automatic telephone dials, which may be chin-controlled or perhaps even voice-controlled, are most useful to such severely disabled individuals.

In our modern, technological society, some means of transportation from home to place of employment is virtually a necessity. There are few rewarding occupations one may engage in at home. To provide himself with the necessary mobility, the spinal cord injured person must learn to drive a car that is equipped with specially adapted devices such as hand controls instead of foot pedals. Today, practically all states recognize that it is essential for the disabled to drive, and extensive experience has shown that the handicapped driver, properly trained, is no more hazardous on the road than the average non-disabled individual.

Adjustments in the family attitude towards acceptance of the disabled individual into the home setting can often be accomplished with the help of the social worker. Once over this hurdle, the family can make the physical changes in the home that may be required to provide these individuals with mobility and free access to all rooms. Structural alterations involving doors, bathrooms, closets, and even kitchen facilities may be necessary.

FOLLOW-UP CARE

There is no cure for spinal cord injury and an individual so afflicted remains a "patient" for the remainder of his life. Periodic follow-up examinations are an absolute necessity if the well-being of the individual

Functional Goals in Spinal Cord Lesions

Spinal Cord Level	Key Muscle Control	Functional Goals
C5	Neck Upper trapezius	Manipulate electric wheelchair with mouth stick Limited self-care (feeding, make-up) using arm supports and externally powered hand splints
C6	Shoulder muscles Elbow flexors	Turn self in bed with overhead arm slings Transfer to and from bed with assistance Propel wheelchair with hand rim projections Self-feeding with externally powered hand splints or clip-on equipment Light hygiene (make-up, brushing teeth) Dress upper trunk
C7	Wrist extensors Supinators	Transfer to and from bed and auto without assistance Transfer to commode chair with assistance Propel chair with hand rim projections Self-feeding, hygiene (shaving and grooming hair), dressing, writing, and skin inspection, using wrist-driven flexor hinge hand splints where prehension is required Drive auto with hand controls
C8	Elbow extensors Weak hand	Transfer independence to and from bed, car, toilet Propel wheelchair without hand rim projections Wheelchair in and out of car Independent in all self-care without hand splints or adapted equipment except catheter Household activities from wheelchair
T1 - T8	Hand muscles	Wheelchair up and down curb Transfer to and from tub Wheelchair to floor and return Therapeutic standing with posterior leg splints Care of catheter
T9 - T12	Trunk stability	Wheelchair independence Physiological ambulation with bilateral long leg braces and crutches Complete self-care
L1 - L5	Pelvic stability	Ambulation with bilateral long leg braces and crutches
S1 - S2	Knee extension Hip flexion	Ambulation with short leg braces, crutches or canes

is to be assured. It is good clinical practice to examine a patient after his discharge from the hospital every three to four months during the first year and every six to twelve months thereafter, provided no problems of consequence develop in the interim.

In addition to eliciting an interval history and performing a complete physical examination, the patient's progress, physical and vocational activities, and adjustment to his home environment are evaluated. The skin especially is examined carefully for signs of incipient breakdown. Immediate re-hospitalization is advised if any but the most superficial lesion is discovered.

The nutritional status of the patient is noted and the weight recorded. The blood pressure is checked and laboratory tests, including a complete blood count, hemoglobin and/or hematocrit, blood urea nitrogen, serum protein and A/G ratio, urinalysis and urine culture performed. A creatinine clearance study is recommended at least once a year.

An x-ray examination of the chest and a scout film of the abdomen followed by an intravenous pyelogram are probably advisable at each examination. It is thereby possible to detect early stone formation in the kidneys or bladder and to take appropriate action. Cystography, measurement of bladder capacity and residual urine determination (in catheter-free cases) are regularly performed. It is important to be on the lookout for evidence of reflux and/or hydroureter or hydronephrosis, particularly in patients who do not require the use of a catheter.

A brief interview with the vocational counselor, psychologist, or social worker may be indicated, depending upon circumstances.

The authors are indebted to Dr. A. S. Abramson and the editor of the Bulletin of the Hospital for Joint Diseases, to Dr. N. B. Kurnick and the editor of the Annals of Internal Medicine, and to Dr. E. Ejercito for permission to reproduce Figures 2, 3, and 7, and the table on page 822, respectively.

BIBLIOGRAPHY

Abramson, A. S. Bone Disturbances in Injuries to the Spinal Cord and Cauda Equina (Paraplegia). *J. Bone Joint Surg.*, *30A*, 982-987, 1948.

Abramson, A. S. Paraplegia Retrospect and Prospect. The Albee Memorial Rehabilitation Lecture, Kessler Institute for Rehabilitation. West Orange, N. J., Oct. 24, 1964.

Abramson, A. S. and Delagi, E. F. Influence of Weight-bearing and Muscle Contraction on Disuse Osteoporosis. *Arch. Phys. Med & Rehab.*, *42*, 147-151, 1961.

Abramson, A. S. and Hirschberg, G. G. Studies on Spasticity. *Bull. Hosp. Joint Dis.*, *13*, 164-172, 1952.

Armstrong-Ressy, C. T., Weiss, A. A. and Ebel, A. Results of Surgical Treatment of Extraosseous Ossification in Paraplegia. *N. Y. State J. Med.*, *59*, 2548-2553, 1959.

Breasted, J. H. *The Edwin Smith Surgical Papyrus*. Vol. 1. Chicago: University of Chicago Press, 1930. P. 326-327.

Burke, M. H., Hicks, A. F., Robins, M., and Kessler, H. Survival of Patients with Injuries of the Spinal Cord. *J.A.M.A.*, *172*, 121-124, 1960.

Connors, J. F. and Nash, I. E. The Management of Urological Complications in Injuries to the Spine. Report of 54 Cases without a Single Infection in the Urinary Tract. *Am. J. Surg.*, *26*, 159-167, 1934.

Conway, H. and Griffith, B. H. Plastic Surgery for Closure of Decubitus Ulcers in Patients with Paraplegia; Based on Experience with 1000 Cases. *Am. J. Surg*, *91*, 946-975, 1956.

Ebel, A. Electromyography for Determining Trigger Muscles in Spasticity. Proceedings, First Caribbean Congress in Physical Medicine and Rehabilitation, San Juan, May 1966. P. 243-246.

Ebel, A. Restorative Management of Paraplegic Patient; Philosophy and Concept of Bracing. *N. Y. State J. Med.*, *68*, 2037-2040, 1968.

Eichenholtz, S. N. Management of Long-bone Fractures in Paraplegic Patients. *J. Bone Joint. Surg*, *45A*, 299-310, 1963.

Freehafer, A. A., Yurick, R., and Mast, W. A. Para-Articular Ossification in Spinal Cord Injury. *Med Serv. J. Can.*, *22*, 471-477, 1966.

Gordon, E. E. and Vanderwalde, H. Energy Requirements in Paraplegic Ambulation. *Arch. Phys. Med. & Rehab.*, *37*, 276-285, 1956.

Guttmann, L. The National Spinal Injuries Center Stoke Mandeville Hospital, Aylesbury, Bucks. *Mon. Bull. Minist. Hlth. Lab. Serv.*, *21*, 60-71, 1962.

Kaplan, L. I., Grynbaum, B. B., Rusk, H. A., Anastasia, T. and Gassler, S. A Reappraisal of Braces and other Mechanical Aids in Patients with Spinal Cord Dysfunction: Results of a Follow-up Study. *Arch. Phys. Med. & Rehab.*, *47*, 393-405, 1966.

Khalili, A. A. and Betts, H. B. Peripheral Nerve Block with Phenol in the Management of Spasticity. *J.A.M.A.*, *200*, 1155-1157, 1967.

Kurnick, N. B. Autonomic Hyperreflexia and its Control in Patients with Spinal Cord Lesions. *Ann. Int. Med. 44,* 678-686, 1956.

Lewis, Sir T. *Vascular Disorders of the Limbs,* 2nd ed. London: Macmillan, 1949.

Long, C. II and Lawton, E. B. Functional Significance of Spinal Cord Lesion Level. *Arch. Phys. Med & Rehab., 36,* 249-255, 1955. (Modified by E. M. Ejercito).

Meinecke, F. W., Rehn, J., and Leitz, G. Conservative and Operative Treatment of Fractures of the Limbs in Paraplegia. Proceedings of 16th Annual Clinical Spinal Cord Injury Conference, Veterans Administration, Long Beach, Calif., Sept. 27-29, 1967.

Miglietta, O. Motorneuron Excitability in Spasticity. Presented at 17th Clinical Spinal Cord Injury Conference, Veterans Administration, New York, Sept. 30, 1969.

Nathan, P. W. Intrathecal Phenol to Relieve Spasticity in Paraplegia. *Lancet, 2,* 1099-1102, 1959.

Paget, J. Clinical Lectures on Bedsores. *Student's J. & Hosp. Gaz. 1,* 144, 1873.

Poer, D. H. Newer Concepts in the Treatment of the Paralyzed Patient due to War-time Injuries of the Spinal Cord. *Ann. Surg., 123,* 510-515, 1946.

Rofini, R. G. Extraosseous Ossification in Spinal Cord Injury in a Prospective Study. Presented at New York Society of Physical Medicine and Rehabilitation, May 6, 1970.

Rosen, J. S., Lerner, M., and Rosenthal, A. M. Electromyography in Spinal Cord Injury. *Arch. Phys. Med. & Rehab., 50,* 271-273, 1969.

Sheldon, C. H. and Bors, E. Subarachnoid Alcohol Block in Paraplegia; Its Beneficial Effect on Mass Reflexes and Bladder Dysfunction. *J. Neurosurg., 5,* 385-391, 1948.

Stewart, W. B., Hughes, J., and McCouch, G. P. Cord Potentials in Spinal Shock. *J. Neurophysiol., 3,* 139-155, 1940.

Thompson-Walker, J. W. The Treatment of the Bladder in Spinal Injuries in War. *Br. J. Urol., 9,* 217-230, 1937.

Veterans Administration Technical Bulletin TB10-503. *Spinal Cord Injuries.* December 15, 1948.

Weinstein, J. D. and Davidson, B. A. A Fluid-support Mattress and Seat for the Prevention and Treatment of Decubitus Ulcers. *Lancet, 2,* 625-626, 1965.

Wilcox, N. E., Stauffer, E. S., and Nickel, V. L. A Statistical Analysis of 423 Consecutive Patients Admitted to a Spinal Cord Injury Center. Presented at 46th Annual Session, American Congress of Rehabilitation Medicine, Chicago, Aug. 14, 1969.

825

CHAPTER 27

BIRTH INJURIES OF THE SPINAL CORD

RANDOLPH K. BYERS, M. D.
AND
MICHAEL J. BRESNAN, M. D.

"A very brief consideration of breech extraction as it is described in books, shows that it is a unique procedure in obstetrics, in that an entirely unphysiological force is applied to a structure which normally is not subjected to any comparable strain. As far as I know, no other obstetric maneuver, used to deliver living babies, is so illogical or so potentially disastrous" (Crothers, 1922).

The recognition and comprehensive description of obstetrical injury to the spinal cord of the infant, and the clarification of its etiologic relationship to a variety of obstetrical maneuvers by Crothers (1923, 1927) have led to a decline in its occurrence. In 1927, Crothers and Putnam published a description of 28 cases seen at the Children's Hospital in Boston over a period of six years and, subsequently, Crothers (1960) stated that he had seen as many as ten new cases a year. A review of the records of the same hospital for the years 1960-1969 shows two clear-cut examples and in addition, a possible third — a weak child with deformed hands who was admitted for an emergency bronchoscopy because of pulmonary collapse. No further data on her are available. If we accept her as having spinal cord injury, an incidence of 0.3 cases a year obtains. Unfortunately, this vastly improved record is marred by the recognition of two cases (one proven by autopsy and one by surgical exploration) in 1970.

Crothers and Putnam also noted that they had seen 216 uncomplicated examples of brachial palsy and 260 cases of cerebral palsy with "birth trauma, a fair explanation" during the same six years.

Although scattered case reports of obstetrical injury to the infantile spinal cord were published from 1836 on (Crothers, 1927; Parrot, 1870),

826

and Ford reported a series of six cases in 1925, little attention was paid them until Crothers' insistence on the importance of his findings received the recognition of the medical profession.

ETIOLOGY

As pointed out by Crothers (1922), natural labor imposes on the fetus compressive stresses to which it is well adapted anatomically. When obstetrical operations are performed on the infant to hasten delivery, a traction force, i.e., stretching of the spinal axis, is applied. Duncan (1874) showed that the mature human fetus when suspended by the head immediately after death was unable to tolerate a weight of 90 to 120 pounds attached to one leg for one minute. At this level of stress, a loud snap occurred and the fetus increased in length. It seems likely that the loud snap referred to occurred as a result of rupture of the dura. A further increase in weight applied to the feet produced decapitation usually between the fourth and fifth cervical vertebrae. If the spine of a newly dead mature baby is dissected free of all supporting tissue, it is possible, as pointed out by Crothers, for an average man to stretch it a matter of about 5 centimeters (and when this is done, the lengthening is seen to occur in the bodies of the vertebrae). The dura, attached at the foramen magnum and at its sacral end, provides strong protection against such stretching of the spinal axis (beyond 5 cm). Should it rupture, the relatively inelastic spinal cord, anchored superiorly by the structures above the foramen magnum and below by the lower spinal nerve roots, is readily torn, usually in the cervical or dorsal region. Injuries to the region of the lumbosacral cord have been described clinically but no pathological studies are available.

Pierson (1923) called attention to spinal fractures and dislocations, with subsequent gross injury to the spinal cord, affecting most commonly the sixth cervical vertebra, after simple breech extraction and especially following internal podalic version. In 1927, Crothers was able to find approximately 150 such cases in the literature. To this he added another 28 cases. In two of these, details of delivery were not available, but each was "instrumentally delivered with great force." Of the other 26 cases, 19 were delivered by breech extraction and of these, at least seven had had podalic version. Four cases had associated fractures. The remaining seven cases were vertex deliveries, but only in two cases was this described as "easy." One of the seven cases had an associated fracture.

In 1959, Stern and Rand reported two cases of cord injury with autopsy findings and reviewed the literature. They found 53 recorded cases between 1923 and 1959. Of these, 39 had been born by breech extraction or internal podalic version and breech extraction, nine by cephalic delivery, and in five, the method of delivery was unstated. In breech extraction, the injury to the cord occurred at the lower cervical to upper thoracic levels, whereas in vertex deliveries, it tended to be in the upper cervical region.

Spinal cord injury during vertex extractions may occur as a result of traction on the brachial plexus and avulsion of the latter from the spinal cord. In a few instances, such avulsions have been demonstrated by means of myelography, globules of contrast medium escaping from the main column in the subarachnoid space.

In recent years, much has been written concerning the occurrence of spinal cord injury as a result of hyperextension (deflexion) of the fetal head in utero. This malposition of the fetus referred to variously as fetal cervical hyperextension, opisthotonus fetalis, or the "flying fetus," has been associated with spinal cord transection following vaginal delivery, usually breech, and often described as "easy." Hellstrom and Sallmander (1968) in a recent review noted that in no case delivered by Cesarean section, and this included one case with roentgenologically proven cervical subluxation, was there neurological damage to the infant. In contrast, where delivery had been allowed to proceed vaginally, seven of 17 cases sustained cervical cord injuries and only two survived. The etiology of the hyperextension is not known, various causes including uterine abnormalities, special locations of the placenta, and spasm of the neck muscles having been suggested. An opisthotonic posture may persist for months in affected babies who otherwise develop normally.

PATHOLOGY

Pathologic examination, usually after a period of survival, has shown in most instances rupture of the spinal cord with the two ends separated by a thin translucent scar into which the meninges and vessels are incorporated. As one would expect, the ascending fiber tracts of the

828

cord are demyelinated above the injury and the descending fibers below this level (Byers, 1932).

Extensive destruction of the cord by hematomyelia was reported by Beevor (1902) in a case in which hemorrhage extended from C-3 to T-11. The remainder of the cord inferiorly was described as shrivelled and scarred with none of the usual landmarks visible. During life, the infant manifested generalized weakness, suggesting Werdnig-Hoffmann disease, but was unresponsive to pinprick.

Allen et al (1969) reported three cases of obstetrical spinal cord injury, in one of which 8 centimeters of the cord beginning 3.5 centimeters below the olives was softened and infiltrated with blood pigment, and its architecture disrupted. Yates (1959) examined the cervical spine and cord of 60 infants either stillborn or dying in the neonatum and selected at random out of 213 such deaths. Included were eight breech deliveries, three Cesarean sections and 16 stillbirths. While he was primarily interested in lesions of the vertebral arteries, contusion and hemorrhage involving the spinal cord were found in two cases. In one of these the hemorrhage was rather circumscribed, affecting the gray matter preponderantly on one side.

Included in the report of Penry and co-authors (1960) is a well-studied case of cord transection following breech delivery in which increased tone was noted in the upper extremities. The arms were held abducted at the shoulder, flexed at the elbows, wrists and fingers, in the so-called Thorburn posture. Pathologic study revealed a decrease in the neurons of the intermediate gray zone and also of the Renshaw cells in the anterior horns. It was suggested that this unusual posture with rigidity, rather than flaccidity, was due to uninhibited spontaneous discharge of surviving motor neurons.

Recently, Towbin (1964, 1969, 1970) has emphasized that, notwithstanding their frequency, injuries of the spinal cord and brain stem are often not recognized clinically and are even overlooked at necropsy, unless the nervous system is carefully examined. His observations led to the conclusion that spinal epidural hemorrhage is the most frequent manifestation of spinal cord injury. On the whole, there was very little evidence in his material of reaction to the hemorrhages, and one wonders if the bleeding was not agonal (Figs. 1, 2, 3).

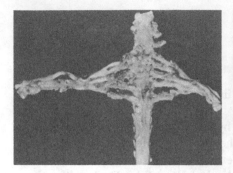
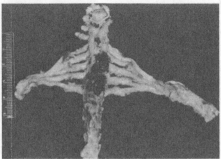

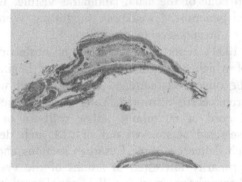

FIG. 1. Anterior aspect of spinal cord showing area of injury extending from lower margin of C-5 nerve roots to T-10. The infant had been born by breech delivery with forceps to the aftercoming head. Mother had toxemia with seizures before and after delivery. Infant quadriparetic at birth with no voluntary movement below deltoids bilaterally. Anesthetic to pinprick below clavicles. Withdrawal reflexes developed at a few weeks in legs. Died of pneumonia at 11 months.

FIG. 2. Posterior aspect of same spinal cord; the hemorrhage shown is a fresh agonal one.

FIG. 3. Section of spinal cord and surrounding dura from between C-7 and C-8. The structure of the cord is completely disorganized; blood vessels, nerve roots, and occasional isolated nerve cells can be identified histologically.

CLINICAL MANIFESTATIONS

Immediate Postnatal Period

The location and extent of the spinal cord injury determine the clinical manifestations. Injuries above the level of the fourth cervical segment are presumably immediately fatal. Lesions of the lower cervical and upper thoracic cord, sometimes associated with injuries to the brachial plexus, are manifested usually by flaccidity of the arms and hands, occasionally by the Thorburn posture, difficulty in breathing, and severe prostration; a Horner's syndrome may be noted. Midthoracic ruptures produce paralysis of the abdominal wall and lower limbs. Paralysis of the lower extremities alone occurs following lesions of the lumbar cord and cauda equina.

During this early period accurate sensory mapping is usually impossible, but gross loss of pinprick perception can be demonstrated as a rule. Bladder paralysis commonly occurs and may be managed in most instances without catheterization. It is usually possible to empty the bladder by gentle suprapubic pressure. Within a few days, most newborns develop more or less effective automatic bladders, save in the rare instances of a lumbar lesion.

Demonstration of injury to vertebral bodies is usually impossible in the neonatal period since the infant's spine is so largely cartilaginous. X-rays of the spine are, however, valuable in excluding congenital anomalies, though occasionally spinal dislocation may be demonstrated. In the immediate postnatal period, motion of the spine should be restricted by a light plaster shell, Bradford frame, or similar device.

Skin lesions are an unusual complication, occurring only in the rare instances of destruction of the lumbosacral cord and nerves. In such cases, bedsores must be anticipated and prevented by utmost skill in nursing.

Surgical intervention is often proposed, and has been employed sporadically with disappointing results. When spinal block is demonstrated by myelography, operation may be justified, but considering the usual pathologic findings, not much improvement should be expected from it. However, since most myelograms and explorations have been done when the infants are several months of age, perhaps earlier attempts should be undertaken.

Later Infancy

Within a few weeks the effects of "spinal shock" are no longer evident, edema subsides, and hemorrhagic extravasations at the site of injury are absorbed. It is then quite possible to make a durable appraisal of the patient's neurologic status. In doing so, it is of extreme importance to differentiate between spontaneous voluntary movement and reflex responses elicited by local noxious stimulation. A period of observation of the undisturbed infant should precede active examination for the

831

purpose of establishing the infant's spontaneous activity, paying careful attention to the face, arms, trunk and legs. Transection of the cord is characterized by the occurrence of reflex responses to painful stimuli over a more or less wide receptive area. The motor responses are quite stereotyped, and do not vary relative to the location of the stimulus; e.g., a pinprick on the sole of the foot produces flexion of the hip and knee with dorsiflexion of the ankle (an appropriate withdrawal), as does also a pinprick on the dorsum of the foot (an inappropriate response to this stimulus). The baby's facial response to such stimuli must be observed for evidence of failure to perceive pain and the extent of the area of analgesia estimated.

The distribution of flaccid paralysis is determined by the level of spinal cord injury. Because of the usual thick layer of subcutaneous fat in the infant, fasciculations are not seen though they may be demonstrated by electromyography.

Spasticity of the sort leading to contractures is unusual. Occasionally, contractures of the hip flexors supervene in infants with lower spinal cord injuries, and are often accompanied by contracture of the femoral fascia. Good orthopedic care is important in such cases to prevent severe deformity of the spine.

In a few instances, the clinical picture suggests that the gray matter of the cord has sustained the bulk of the injury. Such lesions are usually in the cervical and upper thoracic segments and produce weakness and deformity of the hands or chest or both, sometimes with localized sensory loss. Below the lesion evidence of injury to the long tracts may be minimal.

Reflex emptying of the bladder may become well established, usually in response to tactile or painful stimuli applied to the inner aspect of the thighs, and may long postpone the almost inevitable urinary tract infection.

Later Childhood

The diagnosis is usually quite obvious in older children. The history is one of persistent disability following dystocia, but various complications may confuse the picture and suggest progressive disease. Scarring of the meninges may result in spinal block, and either gliosis or occasionally frank hydromyelia may supervene with progressive loss of function, requiring myelography and surgical intervention.

Uneven growth of the body may produce progressive deformities, especially of the spine, which become increasingly evident as the child sits or stands. Ataxia, previously not appreciated, may also become apparent with the attainment of the erect position.

The treatment of older children depends on the extent of neurologic disability. Skillful orthopedic care is essential. The neurologic status of the patient should be reviewed from time to time, especially if any suggestion of deterioration appears.

In general, the diagnosis of spinal cord injury as the result of an obstetrical accident is easy if the possibility is considered. The obstetrical history, the persistence of disability since birth, and the absence of congenital anomalies usually establish the diagnosis. Coincident trauma to the brain may obscure the diagnosis in patients with diffuse injury to the nervous system. Mental impairment is of course not a feature of spinal cord injury and, when present, is indicative of cerebral damage.

DIFFERENTIAL DIAGNOSIS

Only a few conditions need be considered in the differential diagnosis. Myelodysplasia is probably the most important cause of paraplegia in infancy, and this possibility should always be entertained. Spinal cord tumor is more common in infancy than usually appreciated and must be carefully considered. Myelitis of various types can usually be identified by the history, as can osteomyelitis of the spine and postnatal injuries.

PROGNOSIS

A consideration of prognosis from a statistical standpoint will only be possible when postmortem examinations, including the entire spinal cord, are done of all babies dying in the neonatum. A few random observations may be made. A very small number of newborns who appear to have spinal cord injuries recover astonishingly well. One young lady who was admitted a day or two after birth flaccid from the hands down, now makes her living exercising saddle horses on her father's ranch. She has mild weakness and flexion contractures of the second, third, and fourth fingers of the left hand, and a suspicion of ataxia of gait. Another girl with a very complete transection of the cord, as shown by persistent mass reflexes in her legs and anesthesia to the upper chest, made her living as a telephone operator until

833

age 31. She learned to ambulate on crutches without touching her feet to the ground and could stand still and converse while doing so. She had a reflex bladder which she emptied by pinching the inner aspect of one thigh. She succumbed to urinary tract infection in her thirties. Some of the patients reported by Crothers (1923, 1927) and by Ford (1925) in the pre-antibiotic era were older children, though in those days, most infants with spinal cord injuries died early of respiratory infection. Leventhal's series reported in 1960 included patients who ranged in age up to 12 years, with two early deaths, one following laminectomy.

SUMMARY

Obstetrical injury to the spinal cord usually produces immediate and permanent disability, but progressive changes may occur, necessitating further study and perhaps surgical intervention. Early investigation by means of myelography may be worthwhile.

OBSTETRICAL IMPLICATIONS

The incidence of birth injuries at present compared to that encountered by Crothers and Putnam in 1927 is considerably less. Permanent brachial plexus injury is now uncommon, and cord injury, though occasionally encountered, is quite rare. No doubt the introduction of obstetrical analgesia has contributed to the improvement that has been achieved, but the realization by obstetricians that traction on the infantile spinal axis imposes an unphysiologic force and that no emergency exists in breech delivery after birth of the infant's umbilicus, has been especially salutary.

It is becoming apparent that greater use of elective Cesarean section in cases of hyperextension of the fetus in utero may prevent transection of the cord which may otherwise occur in such babies born by breech delivery.

BIBLIOGRAPHY

Allen, J. P., Meyers, G. L., and Condon, V. R. Laceration of the Spinal Cord Related to Breech Delivery. *J.A.M.A.*, *208*, 1019, 1969.

Beevor, C. E. A Case of Spinal Muscular Atrophy (Familial Type) and a Case of Hemorrhage into the Spinal Cord at Birth Giving Similar Symptoms. *Brain*, *25*, 85, 1902.

Byers, R. K. Transection of the Spinal Cord in the Newborn. *Arch. Neurol. & Psychiat.*, *27*, 585, 1932.

Crothers, B. The Effect of Breech Extraction upon the Central Nervous System of the Foetus. *Med. Clin. North Am.*, *5*, 1287, 1922.

Crothers, B. Injury of the Spinal Cord in Breech Extractions as an Important Cause of Fetal Death and Paraplegia. *Am. J. Med. Sci.*, *165*, 94, 1923.

Crothers, B. and Putnam, M. C. Obstetrical Injuries of the Spinal Cord. *Medicine*, *6*, 41, 1927.

Crothers, B. Birth Injuries of the Spinal Cord. In S. Brock (Ed.), *Injuries of the Brain and Spinal Cord*, 4th ed. New York: Springer, 1960.

Duncan, J. M. Laboratory Note on the Tensile Strength of the Fresh Adult Human Fetus. *Br. Med. Jr.*, *11*, 763, 1874.

Ford, F. R. Breech Delivery and its Possible Relations to Injury of the Spinal Cord. *Arch. Neurol. & Psychiat.*, *14*, 742, 1925.

Hellstrom, B., and Sallmander V. Prevention of Spinal Cord Injury in Hyperextension of the Fetal Head. *J.A.M.A.*, *204*, 1041, 1968.

Kennedy, E. Cerebral and Spinal Apoplexy in the New Born. *Dublin J. Med. Sci.*, *419*, 1836.

Leventhal, H. R. Birth Injuries of the Spinal Cord. *J. Pediatr.*, *56*, 447, 1960.

Parrot, J. Note sur un Cas de Rupture de la Moelle Chez un Nouveau Né Par suit de Manoeuvres Pendant l'Accouchement. *L'Union Med.*, *9*, 137, 1870.

Penry, J. K., Hoefnagel, D., van Den Noort, S., and Denny-Brown, D. Muscle Spasm and Abnormal Postures Resulting from Damage to Interneurones in Spinal Cord. *Arch. Neurol.*, *3*, 500, 1960.

Pierson, R. N. Spinal and Cranial Injuries of the Baby in Breech Delivery. *Surg. Gynec. Obstet.*, *37*, 802, 1923.

Stern, W. E., and Rand, R. W. Birth Injuries to the Spinal Cord. *Am. J. Obs. Gyn.*, *78*, 498, 1959.

Towbin, A. Spinal Cord and Brain Stem Injury at Birth. *Arch. Path.*, *77*, 620, 1964.

Towbin, A. Latent Spinal Cord and Brain Stem Injury in New Born Infants. *Devel. Med. Child. Neur.*, *11*, 54, 1969.

Towbin, A. Central Nervous System Damage in the Human Fetus and New Born Infant. *Am. J. Dis. Child.*, *119*, 529, 1970.

Yates, P. O. Birth Trauma to the Vertebral Arteries. *Arch. Dis. Childh.*, *34*, 436, 1959.

835

HERNIATION AND PROTRUSION OF INTERVERTEBRAL DISCS AND SPONDYLOTIC MYELORADICULOPATHY

FRANCIS A. ECHLIN, M. D.

AND

EMANUEL H. FEIRING, M. D.

In this new edition little has been added to the section on herniated discs in the lumbar region, since the fundamental ideas regarding the pathology, diagnosis, and treatment of this condition have not changed radically. Some of the more recent contributions on this subject, however, are reviewed and are included in the bibliography, especially those dealing with end results (Barr, 1967; Bradford, 1960; Gurdjian et al, 1961; Raaf, 1959; Semmes, 1964; White, 1966); with the value of foraminotomy (Shenkin and Haft, 1966); and with the treatment of midline and bilateral herniations (Haft and Shenkin, 1966; Uihlein and Baker, 1968).

The diagnosis and treatment of posterolateral herniations of disc tissue in the cervical region with compression of a solitary nerve root have been the subject of much controversy (Haft and Shenkin, 1963; McGinnis and Eisenbrey, 1964; Raaf, 1958; Scoville, 1966). Considerable difference of opinion also exists regarding the pathogenesis, diagnosis, and management of the myeloradiculopathy resulting from spondylosis in the cervical region (Brain and Wilkinson, 1967; Burrows, 1963; Clarke and Robinson, 1956; Cloward, 1958, 1958, 1963; Connolly et al, 1966; Epstein and Davidoff, 1951; Epstein et al, 1963; Epstein et al, 1969; Frykholm, 1951; Galera and Tovi, 1968; Herzberger et al, 1963; Logue, 1959; Mayfield, 1955, 1965; Raaf, 1958; Riley et al, 1969; Robinson and Smith, 1955; Robinson et al, 1962; Rogers, 1961; Rosomoff and Rossman, 1966; Scoville, 1961; Smith and Robinson, 1958; Stoops and King, 1965; Wilkinson, 1971). These subjects will, therefore, be considered in some detail. Herniated discs in the thoracic region will also be discussed.

Through the years there have been innumerable articles dealing with herniations or protrusions of intervertebral disc tissue into the spinal canal. The essential features of the syndromes produced by many of these disc lesions, especially the syndrome of sciatica, were described long ago by the great neurologists, but the herniated intervertebral disc as a causative factor remained unrecognized. Isolated reports of severe compression of the cauda equina due to sudden traumatic rupture of an intervertebral disc appeared in the literature at an early date (Kocher, 1896; Middleton and Teacher, 1911; Goldthwait, 1911) but it was not yet suspected, except perhaps by Goldthwait, that the intervertebral disc might be a common cause of nerve root compression. As reported by Elsberg (1916, 1925), Steinke (1918), Clymer, Mixter and Mella (1921), Adson and Ott (1922), Stookey (1928), Bucy (1930), and others, herniations of disc tissue were found at operation to have compressed neural structures within the spinal canal but these herniations were considered to be chondromata. According to Elsberg (1931), Stookey (1928) deserves the credit for first calling attention to the fact that the "chondromata" are derived from the intervertebral cartilages.

A new insight into the problem was provided by the studies of Schmorl (1927-30) and his pupils on the pathology of the intervertebral disc and spinal column. Schmorl (1929) demonstrated that posterior herniations of the nucleus pulposus through the annulus fibrosus are common autopsy findings, and Andrae (1929) was able to find such herniations in 15 percent of 368 spinal columns examined routinely at autopsy.

Alajouanine and Petit-Duatillis (1928, 1930) and Mauric (1933) recognized that most chondromata are in reality nucleus pulposus tissue which has herniated through the posterior annulus fibrosus, and in 1929 Dandy reported two cases of loose cartilage from the intervertebral disc simulating tumor of the spinal cord.

It remained for Mixter and Barr (1934) to demonstrate that herniation of the nucleus pulposus is a common cause of low back pain and sciatica, and that the lesion can be diagnosed clinically. This important report in 1934 was followed by an ever increasing number of articles on the physiological, pathological, clinical, roentgenographic, and surgical aspects of the herniated disc. As a result, the syndrome of the herniated disc in the lumbar region became established as a major clinical entity.

The contributions on this subject are so numerous that only a few may be mentioned in the ensuing pages, but in the monographs by Bradford and Spurling (1945), Spurling (1953), Semmes (1964), Armstrong (1965), and DePalma and Rothman (1970), a thorough review of the subject of the herniated lumbar disc may be found. In addition recent articles by the following authors may be consulted: Aronson, 1963; Barr, 1967; Bradford, 1960; Bucy, 1961, 1963; Davidson and Woodhall, 1959; Epstein et al, 1967; Gurdjian et al, 1961; Haft and Shenkin, 1966; Raaf, 1959; Shenkin and Haft, 1966; Uihlein and Baker, 1968; and White, 1966. The radiologic aspects of the subject are well covered in the texts by Taveras and Wood (1964) and by Epstein (1969).

The first part of the present chapter is concerned chiefly with posterior herniations or protrusion of disc tissue in the lumbar region, but some consideration is also given to anatomy, physiology, and pathology as applied to all intervertebral discs. The remainder of the chapter deals with herniated discs in the thoracic and cervical regions and the problem of myeloradiculopathy due to spondylosis.

ANATOMICAL CONSIDERATIONS

Anatomical studies of the intervertebral disc date back at least as far as Vesalius (1555). According to Keyes and Compere, however, it was von Luschka (1858) who first gave an accurate description of its structure and embryology. The essentials of the anatomy of the intervertebral disc may be found in the first edition of Gray's Anatomy (1858) and it is interesting to note that this original description has stood the test of time to the degree that it is used almost verbatim in the modern editions of the same book. Other studies on the developmental and structural anatomy of the intervertebral disc have been reported by Virchow (1857), Kölliker (1860), Dursy (1869), Löwe (1879), Bardeen (1905), and Williams (1908). Among the more recent contributions on this subject are those of Schmorl (1927 to 1930), Calvé and Galland (1930), Beadle (1931), Keyes and Compere (1932), Bradford and Spurling (1945), Coventry, Ghormley, and Kernohan (1945), Inman and Saunders (1947), Prader (1947, 1947), and Compere (1961).

838

The Spinal Column and Intervertebral Discs

The intervertebral fibrocartilages or discs are situated between the opposing surfaces of the bodies of the vertebrae from the axis to the sacrum and are 23 in number. They firmly bind the vertebral bodies together. Articulations thus formed between the vertebrae are amphiarthrodial, or slightly movable and of the symphysis form.

The intervertebral discs make up approximately one fourth of the length of the vertebral column, if the first two vertebrae are excluded. Proportionate to the length of the column, in the cervical and lumbar regions the intervertebral discs occupy more space than in the thoracic region, and allow greater freedom of movement. They are largest and highest in the lumbar region. The cervical and lumbar discs are higher in front than behind, thus contributing to the cervical and lumbar convexities.

The superior and inferior surfaces of the intervertebral discs are intimately adherent to thin plates of hyaline cartilage which cover the bony surfaces of the opposing vertebral bodies. Each cartilaginous plate is cemented to the spongiosa, or cancellous bone of the vertebral body, by a thin layer of calcified cartilage. At its periphery the plate abuts on the elevated epiphyseal ring of the body of the vertebra. These cartilaginous plates are not part of the intervertebral disc proper, although they have frequently been regarded as such for convenience of description.

Structure of the Intervertebral Disc

Each fibrocartilage or disc is made up of two parts, a firmer tougher circumferential part, the annulus fibrosus, and a central softer portion, the nucleus pulposus (Figs. 1 and 2).

The annulus fibrosus consists of laminae of dense connective tissue arranged concentrically in an interwoven fashion. The deeper layers are less sharply separated and alternate with layers of very soft fibrocartilage. The outermost fibres of the annulus are blended with the ligaments surrounding the spine, especially the anterior and posterior longitudinal ligaments, and may be firmly attached to the periosteum. Fibres about the periphery are embedded in the epiphyseal ring of the vertebral body. The annulus is thicker anteriorly and thinner posteriorly where it lies between the nucleus pulposus and the vertebral canal.

839

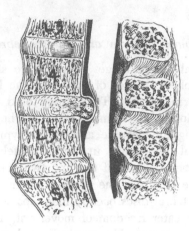

Fig. 1. Diagram of Vertical Section through the Spinal Column Showing
a Normal Intervertebral Disc between the Bodies of the 3rd and
4th Lumbar Vertebrae

Between lumbar four and lumbar five, the nucleus pulposus is fragmented
and a large portion of it has herniated through the annulus fibrosus into the spinal
canal where it is compressing the thecal sac. When the nucleus pulposus herniates in this fashion it no longer serves any normal function but acts only as a
foreign body, the removal of which does not further weaken the intervertebral
disc. Between lumbar five and sacral one, the intervertebral disc is degenerated
and softened, and the annulus fibrosus is bulging posteriorly into the spinal canal.

Compressed within the central portion of the annulus fibrosus and
intimately adherent to it is the gelatinous or pulpy nucleus pulposus.
The nucleus varies in size and occupies a position slightly posterior
to the center of the disc. When the vertebral column of a young individual is divided horizontally the nucleus rises up considerably above
the surrounding level (Gray, 1858), and has a glistening, pearly
white appearance. To palpation the nucleus is plastic but moderately
tough and elastic. There is no sharp line of division between the
nucleus and the annulus fibrosus as one fades off gradually into the
other. The distinction between them, however, is by no means artificial
as they are quite different both in structure and function.

Microscopically the nucleus pulposus consists of a loose irregular
meshwork of connective tissue, poor in elastic fibres, interspersed with
cartilage cells, and at times, clear vacuolated cells; the latter are
considered by some to be surviving remnants of the notochord. The
nuclear tissue contains a highly fluid matrix, the water content of
which is high.

840

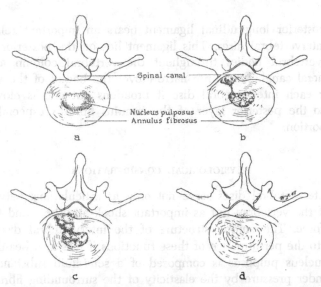

FIG. 2. Diagram to show: a. normal intervertebral disc, b. fragmentation of the nucleus pulposus with herniation of nuclear material into the spinal canal through a small tear in the annulus fibrosus, c. herniation of nuclear material through a wide gap in the annulus fibrosus, and d. degeneration of the intervertebral disc with posterior protrusion of the annulus fibrosus, but without herniation of the nucleus pulposus. Note that in b, c, and d, there is compression of the adjacent nerve root.

The adult intervertebral discs have no blood vessels, but Uebermuth (1929), Böhmig (1930), and Camera (1934) describe blood vessels arising from the marrow spaces which perforate the cartilaginous plates in early life. These undergo progressive obliteration and disappear by the end of the growth period.

Jung and Brunschwig (1932) were able to demonstrate nerve fibres in the anterior and posterior longitudinal ligaments, and Roofe (1940) has described nerve fibres within the posterior annulus fibrosus. These fibres apparently originate from the posterior root ganglion two segments above their final distribution. The type of terminal arborization which they possess suggests that they are pain fibres. Nerve fibres in the anterior and posterior longitudinal ligaments and in the superficial layers of the annulus fibrosus have also been demonstrated by Ferlic (1963) and Hirsch et al (1963). The anatomy of the sinuvertebral nerves, believed to be of importance in the transmission of sensation from structures involved in low back pain, is the subject of a report by Pedersen et al (1956).

841

The posterior longitudinal ligament bears an important relationship to the intervertebral discs. This ligament lies on the posterior surfaces of the vertebral bodies throughout the vertebral column and ends in the sacral canal. It is quite narrow over the bodies of the vertebrae but over each intervertebral disc it broadens out and is closely connected to the posterior layer of the annulus fibrosus especially in its medial portion.

PHYSIOLOGICAL CONSIDERATIONS

The intervertebral discs serve not only as articulations between the bodies of the vertebrae but as important shock absorbers and transmitters of force. The unique structure of the intervertebral disc is well adapted to the performance of these functions if it is in a healthy state.

The nucleus pulposus is composed of a semi-fluid substance maintained under pressure by the elasticity of the surrounding fibres of the annulus fibrosus, by muscle tone and by the pressure of the weight of the body on the spinal column. The nucleus pulposus obeys the laws of fluids and, although non-compressible, under pressure (whether static or sudden) it becomes flatter and broader and distends the fibres of the annulus in all directions. In this manner the intervertebral disc absorbs the numerous shocks to which the vertebral column is subjected. It is the elasticity of the annulus fibrosus which permits an increase in the radius of the disc (Horton, 1958).

Because the nucleus obeys the laws of fluids, forces applied to the vertebral column are transmitted equally over the entire opposing surfaces of adjacent vertebrae. In thus equalizing the forces between adjacent vertebrae, the nucleus serves to protect any one portion of an opposing vertebral surface from bearing the brunt of a given trauma (Bradford and Spurling, 1945).

Formerly it was thought that the nucleus possessed an inherent elastic turgor (Schmorl, 1927b) and that this explained why the nucleus protrudes or bulges above the surrounding level of the disc when the spine is sectioned in the sagittal plane. Actually this apparent expansile quality of the nucleus is due to the pressure exerted upon it by the elasticity of the fibres of the annulus (Donohue, 1939).

Movement is slight between any two vertebrae but when it occurs in all the joints of the vertebral column the total range of motion is very considerable. When the vertebral column is flexed, or bent forward, there is relaxation of the anterior longitudinal ligament, compression of the intervertebral disc in front, and posterior displacement of the nucleus pulposus. At the same time the posterior longitudinal ligament, ligamenta flava, and posterior fibres of the annulus fibrosus are stretched.

Extension of the spine produces an effect opposite to that of flexion on the disc and spinal ligaments; extension is limited in the lumbar region, but relatively free in the cervical area.

Flexion is the most extensive of all the movements and is most freely performed in the lumbar region. The greatest range of flexion occurs at the levels of the fourth lumbar and lumbosacral discs.

It has been demonstrated that the load on lumbar discs is related both to body weight and position (Nachemson, 1966). In lifting a weight from the floor with the spine flexed, the region of the fourth and fifth lumbar discs acts as the fulcrum and these discs are subjected to enormous pressures. Bradford and Spurling (1945) have estimated that a man of average height lifting 100 pounds from the floor brings a force of 1600 pounds to bear upon the lumbosacral disc. (See also Morris et al, 1961.) For the intervertebral discs to withstand such forces and to perform their functions in a normal manner, it is obvious that they must be unique structures. At the same time it is not surprising that the intervertebral discs, especially in the lower lumbar region, may show degenerative changes.

A normally functioning nucleus pulposus has a high water content. Upon this factor depends in large part the ability of the nucleus to transmit forces equally between the vertebrae. Progressive diminution of the water content of the nucleus with age has been described by Püschel (1930), and Keyes and Compere (1932). Evidence presented by de Puky (1935) suggests that there may even be a daily fluctuation in the water content of the nucleus. In examining 1,200 people he found the height, especially of the younger individuals, to be greater in the morning on arising than in the evening. The normal fluid exchange of the intervertebral disc depends probably on the nucleus pulposus possessing the properties of a gel. The imbibition index, a measure of the hydration capacity, was found to be much less in degenerated discs (Hendry, 1958).

Biochemical alterations in herniated intervertebral discs have been reported by Davidson and Woodhall (1959), Mitchell, Hendry and Billewicz (1961) and Naylor (1962, 1971). The mucopolysaccharides, by virtue of their effect on the maturation of collagen and on the water content of the nucleus pulposus, appear to be of fundamental importance in relation to disc degeneration and herniation.

843

Since there are no blood vessels in the adult intervertebral disc, its nourishment is apparently derived from the marrow by diffusion through the perforated bony end plate of the vertebral body (Uebermuth, 1939; Böhmig, 1930; Donohue, 1939).

PATHOLOGICAL CONSIDERATIONS

It is now firmly established that a posterior herniation of nucleus pulposus tissue through some or all of the fibres of the annulus fibrosus (Figs. 1, 2b, 2c) (Mixter and Barr, 1934; Peet and Echols, 1934; Love, 1936; Simonds, 1937; Fincher and Walker, 1938; Furlow, 1938; Naffziger, Inman, and Saunders, 1938; Poppen, 1938; Adson, 1939; Spurling and Bradford, 1939; Craig and Walsh, 1939; Semmes, 1939; et al), or, less often, a protrusion of the annulus fibrosus into the spinal canal without herniation of the nucleus pulposus (Figs. 1, and 2d) (Love, 1936; Love and Camp, 1937; Love and Walsh, 1938; Saunders and Inman, 1940; Naffziger and Boldrey, 1946), are common causes of nerve root compression, and more particularly of low back and sciatic pain.

A sudden excessive force or trauma applied through the spinal column to the normal intervertebral disc may be instrumental in producing its rupture. There is increasing evidence, however, that so-called "degenerative" lesions of the intervertebral disc and adjacent cartilaginous plates are in many cases predisposing factors in the eventual posterior herniation or protrusion of disc tissue (Schmorl, 1929; Mixter and Barr, 1934; Saunders and Inman, 1940; Bradford and Spurling, 1945; Naffziger and Boldrey, 1946; Hyndman, 1946; Steindler, 1947; Armstrong, 1965; and DePalma and Rothman, 1970).

Since man assumed the upright posture, the intervertebral discs and cartilaginous plates have been subjected to more constant and greater degrees of pressure and shocks than perhaps they were originally designed to bear. According to Donohue (1939), the wear and tear (minor traumas) of everyday life, without sudden excessive injury, can bring about widespread structural changes, so much so that lesions which are associated with the decrescence of life are present in the intervertebral disc and spinal column to a degree surpassed in no other organ of the body. These degenerative lesions destroy the normal function of the disc. As a result the annulus may no longer be able to

844

resist forces it could normally withstand, and a minor trauma may cause its rupture and the release of nuclear tissue into the spinal canal. In other cases the disc is softened, the intervertebral space narrows and the annulus bulges posteriorly against the neighboring nerve root.

The physiological and pathological changes which commonly involve the intervertebral disc have been described by many observers (Schmorl, 1927, 1928, 1929; Uebermuth, 1929; Böhmig, 1929; Calvé and Galland, 1930; Beadle, 1931; Keyes and Compere, 1932; Joplin, 1935; Saunders and Inman, 1940; Bradford and Spurling, 1945; Coventry, Ghormley, and Kernohan, 1945; Friberg and Hirsch, 1949; Hirsch and Schajowitz, 1952; Rissanen, 1964; Armstrong, 1965; and Harmon, 1966.)

In this chapter we are primarily concerned with lesions of the intervertebral disc which cause nerve root compression. For a proper understanding of these lesions, however, other pathological changes of the intervertebral disc which predispose to eventual herniation of the nucleus pulposus or protrusion of the annulus fibrosus will also be considered.

Posterior Herniation of the Nucleus Pulposus through the Annulus Fibrosus

If the fibres of the annulus fibrosus become weakened whether as a result of trauma, "degenerative" processes or both, they may give way allowing the nucleus pulposus tissue to herniate posteriorly with resulting pressure on neural structures (Figs. 2, 4). This escape or herniation of nuclear substance is facilitated by the fact that the nucleus is normally maintained under tension by the fibres of the annulus. Experimentally it has been shown that when the posterior fibres of the annulus are incised or pierced nuclear tissue spontaneously herniates or extrudes itself through the artificial opening or tear (Keyes and Compere, 1932; Barr, 1937).

The annulus fibrosus is thinner posteriorly where it borders the spinal canal and it is here that the great majority of herniations occur. There are other reasons, already mentioned, why the annulus is prone to rupture posteriorly. When the spine is flexed the posterior aspect of the intervertebral disc is widened, the annulus fibrosus stretched, and the nucleus pulposus displaced posteriorly, exerting additional pressure on the annulus. In this manner the annulus is subjected to marked stress and strain by a powerful force, especially in the lower lumbar region. Exclusive of the cervical region it is estimated that approximately 96 percent of the herniations of the intervertebral discs occur in the lower lumbar region. Over 90 percent of the lumbar herniations are from the fourth lumbar and lumbosacral discs, with the third lumbar disc contributing about 8 percent. Herniation of a thoracic disc is rare.

Herniations of the nucleus pulposus usually take place to one side of the spinal canal where the disc is not covered by the full thickness of the posterior longitudinal ligament. Laterally the ligament fans out over the intervertebral disc contributing only a few fibres to the posterior layers of the annulus. In the midline of the canal the posterior longitudinal ligament is thicker and by reinforcing the annulus fibrosus aids in the prevention of posterior herniations at this site.

Posterior herniations of disc tissue may be small and cause no symptoms. Frequently, however, they compress the fibres of the adjacent nerve root crossing the disc in this region (Fig. 2). The dome of the herniation may lie directly anterior to the nerve root (Fig. 4 C) or between the root and the thecal sac proper (Fig. 4 B). The nerve root may be compressed before its fibres have emerged completely from the thecal sac (Fig. 4 A). Occasionally the herniation lies far lateral and exerts pressure on the nerve root as it leaves the intervertebral foramen. At times a herniation occurs bilaterally on each side of the posterior longitudinal ligament, or it may even be located in the midline beneath the thecal sac. In some cases the herniated tissue extends or migrates upward or downward to overlie the body of the vertebra at some distance from the intervertebral disc.

Herniations may take place through a small fissure-like tear in the annulus (Fig. 2 b). The herniated material then lies posterior to the annulus and the aperture in the annulus through which it escaped is sometimes hard to find and may even heal over. In other cases a wide tear in the annulus is present (Fig. 2 c) and the herniated portion of the nucleus is directly continuous over a wide base with the remainder of the nucleus in the depths of the intervertebral disc. The herniated material is usually covered with a membrane which may be transparently thin or as much as a few millimeters in thickness. Bradford and Spurling (1945) believe that this capsule covering the herniation is derived from the loose connective tissue of the anterior part of the spinal canal.

The findings at operation (see under operative technique) indicate that when herniation of disc tissue has occurred the nucleus pulposus rarely remains intact but has already become fragmented into several separated pieces. Less often the nucleus pulposus remains as one piece of tissue but no longer maintains its intact globular shape, and obviously is incapable of carrying out its normal functions.

The extruded material is composed mostly of nucleus pulposus tissue but there is no doubt that the inner layers of the annulus fibrosus may also be included. In some cases when traction is applied to a small piece of herniated disc tissue, a mass of material is withdrawn from the depth of the disc which is so large that it must include portions of annulus fibrosus as well as nucleus pulposus. Occasionally even a piece of the cartilaginous plate may be attached to this tissue which can be withdrawn from the opening in the annulus.

Microscopic examination of the intervertebral disc tissue removed at operation reveals chiefly nucleus pulposus material and also portions of inner, less well organized layers of the annulus fibrosus. Cellular degeneration, with loss of fibrillar structure and fibroblastic proliferation, with or without vascularization is usually present in both the nucleus and annulus tissue. Edema may be present in the herniated material, especially in younger age groups (Deucher and Love, 1939).

After thorough removal of the intervertebral disc tissue and cartilaginous plates at operation it is probable that the disc space is narrowed and invaded by granulation tissue. In time fibrous union between the neighboring vertebral bodies may take place. Even bony union is possible between some areas of the adjacent vertebrae if the cartilaginous plates are curetted away at operation.

Posterior Protrusion of the Annulus Fibrosus without Herniation of the Nucleus Pulposus

Nerve root compression or irritation may be caused by a posterior protrusion of the annulus fibrosus without herniation of the nucleus pulposus (Figs. 1 and 2 d). This type of pathological lesion of the intervertebral disc has been included by Love and Walsh (1938) under the term "Protruded Intervertebral Disc," and Dandy (1941) has described the condition as a so-called "concealed disc." Naffziger and Boldrey (1946) have given a clear description of the pathological mechanism by which the annulus may protrude and compress a nerve root.

Posterior protrusion of the annulus fibrosus occurs following degeneration of the disc structure. As a result of degenerative processes within

847

the intervertebral disc and cartilaginous plates (see below), the nucleus pulposus loses its normal water content. Large fissures appear in its substance. It no longer serves its normal function. The degenerative process spreads to the inner portions of the annulus, but a ring of more or less well preserved annulus tissue may remain around the periphery in the region of its attachment to the epiphyseal ring.

With these changes the intervertebral disc loses volume as a whole. The disc space may become narrowed and the annulus fibrosus protrudes outward in all directions around the margin of the disc. The protrusion of the posterior annulus, in some cases, is sufficient to irritate or compress the overlying nerve root with resultant radicular pain.

On palpation of such a disc lesion at operation, the protruding annulus is soft and boggy. It is considerably thinner than normal and at times can be ruptured by pressure with the point of a bayonet forceps. When this is done, or when the pathological annulus is incised, nuclear material, in most cases, does not herniate spontaneously through the artificial opening. Exploration of the intervertebral disc space reveals variable amounts of soft degenerated material, but this is usually much less than is found in cases of true herniation of the nucleus pulposus.

A posterior protrusion of the annulus of this type is usually apparent when the patient's spine is in the anatomical position, or when it is extended. At operation on such cases, however, if the patient's back is in flexion on the table the annulus fibrosus is stretched and in some instances may not bulge posteriorly. The operator may regard the disc as normal and describe the operation as a negative exploration. With lesions like this, if the nerve root is decompressed posteriorly by the removal of bone and ligamentum flavum, the patient may be relieved of his symptoms of nerve root compression. It is believed that posterior protrusions of this kind explain why some patients are relieved of symptoms following a so-called negative exploration for a herniated disc.

Hypertrophy of the Ligamentum Flavum

Thickening or hypertrophy of the ligamentum flavum commonly occurs in association with a herniation of disc tissue (Love, 1939; Love and Walsh, 1940) or protruded annulus. In some cases this hypertrophy has been described as an isolated phenomenon (Naffziger and Boldrey, 1946).

The ligamentum flavum is firmly adherent to the upper posterior border of the lamina below each interspace and is attached to the under (anterior) surface of the lamina immediately above, where it extends far laterally into the canal. In this lateral position the ligamentum flavum lies beneath the shelf of bone which overhangs the nerve root. When herniations of disc tissue are present they will force the nerve root backward, compressing it against the ligamentum flavum and the overlying shelf of bone. If the ligament is thickened, compression occurs more easily. When overstretched the ligament is sometimes torn away from its laminar attachments. The detached yellow elastic fibres tend to retract, curl up and are replaced in part by scar tissue. In this manner the ligament may become thickened and occasionally may be partially calcified.

The syndrome of root compression from hypertrophy of the ligamentum flavum alone is probably much rarer than previously supposed. Bradford and Spurling (1945) point out that herniations of the nucleus pulposus or posterior protrusions of the annulus fibrosus may have been overlooked in some of the earlier cases where symptoms were considered to be entirely due to hypertrophy of this ligament.

Lesions of the Intervertebral Disc, Cartilaginous Plates, and Vertebral Bodies which may Predispose to Herniation or Protrusion

Normal functioning of the intervertebral disc depends upon the integrity of the nucleus pulposus, annulus fibrosus, and adjacent cartilaginous plates. A lesion in any of these structures will lead to changes in the others with the ultimate possibility of rupture or protrusion of the annulus fibrosus.

The so-called "degenerative" lesions of the intervertebral disc are the most important pathological changes which may predispose to herniation of nuclear tissue or protrusion of the annulus. For a proper appreciation of the pathology to which the intervertebral disc is subject, two other lesions deserve mention, namely expansion of the nucleus pulposus into the spongiosa of the vertebral body with thinning of the adjacent cartilaginous plates and ruptures of the cartilaginous plates with prolapse of the nuclear tissue into the spongiosa.

So-called Degenerative Lesions of the Intervertebral Disc

Degenerative lesions of the intervertebral disc are very common and frequently accompanied by similar changes in the cartilaginous plates.

849

Changes begin to appear in the intervertebral disc at a comparatively early age. The disc gradually loses its elasticity and becomes softer. By middle age the nucleus loses its transparent appearance and does not swell upon section as does the normal disc. The disc loses volume and is narrowed. Horizontal fissures frequently appear within the nucleus. So common are these changes that it is hard to determine which are pathological and which the normal accompaniment of advancing years. Microscopically the intervertebral disc in older people shows a gradual obliteration of cellular elements and fibrillar structure.

In some cases swelling of the nucleus occurs in young individuals and this spreads to involve the inner fibres of the annulus. An outer ring of annulus tissue, however, is not infrequently well preserved around the periphery where it is attached to the epiphyseal ring. The disc becomes softer and the annulus friable. Microscopically this type of degenerated disc also shows gradual obliteration of cellular elements. The fibres become more scanty and blurred, at times disappearing completely, and areas of brownish pigmentation may appear.

The pathological changes which have just been described in the intervertebral disc proper are frequently accompanied by degenerative changes in the adjacent cartilaginous plates. With destruction of the plates the normal physiology of the nucleus is disturbed, especially its water metabolism, which is dependent upon diffusion processes from the marrow of the vertebral bodies.

Degenerative lesions of the intervertebral disc abolish normal function. The disc no longer acts as a shock absorber nor does it serve to transmit forces equally between the adjacent vertebral bodies. Abnormal mobility may take place between adjacent vertebrae at the site of the pathological disc and even actual narrowing of the disc space occurs. The vertebral bodies and intervertebral articulations are subjected to abnormal forces and may show arthritic changes. The ligamenta flava, longitudinal and other spinal ligaments must sustain abnormal stresses and thus may themselves become the source of recurrent pain in the back.

Expansion of the Nucleus Pulposus into the Spongiosa of the Vertebral Body

These expansions of the nucleus pulposus are a common pathological finding in young people, and are regarded as congenital or developmental in origin (Schmorl, 1930). The enlargement is not due to the formation of new tissue but to the taking up of additional water

850

(Donohue, 1939). The expansions are hemispherical in shape and lead to a thinning out of the overlying cartilaginous plates as they bulge into the spongiosa of the adjacent vertebral bodies. The thinning of the plates may predispose to their rupture.

Bulging of the nucleus into the bodies of the vertebrae is also seen in other conditions where there is softening or destruction of bone (senile osteoporosis, multiple myeloma, Paget's disease, osteomalacia, osteoclastic tumor, metastases). Under these circumstances the bulging occurs because of the lack of resistance offered by the softened bone and also as a result of the tensile force applied to the nucleus by the annulus.

Prolapse of the Nucleus Pulposus into the Spongiosa of the Vertebral Bodies

When a break or tear occurs in the cartilaginous plates, nucleus pulposus tissue not uncommonly escapes or prolapses through the tear into the spongiosa of the body of the vertebrae. Von Luschka in 1858 described prolapses of intervertebral disc tissue into the spongiosa. Schmorl (1930) and his pupils made an extensive investigation of these lesions.

In young individuals expansion of the nucleus pulposus may play a part in bringing about breaks in the cartilaginous plates. In such cases prolapse of disc tissue typically occurs at several levels in the spinal column. Schmorl (1939 b) and Beadle (1931) have described jagged fissure-like tears in apparently otherwise normal cartilaginous plates. They regard these lesions as possibly developmental in origin and they serve as a plausible explanation for the weakening of the cartilage plates and prolapse of disc tissue.

In middle aged and elderly people breaks in the cartilaginous plates are usually the result of senile degenerative changes in the cartilage. It is more common for isolated discs to be involved in this age group rather than a whole series as in young people. With loss of areas of the cartilaginous plates, nuclear tissue penetrates into the exposed spongiosa. The nucleus loses its water content and degenerates. The disc space becomes narrowed and is invaded by granulation tissue which may result in solid fibrous union between the adjacent vertebrae.

Schmorl (1927 b) found prolapses of disc tissue into the spongiosa in 38 percent of autopsies performed on a mixed age group.

851

The role of trauma as an etiologic factor in posterior herniation of disc tissue in the lumbar region probably cannot be overemphasized; that a single injury is the primary cause of herniation in most cases is more debatable.

It is true that a relatively severe injury has coincided with the onset of symptoms in about 50 percent of the reported cases, and that in these patients one must conclude that the herniation was precipitated by the injury. Even in this group, however, the degree of trauma commonly does not appear of sufficient magnitude to rupture a normal disc.

Repeated mild trauma (the wear and tear of everyday life) seems to be more important as a cause of herniations in the lumbar region, than a single severe injury. There is considerable evidence (see under pathology) to show that degenerative changes in an intervertebral disc predispose to its herniation, that such changes frequently precede any herniation or protrusion, and that repeated mild trauma is the most important cause of these degenerative changes.

The thesis that degenerative changes usually precede a posterior herniation in the lumbar region is supported by the fact that no history of a single severe trauma is obtained in about 50 percent of cases and that, according to pre-war statistics, about 75 percent of patients with a herniation are in or beyond the fourth decade (Bradford and Spurling, 1945). The role of trauma in the production of degenerative changes is indicated by the observations of Beadle (1931) and of Schmorl and Junghanns (1932) that degenerative lesions of the disc are more pronounced in people who have done hard manual labor than in those who have led a more sedentary life. Trauma as a causative factor in herniation is emphasized by the fact that about 75 percent of patients with a lumbar herniation are males and that during the last war, when trauma was prevalent, there was a much higher incidence of herniation among the younger age groups (3rd decade) than is seen in civilian life. Woodhall (1947) reported that 2858 cases of rupture of the intervertebral disc were treated by operation in the neurosurgical centers of the Zone of the Interior between the early part of 1942 and September 1st, 1945.

Armstrong (1965) believes that "it is the intrinsic quality of the nuclear tissue which determines whether or not it will stand up to the widely varying mechanical stresses to which a lumbar disc is constantly subjected during life and that it is the inborn durability of the disc rather than the nature and magnitude of these stresses which determine whether or not degenerative changes occur."

THE CLINICAL DIAGNOSIS OF A POSTERIOR HERNIATION
OR PROTRUSION OF DISC TISSUE IN THE LUMBAR REGION

A herniated disc may be completely asymptomatic. On the other hand, when a herniation or protrusion of disc tissue into the spinal canal is sufficiently large to cause relatively severe pressure on a nerve root, or roots, characteristic signs and symptoms of the disc syndrome will appear. Such a lesion of an intervertebral disc is by far the most common cause of low back pain with sciatica and the correct diagnosis can be made clinically in a high percentage of cases (Mixter and Barr, 1934; Peet and Echols, 1934; Love, 1936; Brown, 1937; Fincher and Walker, 1938; Furlow, 1938; Love, 1938; Naffziger, Inman, and Saunders, 1938; Poppen, 1938; Adson, 1939; Semmes, 1939; Spurling and Bradford, 1939; Love and Walsh, 1940; Pennybacker, 1940; Symonds, 1943; Munro, 1945; Mixter, 1951; Semmes and Murphey, 1954; Bucy, 1961; Semmes, 1964; Armstrong, 1965; DePalma and Rothman, 1970). There are, however, many other conditions which may at times cause pain in the back and along the sciatic nerve, and these conditions must be considered in the differential diagnosis.

When only a small herniation or protrusion of disc tissue has occurred and nerve root pressure is slight or lacking, the clinical diagnosis of a herniated disc becomes very difficult. The patient with a lesion of this type may have pain in the back alone or in addition vague sciatic pain unaccompanied by paresthesiae, objective sensory, motor, or reflex changes. The clinical differential diagnosis between such a disc lesion and a multitude of orthopedic conditions which may involve the low back can be almost impossible. Orthopedists, notably Steindler and Luck (1938) and Hyndman, Steindler, and Wolkin (1943) have called attention to patients with low back pain, in whom one finds a local point of tenderness due to deep ligamentous injury or myositis or fascitis. Reflex sciatic pain may occur in these cases but is unassociated with muscle wasting, reflex abnormalities, or sensory defects. Novocaine injection of the focal painful area causes temporary disappearance of the local tenderness and sciatic or other pain radiation.

The controversy which has arisen concerning the accuracy of clinical diagnosis in herniated disc is, perhaps, partly due to the fact that the findings reported by most neurosurgeons have been derived from severe, often relatively intractable cases, whereas orthopedic surgeons and others have had a wider contact with the disc syndrome in its milder form.

Statistics reported in the literature (Bradford and Spurling, 1945; Love and Walsh, 1940) and in this chapter, on the accuracy of clinical diagnosis and on the relative incidence of the various symptoms and clinical signs in patients with posterior herniation or protrusion of disc tissue have been based chiefly on the findings in cases with evidence of nerve root involvement and symptoms severe enough to warrant surgery. In this group of patients with a herniated disc the correct clinical diagnosis is possible in about 80 percent of the cases. In about 90 to 95 percent (of this 80 percent) the lesion can be accurately localized clinically to the level of the fourth lumbar or lumbosacral disc. Clinical differential diagnosis between a lesion at these two levels, however, is much more difficult. It is true that in perhaps 60 percent of cases the preoperative diagnosis of the exact level of the lesion will prove correct. Preoperatively, however, one cannot separate out this 60 percent and say confidently that in these cases further diagnostic information (as supplied by myelography) is not indicated since the exact level of the lesion is known. Also multiple herniations cannot be excluded on clinical evidence alone.

Symptoms and Signs

Pain in the low back is the first symptom in approximately 70 percent of cases of herniation of an intervertebral disc in the lower lumbar region. In about 50 percent of patients, the symptoms are initiated by trauma. In most instances the pain in the back comes on suddenly, but the onset may be gradual, or there may be a latent interval between trauma and the commencement of symptoms. The pain frequently follows undue exertion especially when the patient has been suddenly forced to lift an excessive weight while his lumbosacral spine is in a flexed position. At the onset the patient sometimes feels a sudden click in the back or complains that he felt something give way and he may be unable to straighten up for a short period following the onset of pain. Other forms of trauma commonly precede the symptoms. There may be no history of trauma but the patient experiences sudden low

854

back pain merely on stooping forward to lift a handkerchief from the floor or to lace his shoes.

The pain at first is usually confined to the low back. Less often (in about 30 percent of cases) in the first attack it also radiates to the buttock or down the lower limb in the sciatic nerve distribution. In occasional cases the first symptom is pain along the course of the sciatic nerve.

These initial symptoms are often regarded as due to a low back strain unless typical sciatic pain is present.

Course

One of the characteristic features is the recurrent nature of the attacks alternating with remissions in which the patient is relatively or completely free of pain (symptoms were intermittent in 84 percent of 500 cases reported by Love and Walsh, 1940). The first attack may be slight and of short duration, or it may confine the patient to bed for weeks. A second attack, which may be of much greater severity than the first is commonly precipitated by the most trivial injury. In some cases the recurrent pain is confined to the low back for months but during this interval it is usually severe enough on many occasions to incapacitate the patient for work.

Sooner or later symptoms of nerve root compression frequently appear and pain begins to radiate down the distribution of the sciatic nerve on the same side as the herniation. In perhaps 10 percent of cases the pain is referred down both lower limbs. In many cases the back pain disappears and the sciatic pain becomes more severe. The attacks tend to occur more often and to become more incapacitating until frequently the patient is bedridden with pain.

Special Features

Pain. The most characteristic features of the low back or sciatic pain is its aggravation or precipitation by certain mechanical factors. Various postures or fluctuations in spinal fluid pressure cause a change in relationships between the herniated disc, neighboring nerve root and surrounding tissues with a resulting increase in compression or stretching of pain fibres.

Effect of Posture. Accentuation of low back or sciatic pain occurs in most patients on bending forward at the waist with the knees extended.

855

Some, however, remain in a stooped over position and are unable to straighten up. Extension of the lumbosacral spine may increase low back pain but less often causes it to radiate to the lower limb. The pain is frequently brought on or made worse by standing or by prolonged sitting in one position, or by movements such as turning over in bed or changing position in a chair. The jarring in a subway may be intolerable. The pain is usually less severe on rising in the morning and increases with exercise.

Temporary relief of pain occurs in some patients when standing or moving about. When sitting, a slight shift in position may bring momentary improvement. Lying recumbent in bed with boards beneath the mattress frequently gives relief but in some only serves to aggravate the condition. Certain patients move about in bed until they find a comfortable position. Relief is not infrequently obtained by lying on the unaffected side with the painful lower limb flexed at the hip and knee.

Effect of Changes in Spinal Fluid Pressure. Sneezing or coughing, by producing a sudden rise in spinal fluid pressure, very commonly (in over 50 percent of cases) causes an increase of the pain in the low back which may shoot down the leg if nerve root pressure exists. Straining at stool or exertion of other types that cause an elevation of cerebrospinal fluid pressure may likewise cause an exacerbation of the pain.

Distribution of the Pain and Paresthesiae

The pain in the back is rarely diffuse and is low down below the level of the pelvic brim in the great majority of cases when the fourth or fifth lumbar disc is involved. It is sometimes in the midline, or bilateral, but is frequently lateralized to the side of the lesion. In a unilateral herniation of the fourth lumbar or lumbosacral disc the pain at first may radiate only to the gluteal region on the involved side. Later the pain is felt along the course of the sciatic nerve, but is most severe in the buttock, posterior thigh, behind the knee and in the calf. Aching pain may radiate to the region of the malleoli but rarely into the foot or toes. Burning pain and especially paresthesiae are, however, commonly felt in the foot and toes.

The pain in the thigh and leg is for the most part due to involvement of fibres from deep receptors and is usually aching in character. The burning or stinging pain which is felt over the calf and foot is of a more superficial type.

Pain and paresthesiae which radiate below the knee when the patient flexes his spine anteriorly, or when the Lasègue (1864) test is performed, or when the patient changes his posture in other ways, indicate mechanical compression of the nerve root; this is seen in the presence of a herniated disc more often than in any other condition.

The location of the pain is of little value in distinguishing between a herniation of the fourth lumbar and a lumbosacral disc, but paresthesiae, present in about 50 percent of the cases, are often of considerable value in localization. Paresthesiae are most frequently described as tingling, numbness, or a feeling of pins and needles. When these sensations radiate into the great toe the fifth lumbar nerve root is usually involved by a herniation of the fourth lumbar disc (Figs. 3, 4A). Paresthesiae over the lateral aspect of the dorsum and lateral

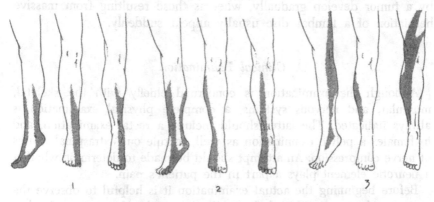

Fig. 3. 1. Approximate dermatome of the 5th lumbar nerve root, according to Bradford and Spurling (1945) and K. G. McKenzie (as illustrated by Bradford and Spurling 1945). 2 and 3. Approximate dermatomes of the 1st and 2nd sacral nerve roots respectively, according to Bradford and Spurling (1945).

portion of the sole of the foot extending into the lateral toes occur in herniations of the lumbosacral disc when the first sacral nerve root is compressed (Figs. 3, 4C). On the lateral aspect of the calf, paresthesiae accompanying involvement of the first sacral root, are felt more posteriorly than those with fifth lumbar root involvement.

The location of the pain is of distinct value in determining whether a herniation lies in the upper lumbar region or in the lower lumbar region. Pain over the anterior upper thigh in the distribution of the second lumbar dermatome occurs in herniations of the first lumbar disc, and over the lower anterior thigh and around the knee in herniations of the disc between the second and third lumbar vertebrae.

857

Pain on the medial aspect of the leg and in the region of the knee accompanies herniations of the third lumbar disc. In some cases the distribution of the pain will lie a segment higher than that just mentioned. For instance, herniation of nuclear material from the third lumbar disc may migrate upward over the body of the vertebra and compress the third lumbar nerve root rather than the fourth as is usual. Paresthesiae also may be present over the respective dermatomes.

Marked loss of motor power, extensive sensory impairment or loss of sphincter control do not occur in lesions of a lumbar disc unless an unusually large herniation of the nucleus pulposus has taken place with compression of the cauda equina. Such signs and symptoms should immediately make one suspect the presence of a cord tumor, or some lesion other than a herniated disc. As a rule the manifestations caused by a tumor develop gradually, whereas those resulting from massive herniation of a lumbar disc usually appear suddenly.

Clinical Examination

Although the examination is concerned chiefly with the skeletal, muscular, and nervous systems, a complete physical examination is always indicated. The latter should include a rectal examination, and in females a pelvic examination as well, to rule out extraspinal causes of nerve compression. An attempt should be made to determine whether a neurotic element plays a part in the patient's pain.

Before beginning the actual examination it is helpful to observe the patient as he removes his clothes. A patient with a herniation of a low lumbar disc sits down with care, avoiding flexion of the lumbar spine. All the patient's movements are guarded and there is particular difficulty in removing the shoes because of the necessity of keeping the lumbar spine rigid.

It is well to begin the examination proper with the patient standing in the erect position with the heels and toes together. Many patients will stand with the painful lower limb flexed, bearing most of their weight on the good limb. A pelvic tilt is commonly present. This tilt is usually away from the side of the lesion, less often toward it, and frequently accompanied by a compensatory scoliosis. There is flattening or obliteration of the normal lumbosacral curve in at least 60 percent of cases. Splinting (spasm) of the erector spinae muscles may be marked and this becomes more evident as the patient bends forward or to the side.

Flexion of the lower lumbar and lumbosacral spine is usually limited and often to a marked degree. This maneuver as a rule accentuates low back pain, and where nerve root compression is already present, pain may radiate toward the buttock and down the distribution of the sciatic nerve on the involved side. At times the pain does not appear to the patient to radiate, but he experiences an accentuation of the pain in the gluteal region, posterior thigh, or calf.

Lateral flexion of the spine is limited in the lower lumbar region and sometimes causes pain in the low back especially on flexion toward the side of the herniated disc. Extension of the lumbosacral spine may or may not accentuate pain.

Heavy percussion over the lumbar region at the site of the herniation, especially when the patient is bending forward, frequently (i.e., in over 50 percent of cases) causes sudden pain to shoot down the compressed sciatic nerve root. Tenderness, with radiation of pain to the lower limb, may be induced by deep pressure just lateral to the midline near the site of the herniated disc. Diffuse tenderness is rarely caused by herniated disc alone.

With the patient in the standing position it is well to observe the size of the calves and thighs, as atrophy may be visible on the side of the herniation especially in the calf. The muscles should be palpated and may be tender in the calf and posterior thigh of the painful limb. Some tenderness is commonly found along the course of the sciatic nerve.

Tests for *muscle weakness* can be carried out at this point. Weakness is usually slight but may be present in the anterior tibial or Achilles group of muscles. The patient is asked to stand and to walk on his heels. This may reveal impairment of dorsiflexion of the foot or toes due to weakness of the anterior tibial group of muscles. Weakness of dorsiflexion of the great toe is seen in herniations of the fourth lumbar disc. Weakness of the Achilles group of muscles which is occasionally present in herniations of the lumbosacral disc is tested by having the patient walk and hop on his toes.

Careful observation of the patient's gait should be made. The patient usually limps to some degree with the painful limb.

The patient is now asked to lie recumbent on the examining table. He usually does this with difficulty because of pain and limitation of movement in the lumbar spine.

Straight leg raising on the side of the herniated disc is almost always limited when nerve root compression exists. The test is performed by flexing the thigh at the hip with the knee extended. The maneuver stretches the sensitive sciatic nerve. When the test is positive, pain radiates down into the distribution of the involved dermatome. There is frequently accentuation of pain in the calf and tingling may radiate into the foot. The patient is questioned carefully during the maneuver to determine the exact distribution of his pain and paresthesiae, for, as already mentioned, this may give a clue as to which nerve root is compressed, i.e. to the level of the herniated disc. When the patient experiences only a pulling or taut sensation in the posterior thigh, the test is not considered positive. Straight leg raising on the side opposite the herniation may also be limited and frequently causes low back pain and at times some radiation down into the involved dermatome of the lower limb on the side of the herniation. During the performance of the straight leg raising test, accentuation of pain may be produced in some patients by dorsiflexing the foot and thus further stretching the sciatic nerve.

The Lasègue (1864) test, although similar to the straight leg raising test, is worth performing. The thigh is first flexed at the hip and the leg is then gradually extended at the knee. The latter maneuver stretches the sensitive sciatic nerve and gives rise to pain in its distribution.

Patrick's test is performed by abducting the thigh at the hip after placing the heel on the opposite knee. This sign is positive in disease of the sacroiliac joint, but essentially negative in herniated disc.

The jugular compression test may now be done with the patient lying or preferably standing. A blood pressure cuff can be used around the neck or digital pressure applied bilaterally to the jugular veins. Compression of the jugular veins causes a rise in cerebrospinal fluid pressure which distends the dural sac in the lumbar region. In some manner the sensitive nerve root, already compressed by the herniation, is further irritated and pain may be felt in its distribution or in the low back. The test is frequently positive in intraspinal disease.

A complete *neurologic examination* should be carried out. The cranial nerves will be found negative. Deep reflexes in the upper extremities are normal. In low lumbar herniations the abdominal reflexes are equal and active and so are the cremasteric. Plantar stimulation produces a normal flexion response of the toes. The deep reflexes in the lower extremities are very important. The knee jerks will be essentially normal when the herniation is below the third lumbar disc. Occasionally, however, in herniations of the fourth or fifth lumbar disc, pain will give rise to muscle spasm which influences the knee jerk; as a result of this the knee jerk may be increased and occasionally may appear diminished. In a herniation of the intervertebral disc between the third and fourth lumbar vertebrae, the knee jerk is frequently diminished on the side of the lesion. Craig and Walsh (1941) found the knee jerk diminished or absent in 49 percent of their cases of herniation at the third lumbar disc.

The ankle jerk is diminished or absent in about 80 percent of frank herniations of the lumbosacral disc and is diminished in approximately 25 percent of cases of herniation of the disc between the fourth and fifth lumbar vertebrae (Bradford and Spurling, 1945). To reveal a slight diminution of an ankle jerk, the test should be carried out with the patient in different positions. The ankle jerks may be tested with the patient kneeling on a chair with his back to the examiner, lying prone with the lower limbs extending over the end of the examining table, or with legs flexed at the knee, or lying supine with the lower limbs flexed at the knee and hip.

Motor power is usually grossly normal although there may be some weakness of dorsi- or plantar flexion of the foot or toes on the involved side. More extensive weakness, especially of the proximal musculature may appear to be present due to pain.

Careful observation and measurements of the calves and thighs for atrophy should be made. Some atrophy of the calf muscles is frequently present in a herniated disc at lumbar 4 or 5 levels, and slight atrophy of the thigh may also be found probably due to disuse. Fascicular twitchings are occasionally seen in the muscles of the involved extremity, especially in the gluteus maximus muscle in herniations of the lumbosacral disc. Some loss of tone occasionally is present in this muscle.

Coordination tests are normal except in that small group of cases where a large herniation has compressed the cauda equina or spinal cord.

Sensory Examination. A careful sensory examination is of great importance. Slight, rarely marked diminution of sensation involving touch, pinprick and temperature perception over the lateral calf or foot is frequently demonstrable (in approximately 75 percent of cases according to Bradford and Spurling, 1945) in symptomatic herniations of the fourth lumbar or lumbosacral intervertebral discs. The finding of such diminished sensation is pathognomonic of involvement of nerve fibres and is not seen in lumbosacral strain or arthritis of the sacroiliac joint.

There is a difference of opinion among the best observers concerning the exact distribution of the various lumbosacral dermatomes. Differentiation between a herniation of the fourth and fifth lumbar (or lumbosacral) disc on the basis of the sensory findings is, therefore, often unreliable.

Impaired sensation over a small strip on the anterolateral aspect of the calf, which may extend downward over the dorsum of the foot to involve the base of the great toe, is seen in herniations of the fourth

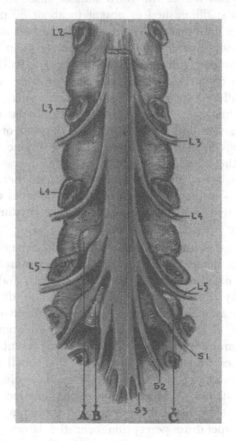

Fig. 4. Diagram to Illustrate Compression of Nerve Roots by Herniations of Nucleus Pulposus Tissue at Different Levels and Sites

A herniation of the 4th lumbar disc on the left side is shown compressing the 5th lumbar nerve root at A. At the level of the lumbosacral disc a herniation on the left side is compressing the 1st and 2nd sacral nerve roots only at B. On the right side at this level a herniation is seen compressing the 1st sacral root only at C.

862

lumbar disc, when the fifth lumbar nerve root is compressed (Figs. 3 and 4A). Sensory impairment over the lateral calf, and over the lateral aspect of the dorsum and sole of the foot extending into the lateral three toes occurs in herniations of the lumbosacral disc that compress the first sacral root (Figs. 3 and 4C). In a small number of cases a narrow strip of sensory impairment will be found over the posterior thigh in the distribution of the second sacral dermatome. This is most commonly present in herniations of the nucleus pulposus of the lumbosacral disc. Perianal anesthesia is occasionally seen but saddle anesthesia very rarely. Sensory loss over the second or third lumbar dermatomes on the anterior thigh indicates a lesion at a level higher than the lower two lumbar discs.

DIFFERENTIAL DIAGNOSIS

Investigation of a patient suspected of having a herniated disc is not limited to a neurological and musculoskeletal examination. X-rays of the lumbosacral spine and pelvis should be taken in all cases and preoperative myelography performed in selected cases. Spinal fluid and manometric studies are of value particularly in cases suspected of having an intraspinal tumor or inflammatory lesion, although the spinal fluid protein is elevated in over half the cases of herniated disc (in 70 percent of cases according to Bradford and Spurling, 1945). Finally a combined orthopedic and neurosurgical opinion has become almost routine in many hospitals.

Some Conditions Which May Simulate the Disc Syndrome

Orthopedic Conditions Involving the Low Back. Acute ligamentous and muscle strains, postural defects, congenital abnormalities of the lumbosacral joint, degeneration of an intervertebral disc with narrowing, narrowing of an intervertebral foramen, hypertrophic arthritis involving especially the articular facets, instability of the lumbosacral joint, sacroiliac arthritis, and other orthopedic conditions may cause pain in the back with radiation of pain to the lower limb. With the exception of hypertrophic arthritis, these conditions rarely cause typical radiation of pain or paresthesiae over the distribution of the sciatic nerve below the knee, either spontaneously or on the straight leg raising test, as is so commonly noted in a herniated disc. In addition, these orthopedic conditions (except for hypertrophic arthritis) do not give rise to other signs of a disc lesion such as a diminished ankle jerk, atrophy of the

863

calf (except rarely as a result of disuse) or diminished sensation over the lower lumbar and sacral dermatomes.

Roentgenograms will be of aid in ruling out a number of the conditions mentioned and myelography will usually establish the diagnosis in cases where operation is considered.

Spondylolisthesis. Roentgenographic studies will affirm the diagnosis. Spondylolisthesis is sometimes accompanied by anterior compression of the caudal roots by a prominent edge of the body of the L-5 or S-1 vertebra or even by a protruding or herniated disc. A myelogram may be necessary to demonstrate such a lesion and laminectomy at the time of fusion is occasionally required to decompress the nerve roots.

Narrowed Spinal Canal. Nerve root and cauda equina compression may occur as a consequence of minimal disc or osteophyte protrusion in cases of narrowing (stenosis) of the lumbar spinal canal and intervertebral foramina caused by developmental or other (e.g., spondylosis) factors (Verbiest, 1954; Epstein et al, 1962; Pennal and Schatzker, 1971). In cases of developmental stenosis the pedicles, laminae and facets are thickened. The changes may be apparent on plain roentgenograms; myelography discloses varying degrees of encroachment on the spinal canal at one or multiple levels.

Intraspinal Tumors. An intraspinal tumor and particularly an intradural perineurial fibroblastoma (neurofibroma) can produce symptoms that will lead to the tentative diagnosis of herniated disc by the best of neurologists (Raney, 1943; Love, 1944; Ray, 1946). These perineurial fibroblastomas are small, encapsulated, attached to a nerve root, and not uncommonly are present within the subarachnoid space for three or four years before any severe signs of compression of the cauda equina appear. Because they may lie almost free in the subarachnoid space, they become displaced upward or downward and give rise to intermittent bouts of pain along the nerve root to which they are attached.

Other intra- or extradural tumors, and varicosities of the spinal vessels also occasionally simulate a herniated disc and must constantly be kept in mind if unfortunate results are to be avoided. Perhaps the most helpful piece of information in recognizing an intraspinal tumor that has not grown to sufficient size to make its presence manifest in the neurological examination is the almost constant finding of an elevated protein (usually over 100 mgm per 100 cc) in the spinal fluid. A herniated disc may be accompanied by protein of over 100 mgm per 100 cc, but in not more than 10 percent of cases. A finding of such a high protein, therefore, should always call for manometric studies and a myelogram.

Bilateral sciatic pain may occur in a large bilateral or midline disc herniation but it is also a symptom seen in intraspinal tumors. A large herniation can occasionally cause extensive motor and sensory impairment with sphincteric disturbances but such findings always necessitate the exclusion of neoplasm. In fact, the presence of even a mild degree of bilateral motor or sensory deficit in any case of suspected disc herniation indicates a full investigation for tumor.

It is well to remember that a tumor may lie as high as the twelfth thoracic vertebra and yet give pain along a single nerve root such as the fifth lumbar or first sacral. Neoplasms lying low in the spinal canal are prone to cause diminished or absent sensation bilaterally over the saddle area.

X-rays of the spine in cases of tumor may reveal widening of the interpedicular spaces or erosion of pedicles adjacent to the neoplasm. Lumbar puncture may demonstrate a partial or complete block and myelography discloses a characteristic filling defect.

Tuberculous ("Cold") Abscess. Extradural cold abscess has on a number of occasions been diagnosed as a herniated disc preoperatively. X-rays of the spine and chest may give no clue to the diagnosis. When an extradural fluctuant mass is encountered on exploring for a herniated disc, one must avoid opening the dura. Otherwise in the presence of a cold abscess a tuberculous meningitis may result.

Primary and Metastatic Neoplasms of the Spine. In known cases of extraspinal neoplasm, metastatic lesions should obviously be suspected. Roentgenographic studies will rule out many primary and secondary vertebral lesions (e.g., primary sarcoma of sacrum or chordoma).

Fractures of the Spine. Old spinal injuries may be accompanied by a herniated disc or may in themselves cause pain and other neurologic manifestations. Roentgenograms and myelography will usually establish the diagnosis.

Abdominal, Pelvic, and Peripheral Neoplasms. Abdominal, pelvic, and prostatic neoplasms, as well as peripheral nerve and soft tissue tumors in the extremities may give rise to pain along the sciatic nerve. Investigation should, therefore, include examination of the abdomen, pelvis, and prostate, and palpation along the sciatic nerve.

Radiculitis. Herpes Zoster: The course of the condition, the relative constancy of the symptoms, the presence of vesicles and the absence of pelvic tilt, scoliosis, and limitation of movement of the lumbosacral

865

spine aid in differentiation. The distribution of the pain may be very difficult to distinguish from that occurring in a herniated disc.

A localized leptomeningitis and radiculitis is sometimes seen in syphilis and following spinal anesthesia. Careful history and serological studies as well as other signs in case of syphilis should help in the differentiation.

Lumbar arachnoiditis may be associated with herniated disc or occur alone and offer difficulty in the differential diagnosis. It may be the cause of persistent symptoms after herniated disc excision (French, 1946.)

Gluteal Injections. Some patients with pain in the back and vague reference to the sciatic nerve (who do not have a herniated disc) have received therapeutic injections into or alongside the sciatic nerve. Such an injection may be followed by a diminished ankle jerk, thereby adding one more sign which helps to confuse the diagnosis. Other patients have developed sciatic pain for the first time as a result of gluteal injections for various reasons.

The above list includes some of the conditions which may at times simulate a herniated disc. There are other conditions but, these like the ones mentioned, can usually be eliminated following adequate investigation.

SPECIAL EXAMINATIONS

Roentgenological Examination

Routine anteroposterior and lateral roentgenograms should be taken of the lumbosacral and lower thoracic spine and of the pelvis in all cases suspected of having a posterior herniation of the nucleus pulposus or protrusion of the annulus fibrosus in the lower lumbar region. Roentgenograms alone are of very little value in making a diagnosis of a herniated lumbar disc. They are of great value, however, in demonstrating or ruling out other lesions which may simulate a herniated disc. Among the lesions which may be so demonstrated are anomalies of the vertebrae, osteoarthritis of the lumbosacral spine or sacroiliac joint, calcified lesions, decalcifying vertebral disease, spondylolisthesis, primary or secondary bone tumors, infectious processes, fractures, etc.

Narrowing of an intervertebral disc is a relatively common finding in the x-ray films but is by no means diagnostic of herniation of the nucleus pulposus. Narrowing of a disc may result from other causes, including degenerative and inflammatory (e.g., tuberculous) disease.

Hampton and Robinson (1936) found that narrowing of the fifth disc was more commonly seen in herniations of the fourth disc than when there was a herniation of the fifth (lumbosacral) disc itself. This finding indicates that disc narrowing does not necessarily mean herniation, and also that herniation of one disc is not uncommonly associated with a degenerative lesion in a neighboring one. Hampton and Robinson (1936) did find, however, that the fourth disc was narrowed in one third of the herniations at that level. Significant narrowing of the fourth lumbar interspace was observed by Epstein (1969) in 25 percent of herniations at this level.

Lumbar Puncture

Lumbar puncture should probably be performed in all cases of suspected herniation of an intervertebral disc. The level of the puncture and whether it should be carried out at the time of myelography or some time before the latter test is dependent upon the nature of the individual case.

If a space-occupying lesion other than herniated intervertebral disc is suspected, manometric studies are usually imperative. The lumbar puncture is best performed about a week before myelography or at the same time. In such a case the patient is placed on his side and the lumbar puncture needle inserted as low as possible, viz., at the lumbosacral interspace, so that it will be below any block which may be present in the subarachnoid space.

Manometric tests with water manometer and jugular compression with a blood pressure cuff around the neck (Grant and Cone, 1934) are then carried out in the usual fashion. The spinal fluid protein will also be assessed, a knowledge of which is of course of diagnostic aid (see under diagnosis).

If there is any suspicion of lues or other intraspinal disease complete studies of the spinal fluid are indicated and should include serologic and colloidal gold tests and cell count.

When the diagnosis of a herniated disc is reasonably certain the lumbar puncture is best performed at the same time as myelography. This spares the patient the discomfort of two lumbar punctures. Also a previous recent needle puncture of the arachnoid may allow spinal fluid to escape into the subdural space. The presence of this fluid not only renders a second puncture more difficult at this level, but facilitates the injection of Pantopaque into the subdural, rather than into the subarachnoid space. Subdural fluid in addition may produce an artifact in the myelogram.

Myelography

The indications for the use of myelography and its value in the diagnosis of herniations of the nucleus pulposus or protrusion of the annulus fibrosus are still matters of controversy. A large number of articles have been published, however, attesting to the value of myelography with Pantopaque (ethyl iodophenylundecylate) as an aid in the preoperative diagnosis of these lesions of the intervertebral discs (Spurling and Thompson, 1943) and many authors (Childe, 1945; Soule et al, 1945; Echlin et al, 1945, 1946; Begg et al, 1946; Brown and Pont, 1963; White, 1966; Epstein, 1969; and Raaf, 1970) are of the opinion that the test should be used as a routine preoperative procedure in all suspected cases, provided operation is contemplated.

Four different contrast media have been used in myelography: Lipiodal, Thorotrast, air or oxygen, and Pantopaque.

Before the development of Pantopaque by Strain et al (1942), Plati et al (1943) and Steinhausen et al (1944), myelography had been lergely abandoned by some surgeons. This had been done partly on the basis that clinical diagnosis is sufficiently accurate (Dandy, 1941), that myelography may fail to demonstrate the presence of a herniation (Semmes, 1939; Bradford and Spurling, 1941; McKenzie and Botterell, 1942) and because the older contrast media were deemed unsatisfactory. Lipiodal was used with caution since it could not be easily removed from the subarachnoid space (before the report of Kubik and Hampton, 1941, on a method of removing Lipiodal by aspiration), and if left in situ might at times give rise to irritative phenomena in the leptomeninges. The objections to the use of air (or oxygen) have been that it frequently fails to show the presence of a small disc herniation and that severe headache may temporarily follow its use. Thorium dioxide solution (Thorotrast) was considered dangerous since it is radioactive and an irritant.

Pantopaque has made myelography a simpler and more justifiable procedure than it was in the past. It is of lower viscosity than Lipiodal and more easily removed from the subrachnoid space. If left in the subarachnoid space it is gradually absorbed at the rate of about two-thirds of its volume in a year (Begg et al, 1946). Serious reactions following the use of Pantopaque are of rare occurrence, even when it is left in the spinal canal. Occasionally it causes a mild irritation of the leptomeninges and produces a slight rise in temperature and mild bilateral sciatic pain for about 24 hours. Pantopaque should be removed whenever possible at the termination of the myelographic examination. This can be accomplished with ease in most cases by aspiration through a 17- or 18-gauge needle as described by Kubik and Hampton (1941).

The Value of Pantopaque Myelography as an Aid to Clinical Diagnosis

A posterior herniation of the nucleus pulposus or protrusion of the annulus fibrosus in the lumbar region can be diagnosed clinically in at least 75 to 80 percent of cases. In about 60 percent of patients the clinical localization of the level of the lesion will prove correct at operation. In only about 30 to 40 percent of cases, however, can a preoperative clinical diagnosis of the exact level of the lesion be made with assurance and even in these cases multiple lesions cannot be excluded; in the remaining 60 to 70 percent of patients myelography will be of great aid in precise localization.

It is undoubtedly very reassuring to the surgeon to have positive evidence of the presence and level of a herniation. Otherwise it is often difficult to know how thoroughly an interspace should be explored if the lesion is not apparent on first retracting the nerve root in the usual fashion. Myelography will usually show the exact level of the lesion and limit the necessity of surgical exploration to this site. The length of the operation is thus shortened and unnecessary sacrifice of bone is avoided.

In addition myelography will indicate whether the lesion is centrally or laterally placed or whether it has extended over the body of the vertebra. It will demonstrate the presence of bilateral herniations (Echlin, et al 1946) and also of multiple herniations, which occur in about 16 percent of individuals with a herniated disc (Camp (1939), 12 percent; Soule et al (1945), 14.2 percent; Echlin et al (1946), 16.6 percent; Begg et al (1946), 17 percent). Spinal cord tumors which clinically may simulate a herniated disc will also be detected in the myelogram.

All of this information obtained from myelographic studies is helpful to the surgeon. It is true the surgeon will find most herniations if he thoroughly explores both the fourth lumbar and lumbosacral discs in all cases. Such exploration, in the absence of a myelogram, however, if performed through the usual small unilateral approach may fail to expose a midline herniation or a bilateral one. Small herniations which have migrated upward or downward away from the interspace and which ordinarily would produce a filling defect in the myelogram, may not be found. A protrusion of the annulus fibrosus, which may show up in the myelogram when the patient lies flat on the x-ray table, may also be overlooked at operation, when the patient usually lies in a flexed position. Herniations of both the fourth and the fifth lumbar discs may produce clinical symptoms of a herniation at the fifth disc. Without the information supplied by a myelogram the fifth disc (lumbosacral) would probably be explored first and if a herniation were found there the surgeon would more than likely be content with his findings and fail to explore for a herniation at the level directly above.

There are several objections to the use of Pantopaque myelography. Certainly it is not an ideal method and takes time to perform but until a better one is found it will serve a valuable purpose. The incidence of adverse reactions is low; earlier reported untoward effects were probably caused by impurities. The two most serious objections are that Pantopaque may fail to reveal the presence of a herniation in perhaps 12 percent of cases and that artifacts may be misleading (Arbuckle et al, 1945; Begg et al, 1946; Raaf, 1959; Gurdjian et al, 1961; Brown and Pont, 1963). The occasional occurrence of a negative myelogram in the presence of a herniated disc is no more a contraindication to the future use of the procedure than is a negative x-ray of the chest in pulmonary tuberculosis, or a negative barium meal in carcinoma of the stomach a reason for discontinuing roentgenograms in such cases. When myelographic studies fail to demonstrate a herniation or protrusion of disc tissue in a patient in whom the clinical picture is typical of such a lesion, the decision to operate and the level at which this should be performed must be based on the clinical findings alone. Artifacts in the myelogram will be mentioned later. In most instances they are recognizable as artifacts but occasionally they will lead to the erroneous diagnosis of a herniated disc.

The writers believe that myelography with Pantopaque should be performed preoperatively in all cases suspected of having a posterior herniation or protrusion of disc tissue. The myelogram should not be done until the patient has failed to respond to conservative orthopedic measures, or in other words until such time as operation is indicated.

870

The procedure is carried out with the patient lying prone on the x-ray tilt table, with his feet resting on a foot board attached to the bottom of the table. A folded pillow is placed beneath the abdomen to obtain flexion of the spine. The head of the tilt table is then raised to about 30 degrees. This elevates the patient's head and causes a rise in spinal fluid pressure which distends the dural sac and facilitates lumbar puncture. Alternatively the procedure may be performed with the patient lying on his side with his trunk flexed, or else in the sitting position.

In choosing the level of lumbar puncture it should be kept in mind that artifacts in the myelogram may be produced at the site of puncture. It is advisable therefore, not to insert the needle at the suspected level of the herniation. Herniations are most common at the level of the fourth lumbar or lumbosacral disc and it is frequently impossible to distinguish clinically between lesions at these two levels. In some cases a herniation of both the fourth and fifth intervertebral disc is present in the same patient. In suspected herniations at these levels, the needle is therefore inserted between the third and fourth lumbar spinous processes. If the herniation is probably at the third lumbar level the needle is inserted at the interspace below or above.

The interspace to be punctured is identified by palpation. The interspace between the third and fourth lumbar spinous processes usually lies just above the level of the brim of the pelvis.

The entire lumbosacral region is prepared with Betadine or other suitable solution. A half cubic centimeter of 1 percent novocaine is injected into the skin and subcutaneous tissue at the desired level, and a 17 or 18 gauge lumbar puncture needle with a short bevel directed into the subarachnoid space. The needle is advanced slowly in an attempt to determine when it penetrates the dura. It is then advanced about 1 mm further and the stylet withdrawn. If spinal fluid escapes the needle is advanced several more millimeters so as to be sure that it is well within the subarachnoid space. In some cases if the needle transmits no sensation as it passes through the dura it may be advanced until it contacts the anterior spinal wall and then withdrawn a few millimeters. A perfectly free flow of spinal fluid should be obtained from the needle before injecting any Pantopaque. A specimen of spinal fluid may now be taken for examination. Six cubic centimeters of Pantopaque are slowly injected into the subarachnoid space, the stylet

871

replaced in the needle and the field covered with a sterile towel, which may be held in place with two small pieces of adhesive. The pillow is withdrawn from beneath the abdomen and fluoroscopy carried out.

The tilt table is raised almost to the vertical position so that the Pantopaque flows downward to the bottom of the thecal sac. The head of the table is then lowered very gradually, allowing the Pantopaque to ascend as an intact column toward the patient's head.

Great care should be taken to note any deviation of the head of the column which usually occurs as it passes a herniation. This information is very important, especially in small herniations that indent only the anterior wall of the thecal sac. When the center of the column is opposite the lumbosacral disc, anteroposterior films are taken with the spot film device. Lateral views are also made with the patient in the prone position. Additional information may be obtained from films taken when the patient is rotated into an oblique position.

The Pantopaque is then allowed to flow upward and similar x-ray films taken at the level of the fourth lumbar disc and also at the third, if there is any suspicion of a filling defect. The lower thoracic region should be routinely visualized in all cases of suspected disc herniation. This is especially important if no lesion has been demonstrated at the expected levels. If there is any question of pathology at a higher level in the spine, the flow of Pantopaque may be continued upwards as high as necessary. It is always advisable to repeat the above procedure by allowing the Pantopaque to migrate gradually downward toward the lower end of the thecal sac. In this way any filling defects that may have been present will be reproduced, particularly if they are genuine.

The Pantopaque is now removed by placing the column directly beneath the tip of the lumbar puncture needle. A two cc syringe is attached to the needle and the solution is gently aspirated. Repeated fluoroscopy to place the center of the column beneath the tip of the needle may be necessary before all the Pantopaque can be aspirated. With a little patience this is usually possible if the patient is cooperative.

The patient should remain in bed for at least a day after myelography as post-lumbar puncture headace may otherwise occur. This is one reason for performing the procedure preoperatively.

872

Interpretation of the Myelogram

The diagnosis of a herniation or protrusion of disc tissue is primarily a clinical problem. The myelogram only serves as an aid in evaluating the clinical findings and must be interpreted in that light (Taveras and Wood, 1964; Epstein, 1969).

Filling defects in the myelogram characteristic of a herniated lumbar disc have been found in individuals who have had no symptoms of such a lesion. On the other hand minimal filling defects, even of a root pouch alone, may be strongly indicative of a herniation when the myelographic and clinical findings correspond.

Abnormalities in the myelogram due to herniations or protrusions of disc tissue in the lumbar region may be divided into filling defects produced by disc tissue which lies laterally, medially or bilaterally in the spinal canal. These defects are almost always at the level of the intervertebral disc but may extend upward or downward over a neighboring vertebral body. They must be distinguished from artifacts and from normal variations in the size, shape and position of the theca and nerve root pouches. Complete block to the flow of opaque material occurs with some disc herniations and is to be differentiated from an obstruction due to a tumor, adhesions, or a bony lesion.

Filling Defects Due to Lateral Herniations or Protrusions of Disc Tissue

Filling defects due to posterolateral herniations or protrusions are the most common and vary according to the size and position of the disc material which projects into the spinal canal. The size of the filling defect, however, frequently does not give accurate information as to the size of the lesion, since it outlines only its medial border.

If the herniation or protrusion extends far medially it will cause an indentation of the lateral border of the theca and hence of the column of Pantopaque, and at the same time compress the root pouch or displace it and prevent its filling (Fig. 5 c, d, e). Filling defects of this type may be caused by large lateral herniations or protrusions or by smaller lesions which lie more medially.

When the herniation or protrusion does not extend far medially and lies anterior or lateral to the nerve root it may merely cause an obliteration or displacement of the root pouch producing no or little filling defect in the column of Pantopaque proper (Fig. 5 a, b). In some cases (about 5 percent) a herniation may occur far laterally and

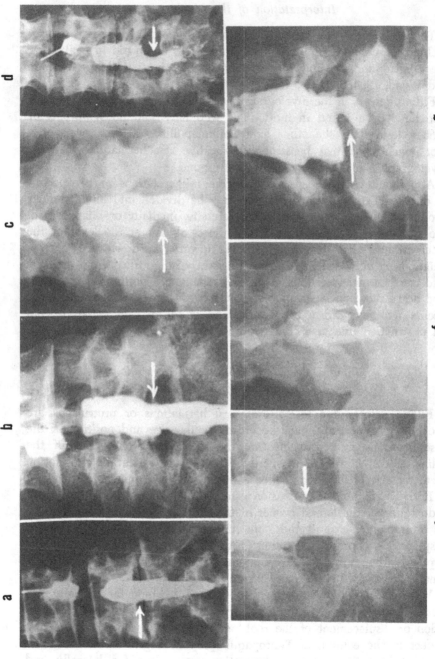

Fig. 5. Seven x-rays Are Shown of Different Types of Filling Defects in the Pantopaque Column (Myelogram)
As a Result of Unilateral Herniation of Nucleus Pulposus Tissue from the Lumbosacral Disc

compress the nerve root without giving rise to any defect in the thecal column or in the root pouch. Lateral herniations that are accompanied by a normal myelogram occur at the lumbosacral disc and are rarely seen at higher levels. This happens because the first sacral nerve root may be compressed by a herniation of the lumbosacral disc after the nerve has passed some distance beyond the dural sac. A herniation or protrusion of the fourth lumbar disc (Fig. 6a), on the other hand, will compress the fifth lumbar nerve root before it has left the dural sac and hence will simultaneously give rise to a filling defect in the thecal column which is almost always detectable in the myelogram.

Rarely myelography may reveal protrusion of the intervertebral disc contralateral to the side of the clinical symptoms (Murphy, 1949; Epstein, 1969).

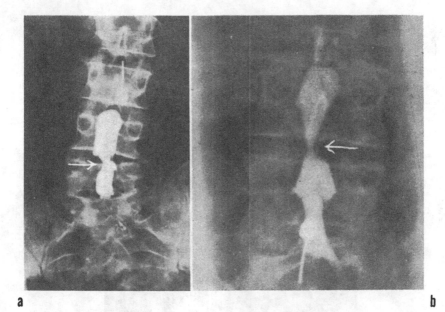

a   b

FIG. 6 a. Typical example of a large unilateral herniation of nucleus pulposus tissue from the 4th lumbar disc (at the arrow). b. Unusually large herniation from the 3rd lumbar disc. The herniated material extends upward over the body of the vertebra, where it compresses the 3rd lumbar root against the pedicle. The 4th lumbar root was compressed at the level of the intervertebral disc proper.

Filling Defects Due to Central or Bilateral
Herniations or Protrusions

A bilateral or midline herniation will cause an hourglass type of defect in the Pantopaque column (Echlin et al, 1946; Haft and Shenkin, 1966) (Fig. 7 b) or it may result in a complete or almost complete block (Fig. 7 a). A subarachnoid block due to a herniation is to be distinguished from that caused by a tumor or other compressing or expanding lesion (Figs. 7 c, d).

A midline herniation produces an hourglass type of defect, according to Begg et al (1946) because the protrusion of disc tissue in the midline displaces the roots of the cauda equina to either side allowing the Pantopaque to flow only in the midline over the dome of the lesion.

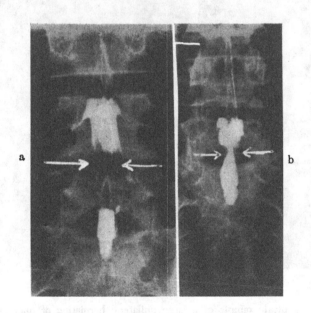

Fig. 7 a. An almost complete block in the flow of Pantopaque is demonstrated at the level of the 4th lumbar disc due to a bilateral herniation of the nucleus pulposus. b. An hour-glass type of filling defect is present in the myelogram opposite the lumbosacral disc as a result of a bilateral herniation of the nucleus pulposus.

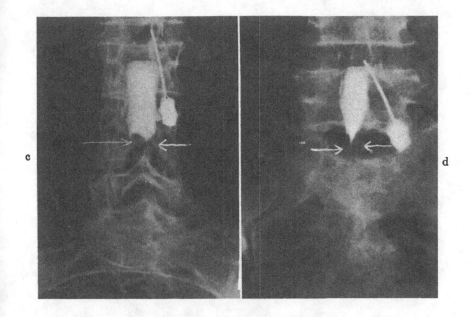

c   d

FIG. 7   (Cont.)

c. This roentgenogram was taken with the patient in the erect position and shows a
complete block to the flow of Pantopaque at the level of the body of the 4th
lumbar vertebra, due to a tumor (perineurial fibroblastoma). The patient had
unilateral sciatic pain almost typical of herniated disc. Note the dome-like defect
in the head of the column of Pantopaque characteristic of this type of tumor. d.
The Pantopaque in this case was injected at the 4th lumbar interspace and the
patient placed in the erect position. The Pantopaque fails to descend below the
level of the 5th lumbar disc and the head of the column is markedly constricted
bilaterally. The pathology in this case was a metastatic carcinoma involving the
epidural space. A herniated disc rarely if ever produces this type of defect.

Intermittent Protrusion of the Annulus Fibrosus

Occasionally what appears to be a filling defect due to a herniated
disc will be present in the myelogram (Fig. 8) but at operation no
evidence of herniation or protrusion of disc tissue will be found. In
some of these cases, a true posterior protrusion of disc tissue is present
when the patient lies prone on the x-ray table during myelography.
However at operation with the patient's back in flexion, the posterior
aspects of the vertebral bodies are separated, the intervertebral disc
space widened posteriorly and the posterior annulus stretched, thus
reducing the protrusion. A contributing factor in the reduction of the
protrusion may also be the lessening of pressure on the disc by
relaxation of the musculature under anesthesia. As Begg et al (1946)

877

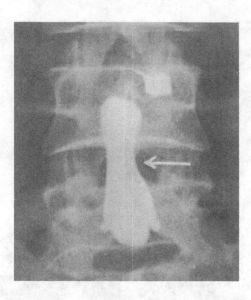

FIG. 8. THIS IS AN EXAMPLE OF A DEFECT IN THE PANTOPAQUE COLUMN PRO-
DUCED BY A PROTRUSION OF THE ANNULUS FIBROSUS OF THE 4TH LUMBAR
INTERVERTEBRAL DISC, WITHOUT HERNIATION OF THE NUCLEUS PULPOSUS.

The patient gave a history of low back and left sciatic pain typical of that obtained in cases of herniation of the 4th lumbar disc. The findings also indicated such a diagnosis. At operation there was no herniation of the nucleus pulposus, but at the site of the filling defect, the annulus fibrosus was thin and the intervertebral disc grossly degenerated. The patient has been free of symptoms since operation.

point out, a lesion of the intervertebral disc of this type is probably identical with the so-called "concealed" disc of Dandy (1941). It has been discussed in this chapter under the term posterior protrusion of the annulus fibrosus.

Multiple Herniations or Protrusions

The abnormalities in the myelogram resulting from multiple herniations or protrusions are similar to those described for solitary lesions except that filling defects may be present at the level of more than one disc (Figs. 9, 10).

Multiple defects in the myelogram must always be interpreted in the light of the clinical findings. A herniation or protrusion does not always produce symptoms and in any one case not all the demonstrable lesions need be clinically significant.

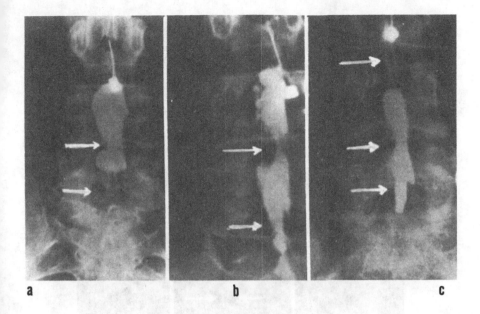

a   b   c

Fig. 9. Multiple Herniations

a. Myelography showed a large filling defect at the level of the fourth lumbar disc on the right side (top arrow). The lower arrow points to an area of bone removal where a herniated disc (fifth lumbar) was reported to have been extirpated previously. The patient had persistence of symptoms on the right side following the initial operation. At a second operation a large herniation of the disc was found at the site of the filling defect. b. The filling defect noted at the level of the 4th lumbar disc (top arrow) outlines what proved at operation to be a large herniation of the disc. The patient on whom we performed this myelogram had had a protruded disc removed elsewhere from the 5th lumbar interspace (bottom arrow). c. Filling defects are present in the Pantopaque column at the level of the 4th (middle arrow) and the 5th lumbar discs (bottom arrow). Herniated discs were found at the site of each filling defect. The patient had had a negative operative exploration done elsewhere at lumbar three level (top arrow). By permission of *Surgery, Gynecology and Obstetrics* (Echlin et al, 1946).

It is not surprising that multiple herniations or protrusions are relatively common in view of the fact that "degenerative" lesions of the intervertebral discs, which are rarely confined to one disc, are an important causative factor in most herniations.

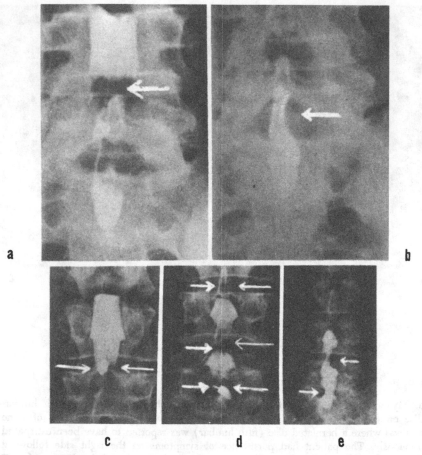

a   b

c   d   e

FIG. 10. MULTIPLE HERNIATIONS

a and b. The patient on whom this myelogram was performed had a large herniation of the disc at lumbar four (a), and at lumbar five level (b). Fluoroscopy
demonstrated an almost complete block at lumbar four interspace and a large
unilateral filling defect at lumbar five (arrows). His clinical symptoms indicated a
herniation of only the fifth disc. c. The column of Pantopaque stops abruptly at the
3rd lumbar disc, where an apparently complete block exists (arrows). The material
was injected at the second lumbar interspace and the patient during fluoroscopy
was left in the upright position for about 20 minutes but the Pantopaque failed to
descend below the 3rd lumbar interspace. d. This is a myelogram done on the same
patient (as in c) several days later. The material was injected at lumbar five interspace and ran upward slowly. When the patient was again tilted into the erect
position the pantopaque remained very nearly stationary, as shown, indicating
an almost complete block at the 3rd, 4th, and 5th lumbar discs (arrows). A large
herniation of the disc was found at lumbar three, four, and five levels on the right
(the side of the sciatic pain). The left side was not explored. Clinically the patient

Anatomical Variations

There is considerable variation in the normal width of the thecal column in the lumbar region but this variation does not usually cause confusion in the interpretation of the myelogram. A very narrow thecal tube, however, is less likely to show a filling defect than a wide one when a herniation of a disc is situated far laterally in the spinal canal.

Posterior protrusions of the intervertebral discs within normal limits may produce an hourglass type of deformity in the myelogram (Fig. 11 a). When the column of Pantopaque arrives at such a disc it hesitates, then trickles over the central portion of the disc, which is its lowest point and spreads out on either side, producing an hourglass deformity (Bradford and Spurling, 1945). A deformity of this type cannot always be distinguished from one due to a bilateral or midline pathological

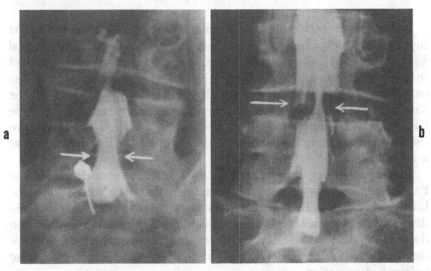

a   b

FIG. 11. a. and b. illustrate examples of "corsetting" (bilateral constriction — at the level of the 4th lumbar disc) of the Pantopaque column, not due to a demonstrable pathological lesion. Case a had a herniation of the nucleus pulposus from the 3rd lumbar disc illustrated in Fig. 6, b. The 4th lumbar disc space was also explored and appeared normal. The 4th lumbar disc appeared normal at operation in case b.

Legend for Fig. 10 (Cont. from p. 880).
was thought to be suffering from a herniation of the 5th disc on the right. e. Two large filling defects in the column of Pantopaque are evident, one at the 4th lumbar interspace on the left side and the other at the lumbosacral junction on the right as indicated by the arrow. At operation two herniated discs were removed, one from the site of each filling defect. Clinically, this patient presented signs and symptoms of a protruded disc only on the left side. By permission of Surgery, Gynecology and Obstetrics (Echlin et al, 1945; 1946).

881

herniation or protrusion of the disc (see above). A lateral projection may be helpful in resolving this problem.

In a small percentage of patients the thecal column terminates above the lumbosacral disc. In these cases a myelogram may be of no value in the diagnosis of a lesion of the lumbosacral disc.

Normally the root pouches of the lumbar and upper sacral nerves are symmetrical but filling is not always uniform, especially if the examination is carried out immediately after injection of the contrast medium. Occasionally, however, there is normal asymmetry of the axillary pouches which may simulate that seen as a result of herniation of the disc tissue.

Artifacts in the Myelogram

In a small percentage of cases a unilateral filling defect is seen in the myelogram which cannot be explained at operation on a pathological basis (Fig. 12 d). Careful inspection at the level of the filling defect in some of these cases has failed to reveal any softening of the disc or bulging of the annulus, even with the patient in extension at the time of operative exploration. In our experience artifacts of this type have usually been at the level of the first to the third disc and have been accompanied by an additional defect due to a true herniation at a different level.

Another confusing type of artifact is a bilateral constriction of the Pantopaque column (Fig. 11 b) simulating that seen in a midline or bilateral herniation. In some cases an asymptomatic prominence of the disc may be responsible, as already mentioned. This latter explanation does not appear satisfactory, however, in the occasional case where the constriction is marked (Fig. 11 b) and no prominence of the disc is found at operation.

A third variety of artifact is that caused by the lumbar puncture needle itself, which may, as it passes through the arachnoid or dura, draw these membranes with it and thus indent the subarachnoid space and hence the column of Pantopaque (Fig. 12 a, b, c).

Finally a further cause of artifacts in the myelogram is the presence of spinal fluid or Pantopaque in the subdural or epidural space. When spinal fluid escapes into the subdural space it may spread upwards and downwards and produce a more or less uniform narrowing of the Pantopaque column. In other instances, only a small amount of spinal fluid collects in the subdural or epidural space and gives rise to an irregular localized filling defect.

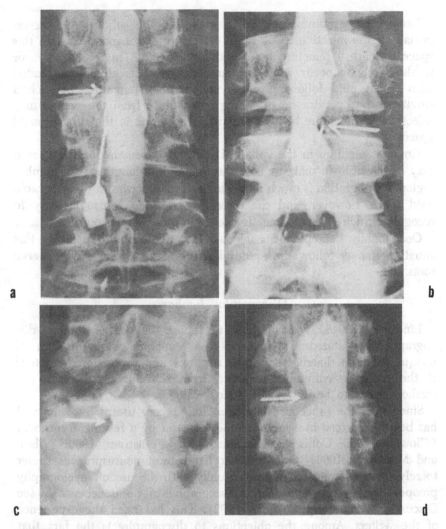

a

b

c

d

FIG. 12. ARTIFACTS IN THE MYELOGRAM

a. In this roentgenogram the Pantopaque column is of normal width at the level of the 3rd and 4th lumbar discs. The Pantopaque shadow is less dense at the point of the needle than elsewhere due to apparent "indenting" of the arachnoidal space. b. A defect is seen in the Pantopaque column at the point of the needle (arrow) due to an artifact produced by "indenting" of the arachnoid or dura and arachnoid by the needle. c. In this myelogram the needle (arrow) has produced an artifact at the 5th lumbar interspace, apparently by "indenting" of the arachnoid or dura and arachnoid. d. A filling defect, due to an unexplained artifact, is present at the level of the 3rd lumbar interspace (arrow). This type of artifact is most commonly seen at the level of the 2nd or 3rd lumbar discs.

883

Pantopaque at times may be injected into the subdural space, especially if the injection is too rapid or forceful, or it may leak into this space through a puncture hole in the arachnoid. This technical error is also likely to occur when the subdural space is already distended with spinal fluid following a previous lumbar puncture. In such a situation, the operator on obtaining spinal fluid from the needle may inject the Pantopaque believing that the needle is in the subarachnoid space.

Contrast medium in the subdural space may remain localized, or it may be possible to make it flow throughout the length of the lumbar region. Its migration is much more sluggish than occurs in the subarachnoid space, however, and the error in technique is usually easy to recognize. Such a myelogram is useless for diagnostic purposes.

Occasionally Pantopaque is injected into the epidural space. In this situation it may follow the epidural spaces even out along the nerve roots.

Discography - lumbar

Lindblom (1948) was the first to report the use of lumbar discography. He stated: "Diagnostic disk puncture with injection of opaque medium demonstrates disk ruptures and protrusions and tells if the patient's symptoms originate from the punctured disk. The method seems to be of great practical value."

Since then the procedure has been found very useful by some and has been performed in a large number of cases by a few neurosurgeons (Cloward, 1962; Collis and Gardner, 1962; Fernstrom, 1960; Wilson and MacCarty, 1969). On the other hand, most neurosurgeons prefer to rely upon the clinical picture, usually with the use of myelography preoperatively, and have found discography to be unnecessary (see Discussion, Collis and Gardner, 1962). This has been the experience of the writers. Among the objections to discography is the fact that it does not give a clear picture of the intraspinal problem and, of course, does not rule out other, at times unsuspected lesions, such as tumors. For a description of the technique of discography the reader is referred to the publications of Collis and Gardner (1962), Collis (1963), and Lindblom (1948).

Electromyography

In the presence of a herniated disc, electromyography may at times be of some value in determining which nerve root (or roots) is involved (Flax et al, 1964; Maranacci, 1955). A diagnosis of herniated disc cannot be made on the basis of electromyography, nor does it provide information of a differential nature.

The treatment of patients suspected of having a herniation or protrusion of disc tissue into the spinal canal may be divided into two categories — conservative and surgical.

Conservative Treatment

Pain in the back may be caused by a multitude of conditions other than a herniated disc. Treatment of such cases is primarily orthopedic and conservative. Myelography or surgical exploration for a herniated disc on the basis of back pain alone is very rarely indicated. Undoubtedly back pain can be the first symptom of a herniation or protrusion of disc tissue. However it seems certain that many patients with a pathological disc who have been treated conservatively at this stage of the condition before nerve root pressure has occurred have been relieved of symptoms. Certain patients with back pain who fail to respond to conservative therapy may be benefited by spinal fusion. Before fusion is considered a herniated disc or other intraspinal lesion must be excluded. After this has been done the decision concerning the advisability of fusion and its performance are orthopedic problems.

Conservative treatment is also indicated as a primary measure in almost all cases of herniated discs even when sciatic pain is present. Prolonged, or even permanent, improvement may be expected in some patients in whom the annulus fibrosus is protruding posteriorly but has not completely ruptured. In these cases conservative measures may reduce the protrusion. Little more than temporary relief, however, can be expected in patients in whom a fragment of nucleus pulposus has herniated completely through a small tear in the annulus and is compressing a nerve root.

A Possible Explanation of the Remissions and Exacerbation of Symptoms

It is true that remissions do occur even when a true herniation is present and in fact this is one of the characteristics of this condition.

We have seen patients with a typical history and clinical signs of a herniated disc, in whom a large herniation has been demonstrated by myelography, who have become free of symptoms (except for slight low back discomfort) for several months. Recurrence of symptoms practically always occurs in these cases however, and the recurrence is frequently precipitated by a minor strain such as stooping over to lace the shoes, or merely turning over in bed. The conclusion seems inescapable that a nerve root subjected to a constant, non-fluctuating pressure (from a piece of intervertebral disc tissue) may in time become adjusted to this pressure and pain in the distribution of the involved nerve root may subside. This hypothesis is strengthened by the fact that some patients, with very large herniations, proved at operation to be causing continuous pressure on a nerve root, are nevertheless free of sciatic (root) pain when they avoid certain movements and postures.

An important factor in the production of root pain is apparently changing (i.e., fluctuating) pressure on nerve fibres. If the herniated material is so placed that the degree of pressure on nerve fibres increases with certain movements of the spinal column or with stretching of the nerve roots (as in straight leg raising), then pain occurs each time this increase in pressure takes place.

With regard to a sudden recurrence of symptoms following a prolonged remission, this may be explained by an increase of pressure on a nerve root from a slight additional herniation of nuclear material, or to a minor shift in the position of the already herniated portion of disc tissue.

Methods of Conservative Treatment

The methods of conservative therapy for low back and sciatic pain are widely known and include avoidance of stooping or lifting and immobilization of the lumbar spine in mild cases, to complete bed rest when the symptoms are acute. During an acute attack of sciatic and back pain, many surgeons prefer to keep the patient flat on his back in bed with boards beneath the mattress. Other surgeons have found that greater immediate, as well as prolonged relief is obtained by placing the patient in bed with the lumbar spine, hips, and knees in a slightly flexed position (Barr, 1947). Such a position can be obtained by elevating the head and knee rests of the bed. Manipulative therapy has also given relief in many cases with back pain but it seems doubtful if a herniated disc can be benefited by such a procedure. Associated muscle spasm, however, may be relieved temporarily. It should be borne in mind that manipulation has been known to produce harmful and even catastrophic effects. Traction with Buck's extension has been of value in certain patients. Analgesics such as codeine, or even morphine, are very helpful during the acute phase in relieving pain and muscle spasm. Massage and diathermy give temporary relief in some cases but aggravate the symptoms in others.

When the acute phase of the attack has subsided and the patient is ambulatory, a properly fitted corset or brace may be used to obtain immobilization of the lumbar spine. Postural defects should be corrected and the patient should be instructed to avoid stooping, or lifting with the spine in a flexed position.

SURGICAL TREATMENT

Selection of Patients for Surgical Treatment

In selecting patients for operation the surgeon must satisfy himself that adequate conservative therapy has been attempted and has failed to produce sufficient relief. Characteristic signs and symptoms of a herniated disc must be present. The degree of pain should be carefully evaluated, especially regarding its interference with the patient's activities, earning capacities, and comfort. The most careful evaluation should be made of neurotic patients and those in whom compensation may be a motive. The surgeon should refuse operation when the symptoms do not appear (to the surgeon) to be of sufficient severity, and operation should not be urged upon a patient who does not feel that his symptoms are severe enough to require surgical intervention.

Patients with motor deficits should be operated upon without delay, and cases of massive disc extrusion with cauda equina compression are surgical emergencies.

The value of preoperative myelography has already been discussed.

Patients who have recurrence of symptoms following a previous operation for a herniated disc require special evaluation as the symptoms may be due to further herniation of disc material at the site of the original exploration (recurrence) or the presence of bilateral or multiple herniations, or adhesions or other pathologic changes involving the musculoskeletal structures.

887

Initially, the operation for removal of a herniated disc involved performing a classical laminectomy. Two or three spinous processes with their laminae were removed and the herniation was exposed through a transdural approach.

Improvement in the operative approach has developed in stages. It soon became evident that most herniations could be exposed extradurally and for a time this was accomplished through a hemilaminectomy. Such an extensive removal of bone was found unnecessary (Love and Walsh, 1940). At present an interlaminar approach is used in most cases, and requires stripping of the muscles from their vertebral attachments on one side only.

In extirpating herniations of the lumbosacral disc it is, in some cases, unnecessary to remove any bone. With most herniations of the fourth or the lumbosacral disc, however, a small amount of bone is usually removed from the inferior lateral margin of the lamina above the interspace to be explored, and from the superior lateral margin of the lamina

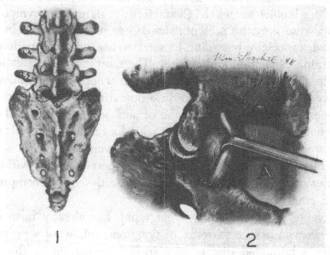

FIG. 13.   1. The lower three lumbar vertebrae and sacrum. The dotted lines on the laminae of the 4th and 5th lumbar and 1st sacral vertebrae indicate the areas of bone removed in the surgical approach to a herniation from the 4th lumbar or lumbosacral disc on the left side. 2. Illustrates the surgical exposure of a herniation of nucleus pulposus tissue from the lumbosacral disc on the left side. The thecal sac is marked A. The 1st sacral nerve root is being retracted medially exposing the underlying herniation.

below (Fig. 13). When operating in the lower lumbar region it is rarely necessary to remove enough of the lamina to interrupt entirely the neural arch, unless an unusually large or midline lesion is present. When a herniation is present at the level of the third lumbar disc or above, however, hemilaminectomy is more frequently required to obtain adequate exposure.

Operative Technique

Under general or spinal anesthesia the patient is placed in the prone position on the operating table. The table is "broken" so as to produce some flexion in the lower lumbar region. Additional flexion may be attained by elevating the kidney rest, and if used, this should be placed beneath the pelvis, rather than the abdomen, so as to avoid pressure on the abdominal veins with its attendant venous engorgement. To relax the sciatic nerve the lower limbs are flexed acutely at the knees and supported in this position with several pillows. The crouch position is favored by some surgeons; the hips and knees are flexed and the buttocks rest on a support.

The back is prepared from the lower buttock to the mid-thoracic region with alcohol, ether, and Betadine. The interspace or interspaces to be explored are identified by palpation (as described under technique of myelography), and these marked by scratching the skin with a scalpel. Alternatively, a drop of methylene blue injected intracutaneously at the site of the myelographic defect to one side of the midline provides a useful guide to the level of the lesion. This is done at the time myelography is performed.

The patient is draped. An incision is made in the midline of the back centered over the interspace to be explored. The lumbodorsal fascia in the midline is incised and by sharp dissection the tendinous attachments to the spinous processes are divided on the side of the herniation. Using a wide, sharp periosteal elevator the muscles are now stripped laterally by subperiosteal dissection. Gauze packing is used to control bleeding. This is withdrawn and an automatic retractor inserted to provide exposure of the spinous processes, laminae and articular facets. Remaining soft tissue, overlying the ligamentum flavum and laminae, above and below the interspace exposed, is now removed with a small periosteal elevator, or with tissue forceps and scissors. The ligamentum flavum is gently stripped from the undersurface of the lamina above. With a rongeur several millimeters of bone are now removed from the inferior lateral surface of the lamina above the interspace to be explored (Fig. 13) although this is not always necessary at the lumbosacral interspace.

A small incision in the ligamentum flavum is made with care. As soon as epidural fat is exposed a flat blunt director is passed beneath the ligamentum flavum as a guide. This ligament may then be divided in elliptical fashion and turned laterally as a flap. The base of the flap is divided on the director which is kept beneath it. With a Spurling-Kerrison rongeur further bone, with its underlying ligamentum flavum, is then usually removed laterally. A small portion of the upper lateral border of the lamina below the interspace is removed in similar fashion. A wide foraminotomy may be performed at this stage of the operation (Shenkin and Haft, 1966).

The dural sac is gently retracted medially to expose fully the nerve root. At the fourth lumbar interspace the nerve root is still incorporated in the dural sac, but at the level of the lumbosacral disc it lies separate within its own dural sleeve. The nerve root is examined for evidence of pressure anteriorly. With care it is then retracted medially, or at times laterally (in exploring the fifth lumbar interspace), to uncover the underlying intervertebral disc. Small pledgets of cotton rolled into the shape of a cylinder and to which are attached long silk threads, are carefully packed into the epidural space upward and downward, lateral to the nerve root. These are very helpful in controlling bleeding from the epidural veins. Narrow strips of cottonoid may also be used to control epidural bleeding. The herniated disc is now brought into view. Epidural tissue or veins which often lie on its surface are gently displaced. They may be coagulated with a bayonet forceps (bipolar current) if the field is dry and great care is taken to avoid any spread of the current to neural structures.

The herniated material may lie entirely free in the spinal canal or may communicate with the remainder of the intervertebral disc through an opening in the posterior longitudinal ligament and annulus. In other cases the herniated material may be covered by a thin or thick layer of annulus and connective tissue (see Pathological Considerations). Any herniated material free in the spinal canal is removed by gentle traction without fragmenting it, if possible, as it may extend some distance beyond the disc space and a portion could conceivably be overlooked. Following removal of free extruded disc, the posterior longitudinal ligament and annulus fibrosus are exposed and the opening further enlarged by an incision parallel to and over the disc space. In the event the annulus is intact, after the field is completely dry and the lesion adequately exposed, the dome of the herniated or protruding portion of disc tissue is incised in a cruciate fashion. Nucleus pulposus material may now spontaneously herniate through the opening. It is grasped with a nasal forceps and in stages teased from its bed. A large amount of nucleus pulposus material may be obtained in this fashion. The Cushing pituitary rongeur is now inserted into the depths of the intervertebral disc. Its blunt point will encounter firm resistance as it makes contact with the annulus anteriorly in the interspace. It is withdrawn one or two millimeters, opened, and further nucleus pulposus material grasped and withdrawn. The rongeur is directed laterally (and against the opposing surfaces of the vertebral bodies) at first and all loose material removed from this region. After reversing the rongeur, it is reinserted toward the midline and further removal accomplished in this region. A grooved director, bent to a right angle, may now be inserted through the opening in the annulus and passed medially beneath (anterior to) the posterior longitudinal ligament, and any nucleus pulposus material in this region gently pushed anteriorly and outward in the intervertebral disc space. The grooved director is withdrawn, a Cushing pituitary rongeur reinserted and a search made for further loose fragments of tissue. An angled pituitary rongeur may be used in place of a grooved director. Curettage of the interspace, cautiously performed, may yield additional fragments of disc tissue. When all possible nucleus pulposus material and cartilaginous plate have been obtained and the nerve root appears adequately decompressed, the cotton pledgets are withdrawn from the epidural space after irrigation with warm saline. Brisk bleeding may occur at this point and can usually be controlled with ease by inserting temporarily a small piece of cottonoid or Gelfoam into the epidural space. If Gelfoam is used it can usually be removed completely in a few minutes without starting any fresh bleeding. A small piece may be left in the epidural space if necessary to assure hemostasis.

When all bleeding has been controlled closure is commenced. The table is flattened and the wound thoroughly irrigated with warm saline. Bleeding points, unless immediately under the skin, are controlled by coagulation applied via a bayonet forceps. The ligamentous attachments are resutured to the spinous processes. It is not necessary to suture muscle unless a laminectomy has been done or the dura opened. Subcutaneous tissue and skin are closed with interrupted silk sutures. A sterile dressing is applied to the wound and held in place with adhesive strips which should be applied firmly in order to take tension off the wound and give firm support to the back.

An excellent article, well illustrated, on surgical treatment of herniated lumbar intervertebral discs was recently published by Raaf (1970).

Special Points in the Operation

Identification of the interspace leading to the fourth lumbar or lumbosacral disc is usually easy by palpation through the skin, providing a bony anomaly does not exist, and the patient is not unduly obese. The fourth interspace in most cases lies just below the pelvic brim and this supplies the relative position of the interspace below. When the muscles have been stripped from their attachments, direct visualization or palpation of the sacrum will further accurately localize the desired interspace.

Before operation, however, careful check of the x-rays should always be made to determine the level of the fourth interspace in relation to the pelvic brim and to rule out anomalies. Not infrequently lack of fusion of the first sacral vertebra will give rise to an interspace at this level which may be mistaken for the lumbosacral interspace. Occasionally a patient will have six or four lumbar vertebrae and the wrong level may be explored.

When there is a herniation of the third lumbar disc or one at a higher level, the sacrum is not usually directly visualized at operation and localization of the level of the lesion may be difficult. This is particularly true in the presence of four or six lumbar vertebrae. In such cases one or two interspaces which are palpable can be marked with an indelible pencil and a lead marker, and an x-ray taken. By examining the x-ray and comparing it with the myelogram (which is almost always necessary to localize accurately these higher lesions in the first place) the interspace to be explored can be identified.

As already indicated, the level to be explored may also be readily identified by injecting a drop of methylene blue intracutaneously at the time of myelography directly overlying the defect in the column of Pantopaque.

During exposure of the herniation it is preferable to remove the bone and ligamentum flavum which immediately overlies the nerve root, taking care at the same time to avoid entering the articular facet. This removal of bone and ligamentum flavum serves two purposes. First, it decompresses the root posteriorly which renders it less susceptible to any further compression anteriorly. Secondly, such a lateral exposure will permit removal of the herniation with a minimum of trauma to the nerve root from retraction, and it will provide sufficient room for the Cushing pituitary rongeur to be passed easily into the depth of the interspace. A foraminotomy should be carried out in some cases prior to excision of the disc if this facilitates manipulation and helps to avoid injury to the root (Shenkin and Haft, 1966). It is sometimes preferable to perform a foraminotomy following the disc removal.

It is rarely sufficient to remove only that portion of a disc which has herniated or protrudes into the spinal canal, if further herniation of nuclear material at a later date is to be avoided. All possible nucleus pulposus tissue should be obtained from the depth of the interspace. A Cushing pituitary rongeur is an excellent instrument for this purpose, although a curette may be useful. The Cushing pituitary rongeur has a blunt nose and, if care is taken, there is little danger of thrusting it through the firm thick anterior annulus. A curette on the other hand has been known to penetrate the neighboring abdominal aorta. It is doubtful whether the whole disc could be removed surgically; such an attempt is dangerous and unnecessary.

Not uncommonly at operation, an apparently softened but non-protruding, or only slightly protruding disc will be found (see under myelography — intermittent protrusion of the annulus fibrosus). The surgeon is faced with the decision as to whether or not to incise the overlying annulus and remove the nuclear tissue. If the lesion is at the level suspected clinically and the myelogram has shown a definite filling defect at the same level (and only at this level), the disc as a rule should be attacked surgically. It seems likely that some patients with lesions of this type (and a positive myelogram) can be relieved of symptoms by merely decompressing the nerve root at the involved level.

When bilateral herniations are indicated in the myelogram, whether or not the symptoms are bilateral, the intervertebral disc should probably be explored on both sides. The approach used is the same as described for a unilateral herniation but is bilateral.

Exploration for multiple herniations depends upon an evaluation of both the clinical and myelographic findings and the surgeon's judgment. Failure to remove multiple herniations accounts for the recurrence or persistence of symptoms in some cases.

Occasionally the first sacral nerve root will be compressed by the lower edge of the body of the fifth lumbar vertebra, due either to posterior displacement of the vertebra or to bony lipping. In such a case, pressure on the root can be relieved by decompressing it posteriorly and removing the prominent edge of vertebra which lies anterior to the root, with a Cushing pituitary rongeur.

During the first few days after operation the patient usually has pain in the back and occasionally some pain along the sciatic nerve. This can be relieved by giving morphine 15 mg or Demerol 75-100 mg every four hours, if necessary, for a few days and thereafter codeine 30-60 mg at similar intervals supplemented by a sedative at night.

The patient is kept on his abdomen or side for a few days and thereafter may lie in any position so long as he does not flex the lower lumbar region.

The patient is usually allowed out of bed for a short time on the first or second day postoperatively (unless a complete laminectomy or fusion has been necessary), but should be supported by an attendant. Flexion of the lumbosacral spine is avoided. By the second day the patient can usually take a short walk and sit in a chair for one half to one hour morning and afternoon. As a rule bed rest can be almost eliminated within 5-7 days following operation, and the patient discharged from the hospital two days thereafter.

There are several advantages to getting the patient out of bed as soon as possible. The importance of early ambulation in the prevention of venous thrombosis is, of course, well recognized. In addition, micturition is easier and catheterization, which otherwise is sometimes required for a few days, may be avoided. The patient can more easily get rid of flatus, and disturbed vasomotor tone, evidenced by dizziness on assuming the upright position, is avoided or minimized.

When the patient is ambulatory he is instructed to walk with a good posture and to guard against more than slight flexion of the lower lumbar region for about a month. During the subsequent two months flexion of the lumbar spine is gradually increased but lifting is not permitted. Office workers are allowed to return to their jobs in six weeks, manual laborers to light work in three months, and to heavy work in six months.

All patients who have had a herniated disc removed are instructed to avoid lifting with the lumbosacral spine in a flexed position. This precaution in fact should be observed by normal individuals as well, if undue stress on the lower lumbar intervertebral discs is to be avoided.

There are certain symptoms which may develop during the convalescent period that are worth mentioning. In some patients intermittent bouts of their old sciatic pain may return for a few days toward the end of the first week after operation, presumably as a result of temporary edema or inflammatory reaction about the nerve root. Very occasionally an attack of intense pain in the back with associated spasm and tenderness of the erector spinae muscles occurs several days to a few weeks after the patient is up. These symptoms usually subside with bed rest for a few days to a few weeks.

COMPLICATIONS

A number of complications of varying degrees of severity may occur as a consequence of lumbar disc surgery. These include trauma to nerve roots, postoperative arachnoid cysts, infection of the disc space and, most serious of all, laceration of the major vessels in the lumbar prevertebral space and visceral injuries caused by instruments perforating the interbody joints. Arteriovenous fistulae may develop following vascular injuries. For a detailed account of these complications, the reader is referred to a symposium on the subject which appeared in 1968 in the Journal of Bone and Joint Surgery (Ford et al).

SPINAL FUSION

There is no doubt that spinal fusion is indicated in a certain number of patients following the removal of a herniated disc. It is still a highly debatable question however whether all, or even any patients with a disc herniation require a fusion at the original operation for disc removal unless additional pathology exists.

The Question of Spinal Fusion Following the Removal of a Herniated Disc

Reasons Given in Favor of Fusion. A spinal segment from which a herniated disc has been removed is no longer mechanically and anatomically normal (Barr, 1947; Steindler, 1947). Narrowing of the disc with subluxation of articular facets and impingement of the facets on the pedicles may take place and be the forerunner of traumatic hypertrophic changes, local spur formation (Barr, 1947) and at times of narrowing of the intervertebral foramina. In addition the ligaments

895

Table 1

RESULTS OF OPERATIONS FOR HERNIATED DISC

AUTHOR	YEAR	WITHOUT SPINAL FUSION													WITH SPINAL FUSION												
		Pain in back		Pain in leg		Pain in leg or back		Working		Disability on working		Improved	Cured	No. of cases	Pain in back		Pain in leg		Pain in leg or back		Working		Disability on Working		Improved	Cured	No. of cases
		Yes	No	Yes	No	Yes	No	Yes	No	Yes	No				Yes	No	Yes	No	Yes	No	Yes	No	Yes	No			
Fincher	1939											80–90%		50													
Barr and Mixter	1941	32 cases 52%		42 cases 69%											24 cases 73%		30 cases 91%										
Botterell, Keith and Stewart	1944											85%	56%	51													
Grant	1944							89%		37%	52%	89%	52%	150													
Shinners and Hamby	1944					54%		87%			57%	98%	50%	87													
Smith, Deery and Hagman	1944																							81%	34%	58
Poppen	1945	On heavy lifting 60%		90%				95%				95%	38%	400													
Barr	1947	55%		41%						29%	63%	83% in 483	24% in 147	132									24%	63%			10
Lenhard	1947	39%													40%		25%										
Love	1947			35%							64%	90%	54%	987													
Peyton and Simmons	1947	71%		52%							94%		16% cured- 35% minor symptoms	31	66%		71%							90%	22% cured- 68% minor symptoms	41
Steindler	1947											100%	60%	23	13%									63%	88%	8

TABLE 1 (Continued)
RESULTS OF OPERATIONS FOR HERNIATED DISC

Author	Year	WITHOUT SPINAL FUSION													WITH SPINAL FUSION												
		Pain in back		Pain in leg		Pain in leg or back		Working		Disability on working		Improved	Cured	No. of cases	Pain in back		Pain in leg		Pain in leg or back		Working		Disability on working		Improved	Cured	No. of cases
		Yes	No	Yes	No	Yes	No	Yes	No	Yes	No				Yes	No	Yes	No	Yes	No	Yes	No	Yes	No			
Shinners and Hamby	1949	42%		10%			49%	94%				89%	53%	289	36%		23%			41%	82%				85%	35%	66
Young and Love	1959		48%		53%		44%							555		68%		74%		63%					95%		450
Raaf	1959											96%		430													147
Gurdjian et al	1961											95% P / 88% I		619											91% I		119
Brown and Pont	1963											93% P / 86% I		153											57% I		24
Semmes	1964	52%	48%	46%	53%			92%				98%	54%	1453													
Hirsch	1965	15%		2%		70%	12%					96%		179													
Slepian	1966											98% P / 92% I	85% P / 56% I	267 (14 had fusion)													
White	1966																										
Barr et al Examiners' Rating	1967						28% P / 0% I					70% P / 71% I		57 P / 7 I						37% P / 36% I					78% P / 71% I		73 P / 14 I
Patiens' Rating							68% P / 38% I					90% P / 82% I		159 P / 16 I						76% P / 70% I					94% P / 91% I		210 P / 43 I
Uihlein et al	1968											96%		514											96%		435
DePalma and Rothman (L5–S1)	1970	37%	27%									89%			32%		22%								93%		
Gartland	1971											77%		33											85%		83

I = Industrial   P = Private

lying posterior to the disc may become relaxed (Steindler, 1947). At operation for a herniated disc the ligamentum flavum is excised and the articular facet occasionally damaged or even removed in some cases. All of these changes, which may in some cases follow the removal of a herniated disc, are supposed on theoretical grounds to predispose to recurrent attacks of low back pain.

Some orthopedic surgeons believe that fusion immobilizes the pathological spinal segment and so helps to prevent this predisposition to pain in the back and they have advised spinal fusion in practically all cases following the removal of a herniated disc (Davis, 1947; Barr, 1947; Steindler, 1947).

Another argument in favor of fusion is the belief that it will lessen the possibility of further herniation of nucleus pulposus material from a disc already operated upon, and that it will prevent herniation of other degenerated discs.

Reasons Given against Fusion. After the simple removal of a herniated disc it is estimated that about 50 percent of patients have been completely or almost completely relieved of their back and lower limb pain (Table 1). After removal of a herniated disc plus a fusion operation, the percentage of cases free of back or lower limb pain has been reported by some writers to be 15 to 20 percent higher than in comparable groups of cases operated upon without fusion (Table 1). These reports, although used as an argument in favor of routine fusion, actually indicate that 80 to 85 percent of patients on whom the operation was performed might have done as well without fusion.

Actually there is considerable statistical evidence to question the value of combining disc excision with fusion (Peyton and Simmons, 1947; Shinners and Hamby, 1949; Gurdjian et al, 1961; Barr et al, 1967; Uihlein et al, 1968). In fact, Barr et al state that "with the realization that additional fusion of the spine does not significantly improve the results of lumbar disc surgery, that it greatly lengthens the period of hospitalization and consequent convalescence, and may lead to serious postoperative complications, the use of the combined operation at the Massachusetts General Hospital has decreased progressively."

Before subjecting a patient with a herniated disc to fusion there are other factors to be considered. The operation for removal of a disc is prolonged if fusion is done and this places some strain on the patient. The convalescent period is lengthened. Further, if secondary operation should be necessary it may be a difficult procedure through a previous fusion.

Secondary operation is not uncommonly required following the removal of a herniated disc because of: recurrent herniation of the nucleus pulposus (Figs. 14 a, c), adhesions at the operative site, failure

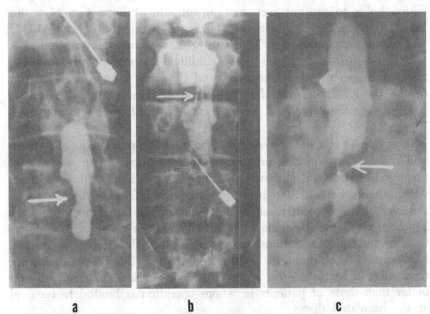

a b c

FIG. 14. RECURRENT HERNIATION WITH AND WITHOUT SPINAL FUSION

a. A large filling defect is shown in the myelogram (at the arrow) due to a recurrent herniation of nuclear tissue from the lumbosacral disc. At a previous operation a herniation from the lumbosacral disc was removed and a spinal fusion performed. At a second operation a large piece of nuclear tissue, which had herniated completely through the annulus fibrosus, was removed from the site of the filling defect in the myelogram. This case illustrates that a recurrent herniation may occur beneath a spinal fusion. b. A large filling defect is shown at the level of the 3rd lumbar disc due to a herniation which occurred many months following a spinal fusion of the 4th and 5th lumbar and 1st sacral vertebrae. After fusion of the two lower lumbar vertebrae the fulcrum in lifting was shifted to the level of the 3rd lumbar disc. Apparently, as a result of the additional forces to which it was subjected, herniation of this disc occurred. c. The filling defect seen at the arrow in the myelogram was due to a recurrent herniation of nuclear material from the 4th lumbar disc on the left side. Three years previously a herniation is reported to have been removed from this site. Originally the sciatic pain was on the left but at the time of this myelogram the patient had bilateral sciatic pain, more on the right. At operation the herniation was on the left, but the 5th lumbar root on the right was adherent to a bulging annulus fibrosus.

to find solitary, multiple or bilateral herniations or protrusions at the first operation, and the occurrence of subsequent herniations above (Fig. 14 b) or below the original operative site. It is likely that adequate fusion helps to prevent recurrent or subsequent herniation of a disc beneath the graft, but such cases have been reported (Love, 1947), and one is demonstrated in Figure 14 a. Love raises the question as to whether a fusion does not place additional stress on the disc just above the upper end of the graft and describes a case of herniation of the third lumbar disc after fusion of the fourth and fifth lumbar vertebrae to the sacrum. A myelogram of a similar case is shown in Figure 14 b.

In any series of cases of herniated disc, a certain percentage of patients will have x-ray evidence, or evidence at operation, of an unstable or abnormal lumbosacral (or fourth lumbar) joint. Many of these patients will probably be benefited by fusion after the offending disc has been removed. Patients who must do heavy work, and in whom the back has been weakened by removal of articular facets or by wide exploration for multiple herniations, will probably also be helped by fusion. Exclusive of such cases it would appear that the results following removal of a herniated disc plus a fusion operation are essentially no better than those of patients in whom operation is limited to removal of the herniated disc.

Present Attitudes Regarding Fusion. The general consensus at present is that patients with an uncomplicated clinical picture of a herniated disc, in whom a herniation is found and removed at operation, should not have a spinal fusion (Spurling and Grantham, 1949; O'Connell, 1950; Res. Comm. Am. Orthop. Assoc., 1952; Semmes, 1964; White, 1966). If such patients should develop pain at a later date, then spinal fusion may be indicated in some instances.

Although some surgeons have had excellent results following the combined operation of disc excision and spinal fusion, Semmes (1964) states, categorically: "Despite the debate that still goes on, it is clear that fusion has no part in the treatment of lumbar disc. In the few cases where fusion of the lumbar spine is indicated, it is for conditions other than ruptured lumbar disc."

In reviewing their experience with the surgical treatment of ruptured lumbar intervertebral discs, Barr et al (1967) indicated that, in general, the results were the same after simple excision as after combined excision and fusion.

Reports published on the end results following operation for a herniated disc indicate that approximately 80 to 90 percent of cases are either cured or improved by surgery, but only 50 to 60 percent are rendered essentially symptom-free (Table 1). It is clear from these reports that surgery has much to offer the patient with severe symptoms that do not respond to conservative treatment. On the other hand, it is no less obvious that the end results are not sufficiently good to warrant removal of a pathological disc, except in those cases in which adequate conservative measures have failed.

HERNIATED DISCS IN THE THORACIC REGION

Excellent reviews of this aspect of the herniated disc problem have been published by Tovi and Strang (1960), Love and Schorn (1965), Fisher (1965), and Reeves and Brown (1968).

Only about 0.5 percent of all herniated discs occur in the thoracic region (Love and Schorn, 1965). They are most common in the fourth to the sixth decade but have been reported at all ages after eighteen years with females being affected almost as often as males. The greatest number operated upon have been at the lower four thoracic levels with the eleventh disc predominating. They are more often central but may be centro-lateral or lateral. Occupation does not seem to play much role but trauma occasionally may be a precipitating or aggravating factor. In the absence of trauma the onset of symptoms is usually gradual over a period of weeks to several years and quite frequently the symptoms are intermittent. However, sudden onset with severe spinal cord involvement does occur.

Pain is a common symptom being radicular in perhaps 60 percent of cases; it may be burning, shooting, cutting, sharp, intermittent or constant, and may be associated with numbness and tingling. There is often back pain referable to the thoracic, thoracolumbar, or even lumbar region, made worse at times by certain movements and frequently improved or absent on lying down. Urinary symptoms in the form of urgency, frequency, or diminished bladder sensation may occur as well as constipation and diminution of normal bowel sensation.

Along with these symptoms varying degrees of sensory loss and weakness involving the legs may appear.

The neurologic signs include bilateral or unilateral weakness of

901

the legs, increased deep tendon reflexes, diminished or absent abdominal reflexes, positive Babinski signs, a spastic, ataxic gait, and sensory impairment with proprioception less often involved. The resulting picture is often one of a progressive paraparesis or, not uncommonly, that of a Brown-Sequard syndrome. When the herniation is at T 11 to L 1 levels the picture may be much more complicated with severe radicular pain, diminished tendon reflexes, and disturbance of bladder function due to conus involvement. Myelography may reveal a complete or partial block (Fig. 15).

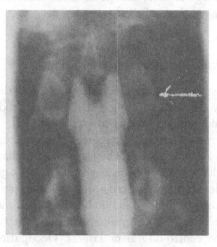

Fig. 15. Myelogram showing a complete block in the flow of Pantopaque at the level of the mid point of the body of the L1 vertebra. The patient had severe pain radiating diffusely throughout both legs and a bladder paralysis. At operation a large piece of herniated disc was found lying in the midline over the mid portion of the body of D 12 and there were two other small pieces of extruded disc over the body of L1 vertebra. After opening the dura, the extruded disc was "milked" laterally and removed extradurally. In this instance the herniated fragments of disc would not have been found if an anterior approach had been used.

Surgical Treatment

A wide bilateral laminectomy extending well above and below the area of protrusion and compressed spinal cord and nerve root has been the surgical procedure of choice in treating these lesions. Unfortunately these herniations are not as easy to treat and the results of surgery are much less gratifying than in the lower lumbar region. The herniation may have already caused infarction of the spinal cord

902

or hematomyelia. It may lie in the midline and not infrequently has eroded the dura and become embedded in the spinal cord. In such cases even the slightest manipulation has only too often been followed by permanent paraplegia. In some cases the protruded disc material lies laterally and can be easily removed extradurally (Feiring, 1967). In others the herniation is more medially placed and is best visualized and excised after opening the dura. In these cases section of the dentate ligaments and possibly even of a root with gentle retraction of the cord may allow transdural removal, or the disc material may be "milked" laterally with a blunt dissector and withdrawn from its bed through an extradural approach. Not infrequently the herniated portion of disc lies over the mid portion of the body of the vertebra above or below the level of herniation and is no longer in continuity with the disc space. An anterior or anterolateral surgical approach to remove such a herniation would be fruitless since it would not even expose it.

The results of surgery have been poor when severe neurologic defects, especially those due to spinal cord involvement, have existed preoperatively. In fact, most of these patients have not shown improvement and many have become worse. When preoperatively there is only root pain with minimal signs of spinal cord involvement, the results have been good to excellent in most instances.

The question always arises as to whether patients with a severe neurologic deficit and evidence of a herniated thoracic disc should be operated on at all. In answer to this query Love and Schorn (1965) point out that the natural course of the condition is progressive. Also, in the presence of a mass lesion demonstrated by myelography one cannot always be sure of its nature until it is exposed at operation.

In view of the hazards involved in the treatment of central thoracic disc protrusions by laminectomy, an anterolateral transthoracic approach has been proposed in cases in which an accurate diagnosis has been established preoperatively (Hulme, 1960; Perot and Munro, 1969; Ransohoff, 1969). The factor of additional surgical trauma to an already compromised and vulnerable spinal cord is thereby lessened, but the procedure is not without its shortcomings and insufficient data have been accumulated to fully establish its value.

Also for the purpose of avoiding retraction of the spinal cord as much as possible, Bucy (1961) recommended a bilateral laminectomy and removal of the articular facets and pedicle on one side as a means of gaining access to the herniated disc and anterior wall of the spinal canal.

903

Forty years ago, in the early thirties, no one suspected that a herniated lumbar intervertebral disc was a common cause of sciatica, and that thousands of operations for its treatment would soon be performed each year. Ten years later, at the onset of the forties, it is doubtful that anyone believed that a lateral herniation of a cervical disc was commonly responsible for nerve root compression with resulting pain in the neck, radiating into the arm and hand (Frykholm, 1951; Scoville et al, 1951; Semmes and Murphey, 1943; Spurling and Scoville, 1944); and it was not until the fifties that the importance of spondylosis as a cause of cervical radiculopathy and myeloradiculopathy was generally realized (Brain et al, 1952; Brain and Wilkinson, 1967; Cloward, 1958; Epstein and Davidoff, 1951; Robinson et al, 1962).

In the cervical region the problems associated with intervertebral disc pathology and treatment are more complicated and less clearly understood than in the lumbar region. This is particularly so because of the presence of the vulnerable spinal cord. The intervertebral disc in the cervical region may herniate posterolaterally or occasionally centrally. Disc degeneration with narrowing may be accompanied by bony lipping of the adjacent vertebral bodies causing a spondylotic ridge to project across the spinal canal and into the intervertebral foramina, or a bony spur to encroach on an intervertebral foramen. As a result of these pathological changes three major syndromes may occur.

1. The syndrome of root irritation or radiculopathy due to pressure on a nerve root by a herniated disc, or by a bony protrusion.
2. The syndrome of spinal cord compression from a central herniated disc (rare) or spondylotic ridge — spondylotic myelopathy.
3. Myeloradiculopathy due to spinal cord and root pressure from spondylosis or herniated disc.

Although radiculopathy and myeloradiculopathy are quite well-established clinical entities, the cause of the pathological changes in the spinal cord and the best form of treatment, especially of the myelopathies, remain controversial. The differentiation between a radiculopathy due to a herniated disc and one caused by a bony osteophyte may be difficult.

As early as 1928, Stookey clearly established that a protrusion of disc tissue in the cervical region, which he referred to as an extradural ventral chondroma, may give rise to three different syndromes: the syndrome of bilateral ventral cord pressure; the syndrome of unilateral ventral cord pressure; and the syndrome of root pressure. His article contained only one case of pure root compression. Other early reports on cervical disc herniation, usually with spinal cord compression, are contained in the papers of Adson and Ott (1922); Elsberg (1925); Stookey (1928); Peet and Echols (1934); Mixter and Ayer (1935); Hawk (1936); Love and Walsh (1940); and Bradford and Spurling (1941). According to Semmes and Murphey (1943), these pre-1940 papers include records of only four cases of operation for nerve root compression by a cervical disc without spinal cord involvement.

In 1943, Semmes and Murphey's description of four cases of rupture of the sixth cervical disc with compression of the seventh cervical root finally raised the curtain on the syndrome of cervical root pressure as an important clinical entity, as had Mixter and Barr's paper in 1934 on lumbar herniations. Since then there have been a series of outstanding articles on the lateral and, to a less extent, midline herniations and protrusions of cervical disc tissue, by Spurling and Scoville (1944), Michelson and Mixter (1944); Bucy and Chenault (1944); Echols (1946); Kristoff and Odom (1947); Scoville, Whitcomb, and McLaurin (1951); Love (1951); Frykholm (1951); Brain, Northfield, and Wilkinson (1952); Allen (1952); Davis, Odom, and Woodhall (1953); Pool (1953); Schlesinger and Taveras (1953); Spurling (1956); Odom, Finney and Woodhall (1958); Bucy (1961); Haft and Shenkin (1963) Murphey and Simmons (1966); and Scoville (1966).

The changing status of the herniated cervical disc, especially from the surgical standpoint, is reflected in the fact that 1768 cases of cervical disc or disc-like syndrome were operated upon in the five-year period 1950–1955 by 33 members of the American Academy of Neurological Surgery (AANS). This information was obtained in answer to a questionnaire sent by one of the writers to the members of the Academy. Over 90 percent of the 1768 cases had pressure on a nerve root without spinal cord compression.

Since the publication of the papers by Epstein and Davidoff (1951) and by Brain, Northfield, and Wilkinson (1952) on the neurologic manifestations of cervical spondylosis and the latter authors' monograph (1967) on cervical spondylosis, there has been an increasing appreciation of the role of this condition in cervical radiculopathy, myelopathy and myeloradiculopathy, and even of its relationship to vertebral (basilar) artery insufficiency.

905

Anatomical and Physiological Considerations

The cervical spinal cord is held relatively immobile by the dentate ligaments and by the nerve roots. The anterior surface of the cord is in close apposition to the cervical discs as are the nerve roots where they pass into the restricted spaces of the intervertebral foramina. These two factors of immobility and apposition to the discs render the nerve roots and the spinal cord susceptible to pressure from a herniated disc or from bony encroachment upon the spinal canal or intervertebral foramina (Fig. 16).

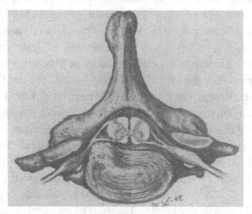

FIG. 16. DIAGRAM TO SHOW A LATERAL HERNIATION OF NUCLEAR TISSUE FROM A CERVICAL INTERVERTEBRAL DISC

The herniation has compressed the nerve root without impinging upon the spinal cord.

In addition if the spinal canal is narrower than normal the spinal cord may be more vulnerable to pathological injury should spondylosis develop (Burrows, 1963; Payne and Spillane, 1957; Reid, 1960; Wilkinson et al, 1969). Indeed many authors believe that narrowing of the anteroposterior diameter of the spinal canal is perhaps the most important predisposing factor in the development of myeloradiculopathy in patients with spondylosis. This perhaps explains why many patients with advanced spondylosis remain essentially symptom-free.

Pathological and Etiological Considerations

The cervical discs are not exposed to the great forces which are operative at the lower lumbar level during lifting, or to the stress resulting from the weight of the body. As in the lumbar region, the wear and tear of movement plays a part, however, in producing degenerative changes in the disc structure which in turn probably predispose to herniation or to hypertrophic bony lipping along the opposing edges of the vertebral bodies, about the posterior articular processes, or lateral intervertebral joints (Jackson, 1966).

The fact that the great majority of herniations occur in the fourth decade or beyond favors the belief that repeated trauma (or a degenerative process) rather than a single trauma is the most important etiological factor in the production of a herniation. There was no patient with herniated cervical disc under 30 years of age among 20 reported by Kristoff and Odom (1947) nor in 115 cases described by Scoville et al (1951). In fact, the average age of these patients was in the late forties. A more recent review of 741 cases by Scoville (1966) indicates that 70 percent occurred between the ages of 40 and 60 years. That an individual trauma may precipitate a herniation or bring on the syndrome of root irritation in an otherwise asymptomatic case is beyond doubt. A history of trauma was obtained in 50 percent of 115 cases reported by Scoville et al, and in over one-third of the 93 lateral disc herniations of Davis, Odom, and Woodhall (1953). Movement is freest in the neck at the level of the fifth and sixth discs, and it is at these levels that the great majority of herniations occur; most frequently the sixth (C 6-7) interspace is the site of rupture.

THE SYNDROME OF CERVICAL NERVE ROOT PRESSURE

This syndrome may be caused by a herniated disc, or by an arthritic bony spur or osteophyte protruding into the intervertebral foramen, often accompanied by spondylosis. The prognosis is excellent after removal of a lateral herniation and frequently only good to fair when the cause is a bony spur. There is a difference of opinion regarding the relative frequency of the two lesions as a cause of root compression, and regarding the possibility of differentiating between them preoperatively. The observations of Scoville and his associates, however, are very important and pertinent to this question.

In 1966 Scoville reported having operated upon 741 cervical discs, 702 of which were lateral in location. Of these 607 were "soft" and 95 'hard" lesions. The results of removal of these lateral herniations through a small posterior "key-hole" partial hemilaminectomy and facetectomy with uncapping and unwalling of the involved root are described as "amongst the most rewarding of all operations in the field of neurosurgery."

907

Clinically the classical syndrome of cervical root compression may be the same whether due to a herniated disc or to a bony spur. The first symptom is usually pain in the lower part of the neck which may come on suddenly, and frequently occurs in intermittent attacks. After a period of days to months or even years, the pain begins to radiate toward the shoulder and into the arm along the distribution of the involved cervical nerve root (usually the sixth or seventh). The radiating pain may become constant but not uncommonly occurs in attacks of great violence. The pain may be referred to the precordium, in which case it may closely simulate that of coronary disease. The points of greatest pain are usually the neighborhood of the shoulder, medial to the scapula, and the posterolateral aspect of the arm as far as the elbow. The pain at times radiates to the dorsum of the forearm or hand but more often paresthesiae are felt in the latter area. Headache, both occipital and temporo-frontal on the side of the root involvement may also occur.

Paresthesiae are felt along the lateral (radial) side of the forearm on its anterior and posterior surface, and extend into the thumb, index, and middle fingers. In lesions of the seventh root, paresthesiae, numbness, and even weakness are most common in the index and middle fingers whereas the thumb and index finger are more often involved when the sixth root is compressed. Some patients complain that the whole hand "goes to sleep" and feels cold. These latter symptoms are not usually due to root compression but to ischemia from pressure on the subclavian artery as a result of associated reflex spasm of the scalenus anticus muscle (Spurling and Scoville, 1944).

As in the lumbar region, the cervical root pain and paresthesiae are aggravated by certain mechanical factors such as movement of the head and neck, and by elevation of cerebrospinal fluid pressure brought on by sneezing, coughing or straining.

Clinical Signs. The patient may hold his head tilted to one side. The neck is often stiff and moved with caution. Splinting (spasm) of the cervical and shoulder muscles is commonly present and there may be tenderness over the rhomboid muscles. In most cases, tenderness is elicited on pressure just lateral to the mid-line on the back of the neck at the level of the herniation. Percussion in this region or manipulation of the neighboring spinous process frequently causes a radiation of pain and paresthesiae along the distribution of the involved nerve root into the forearm, thumb, and fingers. A similar accentuation of the pain and paresthesiae may be produced by movement of the neck. A maneuver described by Spurling and Scoville (1944) seems most likely to cause additional nerve root compression with its attendant radiation of pain and paresthesiae; it consists of applying pressure to the top of the head when the neck has been extended and tilted laterally toward the painful extremity. In some cases complete or partial relief is obtained by applying traction to the neck.

The objective neurological signs are variable. In some cases there are no gross sensory or motor findings, even though the patient complains of subjective weakness of the upper extremity and numbness in the first two fingers or thumb. Paresthesiae on stroking the forearm, hand or fingers over the areas supplied by the sixth and seventh nerve roots may be the only neurological sign. However, when pressure on the nerve root has been pronounced, sensory diminution and, less often, motor and reflex changes are present. There is considerable overlap in the sensory areas innervated by the sixth and seventh nerve roots, and it is therefore often difficult to determine which root is involved on the basis of the sensory findings. If the sixth cervical nerve root is compressed by a herniation of the fifth disc, sensory impairment is usually found over the posterolateral aspect of the forearm, thumb, and index finger. These changes are at times accompanied by hypotonia, fine muscle twitchings, weakness, and even atrophy of the biceps muscle and a diminished biceps jerk. In herniations of the sixth cervical disc which press upon the seventh cervical nerve root, the objective sensory loss and paresthesiae as a rule are on the lateral aspect of the forearm (anterior and posterior surfaces) and in the index and middle fingers. In addition there may be weakness of flexion of the index finger, weakness of the triceps muscle, and a diminished triceps tendon jerk.

When signs and symptoms of root pressure are acute in onset, severe and protracted, and soon lead to neurological changes, a herniated disc is usually the cause. If the history is a long one with mild recurrent attacks and few neurologic signs, encroachment on the foramen by arthritic spurring is more likely. However with the latter lesion a minor trauma, as in a 'whiplash' injury, may at times precipitate an acute episode. Trauma apparently can cause edema of soft tissues sufficient to produce temporary compression of the root within the restricted space of the foramen, especially when the foramen is already narrowed by osteophyte formation. In these circumstances the acute symptoms are usually not prolonged and severe neurologic deficit is unlikely.

Anteroposterior, lateral, and oblique roentgenograms of the cervical spine should be taken in all suspected cases of cervical herniated disc. Roentgenograms are of value in ruling out fractures, arthritic changes, primary or secondary bone tumors, and other lesions.

Roentgen examination will reveal in many cases of lateral herniation (about 30 percent, Davis et al, 1953) a narrowing of the involved disc space and, frequently, associated hypertrophic spurring into the foramen. There will be approximately 25 percent of additional cases in which similar x-ray findings are present at a level adjacent to but not at the level of the herniated disc.

In patients with root compression due to bony encroachment on the foramen, the x-ray findings are frequently similar to those just described. The diagnosis is more likely to be bony compression if a large bony spur projects into the foramen at the suspected level or if spondylosis is present. Moderate narrowing of a disc with minimal spurring favors herniation, as does an absence of x-ray abnormalities other than a reversal of the normal cervical curve. It is, of course, obvious that arthritic changes involving the foramina may be misleading since they occur so commonly without ever giving rise to symptoms.

Lumbar Puncture and Manometric Studies. Examination of the cerebrospinal fluid for protein content and manometric studies are valuable especially in cases where cord compression is present. In these cases the protein content is frequently elevated and a partial or, rarely, complete block may be demonstrated on jugular compression. The spinal fluid protein is elevated, usually slightly, in about half the cases of nerve root pressure, whether the cause is a herniation or hypertrophic changes.

Myelography

Undoubtedly the myelogram will fail to demonstrate a herniation in some cases, but this does not appear to be an adequate contraindication to its use. In those cases where myelography is negative the clinical findings will have to be relied upon in determining diagnosis and treatment.

The technique of injection and removal of Pantopaque is the same as described for the lumbar region, but a larger quantity (6 to 9 cc) of the contrast medium should be used. The patient is placed prone on the x-ray tilt table with the shoulders in a special support. A folded pillow is placed beneath the abdomen to flex the spine and reverse the lumbar curve. This facilitates upward flow of the dye with lessened tilt of the x-ray table. The head is acutely extended on the neck with a soft padding beneath the chin. With the patient in this position Pantopaque will not enter the cranial cavity, if rotation of the head to either side is avoided at all times and he follows the instruction not to cough. The table is now gradually lowered so that the head becomes dependent and Pantopaque is observed under the fluoroscope to flow upward as a column. Lowering of the head of the table is continued until all Pantopaque has entered the cervical region. The tilt table may now be reversed to some degree, for once Pantopaque has entered the cervical spinal canal it will remain there (unless the head of the tilt table is elevated quite high) because of the lordotic curve in this region of the spine.

Careful fluoroscopic observation of the Pantopaque column should be made. Posteroanterior and lateral roentgenograms are now taken of the cervical spine. The lateral views are made without moving the patient's head. Under the fluoroscope it is permissible to flex the patient's head slowly if the occipital bone is obscuring visualization of the cervical spine. The amount of flexion necessary to accomplish this is usually slight and not sufficient to permit Pantopaque to flow into the posterior fossa of skull. Visualization of the upper end of the Pantopaque column in the roentgenograms may be achieved by having the patient open his mouth widely. Since the head of the column usually lies in the upper cervical region its visualization is not required in cases of herniated disc, though necessary in cases of suspected high cervical cord tumors.

Defects produced in the myelogram vary with the size and position of the herniation and are present in most cases. A lateral herniation frequently causes a discrete rounded lateral indentation of Pantopaque (Fig. 17) or may only prevent filling of the root pouch. The latter is especially true if a bony spur is the cause of the root compression (Fig. 18 a, b). A large herniation compressing the cord may of course give rise to an almost complete block. Knowledge of the size and position of the filling defect is of value to the surgeon, not only in localizing the level of the herniation but in helping him to decide whether a unilateral surgical approach or a bilateral laminectomy is indicated to accomplish removal of the lesion.

In the literature opinions differ as to the necessity and value of

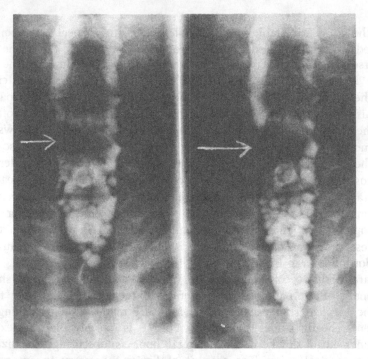

Fig. 17. Cervical myelogram showing a large filling defect due to a herniated disc on the left side between the 6th and 7th cervical vertebra.

myelography. Some do myelograms rarely (Love, 1951) whereas others employ the test routinely and find it "positive" in 99 percent of cases (Scoville, Whitcomb, and McLaurin, 1951). In another large series myelography gave positive results in over two-thirds of the operated cases of herniated cervical disc (Davis, Odom and Woodhall, 1953). Spurling (1956) advocated myelography "regardless of the clarity of the neurologic or plain roentgenologic findings." He pointed out that "we have been misled too often in the past by assuming that localized spurs in a foramen at one level indicated the site of root pressure, only to find, at operation, a soft disc one segment higher or one segment lower." According to Murphey and Simmons (1966), however, "cervical myelography is only indicated or necessary when the clinical findings fail to localize the lesion exactly or when there is a normal cervical curve."

The authors advise myelography and believe that most neuro-surgeons undoubtedly would be reluctant to explore the spine without the benefit of a preliminary myelogram.

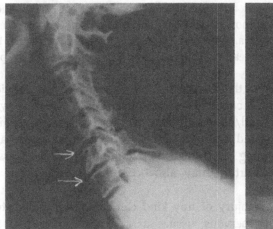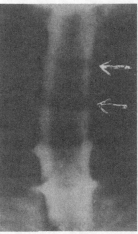

Fig. 18. a and b. Myelogram demonstrating only lack of filling of the root sleeves at C 5-6 and C 6-7 on the left side. Clinically the patient was a left-handed surgeon with severe pain and neurologic changes indicating compression of the 6th, and probably 7th, cervical nerve roots. At operation the roots at C 5-6 and C 6-7 were found to be markedly compressed by bony spurs plus adhesions. A keyhole, partial hemilaminectomy and foraminotomy (facetectomy), with freeing of the root at each level, relieved the patient. Osteoarthritic changes visible on the plain x-ray.

Whiplash and other Injuries to the Cervical Structures, Spinal Cord, and Cervical Nerve Roots

Whiplash injury is a term which has recently come into use to describe the results of sudden extreme movements of extension of the neck, followed by forward flexion or vice versa, less often of lateral flexion of the neck. This kind of injury is usually seen in individuals involved in auto accidents, especially collisions, when the body and head are subjected to different forces of acceleration or deceleration. The word *whiplash* should be confined to a description of the *mechanism* underlying the production of the effects. As often used, the term covers such a wide and variable clinical picture that it has no value as a syndromic designation.

In severe cases, the muscles at the occipitonuchal junction may be stretched or torn, and small hemorrhages may occur; cervical ligaments and small intervertebral joint capsules may also be torn or stretched. Much less frequently the cervical vertebrae and the intervertebral discs are affected, with involvement of sundry anterior and/or posterior cervical nerve roots. Such trauma may aggravate cervical ostéoarthritic disease and so bring about anterior and/or posterior root involvement chiefly as a result of temporary soft tissue swelling in the region of the intervertebral foramina. In the presence of osteoarthritis the spinal cord may also be readily injured as a consequence of hyper-extension.

In severe neck injuries, there may be involvement of the cervical vertebrae in the form of a compression or other type of fracture with or without dislocation and/or disruption of the intervertebral disc. In unusual cases it is stated that stretching of the carotid artery and injury to its intimal lining may lead to thrombosis of the vessel. Damage to the vertebral artery may also occur as a consequence of spinal trauma.

Whether purely nuchal injury of any kind can so stretch and distort the central spinal-bulbar nervous tissues as to cause brain-stem involvement is very questionable, though it is conceivable in quite rare cases of extreme violence with much skeletal (bony and ligamentous) damage.

Associated cerebral concussive effects should be considered separately, not as a necessary part of whiplash nuchal injury. The head injury is usually the result of the impact of the head against such objects as the dashboard of a car; the forces of acceleration and deceleration are usually spent on the nuchal tissues and are not transmitted to the skull in forceful measure.

In actual practice, neck injuries are usually confined to the skeletal structures (muscles, tendons, ligaments, and bone) and are of ortho-pedic interest. For years, the term "cervical sprain" has been used to designate ligamentous and muscular involvement. Some cervical root pains or paresthesiae and mild signs of motor root involvement with reflex signs and muscle wasting and weakness may be noted. These symptoms are usually not permanent.

It must also be recognized that the neck, like the lower back, is a fruitful source of neurotic fixation and elaboration in those who are of neurotic bent. The unnecesssary wearing of a heavy leather collar seems to help fix the neurotic symptoms in a considerable number of cases, in which there are no evidences of any type of organic disease and in which there are often many other associated neurotic complaints.

Hartley (1958) points out that unless some symptoms are present within a few days to a week after injury, it is very difficult if not impossible to prove causal relationship to injury.

For a more detailed description of the effects of hyperextension

914

injuries on the skeletal structure of the cervical region the reader is referred to the recent monograph by DePalma and Rothman (1970).

Differential Diagnosis

The differential diagnosis between the lateral herniation of a cervical disc which compresses a nerve root and a number of other conditions that cause pain in the neck and upper extremity may be difficult. This is particularly true in the early stages of a herniation when it is very small and has not injured the root sufficiently to produce objective sensory or motor changes.

As Semmes and Murphey (1943) point out, it may be that many of the so-called "cricks" in the neck, formerly attributed to sleeping in a draft, a focus of infection, or a fibrositis, are in reality the first symptoms of a herniation.

Pain in the neck referred to the arm is common following a whiplash injury or neck sprain. The pain may be of the referred type due to injury of soft tissues, or it may be caused by temporary nerve-root irritation or compression. Compression of a cervical nerve root can occur in its foramen from soft tissue swelling, with or without sub-luxation of the vertebral bodies or as a result of tearing or stretching of capsular or ligamentous structures.

Cervical arthritis can cause pain in the neck referred to the shoulder and arm. The pain in arthritis does not often follow the distribution of a single nerve root, nor are there usually symptoms of aggravation of pressure on a solitary root when the neck is extended and laterally tilted toward the side of the lesion. When sensory and/or motor symptoms or signs are intractable and severe and confined to the sixth or seventh nerve root, the patient should be investigated completely for herniation or protrusion of disc tissue or narrowing of an intervertebral foramen due to spondylosis.

The scalenus anticus syndrome with its vascular and nervous components may simulate that of herniated disc. In the former condition, however, the pain is referred to the eighth cervical and first thoracic roots, usually to the ulnar part of the palm, ring and little fingers, and occasionally to the whole hand, rather than to the thumb and first two fingers, as in a herniation of the fifth or sixth disc. Symptoms of pressure on the sixth and seventh nerve roots on lateral flexion or compression downward on the cervical spine are absent in the scalenus anticus syndrome. Semmes and Murphey (1943),

915

Spurling and Scoville (1944), and others have drawn attention to the fact that reflex spasm of the scalenus anticus muscle may be an associated phenomenon in cervical disc herniation, and believe that, as a result, many erroneous diagnoses of scalenus anticus syndrome have been made. In fact, since the widespread recognition of the syndrome of the herniated cervical intervertebral disc, it would appear that the incidence of the scalenus anticus syndrome (and of the thoracic outlet syndrome in general) has diminished proportionately.

Other conditions which must be considered in the differential diagnosis are brachial neuritis, subdeltoid or subacromial bursitis, neoplastic, congenital, traumatic or inflammatory disease of the cervical spine, spinal cord tumors involving a nerve root, pressure by a cervical rib or bands, Pancoast tumor (malignant growth of the apex of the lung), and as mentioned previously, coronary disease. Some of these conditions will be ruled out or diagnosed by x-ray and others by a careful examination and interpretation of the history. All but a few of the remaining lesions can be eliminated if the criteria mentioned as diagnostic of a herniated cervical disc are adhered to. Finally Pantopaque myelography may be necessary to confirm the diagnosis.

Disc herniations which compress the spinal cord have to be differentiated from other intraspinal masses that exert pressure on the cord anteriorly. Myelography will be necessary in these cases and the final diagnosis will frequently be made only at operation.

Treatment

A preliminary trial of conservative therapy should be instituted in cases of cervical nerve root compression due to a herniated disc or bony spur. If the symptoms are severe, bed rest, sedation, and halter traction of five to ten pounds may give relief. In milder cases a cervical collar for support and immobilization can be tried. Some cases with acute onset and all the signs and symptoms of a herniated disc will clear up spontaneously, without treatment, except rest, in a period of a few weeks. Patients with severe intractable pain who are not satisfactorily benefited by conservative treatment are candidates for surgery.

Patients with signs of spinal cord compression or with a motor or significant sensory deficit from root compression as a result of a herniated disc, should be treated surgically without delay.

In patients with symptoms of cervical nerve root compression, analysis made by 23 out of 34 members of the AANS showed that 80 to 90 percent of their cases improved sufficiently with conservative

916

measures to obviate surgery. Spurling (1956) reported excellent or good results in 131 out of a total of 184 cases (71 percent) of ruptured cervical disc treated conservatively. DePalma and Rothman (1970) state that "the majority of patients with cervical disc disease, either acute or chronic, will respond to a conscientious program of conservative therapy."

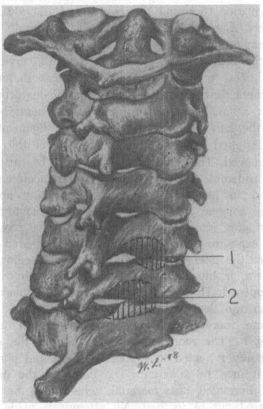

FIG. 19. DRAWING OF THE CERVICAL VERTEBRAE TO SHOW THE AREAS OF BONE REMOVED IN THE SURGICAL APPROACH TO A LATERAL HERNIATION FROM A CERVICAL INTERVERTEBRAL DISC

1. shows the bone removed in exposing a herniation between the 5th and 6th cervical vertebrae on the right side and 2. bone removal in approaching the disc between C6 and C7.

Operative Technique for Removal of a Lateral Herniation Compressing the Nerve Root. The operative approach consists of a partial hemilaminectomy as shown in Fig. 19. Local or general endotracheal anesthesia, preferably the latter, is used. The operation can be performed with the patient in the sitting position, or prone in the usual

917

position for cervical laminectomy. The upright position is favored by many surgeons. A 2-to 3-inch incision is made in the mid-line of the back of the neck centering over the interspace to be explored. The incision is carried to the tips of the underlying spinous processes, and the muscles are stripped laterally by subperiosteal dissection on the side of the herniation, exposing the laminae of the fifth, sixth, and seventh vertebrae. Care should be taken in identifying the correct interspace for exploration. Usually there is a pronounced bifurcation of the tip of the fifth cervical spine; the seventh cervical spine is the longest and most prominent, its tip being smooth and rounded. One may also count down from the prominent spinous process of C-2. With a rongeur a small amount of bone is now removed from the lower edge of the lamina above the lesion. The ligamentum flavum is then gently stripped from the anterior surface of this lamina and further bone removed. The removal of bone must be carried laterally to include a considerable portion of the articular facets and this may be accomplished in many ways (power drill, tiny angulated or Spurling-Kerrison rongeurs, etc). The exposed ligamentum flavum is now excised, bringing into view the underlying nerve root. To obtain more adequate exposure, some bone is usually rongeured away from the lamina below the interspace. Epidural venous bleeding is controlled with Gelfoam or bipolar coagulation. The sheath overlying the dural sleeve is opened. The nerve root as a rule is flattened and tense as it passes over the dome of the herniation which lies beneath it. It usually becomes more relaxed and less flattened after opening the sheath overlying it. The root is gently freed from the surrounding tissues and carefully retracted to expose the herniated portion of the disc to which it may be adherent. The dome of the protrusion is incised and all herniated disc material, which may be very small in quantity, teased out of its bed. No attempt is made to remove disc tissue from the depth of the intervertebral space, as is customary in the lumbar region. When the root is compressed by a bony spur in the foramen, it should be decompressed by unroofing the foramen as completely as possible (foraminotomy) and in certain cases the bony spur or osteophyte may be chiseled away or removed with the ingenious instruments devised by Mayfield (1957) and by Epstein et al (1969).

In recent years many neurosurgeons have used the anterior cervical approach originally reported by Raney about 1948, (Robinson and Smith, 1955; Cloward, 1958; Aronson et al, 1970) in the treatment

918

of nerve-root compression by herniated disc or bony protrusion. At present it is impossible, at least for the authors to determine whether the results with this procedure are as good as those with the posterior approach reported in the next paragraph. The difficulty in evaluating the reports of the good results obtained with the anterior approach is compounded by the fact that patients with solitary root compression from a herniated disc are often lumped together with cases having radiculopathy or myeloradiculopathy due to spondylosis. In a series of cases, specifically of soft cervical disc herniation operated upon by the anterior route, Aronson et al (1970) reported 90 to 100 percent improvement in 23 (65 percent) and 50 to 75 percent improvement in 12 (35 percent).

Prognosis

The prognosis in the treatment of radiculopathy by the posterior approach, especially where a soft herniation is present, has been reported in the literature as uniformly good to excellent (Scoville et al, 1951 and 1966; Davis et al, 1953; Spurling, 1956; Odom et al, 1958; Haft and Shenkin, 1963; Murphey and Simmons, 1966); 21 of 27 neurosurgeons (AANS) stated that their results were either good or excellent in 70 to 100 percent: only two surgeons had "poor" results in 5 percent and one in 10 percent. When the root was compressed by bone the results were less impressive and here the anterior approach may have a place. This may also be true in those patients whose only complaint is pain in the neck. Anterior fusion may. relieve such pain but it should be kept in mind that it puts an added stress on the discs above and below the operative level.

CERVICAL MYELOPATHY AND MYELORADICULOPATHY

Compression of the spinal cord in the cervical region may occur as a result of a central herniation of an intervertebral disc. A much more common cause is cervical spondylosis. The importance of spondylosis in the production of cervical myelopathy and radiculomyelopathy has become increasingly evident in recent years (Brain and Wilkinson, 1967; Smith, 1968; Wilkinson, 1971). The onset of symptoms in cases of disc prolapse may be abrupt or insidious, whereas the clinical picture associated with cervical spondylosis is generally one of gradual onset and progression (Lees and Turner, 1963).

In cases of myelopathy due to spondylosis, there is usually flattening of the cord. Hughes (1966) has stated: "All cases with mye-lopathy show deformity due to indentation of the spinal cord by spon-dylotic protrusions but indentation may occasionally occur without any clinical or pathological evidence of myelopathy." There is fre-quently demyelination of the lateral and posterior columns with cell damage and loss in the gray matter. Cavitation may occur.

The cause of the pathological changes in the spinal cord resulting from spondylosis is the subject of much controversy (Hughes, 1966). Some authors have felt that mechanical compression of the spinal cord by bony ridges or bars may occur (Wilkinson, 1960), perhaps because the cord is "anchored" in close proximity to these ridges by the dentate ligaments and nerve roots (Frykholm, 1951; Kahn, 1947; Wilkinson, 1960) and, as a result, recurrent minor traumas to the cord may take place on extension or possibly flexion of the neck (Allen, 1952; Logue, 1959).

The fact that the cord often shows no sign of compression at operation plus evidence that the level of the neurologic dysfunction may not correspond to that of the spondylotic lesion suggests that a vascular component is important. Brain (1956) thought that the earliest changes were due to compression of veins. Some have considered involvement of the anterior spinal artery to be the cause but others point out that this does not explain the anatomic distribution of the degenerative changes. It has also been suggested that compression of the radicular arteries may contribute to cord ischemia (Brain and Wilkinson, 1967; Smith, 1968).

Based on animal experiments Shimomura et al (1968) concluded that ischemic myelopathy depends upon involvement of the blood vessels of the surface of the spinal cord, including the anterior and dorsolateral spinal arteries, the medullary components of the radicular arteries and the pial plexus.

Symptoms and Signs

The neurologic manifestations of cervical spondylosis result from involvement of nerve roots and/or the spinal cord. As a rule the clinical picture is characterized by an insidious onset and progressive course. There may be radicular pain together with dysesthesiae and weakness corresponding to the nerve root or roots affected. Fre-quently the initial symptoms include numbness and tingling together with clumsiness of the hands and weakness of the lower limbs. Atrophy may involve the intrinsic hand muscles at times as well as the spinati, deltoid, biceps, and triceps muscles. Occasionally fasciculations are present. The deep reflexes are generally exaggerated in the legs and may be either diminished or hyperactive in the arms depending upon the level and degree of root or anterior horn and pyramidal tract involvement. Sensory impairment is variable and may be present in the lower extremities as well as in the upper limbs and involve proprioception as well as touch, pain, and temperature perception. Sphincter control is usually preserved. Pain in the neck is not invariably present. Symptoms indicative of vertebro-basilar insufficiency may occur.

Radiology of Cervical Spondylosis

Spondylosis is a common degenerative disorder which usually begins in middle age and most often remains asymptomatic. Among the characteristic findings are narrowing of one or more intervertebral disc spaces together with varying degrees of sclerosis and osteophytosis affecting the adjacent vertebrae. There may be anterior, posterior and posterolateral osteophytes. The anterior osteophytes may be very large and may buttress the bodies against movement. The posterolateral osteophytes may project into foramina and encroach upon nerve roots, while posterior osteophytes may protrude into the spinal canal and compress the spinal cord. Laterally placed anterior osteophytes can impinge upon the vertebral arteries. The anteroposterior diameter of the spinal canal is an important factor in determining the effects of cervical spondylosis on the spinal cord.

Myelography in Spondylosis

Myelography with 6 to 9 cc of Pantopaque is useful in diagnosis and in determining the level of the lesion, or lesions, prior to surgery. The defects in spondylosis are extradural and either lateral or central, single or multiple. The lateral defect may be merely lack of filling of a root sleeve or else a large round protrusion. The anterior filling defect ranges from a slight indentation of the cord centrally or across the width of the disc to a complete block (Fig. 20 a, b, c).

Discography employing a radiopaque contrast medium has been utilized by some in the diagnosis of cervical disc disease (Cloward, 1958; Klafta and Collis, 1969; Walker, 1958) and has been stated

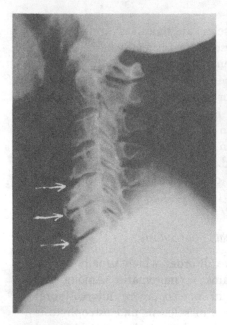
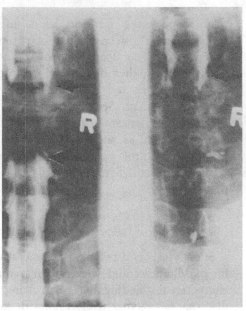

a   b   c

FIG. 20. An example of spondlylosis of the cervical spine with narrowing of the I.V. disc and hypertrophic changes at C 4-5, C 5-6, and C 6-7. There was a hypertrophic bony ridge across the canal with marked foraminal encroachment at all three levels. Clinically the patient had evidence of severe cervical spinal cord involvement plus root compression, manifested by advanced atrophy of the intrinsic muscles of both hands. b and c. The myelogram demonstrated an almost complete block in the flow of Pantopaque at the C 6-7 level in the head-down position (b) and also a similar block at C 4-5 with the patient erect (c).

to be very helpful at the time of operation in localizing the space to be fused when the anterior approach is used (Riley et al, 1969). The interpretation of the findings may be difficult, however, and the procedure has not gained widespread acceptance. Most surgeons are skeptical of its value, and prefer to be guided by the clinical history, examination and myelographic data.

For an account of the technique of cervical discography the reader is referred to the articles by Cloward (1958) and Klafta and Collis (1969).

922

Treatment

Medical treatment is primarily intended to alleviate pain and discomfort in the neck and upper limbs. Bed rest, local heat, and cervical traction together with sedatives and analgesics may be employed for the relief of acute pain. Immobilization by means of a collar with the neck in the neutral or slightly flexed position is often helpful in more chronic cases. Painful muscle spasm may be relieved by heat and massage. Patients with radicular pain who fail to respond to an adequate trial of conservative treatment require operative decompression of the involved roots. Surgical treatment is also indicated in cases of myelopathy with progressive deterioration of neurologic function.

In cases in which progressive cord compression or myeloradiculopathy has resulted from a midline disc herniation or cervical spondylosis, attempts to deal with the lesion by means of a laminectomy have not infrequently proved unsatisfactory. Removal of a central herniated disc involves opening the dura, sectioning several dentate ligaments and incising the anterior dura overlying the protrusion. Decompressive laminectomy for spondylotic myelopathy was at one time combined with division of the dentate ligaments, but the current trend is not to open the dura. Frequently a foraminotomy is performed in conjunction with the laminectomy.

Because the disc protrusion or bony ridge lies anterior to the spinal cord, the anterior approach seemed a logical one and has been used by many surgeons (Brain and Wilkinson, 1967; Cloward, 1958; Riley et al, 1969; Robinson and Smith, 1955; Rosomoff and Rossman, 1966; Smith and Robinson, 1958).

Technique: Detailed accounts of the anterior cervical approach for the removal of ruptured intervertebral discs or osteophytes and vertebral body fusion are available in the publications of Smith and Robinson (1958) and of Cloward (1958). Through an incision in a skin crease to one side of the midline of the neck, usually at about the level of the cricoid cartilage, a plane of cleavage is established between the sternomastoid and paratracheal muscles. The dissection is continued between the carotid sheath laterally and the trachea and esophagus medially, these structures retracted, and the anterior cervical spine exposed. Identification of the appropriate interspace is assured by means of a lateral roentgenogram. The annulus is incised and the disc removed. Utilizing the Cloward technique a hole is

923

drilled between the vertebral bodies and the remaining disc material excised together with spurs from the intervertebral foramina and spinal canal by means of curettes and rongeurs. A dowel cut from the iliac crest or obtained from a bone bank is inserted into the opening to achieve a fusion of the vertebral bodies.

Complications include esophageal trauma, shoulder pain, post-operative hemorrhage, injury to the carotid or vertebral arteries, bone graft displacement, collapse and absorption, recurrent laryngeal nerve damage, wound infection, perforation of the pleura, and nerve root and spinal cord injury (Cloward, 1971).

The results reported in the past few years have varied from 100 percent improvement to 17 percent (Galera and Tovi, 1968). In a recent analysis of 90 anterior cervical discectomies combined with interbody fusion performed for spondylotic radiculopathy, Jacobs et al (1970) reported good to excellent results in 82 percent of patients (51) who returned for follow-up examination two to seven years after operation. Utilizing the anterior cervical spine fusion technique of Robinson and Smith at one or more levels, good to excellent results were achieved by Riley et al (1969) in 72 percent of 93 patients with pain in the neck and upper extremity; posterior neck discomfort was the most common symptom in this group. On the other hand, in a careful study of 46 patients in whom the Cloward procedure of anterior removal of the spondylotic ridge followed by fusion was used in the treatment of cervical spondylosis causing serious neurologic disturbances (root compression and/or cord compression) Galera and Tovi (1968), reported satisfactory results in only 17 percent and poor results in 83 percent one to two years after surgery. In fact they stated that in cases with a classical picture of cervical spondylosis associated with evidence of both cord and root compression (41 percent of their cases), this operation did not halt the progression of the neurologic signs and symptoms. More favorable results of varying degree have been reported by others (Aronson et al, 1968; Cloward, 1963; Connolly, 1966; Herzberger et al, 1963; Robinson et al, 1962; Rosomoff and Rossman, 1966).

In view of these discrepancies, the posterior approach may be more promising in cases with severe myeloradiculopathy (Brain, 1956), especially if an extensive laminectomy with bilateral partial or complete facetectomy (foraminotomy) and uncapping of the root sleeves is employed, as described by Scoville (1961). This would be particularly applicable in cases in which the spondylotic changes involved

924

multiple levels and in which the spinal canal was congenitally narrow. A recently published follow-up study by Bishara (1971) confirms this impression. Of 59 patients who underwent the posterior operation for cervical spondylosis with myelopathy, 36 patients were initially improved; 5 years after operation 33 patients were still improved and 10 years following surgery 30 continued to maintain their initial improvement.

Epstein et al (1969) drew attention to the disagreement regarding the management of cervical spondylotic myeloradiculopathy by pointing out the increasing number of procedures advocated (Brain et al, 1952; Clarke and Robinson, 1956; Crandall and Batzdorf, 1966; Epstein et al, 1963; Fager, 1969; Haft and Shenkin, 1963; Logue, 1959; Stoops and King, 1965). Like others they note that the anterior approach does not allow treatment of problems related to the size of the spinal canal and the posterior elements and believe that the ideal operation should relieve the spinal cord and nerve roots from pressures in all quadrants, including those exerted centrally by osteophytes (Allen, 1952; Epstein et al, 1963; Mayfield, 1965), and dorsally by infolded yellow ligaments, laminae, or osteophytes on the facets. They believe that extensive unroofing of the entire cervical canal to disengage the cord from centrally situated osteophytes does not solve the problem of nerve root entrapment caused by foraminal osteophytes. As a result they suggest circumferential decompression of the spinal cord and nerve roots by laminectomy and foraminotomy augmented by the removal of ridges and spurs from the floor and foramina of the spinal canal with special curettes and rasps. This is the ideal procedure but so far, unfortunately, in the experience of many neurosurgeons, the adequate removal of anterior ridges and spurs has not always been possible without damage to neural structures.

The current status of the surgical treatment of cervical spondylosis with myelopathy is well reviewed in the article by Symon (1971).

SUMMARY

When conservative measures have failed, the surgical treatment of nerve root compression by a lateral herniated disc in the cervical region has been highly satisfactory using the posterior approach. This has apparently also been true with the anterior approach. When the root is compressed by a bony spur or osteophyte, the results have been good but less impressive. On the other hand, it appears that in

925

many cases we do not as yet have the answer to the adequate treatment of myeloradiculopathy caused by an anteriorly placed cervical herniated disc or by spondylosis, especially when multiple levels are involved.

BIBLIOGRAPHY

Adson, A. W. Chronic Recurring Sciatica; Diagnosis and Treatment of Protrusions of Ruptured Intervertebral Disks. *Arch. Phys. Therapy,* 20, 325, 1939.

Adson, A. W. and Ott, W. O. Results of the Removal of Tumors of the Spinal Cord. *Arch. Neur. Psychiat.,* 8, 520, 1922.

Alajouanine, T., and Petit-Dutaillis, D. Le nodule fibrocartilagineux de la face postérieure des disques intervertébraux. Etude anatomique et pathogénique d'une variété nouvelle de compression radiculomédullaire extradurale. *Presse Méd.,* 38, 1657, 1930.

Alajouanine, T., and Petit-Dutaillis, D. Compression de la queue de cheval par une tumeur du disque intervertébral; opération; guérison; présentation du malade. *Bull. et mém. Soc. Nat. de chir.,* 54, 1452, 1928.

Allen, K. L. Neuropathies Caused by Bony Spurs in the Cervical Spine with Reference to Surgical Treatment. *J. Neurol. Neurosurg. Psychiatry,* 15, 20, 1952.

Andrae, R. Ueber Knorpelknötchen am hinteren Ende der Wirbelbandscheiben im Bereich des Spinalkanals. *Beitr. z. path. Anat. u. allg. Path.,* 82, 464, 1929.

Arbuckle, R. K., Shelden, C. H., and Pudenz, R. Pantopaque Myelography; Correlation of Roentgenelogic and Neurologic Findings. *Radiology,* 45, 356, 1945.

Armstrong, J. R. The Causes of Unsatisfactory Results from the Operative Treatment of Lumbar Disc Lesions. *J. Bone Joint Surg.,* 33-B, 31, 1951.

Armstrong, J. R. *Lumbar Disc Lesions. Pathogenesis and Treatment of Low Back Pain and Sciatica.* 3rd. ed. Edinburgh: E. and S. Livingstone, 1965.

Aronson, H. A. and Dunsmore, R. H. Herniated Upper Lumbar Discs. *J. Bone Joint Surg.,* 45-A, 311, 1963.

Aronson, N., Bagan, M., and Filtzer, D. L. Results of Using the Smith-Robinson Approach for Herniated and Extruded Cervical Discs. *J. Neurosurg.,* 32, 721, 1970.

Aronson, N., Filtzer, D. L., and Bagan, M. Anterior Cervical Fusion by the Smith-Robinson Approach. *J. Neurosurg.,* 29, 397, 1968.

Bardeen, C. R. The Development of the Thoracic Vertebrae in Man. *Am. J. Anat.,* 4, 163, 1905.

Barr, J. S. "Sciatica" Caused by Intervertebral Disc Lesions: A Report of Forty Cases of Rupture of the Intervertebral Disc Occurring in the Low Lumbar Spine and Causing Pressure on the Cauda Equina. *J. Bone Joint Surg.,* 19, 323, 1937.

926

Barr, J. S. Ruptured Intervertebral Disc and Sciatic Pain. *J. Bone Joint Surg.*, 29, 425, 1947.

Barr, J. S. and Mixter, W. J. Posterior Protrusions of the Lumbar Intervertebral Discs. *J. Bone Joint.*, 23, 444, 1941.

Barr, J. S., Kubik, C. S., Molloy, M. K., McNeill, J. M., Riseborough, E. J., and White, J. C. Evaluation of End Results in Treatment of Ruptured Lumbar Intervertebral Discs With Protrusion of Nucleus Pulposus. *Surg. Gynec. Obstet.*, 125, 250, 1967.

Beadle, O. A. The Intervertebral Discs: Observations on Their Normal and Morbid Anatomy in Relation to Certain Spinal Deformities. *Medical Research Council. Special report series, No. 161.* London: His Majesty's Stationery Office, 1931.

Begg, A. C., Falconer, M. A., and McGeorge, M. Myelography in Lumbar Intervertebral Disk Lesions; A Correlation of Operative Findings. *Br. J. Surg.*, 34, 141, 1946.

Bishara, S. N. The Posterior Operation in Treatment of Cervical Spondylosis with Myelopathy: A Long-term Follow-up Study. *J. Neurol. Neurosurg. Psychiatry*, 34, 393, 1971.

Böhmig, R. Die Blutgefässversorgung der Wirbelbandscheiben, das Verhalten des Intervertebralen, Chordasegments und die Bedeutung beider für die Bandscheibendegeneration. *Arch. f. klin. Chir.*, 158, 374, 1930.

Botterell, E. H., Keith, W. S., and Stewart, O. W. Results of Surgical Treatmen of Sciatica due to Herniation of Intervertebral Disc in Canadian Soldiers Overseas. *Can. Med. Assn. J.*, 51, 210, 1944.

Bradford, F. K. and Spurling, R. G. *The Intervertebral Disc with Special Reference to Rupture of the Annulus Fibrosus with Herniation of the Nucleus Pulposus.* Springfield, Ill.: Chas. C Thomas, 1941.

Bradford, F. K. and Spurling, R. G. *The Intervertebral Disc.* Second ed. Springfield, Illinois: Chas. C Thomas, 1945.

Bradford, F. K. Ruptured Intervertebral Disc in the Industrial Patient: Diagnosis, Surgical Management, and Prognosis. *Tex. J. Med.*, 56, 274, 1960.

Brain, R. Some Aspects of the Neurology of the Cervical Spine. *J. Fac. Radiol.*, 8, 74, 1956.

Brain, W. R., Northfield, D., and Wilkinson, M. The Neurologic Manifestations of Cervical Spondylosis. *Brain*, 75, 187, 1952.

Brain, W. R. and Wilkinson, M. *Cervical Spondylosis and Other Disorders of the Cervical Spine.* Philadelphia: W. B. Saunders Co., 1967.

Brown, H. A. Low Back Pain with Special Reference to Dislocation of the Intervertebral Disc and Hypertrophy of the Ligamentum Flavum. *West. J. Surg.*, 45, 527, 1937.

Brown, H. A. and Pont, M. E. Disease of Lumbar Discs. *J. Neurosurg.*, 20, 410, 1963.

Bucy, P. C. Chondroma of the Intervertebral Disk. *J.A.M.A.*, 94, 1552, 1930.

Bucy, P. C. Neuroanatomical and Neurosurgical Aspects of Herniated Intervertebral Discs. *Instruct. Lect. Am. Ac. Orthop. Surg.*, 18, 21, 1961.

Bucy, P. C. and Chenault, H. Compression of Seventh Cervical Nerve Root by Herniation of Intervertebral Disc. *J.A.M.A.*, 126, 26, 1944.

Bucy, P. C. and Oberhill, H. R. The Diagnosis and Treatment of Herniated Lumbar Intervertebral Discs. *Chicago Med., 66,* 201, 1963.

Burrows, E. H. The Sagittal Diameter of the Spinal Canal in Cervical Spondylosis. *Clin. Radiol., 14,* 77, 1963.

Calvé, J., and Galland, M. Le nucleus pulposus intervertébral; son anatomie, sa physiologie, sa pathologie. *Presse Méd., 38,* 520, 1930.

Calvé, J. and Galland, M. The Intervertebral Nucleus Pulposus: Its Anatomy, Its Physiology, Its Pathology. *J. Bone Joint Surg., 12,* 555, 1930.

Camera, U. Escursione attraverso la patologia del disco intervertebrale. *Boll. e mem. Soc. Piemontese di chir., 4,* 142, 1934.

Camp, J. D. The Roentgenologic Diagnosis of Intraspinal Protrusion of Intervertebral Disks by Means of Radiopaque Oil. *J.A.M.A., 113,* 2024, 1939.

Childe, A. E. The Role of X-ray in the Diagnosis of Posterior Herniation of the Intervertebral Disc. *Can. Med. Assn. J., 52,* 458, 1945.

Clarke, E. and Robinson, P. K. Cervical Myelopathy. A Complication of Cervical Spondylosis. *Brain, 79,* 483, 1956.

Cloward, R. B. The Anterior Approach for Removal of Ruptured Cervical Disks. *J. Neurosurg., 15,* 602, 1958.

Cloward, R. B. Cervical Diskography. Technique, Indications and Use in the Diagnosis of Ruptured Cervical Disks. *Am. J. Roent., 79,* 563, 1958.

Cloward, R. B. Discussion of Paper by Collis, J. S. and Gardner, W. J. Lumbar Discography; an Analysis of 1000 Cases. *J. Neurosurg., 19,* 452, 1962.

Cloward, R. B. Lesions of the Intervertebral Disks and Their Treatment by Interbody Fusion Methods. The Painful Disk. *Clin. Orthoped., 27,* 51, 1963.

Cloward, R. B. Complications of Anterior Cervical Disc Operation and Their Treatment. *Surgery, 69,* 175, 1971.

Clymer, G., Mixter, W. J., and Mella, H. Experience with Spinal Cord Tumors During the Past Ten Years. *Arch. Neur. Psychiat., 5,* 213, 1921.

Collis, J. S., Jr. Lumbar Discography. Springfield, Ill.: Charles C Thomas, 1963.

Collis, J. S. and Gardner, W. J. Lumbar Discography; an Analysis of 1000 Cases. *J. Neurosurg., 19,* 452, 1962.

Compere, E. L. Origin, Anatomy, Physiology and Pathology of the Intervertebral Disc. *Instruc. Lect. Amer. Acad. Orthop. Surg., 18,* 15, 1961.

Connolly, E. S., Seymour, R. J., and Adams, J. E. Clinical Evaluation of Anterior Cervical Fusion for Degenerative Cervical Disc Disease. *J. Neurosurg., 25,* 57, 1966.

Coventry, M. B., Ghormley, R. K., and Kernohan, J. G. The Intervertebral Disc: Its Microscopic Anatomy and Pathology. Part I. Anatomy, Development and Physiology. *J. Bone Joint Surg., 27,* 105, 1945. Part II. Changes in the Intervertebral Disc Concomittant with Age. *J. Bone Joint Surg., 27,* 233, 1945.

Craig, W. M. and Walsh, M. N. Diagnosis and Treatment of Low Back and Sciatic Pain Caused by Protruded Intervertebral Disk and Hypertrophied Ligaments. *Minnesota Med., 22,* 511, 1939.

Craig, W. M. and Walsh, M. N. Neuro-anatomical and Physiological Aspects and Significance of Sciatica *J. Bone Joint Surg., 23,* 417, 1941.

Craig, W. M. and Witt, J. A. Cervical Disk, Shoulder-Arm-Hand Syndrome. *Postgrad. Med., 17,* 267, 1955.

928

Grandall, P. H. and Batzdorf, U. Cervical Spondylotic Myelopathy. *J. Neurosurg.*, 25, 57, 1966.

Dandy, W. E. Loose Cartilage from Intervertebral Disk Simulating Tumor of the Spinal Cord. *Arch. Surg.*, 19, 660, 1929.

Dandy, W. E. Concealed Ruptured Intervertebral Disks; Plea for Elimination of Contrast Medium in Diagnosis. *J.A.M.A.*, 117, 821, 1941.

Davidson, E. A. and Woodhall, B. Biochemical Alterations in Herniated Intervertebral Discs. *J. Biol. Chem.*, 234, 2951, 1959.

Davis, A. G. Symposium on the Intervertebral Disc. Introduction. *J. Bone Joint Surg.*, 29, 425, 1947.

Davis, C. H., Odom, G. L., and Woodhall, B. Survey of Ruptured Intervertebral Disks in the Cervical Region. *N. C. Med. J.*, 14, 61, 1953.

DePalma, A. F. and Rothman, R. H. *The Intervertebral Disc.* Philadelphia: W. B. Saunders Co., 1970.

DePuky, P. The Physiological Oscillation of the Length of the Body. *Acta Orthop. Scand.*, 6, 338, 1935.

Deucher, W. G. and Love, J. G. Pathologic Aspects of Posterior Protrusions of the Intervertebral Disks. *Arch. Path.*, 27, 201, 1939.

Donohue, W. L. Pathology of the Intervertebral Disc. *Am. J. M. Sci.*, 198, 419, 1939.

Dursy, E. *Zur Entwicklungsgeschichte des Kopfes des Menschen und der höheren Wirbelthiere.* Tübingen: H. Laupp, 1869.

Echlin, F. A., Ivie, J. M., and Fine, A. Pantopaque Myelography as an Aid in the Preoperative Diagnosis of Protruded Intervertebral Discs: A Preliminary Report, *Surg., Gynec. & Obstet.*, 80, 257, 1945.

Echlin, F. A., Selverstone, B., and Scribner, W. E. Bilateral and Multiple Ruptured Discs as One Cause of Persistent Symptoms Following Operation for a Herniated Disc. *Surg., Gynec. & Obstet.*, 83, 485, 1946.

Echols, D. H. Radicular Pain Due to Ruptured Cervical Disk. *South. Surgeon*, 12, 205, 1946.

Elsberg, C. A. *Diagnosis and Treatment of Surgical Diseases of the Spinal Cord and its Membranes.* Philadelphia and London: W. B. Saunders Co., 1916.

Elsberg, C. A. *Tumors of the Spinal Cord and the Symptoms of Irritation and Compression of the Spinal Cord and Nerve Roots.* New York: Paul B. Hoeber, 1925.

Elsberg, C. A. The Extradural Ventral Chondromas (Ecchondroses), Their Favorite Sites, the Spinal Cord and Root Symptoms They Produce, and Their Surgical Treatment. *Bull. Neurol. Inst. New York*, 1, 350, 1931.

Epstein, B. S. *The Spine*, 3rd. ed. Philadelphia: Lea and Febiger, 1969.

Epstein, J. A. and Davidoff, L. M. Chronic Hypertrophic Spondylosis of the Cervical Spine with Compression of the Spinal Cord and Nerve Roots. *Surg. Gynec. & Obstet.*, 93, 27, 1951.

Epstein, J. A., Epstein, B. S., and Lavine, L. S. Nerve Root Compression Associated with Narrowing of the Lumbar Spinal Canal. *J. Neurol. Neurosurg. Psychiat.*, 25, 165, 1962.

Epstein, J. A., Epstein, B. S., and Lavine L. S. Cervical Spondylotic Myelopathy;

929

the Syndrome of the Narrow Canal Treated by Laminectomy, Foraminotomy and the Removal of Osteophytes. *Arch. Neurol.*, *8*, 307, 1963.

Epstein, J. A., Lavine, L. S., and Epstein, B. S. Recurrent Herniation of the Lumbar Intervertebral Disk. *Clin. Orthopaedics*, *52*, 169, 1967.

Epstein, J. A., Carras, R., Lavine, L. S., and Epstein, B. S. The Importance of Removing Osteophytes as Part of the Surgical Treatment of Myeloradiculopathy in Cervical Spondylosis. *J. Neurosurg.*, *30*, 219, 1969.

Fager, C. A. Reversal of Cervical Myelopathy by Adequate Posterior Decompression. *Lahey Clin. Found. Bull.*, *18*, 99, 1969.

Feiring, E. H. Extruded Thoracic Intervertebral Disk. *Arch. Surg.*, *95*, 135, 1967.

Ferlic, D. C. The Nerve Supply of the Cervical Intervertebral Disc in Man. *Bull. J. Hopkins Hosp.*, *113*, 347, 1963.

Fernstrom, U. A Discographical Study of Ruptured Lumbar Intervertebral Discs. *Acta Chir. Scand., Suppl.*, *258*, 1, 1960.

Fincher, E. F. Neurologic Aspects of Low Back Pain and Sciatica. *Ann. Surg.*, *109*, 1028, 1939.

Fincher, E. F. and Walker, E. B. Sciatica and Low Back Pain: A Study of 31 Consecutive Cases in Which 24 Were Due to Displaced Intervertebral Cartilage. *South. Surgeon*, *7*, 97, 1938.

Fisher, R. G. Protrusions of Thoracic Disc. The Factor of Herniation Through the Dura Mater. *J. Neurosurg.*, *22*, 591, 1965.

Flax, H. J., Berrios, R., and Rivera, D. Electromyography in the Diagnosis of Herniated Lumbar Disc. *Arch. Phys. Med.*, *45*, 520, 1964.

Ford, L. T., Holscher, E. C., Stokes, J. M., Thibodeau, A. A., and Morgan, H. C. Symposium: Complications of Lumbar-disc Surgery, Prevention and Treatment. *J. Bone Joint Surg.*, *50-A*, 382-428, 1968.

French, J. D. Clinical Manifestations of Lumbar Spinal Arachnoiditis. *Surgery*, *20*, 718, 1946.

Friberg, S. and Hirsch, C. Anatomical and Chemical Studies on Lumbar Disc Degeneration. *Acta Orthop. Scand.*, *19*, 222, 1949.

Frykholm, R. Cervical Nerve Root Compression Resulting From Disc Degeneration and Root-Sleeve Fibrosis. A Clinical Investigation. *Acta Chir. Scand., Suppl.*, *102*, 158, 1951.

Furlow, L. T. Herniation of the Nucleus Pulposus of the Intervertebral Disc. *Tri-State Med. J.*, *10*, 2073, 1938.

Galera, G. R. and Tovi, D. Anterior Disc Excision with Interbody Fusion in Cervical Spondylotic Myelopathy and Rhizopathy. *J. Neurosurg.*, *28*, 305, 1968.

Gartland, J. J. Judgment in Lumbar Disc Surgery. *Orthop. Clin. North Am.*, *2*, 507, 1971.

Goldthwait, J. E. The Lumbosacral Articulation: An Explanation of Many Cases of "Lumbago," "Sciatica," and Paraplegia. *Boston Med. & Surg. J.*, *164*, 365, 1911.

Gray, H. *Anatomy, Descriptive and Surgical.* London: John W. Parker & Son, 1858.

Grant, F. C. Operative Results in Intervertebral Discs. *J. Neurosurg.*, *1*, 332, 1944.

Grant, W. T. and Cone, W. V. Graduated Juuglar Compression in the Lumbar

Manometric Test for Spinal Subarachnoid Block. *Arch. Neurol. Psych.*, *32*, 1194, 1934.

Gurdjian, E. S, Ostrowski, A. Z., Hardy, W. G., Lindner, D. W., and Thomas, L. M. Results of Operative Treatment of Protruded and Ruptured Lumbar Discs (1176 Cases with 82% Follow-up of Three to Thirteen Years). *J. Neurosurg.*, *18*, 783, 1961.

Gurdjian, E. S., Webster, J. E., Ostrowski, A. Z., Hardy, W. G., Lindner, D. W., and Thomas, L. M. Herniated Lumbar Intervertebral Discs — An Analysis of 1176 Operated Cases. *J. Trauma, 1*, 158, 1961.

Haft, H. and Shenkin, H. A. Surgical End Results of Cervical Ridge and Disk Problems. *J.A.M.A., 186*, 312, 1963.

Haft, H.˙and Shenkin, H. A. Herniated Lumbar Intervertebral Disks with Unilateral Pain and Midline Myelographic Defects. *Surgery, 60*, 269, 1966.

Hampton, A. O. and Robinson, J. M. The Roentgenographic Demonstration of Rupture of the Intervertebral Disk into the Spinal Canal after the Injection of Lipiodol with Special Reference to Unilateral Lumbar Lesions Accompanied by Low Back Pain with "Sciatic" Radiation. *Am. J. Roentgenol., 36*, 782, 1936.

Harmon, P. H. Congenital and Acquired Anatomic Variations Including Degenerative Changes of the Lower Lumbar Spine; Role in Production of Painful Back and Lower Extremity Syndromes. *Clin. Orthop., 44*, 171, 1966.

Hartley, J. Modern Concepts of Whiplash Injury. *N. Y. State J. Med., 58*, 3306, 1958.

Hawk, W. A. Spinal Compression Caused by Ecchondrosis of the Intervertebral Fibrocartilage with a Review of the Recent Literature. *Brain, 59*, 204, 1936.

Hendry, N. G. C. The Hydration of the Nucleus Pulposus and Its Relation to Intervertebral Disc Derangement. *J. Bone Joint Surg., 40-B*, 132, 1958.

Herzberger, E. E., Kindschi, L. G., Bear, N. E., and Chandler, A. Treatment of Cervical Disease and Cervical Spinal Injury by Anterior Interbody Fusion. A Report on Early Results in 72 Cases. *Zentbl. Neurochir., 23*, 215, 1963.

Hirsch, C. Efficiency of Surgery in Low Back Disorders. *J. Bone Joint Surg., 47A*, 991, 1965.

Hirsch, C. and Schajowicz, F. Studies on Structural Changes in Lumbar Annulus Fibrosus. *Acta Orthop. Scand., 22*, 184, 1953.

Hirsch, C., Ingelmark, B., and Miller, M. The Anatomical Basis for Low Back Pain. Studies on the Presence of Sensory Nerve Endings in Ligamentous, Capsular, and Intervertebral Disc Structures in the Human Lumbar Spine. *Acta Orthop. Scand., 33*, 1, 1963.

Horton, W. G. Further Observations on the Elastic Mechanism of the Intervertebral Disc. *J. Bone Joint Surg., 40-B*, 552, 1958.

Hughes, J. T. *Pathology of the Spinal Cord.* London: Lloyd Luke, 1966.

Hulme, A. The Surgical Approach to Thoracic Intervertebral Disc Protrusions. *J. Neurol. Neurosurg. Psychiatry, 23*, 133, 1960.

Hyndman, O. R. Pathologic Intervertebral Disc and Its Consequences; Contribution to Cause and Treatment of Chronic Pain Low in Back and to Subject of Herniating Intervertebral Disc. *Arch. Surg., 53*, 247, 1946.

Hyndman, O. R., Steindler, A., and Wolkin, J. Herniated Intervertebral Disk: A Study of the Iodized Oil Column. The Procaine Test in Differential

Diagnosis from Reflected Sciatic Pain. *J.A.M.A., 121,* 390, 1943.

Inman, V. T. and Saunders, J. B. de C. M. Anatomicophysiological Aspects of Injuries to the Intervertebral Disc. *J. Bone Joint Surg., 29,* 461, 1947.

Jackson, R. *The Cervical Syndrome.* 3rd. ed. Springfield, Ill.: Charles C Thomas, 1966.

Jacobs, B., Krueger E. G., and Lewy, D. M. Cervical Spondylosis with Radiculopathy. *J.A.M.A., 211,* 2135, 1970.

Joplin, R. J. The Intervertebral Disc: Embryology, Anatomy, Physiology, and Pathology. *Surg., Gynec. Obstet., 61,* 591, 1935.

Jung, A. and Brunschwig, A. Recherches histologiques sur l'innervation des corps vertébraux. *Presse méd., 40,* 316, 1932.

Kahn, E. A. The Role of the Dentate Ligaments in Spinal Cord Compression and the Syndrome of Lateral Sclerosis. *J. Neurosurg., 4,* 191, 1947.

Keyes, D. C. and Compere, E. L. The Normal and Pathological Physiology of the Nucleus Pulposus of the Intervertebral Disc. *J. Bone Joint Surg., 14,* 897, 1932.

Klafta, L. A. and Collis, J. S. An Analysis of Cervical Discography with Surgical Verification. *J. Neurosurg,. 30,* 38, 1969.

Kocher, T. (Quoted by Middleton and Teacher). Die Verletzungen der Wirbelsäule zugleich als Beitrag zur Physiologie des menschlichen Rückenmarks. *Mitt. a.d. Grenz. geb. d. Med. u. Chir., 1,* 420, 1896.

Kölliker, A. (Quoted by Keyes and Compere). Uber die Beziehungen der Chorda dorsalis zur Bildung der Wirbel der Selachier und einiger andern Fische. *Verhandl. d. phys.-med. Gessellsch., 10,* 193, 1860.

Kubik, C. S. and Hampton, A. O. Removal of Iodized Oil by Lumbar Puncture. *New Engl. J. Med., 224,* 455, 1941.

Kristoff, F. V. and Odom, G. L. Ruptured Intervertebral Disk in the Cervical Region. A Report of 20 Cases. *Arch. Surg., 54,* 287, 1947.

Lasègue, C. Considérations sur la sciatique. *Archives Générales de Médicine, 2,* 558, 1864.

Lees, F. and Turner, J. W. A. Natural History and Prognosis of Cervical Spondylosis. *Br. Med. J., 2,* 1607, 1963.

Lenhard, R. E. End Result Study of the Intervertebral Disc. *J. Bone Joint Surg., 29,* 425, 1947.

Lindblom, K. Diagnostic Puncture of Intervertebral Disks in Sciatica. *Acta Orthop. Scand., 17,* 231, 1948.

Logue, V. Cervical Spondylosis. R. Nassim and H. J. Burrows (Eds.) *Modern Trends in Diseases of the Vertebral Column.* New York: Paul B. Hoeber, 1959.

Love, J. G. Protrusion of the Intervertebral Disk (Fibrocartilage) into the Spinal Canal. *Proc. Staff Meet., Mayo Clin., 11,* 529, 1936.

Love, J. G. Intractable Low Back Pain and Sciatic Pain due to Protruded Intervertebral Disks; Diagnosis and Treatment. *Minnesota Med., 21,* 832, 1938.

Love, J. G. Protruded Intervertebral Disks with a Note Regarding Hypertrophy of Ligamenta Flava. *J.A.M.A., 113,* 2029, 1939.

Love, J. G. Differential Diagnosis of Intraspinal Tumors and Protruded Discs and Their Surgical Treatment. *J. Neurosurg., 1,* 275, 1944.

932

Love, J. G. The Disc Factor in Low-back Pain with or without Sciatica. *J. Bone Joint Surg.*, *29*, 425, 1947.

Love, J. G. Intractable Pain in the Neck and Upper Extremities with Particular Reference to Protrusion of Cervical Disks. *N. C. Med. Jour.*, *12*, 274. 1951.

Love, J. G. and Camp, J. D. Root Pain Resulting from Intra-spinal Protrusion of Intervertebral Disks; Diagnosis and Surgical Treatment. *J. Bone Joint Surg.*, *19*, 776, 1937.

Love, J. G. and Walsh, M. N. Intraspinal Protrusions of Intervertebral Disks; A Report of 100 Cases in Which Operation was Performed. *J.A.M.A.*, *111*, 396, 1938.

Love, J. G. and Walsh, M. N. Intraspinal Protrusions of Intervertebral Disks. *Arch. Surg.*, *40*, 454, 1940.

Love, J. G. and Schorn, V. G. Thoracic-disc Protrusions. *J.A.M.A.*, *191*, 627, 1965.

Löwe, L. (Quoted by Keyes and Compere.) Zur Kenntniss der Säugetierchorda. *Arch. f. mikrosk. Anat.*, *16*, 597, 1897.

Maranacci, A. A. *Clinical Electromyography*. Los Angeles: San Lucas Press, 1955.

Mauric, G. Le disque intervertébral; pathologie, diagnostic et indications thérapeutic. Paris Thèses, Masson-Mayer, 1933.

Mayfield, F. H. Symposium on Cervical Trauma; Neurosurgical Aspects. *Clin. Neurosurg.*, *2*, 83, 1955.

Mayfield, F. H. New Instrument. *J. Neurosurg.*, *14*, 469, 1957.

Mayfield, F. H. Cervical spondylosis; A Comparison of the Anterior and Posterior Approaches. *Clin. Neurosurg.*, *13*, 181, 1965.

McGinnis, K. D. and Eisenbrey, A. B. Diagnostic Criteria for Distinguishing Cervical Disc Herniation from Spondylosis in the Neural Compression Syndrome. *Radiology*, *83*, 67, 1964.

McKenzie, K. G. and Botterell, E. H. The Common Neurological Syndromes Produced by Pressure from Extrusion of Intervertebral Disc. *Can. Med. Assn. J.*, *46*, 424, 1942.

Michelson, J. J. and Mixter, W. J. Pain and Disability of Shoulder and Arm due to Herniation of the Nucleus Pulposus of Cervical Intervertebral Disks. *New Engl. J. Med.*, *231*, 279, 1944.

Middleton, G. S. and Teacher, J. H. Injury of the Spinal Cord Due to Rupture of an Intervertebral Disc During Muscular Effort. *Glasgow M. J.*, *76*, 1, 1911.

Mitchell, P. E. G., Hendry, N. G. C., and Billewicz, W. Z. The Chemical Background of Intervertebral Disc Prolapse. *J Bone Joint Surg.*, *43-B*, 141, 1961.

Mixter, W. J. Rupture of the Intervertebral Disc. Chap. 16. P. 511-541. In A. Feiling (Ed.), *Modern Trends in Neurology*. New York: P. B. Hoeber, 1951.

Mixter, W. J. and Barr, J. S. Rupture of the Intervertebral Disk with Involvement of the Spinal Canal. *New Engl. J. Med.*, *211*, 210, 1934.

Mixter, W. J. and Ayer, J. B. Herniation or Rupture of the Intervertebral Disk into the Spinal Canal. *New Engl. J. Med.*, *213*, 385, 1935.

Morris, J. M., Lucas, D. B., and Bresler, B. Role of the Trunk in Stability of the Spine. *J. Bone Joint Surg.*, *43-A*, 327, 1961.

Munro, D. The Diagnosis of Posterior Herniation of the Lumbar Intervertebral Disks. *New Engl. J. Med.*, *232*, 149, 1945.

Murphey, F. and Simmons, J. C. H. Ruptured Cervical Disk: Experience with 250 Cases. *Am. Surgeon, 32,* 83, 1966.

Murphy, J. P. Lumbar Intervertebral Disc Protrusion Contralateral to the Side of Symptoms and Signs. *Am. J. Roentgenol., 61,* 77, 1949.

Nachemson, A. The Load on Lumbar Disks in Different Positions of the Body. *Clin. Orthop., 45,* 107, 1966.

Naffziger, H. C., Inman, V., and Saunders, J. B. de C. M. Lesions of the Intervertebral Disc and Ligamenta Flava: Clinical and Anatomical Studies. *Surg., Gynec., & Obstet., 66,* 288, 1938.

Naffziger, H. C. and Boldrey, E. B. Surgery of Spinal Cord. In F. W Bancroft and C. Pilcher, (Eds.) *Surgical Treatment of the Nervous System.* Philadelphia: J. B. Lippincott Co., 1946.

Naylor, A. The Biophysical and Biochemical Aspects of Intervertebral Disc Herniation and Degeneration. *Ann. Roy. Coll. Surg. Eng., 31,* 91, 1962.

Naylor, A. The Biochemical Changes in the Human Intervertebral Disc in Degeneration and Nuclear Prolapse. *Orthop. Clin. North Am., 2,* 343, 1971.

O'Connell, J. E. A. Indications for and Results of Excision of Lumbar Intervertebral Disc Protrusions; Review of 500 Cases. *Ann. Roy. Coll. Surg. Eng., 6,* 403, 1950.

Odom, G. L., Finney, W., and Woodhall, B. Cervical Disk Lesions. *J.A.M.A., 166,* 23, 1958.

Payne, E. E. and Spillane, J. D. The Cervical Spine. An Anatomicopathological Study of 70 Specimens (Using a Special Technique) with Particular Reference to the Problem of Cervical Spondylosis. *Brain, 80,* 571, 1957.

Pedersen, H. E., Blunck, C. F. J., and Gardner, E. The Anatomy of Lumbosacral Posterior Rami and Meningeal Branches of Spinal Nerves (Sinuvertebral Nerves) With an Experimental Study of Their Functions. *J. Bone Joint Surg., 38-A,* 377, 1956.

Peet, M. M. and Echols, D. H. Herniation of the Nucleus Pulposus. *Arch. Neurol. Psychiat., 32,* 924, 1934.

Pennal, G. F., and Schatzker, J. Stenosis of the Lumbar Spinal Canal. *Clinical Neurosurgery.* Vol. 18. Baltimore: Williams and Wilkins Co. P. 86-105, 1971.

Pennybacker, J. Sciatica and the Intervertebral Disc. *Lancet, 238,* 771, 1940.

Perot, P. L., Jr. and Munro, D. D. Transthoracic Removal of Midline Thoracic Disc Protrusions Causing Spinal Cord Compression. *J. Neurosurg., 31,* 452, 1969.

Peyton, W. T. and Simmons, D. R. Herniated Intervertebral Disk: Analysis of 90 Cases. *Arch. Surg., 55,* 271, 1947.

Plati, J. T., Strain, W. H., and Warren, S. L. Iodinated Organic Compounds as Contrast Media for Radiographic Diagnosis. II. Ethyl Esters of Iodinated Straight and Branched Chain Phenyl Fatty Acids. *J. Am. Chem. Soc., 65,* 1273, 1943.

Pool, J. L. Cervical Disc Syndrome. Differential Diagnosis and Management Based on 26 Operated Cases. *Bull. N. Y. Acad. Med., 29,* 47, 1953.

Poppen, J. L. Herniation of Intervertebral Disks. *Surg. Clin. North Am., 18,* 879, 1938.

Poppen, J. L. Herniated Disk: Analysis of 400 Verified Cases. *New Engl. J. Med., 232,* 211, 1945.

Prader, A. Die frühembryonal Entwicklung der Menschlichen Zwischenwirbelscheibe. *Acta Anat., 3,* 68, 1947 a.

Prader, A. Die Entwicklung der Zwischenwirbelscheibe beim Menschlichen Keimling. *Acta Anat., 3,* 115, 1947 b.

Püschel, J. Der Wassergehalt normaler und degenerierter Zwischenwirbelscheiben. *Beitr. z. path. Anat. u. z. allg. Path., 84,* 123, 1930.

Raaf, J. Discussion of Paper by Cloward, R. B.: Anterior Approach for Ruptured Cervical Disks. *J. Neurosurg., 15,* 614, 1958.

Raaf, J. Some Observations Regarding 905 Patients Operated upon for Protruded Lumbar Intervertebral Discs. *Am. J. Surg., 97,* 388, 1959.

Raaf, J. Removal of Protruded Lumbar Intervertebral Discs. *J. Neurosurg., 32,* 604, 1970.

Raney, R. The Similarity of Certain Cauda Equina Tumors to the Ruptured Intervertebral Disc. Read before the American Academy of Neurological Surgery, Battle Creek, September, 1943.

Raney. R. See Discussion by W. B. Scoville in R. B. Cloward: Anterior Approach for Ruptured Cervical Disks. *J. Neurosurg., 15,* 615, 1958.

Ransohoff, J., Spencer, F., Siew, F., and Gage, L., Jr. Transthoracic Removal of Thoracic Disc. Report of Three Cases. *J. Neurosurg., 31,* 459, 1969.

Ray, B. S. Differential Diagnosis between Ruptured Lumbar Intervertebral Discs and Certain Diseases of the Spinal and Peripheral Nervous System. *Surg. Clin. North Am.* (April) P. 272, 1946.

Reeves, D. L. and Brown, H. A. Thoracic Intervertebral Disc Protrusion with Spinal Cord Compression. *J. Neurosurg., 28,* 24, 1968.

Reid, J. D. Effects of Flexion-Extension Movements of the Head and Spine upon the Spinal Cord and Nerve Roots. *J. Neurol. Neurosurg. Psychiatry., 23,* 214, 1960.

Research Committee of Amer. Orthop. Assn.: End Result Study of the Treatment of Herniated Nucleus Pulposus by Excision with Fusion and without Fusion. *J. Bone Joint Surg., 34-A,* 981, 1952.

Riley, L. H., Robinson, R. A., Johnson, D. A., and Walker, A. E. The Results of Anterior Interbody Fusion of the Cervical Spine. Review of 93 Consecutive Cases. *J. Neurosurg., 30,* 127, 1969.

Rissanen, P. M. Comparison of Pathologic Changes in Intervertebral Discs and Interspinous Ligaments of the Lower Part of the Lumbar Spine in the Light of Autopsy Findings. *Acta Orthop. Scand., 34,* 54, 1964.

Robinson, R. A. and Smith, G. W. Antero-lateral Cervical Disc Removal and Interbody Fusion for Cervical Disc Syndrome. *Bull. J. Hopkins Hosp., 96,* 223, 1955.

Robinson, R. A., Walker, A. E., Ferlic, D. C., and Wiecking, D. K. The Results of Anterior Interbody Fusion of the Cervical Spine. *J. Bone Joint Surg., 44-A,* 1569, 1962.

Rogers, L. The Treatment of Cervical Spondylitic Myelopathy by Mobilization of the Cervical Cord into an Enlarged Spinal Canal. *J. Neurosurg., 18,* 490, 1961.

Roofe, P. G. Innervation of Annulus Fibrosus and Posterior Longitudinal Ligament. *Arch. Neurol. Psych., 44,* 100, 1940.

935

Rosomoff, H. L. and Rossman, F. Treatment of Cervical Spondylosis by Anterior Cervical Diskectomy and Fusion. *Arch. Neurol.*, *14*, 392, 1966.

Saunders, J. B. de C. M. and Inman, V. T. Pathology of the Intervertebral Disc. *Arch. Surg.*, *40*, 389, 1940.

Schlesinger, E. B. and Taveras, J. M. Syndromes of Cervical Root Compression — Neurological and Roentgenologic Aspects. *Med. Clin. North Am.*, *37*, 451, 1953.

Schmorl, G. Die Pathologische Anatomie der Wirbelsäule. *Verhandl. d. deutsch. orthop. Gesselsh.*, *21*, 3, 1927a.

Schmorl, G. Zur Kenntnis der Wirbelkorperepiphyse und der an ihr vorkom- und Zerreissungsvorgänge und die dadurch an ihnen und der Wirbelspongiosa hervorgerufenen Veränderung. *Verhandl. d. deutsch. path. Gesselsh.*, *22*, 250, 1927b.

Schmorl, G. Zur Kenntnis der Wirbelkorperephiphyse und der an ihr vorkommenden Verletzungen. *Arch. f. klin. Chir.*, *153*, 35, 1928.

Schmorl, G. Über bisher nur wenig beachtete Eigentümlichkeiten ausgewachsener und kindlicher Wirbel. *Arch. f. klin. Chir.*, *150*, 420, 1928.

Schmorl, G. Zur pathologischen Anatomie der Wirbelsäule. *Klin. Wchnschr.*, *8*, 1243, 1929.

Schmorl, G. Die Pathogenese der juvenilen Kyphose. *Fortschr. a.d. Geb. d. Röntgenstrahlen*, *41*, 359, 1930.

Schmorl, G. and Junghanns, H. *Die Gesunde and kranke Wirbelsäule in Roentgenbild.* Leipzig: Georg Thieme, 1932.

Scoville, W. B. Personal Communication, December, 1947.

Scoville, W. B., Whitcomb, B., and McLaurin, R. L. The Cervical Ruptured Disk; Report of 115 Operative Cases. *Tr. Am. Neurol. Assoc.*, *76*, 222,, 1951.

Scoville, W. B. Cervical Spondylosis Treated by Bilateral Foraminotomy and Laminectomy. *J. Neurosurg.*, *18*, 423, 1961.

Scoville, W. B. Types of Cervical Disk Lesions and Their Surgical Approaches. *J.A.M.A.*, *196*, 479, 1966.

Semmes, R. E. Diagnosis of Ruptured Intervertebral Disc. Without Contrast Myelography and Comment Upon Recent Experience With Modified Hemilaminectomy for Their Removal. *Yale J. Biol. Med.*, *11*, 433, 1939.

Semmes, R. E. *Ruptures of the Lumbar Intervertebral Disc.* Springfield, Ill.: Charles C Thomas, 1964.

Semmes, R. E. and Murphey, F. The Syndrome of Unilateral Rupture of the Sixth Cervical Intervertebral Disk. *J.A.M.A.*, *121*, 1209, 1943.

Semmes, R. E. and Murphey, F. Ruptured Intervertebral Disks: Cervical, Thoracic, and Lumbar, Lateral and Central. *Surg. Clin. North Am.*, *34*, 1095, 1954.

Shenkin, H. A. and Haft, H. Foraminotomy in the Surgical Treatment of Herniated Lumbar Disks. *Surgery*, *60*, 274, 1966.

Shimomura, Y., Hukuda, S., and Mizuno, S. Experimental Study of Ischemic Damage to the Cervical Spinal Cord. *J. Neurosurg.*, *28*, 565, 1968.

Shinners, B. M. and Hamby, W. B. The Results of Surgical Removal of Protruded Lumbar Intervertebral Discs. *J. Neurosurg.*, *1*, 117, 1944.

Shinners, B. M. and Hamby, W. B. Protruded Lumbar Intervertebral Disc. *J. Neurosurg.*, 6, 450, 1949.

Simonds, F. L. Low Back Pain due to Herniation or Rupture of the Intervertebral Disc into the Spinal Canal. *Nebraska Med. J.*, 22, 456, 1937.

Slepian, A. Lumbar Disk Surgery. *N. Y. State J. Med.*, 66, 1063, 1966.

Smith, A. de F., Deery, E. M., and Hagman, G. L. Herniation of the Nucleus Pulposus: A Study of 100 Cases Treated by Operation. *J. Bone Joint Surg.*, 26, 821, 1944.

Smith, B. H. *Cervical Spondylosis and Its Neurological Complications.* Springfield, Ill.: Charles C Thomas, 1968.

Smith, G. W. and Robinson, R. A. The Treatment of Certain Cervical Spine Disorders by Anterior Removal of the Intervertebral Disc and Interbody Fusion. *J. Bone Joint Surg.*, 40-A, 607, 1958.

Soule, A. B., Gross, S. W., and Irving, J. G. Myelography by the Use of Pantopaque in the Diagnosis of Herniations of the Intervertebral Discs. *Am. J. Roentgen. Rad. Ther.*, 53, 319, 1945.

Spurling, R. G. and Bradford, F. K. Neurologic Aspects of Herniated Nucleus Pulposus at the Fourth and Fifth Lumbar Interspaces. *J.A.M.A.*, 113, 2019, 1939.

Spurling, R. G. and Thompson, T. C. Notes on the Diagnosis of Herniated Nucleus Pulposus in the Lower Lumbar Region. *Army Med. Bull.*, 68, 142, 1943.

Spurling, R. G. and Scoville, W. B. Lateral Rupture of the Cervical Intervertebral Discs; A Common Cause of Shoulder and Arm Pain. *Surg. Gynec. Obstet.*, 78, 350, 1944.

Spurling, R. G. and Grantham, E. G. The End Results of Surgery for Ruptured Lumbar Intervertebral Discs. A Follow-up Study of 327 Cases. *J. Neurosurg.*, 6, 57, 1949.

Spurling, R. G. *Lesions of the Lumbar Intervertebral Disc.* Springfield, Ill.: Charles C Thomas, 1953.

Spurling, R. G. *Lesions of the Cervical Intervertebral Disc.* Springfield, Ill.: Charles C Thomas, 1956.

Steindler, A. An Analysis and Differentiation of Low-back Pain in Relation to the Disc Factor. *J. Bone Joint Surg.*, 29, 455, 1947.

Steindler, A. and Luck, J. V. Differential Diagnosis of Pain Low in the Back. Allocation of the Source of Pain by the Procaine Hydrochloride Method. *J.A.M.A.*, 110, 106, 1938.

Steinhausen, T. B., Dungan, C. E., Furst, J. B., Plati, J. T., Smith, S. W., Darling, A. P., Wolcott, E. C., Jr., Warren, S. L., and Strain, W. H. Iodinated Organic Compounds as Contrast Media for Radiographic Diagnosis; Experimental and Clinical Myelography with Ethyl Iodophenylundecylate (Pantopaque). *Radiology*, 43, 230, 1944.

Steinke, C. R. Spinal Tumors: Statistics on a Series of 330 Collected Cases. *J. Nerv. Ment. Dis.*, 47, 418, 1918.

Stookey, B. Compression of the Spinal Cord Due to Ventral Extradural Cervical Chondromas. *Arch. Neurol. Psychiat.*, 20, 275, 1928.

Stookey, B. Compression of Spinal Cord and Nerve Roots by Herniation of the Nucleus Pulposus in the Cervical Region. *Arch. Surg.*, 40, 417, 1940.

937

Stoops, W. L. and King, R. B. Chronic Myelopathy Associated with Cervical Spondylosis. Its Response to Laminectomy and Foraminotomy. *J.A.M.A.*, *192*, 281, 1965.

Strain, W. H., Plati, J. T., and Warren, S. L. Iodinated Organic Compounds as Contrast Media for Radiographic Diagnosis. I. Iodinated Aracyl Esters. *J. Am. Chem. Soc.*, *64*, 1436, 1942.

Symon, L. Surgical Treatment. In M. Wilkinson (Ed.), *Cervical Spondylosis*. Philadelphia: W. B. Saunders Co., 1971. P. 154-171.

Symonds C. P. Sciatica. *Internat. Med. Ann.*, *61*, 310, 1943.

Taveras, J. M. and Wood, E. H. *Diagnostic Neuroradiology*. Baltimore: Williams & Wilkins, 1964.

Tovi, D. and Strang, R. R. Thoracic Intervertebral Disk Protrusions. *Acta Chirurg. Scand. Suppl.*, *267*, 1960.

Uebermuth, H. Die Bedeutung der Altersveränderungen der menschlichen Bandscheiben für die Pathologie der Wirbelsäule. *Arch. f. klin. Chir.*, *156*, 567, 1929.

Uihlein, A. and Baker, H. L. Centrally Herniated Intervertebral Disks. *Minnesota Med.*, *51*, 1229, 1968.

Uihlein, A., Kenefick, T. P., and Holman, C. B. Symposium Low Back and Sciatic Pain. Neurologic Changes, Surgical Treatment, and Postoperative Evaluation. *J. Bone Joint Surg.*, *50-A*, 182, 1968.

Verbiest, H. A Radicular Syndrome from Developmental Narrowing of the Lumbar Vertebral Canal. *J. Bone Joint Surg. 36-B*, 230, 1954.

Vesalius, A. De humani corporis fabrica libri septem, Basilae, per J. Oporinum, 1555.

Virchow, R. Untersuchungen über die Entwicklung des Schädelgrundes im Gesunden und Krankhaften Zustande und über den Einfluss derselben auf Schädelform, Gesichsbildung und Behirnbau. Berlin: G. Reimer, 1857.

Von Luschka, H. *Die Halbgelenke des menschlichen Körpers*. Berlin: G. Reimer, 1858.

Walker, E. Personal Communication to R. B. Cloward. The Anterior Approach for Removal of Ruptured Cervical Disks. *J. Neurosurg.*, *15*, 602, 1958.

White, J. C. Results in Surgical Treatment of Herniated Lumbar Intervertebral Discs: Investigation of the Late Results in Subjects With and Without Supplementary Spinal Fusion: A Preliminary Report. *Clin. Neurosurg.*, *13*, 42, 1966.

Wilkinson, H. A., LeMay, M. L., and Ferris, E. J. Clinical-Radiographic Correlations in Cervical Spondylosis. *J. Neurosurg.*, *30*, 213, 1969.

Wilkinson, M. The Morbid Anatomy of Cervical Spondylosis and Myelopathy. *Brain*, *83*, 589, 1960.

Wilkinson, M. *Cervical Spondylosis. Its Early Diagnosis and Treatment*. Philadelphia: W. B. Saunders Co., 1971.

Williams, L. W. The Later Development of the Notochord in Mammals. *Am. J. Anat.*, *8*, 251, 1908.

Wilson, D. H. and MacCarty, W. C. Discography: Its Role in the Diagnosis of Lumbar Disc Protrusion. *J. Neurosurg.*, *31*, 520, 1969.

Woodhall, B. Discussion of Symposium on Intervertebral Disc. *J. Bone Joint Surg.*, *29*, 470, 1947.

Young, H. H. and Love, J. G. End Results of Removal of Protruded Lumbar Intervertebral Discs With and Without Fusion. *Instruc. Course Lect.*, 16, 213, 1959.

Yuhl, E. T., Hanna, D., Rasmussen, T., and Richter, R. Diagnosis and Surgical Therapy of Chronic Midline Cervical Disc Protrusion. *Neurology*, 5, 494, 1955.

CHAPTER 29

EFFECTS OF ELECTRICAL SHOCK
ON THE NERVOUS SYSTEM

JOHN L. SILVERSIDES, M. D.

INTRODUCTION

Electricity is probably the most potentially dangerous commodity in common use in the community, aside from the automobile. Nevertheless, safety measures imposed by society have kept fatalities from this energy source at very low levels. Deaths from electrical injuries constitute less than 1 percent of accidental fatalities in North America and most European countries, and about one-tenth of these are due to lightning. In areas where both civilian and industrial high-voltage electrical accidents are reportable, only about one in every four or five is fatal. It is from the study of the nonlethal group that we seek to determine the effects of electricity on the human organism, and more particularly on the central nervous system.

ELECTROPHYSIOLOGY

To fully understand an electrical accident, it is necessary to analyze all events leading up to it. Also essential is an understanding of the basic principles of electrical currents. The following factors must be determined in each accident when analyzing electrical current effects on the human organism.

Voltage

A volt is the unit of driving or electromotive force. Any exposure to an electrical energy source of over 25 volts must be considered potentially dangerous. On the other hand, high voltage sources of 50,000 volts or more need not result in fatalities, although 46-60 volt currents have resulted in death. Perhaps up to 70 percent of fatalities result from medium voltage injury (200-250 volts). With low voltage source, current flow is increased by grounding as illustrated in common household accidents with electrical appliances as the source and with the victim grounded in water. In France one-half of the fatal accidents are of this type with the common source the household electrical lamp. In the U.S. domestic fatalities account for one-third of a total of some 1000 lethal accidents per year.

Resistance

This is measured in ohms and is the deciding factor in the amount of current traversing any substance. Ohm's law states that the current in amperes is equal to the voltage divided by the resistance in ohms. In human tissue resistance is highest in the skin and subcutaneous fat. For example, thick calloused skin can have a resistance factor up to 1,000,000 ohms; thin moist skin has one or 400 ohms or less. Resistance is low in other body tissues such as muscle or brain (1000-2000 ohms). It is also higher in bone (4000-10,000 ohms). If skin resistance is less than 1000 ohms, then a 110 volt current can be fatal.

Current

This is expressed in amperes ($A = \frac{v}{o}$). The amount of effective current in any particular accident can be very difficult, frequently impossible, to establish since resistance estimation is so uncertain. Electrical currents are either of an alternating (A.C.) or direct (D.C.) variety. A. C. is three times as dangerous at the same voltage as D.C. Alternating currents of 40-150 cycles can be very dangerous whereas those of higher frequency are much less so (e.g., ultra short-wave diathermy). Other factors concerned with the effects of current on the human body relate to the duration of contact of a particular current, as well as the more important factor of current pathway. It was formerly thought that electrical currents travelled along major nerve pathways and/or major blood vessels from entry to exit. We now believe the current passes through tissues by the shortest path along the points of contact, anatomical landmarks not causing deflection. Current diffusion in tissues is thought to be minimal, perhaps only a centimeter or so outside the direct pathway.

PATHOPHYSIOLOGY

Current Pathway

In many nonfatal electrical accidents, the route taken by the current can be determined by the history and accounts of witnesses or if necessary, by a reconstruction of events aided by the evidence

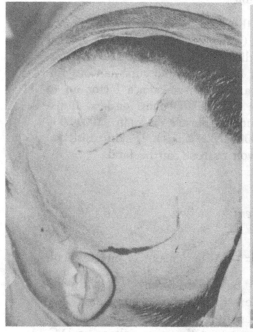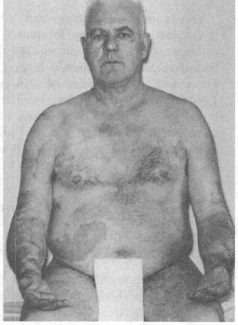

FIG. 1. Scalp to transformer contact; 22,000 volts; immediate unconsciousness with respiratory arrest, responding to artificial respiration. Unconscious four days; posttraumatic amnesia ten days. Aseptic bone necrosis. Severe burns on dorsum of foot. Grafting of scalp and foot. No persisting neurologic sequelae.

FIG. 2. While this man was holding a steel cable and steel sling from a crane the boom struck a cable carrying 44,000 volts. Although he was wearing gloves and safety shoes, there was a small hole in palm of right glove. He was immediately unconscious and his clothes burst into flames. He had transient quadriparesis, was confused and disoriented for several days. Posttraumatic amnesia lasted four days. Characteristic current markings are widespread.

942

of the skin burns at the sites of entry and exit. The effects along a current pathway are dependent on the amount of current and this varies with tissue resistance. With high resistance at the point of contact, electrical energy is converted into heat. This can be sufficiently intense to cause necrosis of skin or bone (Fig. 1). Tissue death is due to coagulation of protein and liquefaction of fat; even tissue water may be vaporized. This thermal reaction is responsible for the peculiar "current markings" of the skin which are frequently seen and are diagnostic of this type of injury (Fig. 2). They appear as greyish-white, painless areas of aseptic necrosis without evidence of surrounding inflammation. As indicated, current passage is direct from entry to exit. Though the effects vary with the current, in hand to hand current passage, the relatively high mortality (up to 60 percent) is due to cervical cord involvement between segments C4-C8. In hand to foot current passage, fatalities, as might be expected, are much fewer (around 20 percent), whereas in cases of scalp to hand or foot passage, the mortality rate is high.

Muscle Reaction

A frequent concomitant of electrical injury in the human is an intense tetanic muscular contraction. Muscles may rupture; one or both humeri or the scapulae have been known to fracture in nonfatal hand to hand current passages. Opisthotonic muscular effects may disrupt vertebrae. Occasionally a severe generalized tetanic reaction may interrupt the contact between the body and the source of the current, saving the patient's life. Prolonged tetanic contraction of respiratory muscles has occasionally been incriminated as a cause of death. As in crush injuries, devitalized muscle calls for early debridement to avoid clostridial infection.

Peripheral Nerve Reaction

Effects of current passage may be direct or indirect, temporary or permanent. The critical level of electrical current causing permanent loss of peripheral nerve conduction is 300 milliamps per 3 millimeters of nerve diameter for a shock duration of 5 seconds. The pathological effects are myelin ballooning and axon fragmentation. This really is nerve necrosis and commonly affects adjacent tissues as well. A few reports suggest that an ascending peripheral neuritis may oc-

943

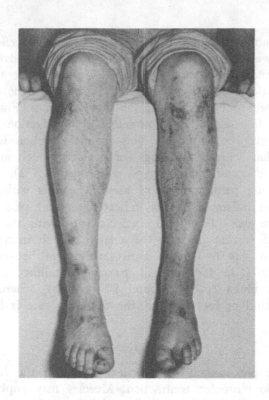

Fig. 3. This man was operating a large auger when the boomer shaft contacted a 20,000 volt source. The patient was immediately unconscious and remained so for 24 hours; thereafter he was amnesic for 10 days. Multiple burns resulted necessitating skin grafting and partial amputation of one toe. The left leg was initially weak, painful and cold, numb, and slightly swollen. This persisted for many months; finally responded to four lumbar sympathetic blocks which resulted in effective rehabilitation.

casionally occur. The nature of such a process can only be surmised.

Autonomic Nervous System

The autonomic nervous system is peculiarly sensitive to electrical shock injury. Regional autonomic dysfunction is most common in the limbs, with edema, discoloration, and sweating resulting from peripheral vascular changes (Fig. 3). Generalized effects, such as transient postural hypotension, may also occur.

944

Causes of Death

These may be primary or secondary. Thus death may occur as a result of injuries sustained in falling. Among the primary causes, prolonged tetanic contraction of respiratory muscles with asphyxia has already been mentioned. Respiratory arrest of central origin has also been suggested but is probably less often responsible. It might be difficult to distinguish between respiratory arrest and the effects of tetanic muscular contraction. The mechanism usually incriminated is ventricular fibrillation, the cerebral effects (or sequelae) being brought about by circulatory insufficiency. It is also stated that in case of death due to ventricular fibrillation, the current must act on the cardiac muscle during the partially refractory period corresponding to the T wave in the ECG complex.

CLINICAL EFFECTS

The clinical effects on the nervous system resulting from electrical shock may be divided into those which are apparent immediately following the accident (immediate stage), those persisting for several days (intermediate stage), arbitrarily defined as a period of five days from the time of injury and, finally, those persisting indefinitely or appearing after a variable delay (late stage). We frequently preoccupy ourselves with voltage in particular cases but these clinical effects have little relevance to this factor, current and current passage being the significant variables.

Immediate Stage Effects

Cerebral Effects

> Loss of consciousness
> Agitation, confusion, amnesia
> Convulsions
> Headache

Motor Effects

> Respiratory irregularity, paralysis
> Weakness (transient limb paresis)
> Tremor
> Myoclonic twitching

945

Sensory Effects

    Pain, paresthesiae, hypesthesia
    Tinnitus, deafness
    Blurred vision, teichopsia

Burns

Causes of death have not been included in the foregoing list of effects. When sudden death occurs, the exact mechanism is frequently in doubt. The absence of trained medical personnel at the scene of the accident makes it difficult to determine precisely what circumstances led to a fatal issue. While ventricular fibrillation is most frequently incriminated, the significance of other factors, such as respiratory paralysis, central nervous system damage, etc., cannot be accurately determined. Also, there is very little correlative pathological material available to guide one in this respect. For this reason, most electrical workers are trained to assume that respiratory paralysis has occurred and are required to institute artificial respiration at once and to continue it until medical help is available. Pending the arrival of professional aid, this procedure has undoubtedly saved lives.

When loss of consciousness occurs, the sequence of events thereafter is similar to what is observed following blunt head trauma, the degree of confusion and agitation varying with the duration of coma and amnesia. The possibility of concomitant (secondary) head injury, separate from electrical effects, must always be considered. Convulsions may be caused by the electrical current but occasionally the exact mechanism responsible for their occurrence is not clear. Headache is commonly present, regardless of the nature of the electrical injury; undoubtedly a number of factors may be responsible for its occurrence. Blood pressure rises appreciably and frequently there is evidence of autonomic dysfunction and peripheral circulatory disturbance. Changes in peripheral capillary permeability and elevation of cerebrospinal fluid pressure have been noted. Head trauma and psychological effects may further complicate the clinical picture.

When consciousness is not lost, patients consistently recall the severely painful tetanic muscle contractions, their vivid fear of death, their inability to call out, the blurring of vision, and the whole catastrophic impact of the events that so frequently contribute to major posttraumatic psychoneurotic developments. Symptoms re-

946

ferable to the motor system are quite variable, though careful questioning will frequently elicit a history of some transient weakness. Temporary quadriparesis in hand to hand currents, transient leg paresis in arm to contralateral leg, or even leg to leg contacts are recorded. Their duration varies from minutes to a few hours. Tremors or muscle twitchings for some time after the contacts are broken have also been reported. Paresthesiae and even hypesthesia in contact limbs are fairly common, again usually transitory, but dependent on the strength of the current, and whether peripheral nerves or the spinal cord have been affected. Burns are caused by heat generated at the contact site and are of varying degree. Usually burns are less severe at the site where the current leaves the body.

Intermediate Stage Effects

Paralysis (Temporary, Usually Legs)

Pain (Trunk and Extremities)

Autonomic Disturbances

 Edema, cyanosis
 Peripheral arterial spasm
 Pupillary abnormalities

Headache

Photophobia

While these phenomena may occasionally persist beyond the five-day period marking the separation between the intermediate and late stages, they not uncommonly disappear within this time limit. Pain and paresis have already been considered. The autonomic effects can be quite marked. They are occasionally overlooked due to local burn effects but become obvious in the course of time.

Late Stage Effects

Cerebral

 Hemiplegia

Aphasia
Epilepsy (posttraumatic?)
Cerebellar dysfunction
Narcolepsy

Basal Ganglia

Parkinsonism — bilateral, unilateral (posthemiplegic)
Choreoathetosis

Cranial Nerve

Optic atrophy; papilledema (transient); pupillary abnormalities
(transient)
Auditory and vestibular damage
Persistent loss of taste
Facial paresis

Brain Stem (Including Multiple Cranial Nerve Involvement)

Spinal Cord

Localized (motor and sensory changes)
Disseminated degeneration (spasticity, flaccidity)
Hematomyelia

Peripheral Nerve

Mononeuritis
Secondary to burns

Autonomic (see Intermediate Stage Effects)

Diffuse aching distress

Functional

Psychoneurosis
Malingering

Because no individual clinician appears to have a large experience
with electrical shock injuries, these late effects are based on data
derived from the author's 23 personal cases and from a review of
the literature. Many effects were, of course, repeatedly recorded. The

cerebral effects, particularly hemiplegia, usually occurred in patients with preexisting cerebral vascular disease or with hypertension. Aphasia, by itself, occurred in patients with a similar background. Epilepsy persisted in a few, not only in those with convulsions immediately following the accident, but also, presumably as a complication, in patients with focal cerebral lesions. Cerebellar dysfunction as an isolated manifestation was a great deal more difficult to explain. In one case, personally observed, it was the predominant, persistent symptom. Several instances of parkinsonism, both bilateral and unilateral following hemiplegia, have been reported. While it is certainly not clear whether vascular changes account for these complications, it is believed that such changes can develop sequentially following electrical shock and may explain some of the late effects. Isolated cranial nerve palsies have been ascribed to direct current passage injury (mononeuritis).

Brain stem phenomena, including on occasion manifestations indicative of corticospinal and perhaps cerebellar pathway involvement, are caused by an unusual type of injury, such as one resulting from a current travelling from occiput to hand. Patients who survive such injuries may exhibit a variety of bizarre signs and symptoms.

Even with seemingly pure spinal cord lesions, the late effects are unpredictable and conform to no specific pattern. There may be flaccidity or spasticity, the tendon reflexes may be exaggerated or depressed and weakness may be mild or severe. Spinal atrophic palsies have been described.

One or more peripheral nerves may be affected.

One of the more common complications is autonomic instability. This may be generalized in distribution or localized to one or more limbs. These effects occasionally respond to sympathetic nerve block and physiotherapy.

A good deal more controversial is the question of possible visceral effects. In one personal case, pancreatitis complicated a severe electrical injury, strongly suggesting a direct relationship. Occasionally renal complications, more in keeping with the crush syndrome than with local tissue heat effects, have appeared.

Another effect of electrical injury is the development of cataracts.

Late effects of a functional type are the rule rather than the exception. The electrical shock experience is psychologically severely traumatic and the late effects frequently resemble those seen following head injury. These run the gamut from functional headache to impotence,

949

fear of electricity and electrical appliances, depression, anxiety, and personality change, psychogenic contracture, etc. Musculoskeletal pain is a common symptom. Sodium Amytal interviews, psychotherapy, change of job, etc., are not always successful in rehabilitation.

NEUROPATHOLOGY

The literature on pathological effects of current passage through brain tissue is relatively meager. Considering the variations in voltage, resistance, and course of the current passage, there obviously is no single combination of parameters. Assuming a mild current, a minimal clinical effect, and no immediate sequelae, there need be no persisting pathological changes. With clinical effects of a minor degree, for example, convulsions only, there may be transient microscopic changes in brain tissue and in the smaller cerebral blood vessels. Reversibility of the pathological changes has been confirmed in laboratory animals. Neuronal vacuolation, swelling and pallor and occasionally neurono-phagia have been described. Demyelination has not been observed. Small ischemic areas are thought to result from arteriolar spasm caused by the electric current.

Persisting neurological deficits, such as hemiplegia, may follow more serious injuries which have initially resulted in convulsions and coma. In these cases preexisting arteriosclerosis or hypertension may have predisposed to the eventual outcome. Again judging from experimental observations, it would seem that current effects on blood vessels result from thermal injury. The muscle fibers of the media are most sensitive, the elastica more resistant. With the media destroyed, a fusiform dilatation of the vessel may occur but rupture is rare; it has, however, been reported in some cases of legal electrocution and occasionally in accidental electrical fatalities. In the latter situation, cortical fissures and wide separation of pia and arachnoid may occur. Peculiar cavities around blood vessels have led to the suggestion of gaseous collections (Figs. 4, 5). Petechial and larger focal hemorrhages in cortex, brain stem and grey matter of the spinal cord have been observed. Chromatolysis of varying severity may be found in pyramidal, Purkinje, medullary, and anterior horn cells. Very occasionally patchy focal demyelination is present. How these pathologic changes are brought about is not clear. Thermal effects are probably the most significant factor. An electrostatic effect with repulsion of similarly charged tissue elements has been postulated. Such a concept might

950

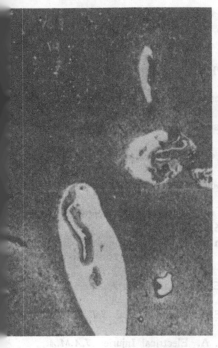
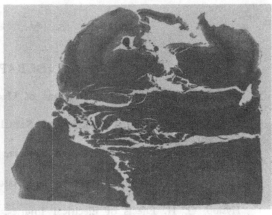

Fig. 4 and 5. A 3200 volt hydro line source of a left parietal, left arm current flow was immediately fatal. Autopsy revealed extensive pontine tissue rupture with one area of focal hemorrhage. Arterial damage plus wide separation of arteries from adjacent tissue was clearly demonstrated. The general appearance of the brain substance suggested widespread small gas bubble formation. This man was not grounded at the time of his injury.

be invoked to explain high voltage injuries in situations in which the patient is not grounded. It might also explain such phenomena as renting of clothing and violent dislodgment of objects or people.

CONCLUSIONS

Persisting severe neurologic sequelae of electrical injuries are fortunately rare. It is astonishing that there are not more residual ill effects. The electrical workers' dictum of death or recovery without serious sequelae usually holds true. Local thermal effects resulting from current passage are probably responsible for most residual deficits while ventricular fibrillation accounts for most fatalities.

The author is indebted to the Editor of the Canadian Medical Association Journal for permission to reproduce Figures 1-5.

BIBLIOGRAPHY

Aita, J. A. Neurologic Manifestations of Electrical Injuries. *Nebraska Med. J.*, *50*, 530-533, 1965.

Farrell, D. F. Delayed Neurological Sequelae of Electrical Injuries. *Neurology*, *18*, 601-606, 1968.

Fisher, H. Pathological Effects and Sequelae of Electrical Accidents. *J. Occup. Med.*, *7*, 564-571, 1965.

Hughes, J. P. W. Electrical Shock and Associated Accidents. *Br. Med. J.*, *1*, 852-855, 1956.

Hyslop, G. H. Effects of Electrical Injuries, with Particular Reference to the Nervous System. *Occup. Med.*, *1*, 199-236, 1946.

Hyslop, G. H. The Effects of Electric Shock on the Nervous System. In S. Brock (Ed.), Injuries of the Brain and Spinal Cord, ed. New York: Springer Publishing Co., P. 680, 1960.

Lee, W. R. The Nature and Management of Electric Shock, *Br. J. Anaesthesia*, *36*, 572-580, 1964.

Lee, W. R. The Mechanisms of Death from Electric Shock. *Med. Sci. Law*, *5*, 23-28, 1965.

Mills, W., Jr., Switzer, W. E., and Moncrief; J. A. Electrical Injuries. *J.A.M.A.*, *195*, 852-854, 1966.

Taussig, H. B. "Death" From Lightning and the Possibility of Living Again. *Am. Scientist*, *57*, 306-316, 1969.

INDEX

956

958